Kriyā Yoga
Bhagavad Gītā

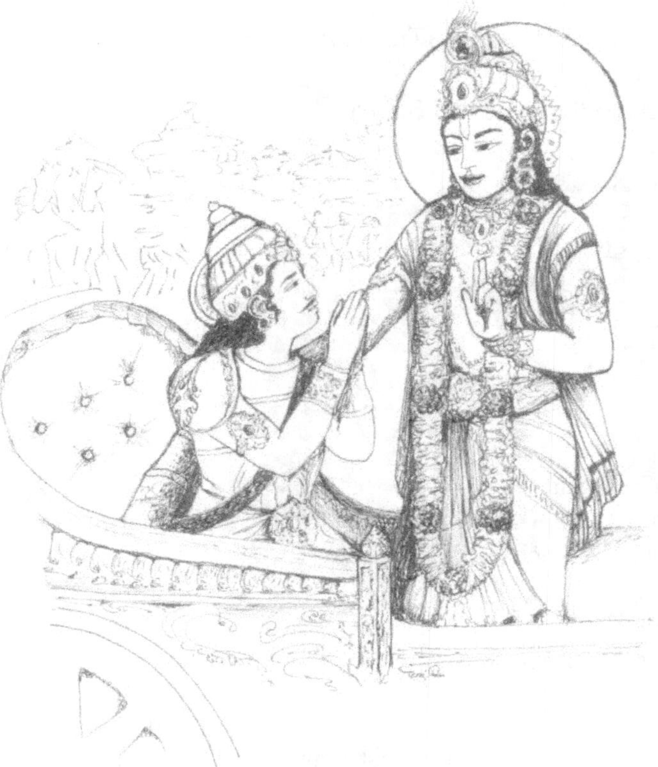

Michael Beloved/ Yogi Madhvācārya

Original Sanskrit text :

- Chapters 23-40 Bhishma Parva, *Mahābhārata*--granted and permitted by John Smith—University of Cambridge, Bhandarkar Oriental Research Institute.

Numbered, four—lined, formatted:

- Marcia & Michael Beloved (April 2008)

Devanagari script:

- Sanskrit 2003 Font

Transliteration:

- URW Palladio ITU font/ ITranslator

Word—for—Word typeset:

- Bernard Adjodha/Michael Beloved

Format assistant:

- Marcia K. Beloved

Proofs Editor

- Dear Beloved

Front Cover: Krishna-Upamanyu Art +
Sri Sri Arjuna-Krishna Line Art:

- Terri Stokes

Mind Diagrams:

- Author

Lord Shiva Art:

- Sir Paul Castagna

Correspondence
Michael Beloved
3703 Foster Ave
Brooklyn NY 11203
USA

Paul Castagna
P.O.Box 150
Iron Belt WI 54536
USA

Email
axisnexus@gmail.com

ISBN
9780979391644

LCCN
2008906544

Kriyā Yoga
Bhagavad Gītā

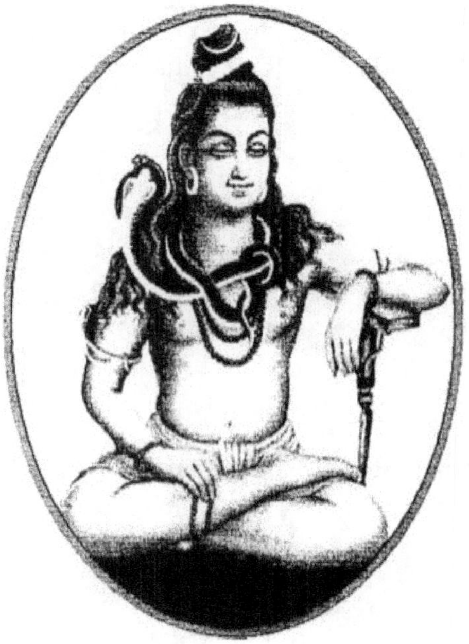

Sanskrit Text

ENGLISH
Transliteration, Word—for—Word Meaning,
TRANSLATION
Kriyā Yoga Commentary

Edited/ Translated
Michael Beloved/ Yogi Madhvācārya

Scheme of Pronunciation

Consonants

Gutturals:	क	ख	ग	घ	ङ
	ka	kha	ga	gha	ṅa
Palatals:	च	छ	ज	झ	ञ
	ca	cha	ja	jha	ña
Cerebrals:	ट	ठ	ड	ढ	ण
	ṭa	ṭha	ḍa	ḍha	ṇa
Dentals:	त	थ	द्	घ	न
	ta	tha	da	dha	na
Labials:	प	फ	ब	भ	म
	pa	pha	ba	bha	ma

Semivowels:

य	र	ल	व
ya	ra	la	va

Numbers:

० १ २ ३ ४ ५ ६ ७ ८ ९

0 1 2 3 4 5 6 7 8 9

Sibilants:	श	ष	स
	śa	ṣa	sa

Aspirate: ह

ha

Vowels:

अ	आ	इ	ई	उ	ऊ	ऋ	ॠ
a	ā	i	ī	u	ū	ṛ	ṝ
ए	औ	ओ	औ	ळ	ॣ	<	:
e	ai	o	au	lṛ	lṝ	ṁ	ḥ

Apostrophe ऽ

Table of Contents

Scheme of Pronunciation 4

Table of Contents 5

How to use this book: 7

A note on the diacritical marks and pronounciation: 7

Introduction 8

*CHAPTER 1 Arjuna's Discouragement** 9

*CHAPTER 2 Divine State** 42

*CHAPTER 3 Cultural Activity and Renunciation** 89

*CHAPTER 4 Disciplines of Accomplishment** 120

Author's Notation: 147

*CHAPTER 5 Disciplined Use of Opportunities by a Yogi** 148

*CHAPTER 6 Yoga Practice** 176

*CHAPTER 7 Krishna: The Ultimate Reality** 226

*CHAPTER 8 Another Invisible Existence** 253

*CHAPTER 9 The Devotional Attitude** 278

*CHAPTER 10 A Fraction of Krishna's Splendor** 308

*CHAPTER 11 The Universal Form** 342

*CHAPTER 12 The Most Disciplined Yogi** 378

*CHAPTER 13 Material Nature The Person The Living Space** 389

*CHAPTER 14 The Extensive Mundane Reality** 417

*CHAPTER 15 Two Types of Spirits** 434

*CHAPTER 16 Two Types of Created Beings** 451

*CHAPTER 17 Three Types of Confidences** 486

*CHAPTER 18 The Most Secret of All Information** 504

Author's Notation on Kriyā Yoga 546

Indexed Names of Arjuna 552

Indexed Names of Krishna 553

Names, Places and Things 556

Index To Verses: Selected Sanskrit Words 557

Index to Translation 565

LIST OF TEACHERS 602

About the Author 603

Publications 604

English Series 604

Meditation Series 606

Explained Series 607

Commentaries 608

Specialty 611

Online Resources 612

How to use this book:

Make a casual reading of the entire text.

Make a second reading taking note of specific interests.

Make a third reading checking carefully for descriptions of kriyā yoga techniques.

Finally, make an indepth study noting how to integrate kriyā yoga into your social life.

A note on the diacritical marks and pronounciation:

Names like Krishna and Arjuna are accepted in common English usage. Their English spellings occur in the translation without diacritical marks.

There is a lettering guide on page 4.

***Here are some hints** on how to use the diacritical marks for near—exact pronunciation:*

*Letters with a **dot** under them, should be pronounced while the tongue touches and is released curling slightly at the top of palate.*

*The s sound for **ś** carries an h with it and is said as the **sh** sound in **she**.*

*The s sound for **ṣ** carries an h with it and is said as the **sh** sound in **shun**.*

*The h sound for **ḥ** carries an echoing sound of the vowel before it, such that **oḥ** is actually **oho** and **aḥ** is actually **aha**.*

*In many Sanskrit words the **y** sound is said as an **i** sound, especially when the y sound preceeds an a. For instance, prāṇāyāma should be praa—**nai**—aa—muh, rather than praa—naa—**yaa**—muh.*

*The **a** sound is more like **uh** in English, while the **ā** sound is like the a sound in **far**.*

*The **ṛ** sound is like the **ri** sound in **ridge**.*

*The **ph** sound is never reduced to an f sound as in English. The **p sound** is maintained.*

*Whenever **h** occurs after a consonant, its integrity is maintained as an air forced sound.*

*If the h sound occurs after a vowel and a consonant, one should let the consonant remain with the vowel which preceeds it and allow the h sound to carry with the vowel after it, such that Duryodhana is pronounced with the d consonant allied to the o before it and the h sound manages the a after it. Say Dur—**yod**—**ha**—na or Dur—**yod**—**han**. Do not say Dur—yo—**dha**—na. Separate the d and h sounds to make them distinct. In words where you have no choice and must combine the d and h sound, as in the word dharma. Make sure that the **h sound** is heard as an **air sound pushed out from the throat**. Dharma should never be mistaken for darma. But adharma should be **ad**—**har**—ma.*

*The **c** sound is **ch,** and the **ch** sound is **ch**—**h**.*

Introduction

Kriya yoga is the practice of mystic actions which bring order and elevation in the psyche. This book is vital to those persons who practice kriyā and who require the grace of Lord Krishna. How does one know if one requires that assistance?

One would know if one ventured to read this book since by doing so one would get in touch with Sri Krishna's contribution to the path of Kriyā yoga. One may need His help and not be aware of the need. For those devotees of Sri Krishna who are kriyā yogins, this book is a boon to free them from biases and negativities to the practice.

Is Śrī Krishna hostile to yogis? Is Krishna against the kriyā yoga path? Is Krishna a personalist who is against all impersonalist yogis? These questions and many more are answered in this commentary which is designed for kriyā yogins and which was direct inspired by Sri Bābāji Mahāśaya.

Kriyā yoga techniques are usually divulged in secrecy and given only to persons who satisfy the requirements of specific gurus who are in a lineage traceable to a famous kriyā master. Generally one must have a physical kriyā teacher. Nonetheless, there are exceptions. If one has keen psychic perception, one may accept kriyās from a spiritual master in the subtle world. In addition, one can check closely in the Bhagavad Gītā for techniques.

The wording of the Gītā may be baffling to a reader but this commentary clarifies a great deal. It explains the application of kriyā yoga and the mystique of it, as discussed by Śrī Krishna.

Regarding the exhaustive Indexes:

All entries, **except** *those for the Commentary, give reference to verse numbers. The last Index which is for the Commentary is the only one which refers to page numbers.*

CHAPTER 1

Arjuna's Discouragement*

धृतराष्ट्र उवाच
धर्मक्षेत्रे कुरुक्षेत्रे
समवेता युयुत्सवः ।
मामकाः पाण्डवाश्चैव
किमकुर्वत संजय ॥ १.१ ॥
dhṛtarāṣṭra uvāca
dharmakṣetre kurukṣetre
samavetā yuyutsavaḥ
māmakāḥ pāṇḍavāścaiva
kimakurvata saṁjaya (1.1)

dhṛtarāṣṭra — Dhritarashtra; uvāca — said; dharmakṣetre — at the place for settling political affairs; kurukṣetre — at Kurukṣetra, a small plain in Punjab, India; samavetā — meeting together; yuyutsavaḥ — being possessed with battle spirit; māmakāḥ — my sons; pāṇḍavāś — the sons of Pāndu; caiva — and indeed; kim — what; akurvata — did so; saṁjaya — Sanjaya

Dhṛtarāṣṭra said: O Sanjaya, being possessed with battle spirit and meeting together, what did my sons and the sons of Pāndu do at Kurukṣetra, the place for settling political affairs? (1.1)

Commentary:

Now here is a man who is not pursuing the course of kriyā yoga. Kriyā yoga concerns itself with personal purification and a personal detachment from family affairs. But here we have the proxy, King Dhṛtarāṣṭra who knew of kriyā yoga but who postponed the practice of it, and instead remained attached to social and cultural affairs.

The battle of Kurukṣetra was an ill—fated occurrence for the Kuru dynasty, because in his youth Bhīṣma took a vow not to become a householder and to be a lifelong celibate. Due to that, complexity developed which evolved into a family crisis that was settled in warfare. This is described in the *Mahābhārata* literature.

The application of this verse to kriyā yogis is this: We should not be like Dhṛtarāṣṭra whereby we know of the kriyā path and do not practice, whereby we are told to desist from the course of social and cultural activities (pravritti marga) and still, we continue with an interest in it.

We should not also engage people like Sanjaya, who are skilled secretaries and kriyā yoga practitioners, in our social and cultural affairs.

Political affairs will be settled with or without our interest because such energies have the power of absorbing valuable time. These incidences are on—going.

Our sons and their sons will fight sometimes, agree sometimes and be indifferent to each other, at other times. This will happen without our participation and interest. Our spiritual development will not occur if we do not take up self—interest in the way of kriyā yoga.

**The Mahābhārata contains no chapter headings. This title was assigned by the translator on the basis of verse 27 of this chapter.*

Political affairs are social and cultural matters which do very little for our purification. Attentiveness to such affairs is actually a distraction. But such distraction has initially caused some of us to take to kriyā yoga in the first place. Becoming disgusted or frustrated with such affairs, especially with their repetitiveness, some of us abandoned that life style to become interested in self purification and ultimate exemption from the course of material existence.

King Dhṛtarāṣṭra had sufficient intelligence to address the place of Kurukṣetra as dharmakṣetra. Kuru is the dynasty. Kṣetra is the property. As it is in the material world, a dynasty is formed. Then there is stress on the land and various assets owned by the family members. King Dhṛtarāṣṭra said dharmakṣetra. Dharma is the responsibility. Kṣetra is the place. Thus the men were at a place where matters of responsibility were settled. Such places are the law courts, council rooms and finally the battlefield, which is the last word in the matter.

The Kurus had family problems. They were unable to settle in the courts. They took to final settlement on a warfield. This system of settlement is not part of kriyā yoga at all. It is not the way of kriyā yogis to settle up social and cultural affairs in the law courts or on the battlefields. King Dhṛtarāṣṭra had a keen interest in such affairs. We could understand that he did not develop in kriyā practice though he was introduced to it by the writer of the *Bhagavad Gītā* and by others.

Due to a lack of practice he was unable to apply kriyā yoga to his life. This applies to each of us as well. As much as we can practice and develop the kriyā habit, that is how much we are exempt from social and cultural affairs. Otherwise our sense of interest will remain endlessly tied to mundane concerns.

संजय उवाच
दृष्ट्वा तु पाण्डवानीकं
व्यूढं दुर्योधनस्तदा ।
आचार्यमुपसंगम्य
राजा वचनमब्रवीत् ॥१.२॥
saṁjaya uvāca
dṛṣṭvā tu pāṇḍavānīkaṁ
vyūḍhaṁ duryodhanastadā
ācāryamupasaṁgamya
rājā vacanamabravīt (1.2)

saṁjaya uvāca — Sanjaya said; dṛṣṭvā — after observing; tu — indeed; pāṇḍavānīkaṁ — Pandava army; vyūḍhaṁ — which was set in battle formation; duryodhanas — Duryodhana, the eldest son of Dhrtarashtra, the crown prince of the Kurus; tadā — at that time; ācāryam — military teacher; upasaṁgamya — approaching; rājā — crown prince; vacanam — remark; abravīt — said

Sanjaya said: Indeed, after observing the Pandava army which was set in a battle formation, the Crown Prince Duryodhana, while approaching the Military Teacher, said this remark: (1.2)

Commentary:

Material existence is supported by the sensual observations of the involved living entities. Thus Sanjaya could see what Duryodhana did and Duryodhana in turn observed the Pandavas army which was before him. Duryodhana formed certain conclusions and decided to consult with his Military Teacher, Droṇāchārya.

That Sanjaya could observe the army is an exhibition of the benefits of kriyā yoga. From that yoga one develops siddhis which are the ability to use the natural powers of a subtle body while one uses a gross form. Generally a spirit using a gross body is at a disadvantage psychically, to the extent that the powers of his subtle form are unavailable for usage. He might experience its powers haphazardly in visions and dreams and then after his gross body dies, he experiences the subtle body in such an awkward and weird way, that he becomes frightened by it and seeks in earnest to take another gross form. By the fear of subtle existence, he takes shelter in the emotion of persons who are using living physical forms. Thus, a spirit using a gross body is unable to use his subtle form independently even though his gross body is powered in part by the same subtle form.

Here, however, Sanjaya exhibited the mystic power of seeing what took place far away without being on the scene. His own kriyā practice was boosted by that of Śrīla Vyāsadeva, the composer of the *Mahābhārata* literature, of which this *Bhagavad Gītā* discourse is an integral part.

Sanjaya was on the battlefield for a time, and when Bhīṣma fell, after being wounded considerably by Arjuna's arrows, Sanjaya went to King Dhṛtarāṣṭra's place to report. At that time, Sanjaya began to narrate all that he saw as well as anything else that he did not witness but which Dhṛtarāṣṭra inquired of Sanjaya, who used the senses of his subtle body, even while having a gross form, to see what transpired on any part of the battlefield.

The use of mystic siddhis for social and cultural purposes is actually not a part of kriyā yoga but we find that in the course of developing kriyā yoga practice, we are sometimes called upon to use these abilities. Even so, the usage detracts from the practice and slows progress.

Duryodhana felt puzzled to observe the Pandava army, but in kriyā yoga the compulsion is to observe those forces in the psyche which block kriyā practice or which cause kriyā practice to be non—productive.

पश्यैतां पाण्डुपुत्राणाम्
आचार्य महतीं चमूम् ।
व्यूढां द्रुपदपुत्रेण
तव शिष्येण धीमता ॥१.३॥
paśyaitāṁ pāṇḍuputrāṇām
ācārya mahatīṁ camūm
vyūḍhāṁ drupadaputreṇa
tava śiṣyeṇa dhīmatā (1.3)

paśyaitāṁ = paśya see + etāṁ — this; pāṇḍuputrāṇām — of the sons of Pāndu; ācārya — sir; mahatīm — great; camūm — army; vyūḍhāṁ — which is set for combat; drupada putreṇa — by the son of Drupada; tava — your; śiṣyeṇa — by a student; dhīmatā — by perception

Sir, see this great army of the sons of Pāndu, which is set for combat by your perceptive student, the son of Drupada. (1.3)

Commentary:

Here Duryodhana brings it to his teacher's attention, that another student used the military training to assist the enemy in their battle formation. By speaking of this Duryodhana insults Droṇa. In kriyā yoga we do not want to insult a teacher. We do not want to put ourselves into a position whereby it becomes necessary to deride a teacher.

In kriyā yoga we do not want to bring anyone's attention to the material world any more than is required. Droṇa was thinking of something when Duryodhana approached and it was not about the battle array before them. Droṇa had his old age to deal with and the unfulfillments in life.

Duryodhana, however, being obsessed with social and cultural affairs was determined to drag the whole world into his complexities and to cause the entire world to work for his benefit. This attitude is against kriyā yoga.

अत्र शूरा महेष्वासा
भीमार्जुनसमा युधि ।
युयुधानो विराटश्च
द्रुपदश्च महारथः ॥ १.४॥
atra śūrā maheṣvāsā
bhīmārjunasamā yudhi
yuyudhāno virāṭaśca
drupadaśca mahārathaḥ (1.4)

atra — here; śūrā — heroes; maheṣvāsā — great bow men; bhīmārjunasamā — equal to Bhima and Arjuna; yudhi — in battle; yuyudhāno — Yuyudhana; virāṭaś — Virata; ca — and; drupadaś — Drupada; ca — and; mahārathaḥ — the great chariot fighter

Here are heroes, great bowmen, who are equal in battle to Bhima and Arjuna. There is Yuyudhāna, Virāṭa, and Drupada, the great chariot fighter. (1.4)

Commentary:

Duryodhana berates the intelligence of his military instructor. This is a continuation of the course of life against kriyā yoga. In kriyā yoga, we take instructions from people for two purposes only. One purpose, the elementary one, is social and cultural education. In order to progress on the course of responsibility we must take instructions in how to make a livelihood and how to be useful in human society.

Teachers who give us information about social and cultural techniques are appreciated. We treat them with respect. We do not, however, take from them their bad qualities and their avaricious attitude towards using up the resources of material nature. At the same time, we do not bring it to their attention that their greedy tendencies could hurt them. We leave them alone, but we make efforts to squelch or destroy such qualities if they arise in us innately or by association.

The other purpose, the advanced one, is to take instructions for spiritual advancement. In order to get our spiritual selves in order we must take advice from others who have mastered certain disciplines and techniques. These are the dearmost of teachers. Some teachers mastered a particular skill. Others bring messages from very advanced teachers.

In kriyā yoga, we are not lazy. We do not want to get anything easily. Experience teaches us that things acquired too easily do not persist. We want a practice, not a boon from the teachers.

Duryodhana berated the intelligence of his military teacher, who was versed in both spiritual and cultural affairs, but Duryodhana never thought of taking spiritual instruction from the teacher. He only valued the man for his skill in warfare. Thus he insulted the teacher by pointing to Bhīma, Arjuna, Yuyudhāna, Virāṭa, and Drupada, all persons who were as versed as Droṇa in certain areas of military strategy. Duryodhana intended to provoke a competitive attitude in Droṇa.

Admittedly, Droṇa did not entirely subscribe to the importance of kriyā yoga but he knew enough of it and had strictly practiced it in his youth. He took partial shelter of it to keep from veering over completely on the competitive cultural path. Droṇa's father was Bharadvāja, a master kriyā yogi.

Droṇa also studied from other kriyā masters like Paraśurāma. However, Droṇa was in an awkward position to be insulted, because he did not take completely to the righteous path.

In order to escape poverty, he took to shelter in the Kuru family, to earn an easy livelihood by selling his military skill. This is why he was now intimidated by Duryodhana.

The lesson for us is this: If we are destined to be poverty-stricken, we should not side-step it by selling a skill to wealthy people, but should, instead, act responsibly under the yoke of that destined poverty. Otherwise, by sidestepping our rightful destiny we will arrive at an impasse and be subjected to intimidation by the stooges of irresponsibility, by people like Duryodhana.

A poverty-stricken kriyā yogi should work honestly under poverty and gradually he may be released from it. If he takes welfare from the government or if he accepts gratuities from wealthy people, pawning his talents for an easy life and position, then he will be intimidated by destiny.

The embarrassment of life is irresponsibility (adharma). It is not poverty. The pride of life is responsibility (dharma). It is not money, wealth or prosperity. A kriyā yogi must account for what he has, not what his relatives and friends think he should have. If one leaves aside the proper usage of the little he has and instead tries to acquire more, thinking that more wealth will bring with it, more proper usages, one will make mistakes.

More wealth means more responsibility but if one cannot manage a little money responsibly, then he will become more inefficient with increasing prosperity. His irresponsibility (adharma) will then increase and he will be ruined.

Generally women and children feel insecure in poverty and for spiritual masters, disciples feel unsuccessful if money does not come easily. Thus a kriyā yoga teacher will fail if he gives in to these insecurities.

धृष्टकेतुश्चेकितानः
काशिराजश्च वीर्यवान् ।
पुरुजित्कुन्तिभोजश्च
शैब्यश्च नरपुंगवः ॥१.५॥
dhṛṣṭaketuścekitānaḥ
kāśirājaśca vīryavān
purujitkuntibhojaśca
śaibyaśca narapuṁgavaḥ (1.5)

dhṛṣṭaketuś — Dhṛṣṭaketu; cekitānaḥ — Cekitāna; kāśirājaś — the king of Kāśi; ca — and; vīryavān — valiant man; purujit — Purujit; kuntibhojaś — Kuntibhoja; ca — and; śaibyaś — Śaibya; ca — and; narapuṅgavaḥ — bull among men

There is Dhṛṣṭaketu, Cekitāna, and the Kāśi ruler, that valiant man. There is Purujit and Kuntibhoja and Śaibya, the bull—bodied man. (1.5)

Commentary:

The sensual mechanism tends to range over any objects before it. In kriyā yoga one tries to control these sensual equipments. Since the spirit is liable for actions committed on the basis of sensual ranging, it is in the spirit's interest to regulate all sensual ranging. This is done by a careful understanding of the sensual mechanism. The senses cannot be controlled merely by desire. One must first get into a position whereby he can exhibit such control. To do so, one must undertake certain austerities in the process of kriyā yoga.

If left to their own devices or urges, the senses will keep on ranging over objects without any regard for any liabilities developed by actions committed on the basis of impulsive responses to objects. The senses are a procuring mechanism and not a discerning force. They procure information by experiences. Generally the experiences are called enjoyments and sufferings. They consist, however, of enjoyments, sufferings and indifferent responses, even though the indifferent feelings are not as keenly noted.

In the business of ranging over objects, the senses are greedy for more. This is why Duryodhana looked and looked and looked, analyzing whatever and whomever he saw before him. All this, being a part of unrestricted social and cultural living, is not kriyā yoga. In kriyā yoga, our development is such that we curtail the ranging power of the senses. We begin to notice less and less of the outer physical world, while increasing subtle perception of the psyche.

युधामन्युश्च विक्रान्त
उत्तमौजाश्च वीर्यवान् ।
सौभद्रो द्रौपदेयाश्च
सर्व एव महारथाः ॥ १.६ ॥

yudhāmanyuśca vikrānta
uttamaujāśca vīryavān
saubhadro draupadeyāśca
sarva eva mahārathāḥ (1.6)

yudhāmanyuś — Yudhāmanyu; ca — and; vikrānta — valiant; uttamaujāś — Uttamauja; ca — and; vīryavān — heroic; saubhadro — the son of Subhadrā; drāupadeyāś — the sons of Draupadī; ca — and; sarve — all; eva — indeed; mahārathāḥ — champions of chariot warfare

There is the valiant Yudhāmanyu and the heroic Uttamauja. There are the son of Subhadrā and the sons of Draupadī, who indeed, are all champions of chariot warfare. (1.6)

Commentary:

Duryodhana has a particular sexual attraction to both Subhadrā, the sister of Lord Krishna, and Draupadī, the wife of the five Pandavas, his opponents.

Being shamelessly driven by sensual preference, Duryodhana does not extend any courtesy to these women. Being vulgar, he mentioned their names here inappropriately. This is not kriyā yoga. In kriyā yoga, one has to be modest, otherwise one irritates the supernatural people who regulate morality. This irritation causes a backlash which manifests in the life of a yogi as social and cultural impediments. We do not need any such impediments since they use up time and cause us to have a less efficient and slower practice.

For a kriyā yogi, the proper thing to do, when mentioning the sons of such sexually—attractive women, is to mention the sons by their own names, or by the names of their respective fathers. Otherwise if one thinks of them in terms of their relationship to their mothers, one may feel sexually—attracted and that would disrupt celibate practice.

Subhadrā is the sister of Lord Krishna and Lord Balarāma and just to think of the sister of these two Lords in a sexual way, is offensive in the least. In addition, Subhadrā was the wife of Arjuna, but Duryodhana hoped to marry her and once, even her brother Lord Balarāma considered her marriage to Duryodhana for the sake of an alliance between their respective dynasties. At the time of the battle of Kurukṣetra, Duryodhana still maintained an attraction to her.

We find that sexual attraction is not easily dropped even by practicing kriyā yogis. Sexual attraction, it may be truthfully said, is the most stubborn impression in the mind. It may remain in a person's psyche for millions of years, in dormancy, and then suddenly flare up to irresponsibly divert him for its fulfillment.

Draupadī was the daughter of Drupada, a king who was offended by Droṇa and she was married to the five Pandavas. Duryodhana was attracted to this lady but providence frustrated his desire. He should not have mentioned the names of those ladies on this occasion, but such behavior is quite natural for one who is under the spell of sexual attraction. Sometimes even a practicing and sincere kriyā yogi, is overpowered by such sexual force in his own psyche. It springs from ancestors who would like to become the children of such women.

When the energy of such ancestors overpowers a man, he will do and say anything even disgracing himself if necessary, in order to achieve a sexual union.

अस्माकं तु विशिष्टा ये
तान्निबोध द्विजोत्तम ।
नायका मम सैन्यस्य
संज्ञार्थं तान्ब्रवीमि ते ॥ १.७॥

asmākaṁ tu viśiṣṭā ye
tānnibodha dvijottama
nāyakā mama sainyasya
saṁjñārthaṁ tānbravīmi te (1.7)

asmākaṁ — our men; tu — but; viśiṣṭā — distinguished; ye — who; tān — them; nibodha — be informed; dvijottama — O best of the initiates; nāyakā — commanders; mama — of my; sainyasya — of the army; saṁjñārthaṁ — for the sake of giving information; tān — them; bravīmi — I mention; te — to you

But, O best of the initiates, be informed of our men who are distinguished. For the sake of giving information to you, I mention the leaders of my army. (1.7)

Commentary:

Droṇāchārya was not the best of the initiates but from Duryodhana's perspective, he was. On one hand, Duryodhana insulted Droṇāchārya and on the other hand, he respected him. As it is with a guru, one finds oneself respecting him at one time and disdaining him at another. It is the same in every other area of human involvement. In the case of husband and wife the same thing occurs. Human existence operates on the basic principle of utility of one individual by another. When a person is no longer useful he or she is regarded in an offensive way.

In kriyā yoga, we make an effort to sort out such things as we begin to clear our path for liberation. If all these twirks of destiny are not worked out, one cannot become liberated, unless he waits for the cosmic dissolution, when all entities will be liberated regardless of their choice.

Dvijottama, the combination of two words, dvija and uttama, means best or foremost (uttama) of the twice born (dvija). Dvija directly means twice (dvi) born (ja). Droṇāchārya was born in two regards, first as the son of a reputed brahmin sage and second by imbibing a high education in yoga, religious doctrine and military science.

Still, he was not the best of the Brahmins. Duryodhana regarded him as a practical and useful brahmin, because Droṇa took a job in the army of the Kurus as a Squadron Commander and Chief Military Instructor. To encourage Droṇa to slaughter the opponents, some of whom were dear students of Droṇa, Duryodhana flatters him with the title of "best of the brahmins." This means that as disciples, we may flatter a teacher just to get his services. Some religious doctrines stipulate that a disciple should rate the teacher as the best but in kriyā yoga we are not required to do this. In fact it is dangerous and detrimental to the kriyā path for us to do this.

Duryodhana acted diplomatically. He intended to show arrogance and show that he supervised all the soldiers including his foremost teacher. He wanted to remind Droṇāchārya, that despite Droṇa's high birth as the son of a brahmin and despite his training in military science, still he was just a hired hand. Thus Duryodhana first saluted him as the best of the initiates and then informed his teacher of the distinguished men on their side. Duryodhana diplomatically said: "First I pointed out to you the important warriors on the other side, taking care to bring to your attention that some were trained by you. Now, I will mention those who favor me. You may be the best of the brahmins because of birth and training, but on the other hand you are deficient; otherwise, how is it that some of your students stand here opposed to you? Therefore be at my service, dear teacher, and do as I would suggest to you."

This tactic of Duryodhana is part of what is called buddhi līlā. In chapter two we will be introduced to the discipline of buddhi yoga, which serves to curb the buddhi organ in the subtle body. Buddhi līlā, or the planning of the buddhi, should be terminated. This occurs by mastery of buddhi yoga, which is a part of kriyā yoga.

भवान्भीष्मश्च कर्णश्च
कृपश्च समितिंजयः ।
अश्वत्थामा विकर्णश्च
सौमदत्तिस्तथैव च ॥१.८॥
bhavānbhīṣmaśca karṇaśca
kṛpaśca samitiṁjayaḥ
aśvatthāmā vikarṇaśca
saumadattistathaiva ca (1.8)

bhavān — your qualified self; bhīṣmaś — Bhishma; ca — and; karṇaśca — Karṇa; kṛpaś — Kṛpaś; ca — and; samitiṁjayaḥ — victorious in battle; aśvatthāmā — Aśvatthāmā; vikarṇaś — Vikarṇa; ca — and; saumadattis — the son of Somadatta; tathaiva — as well; ca — and

There is your qualified self, and Bhishma Karṇa and Kṛpa who are victorious in battle. There is also Aśvatthāmā, Vikarṇa and the son of Somadatta. (1.8)

Commentary:

Despite all the sarcasm, Duryodhana now displays affection by addressing Droṇa as Bhavān, dear qualified teacher. This means that in social and cultural life, one regards a teacher affectionately and unaffectionately. Does this happen also in kriyā yoga?

The answer is no. It does not occur in kriyā yoga, because one's development hinges on practice. His business with the teacher is one of acquiring disciplines to practice. That has little to do with social or cultural connections with the teacher.

If one is like Duryodhana, he will try to take advantage of the spiritual master and that creates a tense relationship. In kriyā yoga we are not concerned with exploiting the teacher. We are so involved with self purification and self reformation to recapture our spirituality, that we have no time to use others even those far below us on the evolutionary scale who could easily become our stooges for one reason or another.

The heroes mentioned in this verse, Droṇa, Bhīṣma, Karṇa, Aśvatthāmā, Vikarṇa and the son of Somadatta, were people more skillful than Duryodhana in warfare. He encouraged them by awarding political favors in terms of giving them rulership over villages, towns or cities and awarding them knightships and regencies. In kriyā yoga, we are not in a position to do such things.

अन्ये च बहवः शूरा
मदर्थे त्यक्तजीविताः ।
नानाशस्त्रप्रहरणाः
सर्वे युद्धविशारदाः ॥१.९॥

anye — other; ca — and; bahavaḥ — many; śūrā — heroes; madarthe — for my sake; tyakta jīvitāḥ — would give their lives; nānā śastra praharaṇāḥ — wielding various weapons; sarve — all; yuddha viśāradāḥ —

anye ca bahavaḥ śūrā
madarthe tyaktajīvitāḥ
nānāśastrapraharaṇāḥ
sarve yuddhaviśāradāḥ (1.9)

being experts in warfare

And many other heroes wielding various weapons, being experts in warfare, would give their lives for my sake. (1.9)

Commentary:

Duryodhana here assures himself, and not Droṇa, that many others of lesser stature would give their lives for his sake. People sacrifice their bodies in a war by patriotism or by being forced to participate. Patriotism is usually drummed up by rulers like Duryodhana. In self—conceit, while perceiving himself as the pinnacle of politics, Duryodhana vaingloriously flatters himself. In kriyā yoga, we are not concerned for others to give their lives for our sake for political or spiritual reasons. We have neither an army nor any set of disciples who would give their lives for us. We do not take ourselves that seriously. If only our mind or life force would sacrifice destructive sensual interest for the sake of spiritual development, then we would be satisfied.

अपर्याप्तं तदस्माकं
बलं भीष्माभिरक्षितम् ।
पर्याप्तं त्विदमेतेषां
बलं भीमाभिरक्षितम् ॥ १.१० ॥
aparyāptaṁ tadasmākaṁ
balaṁ bhīṣmābhirakṣitam
paryāptaṁ tvidameteṣāṁ
balaṁ bhīmābhirakṣitam (1.10)

aparyāptaṁ— inadequate; tad — this; asmākaṁ — of ours; balaṁ — military force; bhīṣmābhi rakṣitam — supervised by Bhishma; paryāptaṁ — sufficient; tvidam = tu — however + idam — this; eteṣām — of these; balam — military power; bhīmābhirakṣitam — protected by Bhīma

Inadequate is this military force of ours which is supervised by Bhishma. Sufficient, however, is their military power which is protected by Bhīma. (1.10)

Commentary:

Some have translated this verse as meaning that Duryodhana thought his own force to be adequate and that of the Pandavas, which he said was protected by Bhīma, to be insufficient. However, a translation which is based on the next verse, in context, shows that Duryodhana was uncertain about his own army which relied on two old men, namely Bhīṣma and Droṇa. The opponents were commanded by younger soldiers. Old men have wisdom but young men have fresh enthusiasm and youthful valor.

Duryodhana's considerations are not part of kriyā yoga. In kriyā yoga, we ensure that our internal military force is adequate. It involves reorganization of the various aspects of the psyche. Certainly, if our inner power is inadequate, nothing we do will improve the psychology. The lower psychological force is insufficient. A kriyā yogi cannot use his teachers, elders, and friends, in the way Duryodhana intended to use Droṇa, Bhīṣma and Karṇa; rather, we take their advice and adopt the disciplines they introduce, but we fight the battles ourselves. We do the supervising, instead of the elders like Bhīṣma. In this way, kriyā yoga is a differs from regular social and cultural affairs.

अयनेषु च सर्वेषु
यथाभागमवस्थिताः।
भीष्ममेवाभिरक्षन्तु
भवन्तः सर्व एव हि ॥१.११॥
ayaneṣu ca sarveṣu
yathābhāgamavasthitāḥ
bhīṣmamevābhirakṣantu
bhavantaḥ sarva eva hi (1.11)

ayaneṣu — in maneuvers; ca — and; sarveṣu — in all; yathā bhāgam — as by assignment; avasthitāḥ — positioned; bhīṣmam — Bhishma; evābhirakṣantu — definitely protect; bhavantaḥ — your honorable master; sarve — all; eva – indeed; hi — certainly

And in all maneuvers, as positioned by assignment, all your honorable masters should definitely protect Bhishma. (1.11)

Commentary:

In this verse we understand, in context, that Duryodhana considered his own force inadequate, first to protect Bhīṣma and second because they lacked what he perceived to be the needed enthusiasm to seize the offensive. As it is in battle, the offended party usually has more zeal than the defensive one. Duryodhana had offended the Pandavas. He was afraid of their retaliation. In such cases, one is always fearful of what the offended party might do.

Duryodhana advised his men to protect his grand uncle Bhīṣma, who is the eldest statesman and military strategist on the warfield. Incidentally Bhīṣma is also the grand uncle of the opponents. This is civil war.

Ironically, even though Duryodhana shows us clearly what is not kriyā yoga, we can also see a similarity between his problem and that of the kriyā yogis. In kriyā yoga, there is an internal struggle between forces of the psyche. Some internal powers are made to rule over other internal energies and there is a death struggle within the nature. That is the similarity.

Duryodhana told his men that they should definitely (eva) protect Bhīṣma the eldest and most capable of the people on his side. Bhīṣma is a person from the generation before Duryodhana's father. In kriyā yoga we look at it in a different way, seeing that the subtle body is the factor which is from the past life. It is more elderly than the physical form. However, we do not trust that subtle body. We do not rely on it and will not try to protect it by putting an army around it for protection.

If anything, we bring the subtle form under control. We curb it. We do not want any advice from it because the inner nature has led us repeatedly down the whimsical path of birth and death without proper consideration for the liabilities. Such a body is not to be positioned as the advisor. We must use it to gain liberation but that does not mean that it is our teacher. So instead, we design our life in a way that in all maneuvers, as positioned by the disciplines of kriyā yoga, the honorable powers in the psyche definitely keep an eye on the subtle body, so that it does not again lead the entire psychology down the path of repeated birth and death.

तस्य संजनयन्हर्षं
कुरुवृद्धः पितामहः ।
सिंहनादं विनद्योच्चैः
शङ्खं दध्मौ प्रतापवान् ॥१.१२॥

tasya — of him (Duryodhana); saṁjanayan — producing; harṣaṁ — happiness; kuruvṛddhaḥ — the eldest Kuru; pitāmahaḥ — the grandfather; siṁha nādaṁ — a lion—like roar; vinadyo ccaiḥ — sounding a loud;

tasya saṁjanayanharṣaṁ
kuruvṛddhaḥ pitāmahaḥ
siṁhanādaṁ vinadyoccaiḥ
śaṅkhaṁ dadhmau pratāpavān (1.12)

śaṅkhaṁ — conchshell; dadhmau — blew; pratāpavān — voluminously

The eldest Kuru, the grandfather, voluminously blew his conchshell, sounding a loud lion—like roar, thus producing great happiness for Duryodhana. (1.12)

Commentary:

This sort of feeling about the support of a grand uncle is outside the scope of kriyā yoga. It is social and cultural support from the ancestral lineage, which is something that fades sooner or later. It hinges on an ongoing link of bodies of spirits who may or may not be related spiritually.

In kriyā yoga we cannot depend on bodily relatives in this way. These relationships lead to rebirth in the same family, life after life, and when we are disenfranchised from that family, we become beggars, having to take birth haphazardly in another family line. Then we quickly amass a set of sinful reactions for irresponsible activities which we enact on the basis of resentments. Thus we pull ourselves down from the same cultural ladder which we were so eagerly ascending.

Śrī Bhīṣma, a great statesman on the cultural plane, a man acclaimed as the most knowledgeable and most experienced human being alive at the time, a man whose word was final, sounded the bugle, a conchshell. Because of his prominence, his shell sounded like the roar of a lion, the king of the jungle.

Duryodhana, hearing that roar and getting an emotional rush from it, could not help but feel happiness at once. It was a hair-raising happiness called harṣam in Sanskrit, a sort of ecstatic emotion. Certainly to Duryodhana, things now seemed favorable for victory. The Pandavas had many warriors, gladiators as it were, but this old man would put them in their place.

From another angle, Duryodhana's excitement was produced by the supernatural support of the ancestors whom Bhīṣma symbolized. They contributed psychological power. If Duryodhana was victorious, they would be assured prominence by birth in his family line. With that subtle support from departed ancestors, Duryodhana was elated (harṣam).

Of course, this is not part of kriyā yoga, and thus we, as students of the art, leave this sort of ancestral support aside.

ततः शङ्खाश्च भेर्यश्च
पणवानकगोमुखाः ।
सहसैवाभ्यहन्यन्त
स शब्दस्तुमुलोऽभवत् ॥ १.१३ ॥
tataḥ śaṅkhāśca bheryaśca
paṇavānakagomukhāḥ
sahasaivābhyahanyanta
sa śabdastumulo'bhavat (1.13)

tataḥ— then; śaṅkhāś— conches; ca — and; bheryaś — kettledrums; ca — and; paṇavānaka gomukhāḥ — cymbals, drums and trumpets; sahasaivā—bhyahanyanta = sahasā— simultaneously + eva – indeed + abhyahanyanta – were sounded; sa — that; śabdas — sound; tumulo — tumultuous; 'bhavat (abhavat)— was

And then the conches and kettledrums, the cymbals, drums and trumpets, were simultaneously sounded. That sound was tumultuous. (1.13)

<u>*Commentary:*</u>

On Duryodhana's side, that subtle power, the joyous fever, spread rapidly to his soldiers. As if in chorus, they elatedly sounded their conches, kettledrums, cymbals, drums, and trumpets. It was tumultuous.

In kriyā yoga we cannot sincerely participate in such events but sometimes circumstantially, we are forced to do so. I remember years ago when I was in a spiritual society, I was sometimes induced to display such emotion even though I was at odds with the basic policies of the society. Sometimes in other purely mundane circumstances, one is circumstantially commissioned by providence to show such support and to join the rallying call of a group of people, but as a kriyā yogi, one knows that it is a false display.

ततः श्वेतैर्हयैर्युक्ते
महतिस्यन्दने स्थितौ ।
माधवः पाण्डवश्चैव
दिव्यौ शङ्खौ प्रदध्मतुः ॥१.१४॥
tataḥ śvetairhayairyukte
mahatisyandane sthitau
mādhavaḥ pāṇḍavaścaiva
divyau śaṅkhau pradadhmatuḥ (1.14)

tataḥ — then; śvetair — with white; hayair — with horses; yukte — harnessed; mahati — in a magnificent; syandane — swift-moving chariot; sthitau — standing; mādhavaḥ — the descendant of Madhu; pāṇḍavaś caiva — and indeed the son of Pāndu; divyau — supernatural; śaṅkhau — two conches; pradadhmatuḥ — blew

Then, standing in a magnificent, swift-moving chariot with white horses harnessed, the descendant of Madhu and the son of Pāndu blew two supernatural conchshells. (1.14)

<u>*Commentary:*</u>

Some kriyā yogis were in this battle, a most unusual occurrence, since normally yogis remain apart from the cultural and social affairs. These two, the descendant of Madhu and the son of Pāndu, referring to Śrī Krishna and Arjuna, were really kriyā yogis, but then again Duryodhana practiced kriyā yoga and so did Bhīṣma, Droṇa, and the blind King Dhṛtarāṣṭra who listened as the first hearer of this narration of Sanjaya, who is also a kriyā yogi.

The technicality is this: Śrī Krishna and Arjuna were genuine kriyā yogis in so far as they practiced and applied the craft without exploiting it just for social and cultural purposes.

Some people, even some devotees of Śrī Krishna, do not regard Him as a kriyā yogi. To them, He is the Supreme Personality of Godhead and nothing else. They also do not acclaim or recognize Arjuna as any sort of practicing kriyā yogi.

Notably, Śrīla Bhaktivedanta Swami, the person from whom I took Vaishnava initiation through his stalwart disciple and agent Kīrtanānanda Swami, wrote in one of his books that there is no history of Arjuna doing yoga austerities. That was an astonishing statement which truly reflects the attitude of the teaching lineage which Śrīla Bhaktivedanta hailed from. It shows their negative attitude towards yoga austerities.

In reality, we know for certain that both Arjuna and Śrī Krishna, the descendant of Madhu, performed yoga austerities and succeeded in invoking Mahādeva, the master of the yogis. This is plainly and clearly described in the *Mahābhārata*.

Since Śrī Nārada, as explained in the Śrīmad Bhāgavatam, berated the *Mahābhārata* literature, his disciple, its author, wrote something else in the form of the Śrīmad Bhāgavatam, which was more directly in line with what Nārada desired. Śrīla Bhaktivedanta

Swami and some of his predecessors did not take care to utilize the *Mahābhārata*. When Śrī Krishna is addressed as a mahāyogī and when Arjuna is addressed as a capable practitioner of yoga, they regard these as honorary rather than actual titles of the two heroes who stood in the magnificent swift-moving chariot with the white horses harnessed.

As kriyā yogis, we cannot afford to overlook the fact that these two accomplished kriyā yogis are involved in such a battle. After all, we want to find out why they were there on the battlefield. It is unusual to find two successful kriyā yogis in such a place. And to boot we are told here that they blew their supernatural (divau) conchshells. This increases our interest.

Two yogis on a battlefield blowing supernatural conchshells? They were accomplished yogis, who mastered the disciplines which we aspire to complete. Somehow they went to a battlefield. They stood on a chariot. They acted as warriors. What sort of successful yogis are these? What do they have to show us about advanced yoga practice?

We are taught that yoga is designed to end material existence. Now we hear that two successful yogis participated in political affairs. We must hear more of this.

पाञ्चजन्यं हृषीकेशो
देवदत्तं धनंजयः ।
पौण्ड्रं दध्मौ महाशङ्खं
भीमकर्मा वृकोदरः ॥ १.१५ ॥
pāñcajanyaṁ hṛṣīkeśo
devadattaṁ dhanaṁjayaḥ
pauṇḍraṁ dadhmau mahāśaṅkha
bhīmakarmā vṛkodaraḥ (1.15)

pāñcajanyaṁ — the conch named Pāñcajanya; hṛṣīkeśo — Krishna; devadattaṁ — a conch named Devadatta; dhanaṁjayaḥ — conqueror of wealthy countries; pauṇḍraṁ — conch named Paundra; dadhmau — blew; mahāśaṅkha — great conch; bhīma karmā — one whose actions are terrible; vṛkodaraḥ — wolf—bellied man

The conchshell named Pāñcajanya was blown by Hṛṣīkeśa, Krishna. The Devadatta conch was sounded by the conqueror of wealthy countries, Arjuna. Bhīma, the wolf—bellied man whose actions are terrible, blew the great conch named Paundra. (1.15)

Commentary:

These three mentioned, namely Krishna, Arjuna, and Bhīma all did kriyā yoga. Śrī Krishna was foremost in that accomplishment, followed next by Arjuna. All three were expert in the social and cultural ways of life. Cool-headedly they responded to the call by Bhīṣma. They are followed by others on their side:

अनन्तविजयं राजा
कुन्तीपुत्रो युधिष्ठिरः ।
नकुलः सहदेवश्च
सुघोषमणिपुष्पकौ ॥ १.१६ ॥
anantavijayaṁ rājā
kuntīputro yudhiṣṭhiraḥ
nakulaḥ sahadevaśca
sughoṣamaṇipuṣpakau (1.16)

anantavijayaṁ — name of a conchshell; rājā — king; kuntī putro — son of Kunti; yudhiṣṭhiraḥ — Yudhishthira; nakulaḥ — Nakula; sahadevaś — Sahadeva; ca — and; sughoṣa maṇipuṣpakau — names of two conchshells: Sughosha and Manipushpaka

The King, Kuntī's son, Yudhishthira, blew the Anantavijayam. Nakula and Sahadeva blew the Sughosha and Manipushpaka respectively. (1.16)

Commentary:

This prince Yudhiṣṭhira was supposed to be the king but Duryodhana and his father, Dhṛtarāṣṭra, held the throne. They are now at Kurukṣetra to settle the matter either in favor of Duryodhana or Yudhiṣṭhira. Nakula and Sahadeva are the youngest of the five Pandavas. The eldest of the five in order of age are Yudhiṣṭhira, Bhīma and Arjuna. Śrī Krishna is a cousin of the brothers. He made an agreement with them, that He would advise while driving Arjuna's chariot. He would not wield weapons.

All five Pandavas, just as in the case of their opponents, were to varying extents practiced in kriyā yoga. Exactly how it is that a person takes up the practice and still remains involved in social and cultural life, will be explained in the *Bhagavad Gītā*. Some people are sincere to the path of kriyā yoga and some are not. However sincerity does not necessarily alter a person's destiny. A sincere practitioner may have to participate in social and cultural activities. This is the lesson of the *Bhagavad Gītā*. Arjuna sincerely practiced but he was guided by Śrī Krishna, the supreme master of kriyā yoga; guided in how to maintain kriyā yoga practice while being involved in the social and cultural affairs. The *Bhagavad Gītā* is essential for those kriyā yogis who must be involved in worldly affairs.

काश्यश्च परमेष्वासः
शिखण्डी च महारथः ।
धृष्टद्युम्नो विराटश्च
सात्यकिश्चापराजितः ॥१.१७॥
kāśyaśca parameṣvāsaḥ
śikhaṇḍī ca mahārathaḥ
dhṛṣṭadyumno virāṭaśca
sātyakiścāparājitaḥ (1.17)

kāśyaś — King of Kāśi; ca — and; parameṣvāsaḥ — superior bowman; śikhaṇḍī — Śikhandī; ca — and; mahā rathaḥ — great chariot fighter; dhṛṣṭadyumno — Dhṛṣṭadyumna; virāṭaś — Virata; ca — and; sātyakiś cā 'parājitaḥ = sātyakiś — Satyaki + ca — and + aparājitas — unconquered one

The King of Kāśi, the superior bowman, and Śikhandī, the great chariot fighter, Dhṛṣṭadyumna and Virata and Sātyaki, the unconquered one, (1.17)

Commentary:

This is being narrated by Sanjaya to King Dhṛtarāṣṭra. Sanjaya was a disciple of Śrīla Vyāsadeva, a masterful kriyā yogi. Dhṛtarāṣṭra was also a disciple and so was King Yudhiṣṭhira, the eldest Pandavas. All these heroes, including the ones mentioned in this verse, are knowledgeable about the kriyā path. Yet we see that they all were involved in political affairs.

This tells us something about the kriyā path — that one may not get exemption from such affairs just because one took to the path. However it does not mean that politics is part of the path. It is not. It should be enacted in such a way as to get one back to the full course of the kriyā path, as quickly as possible. A person whose destiny dictates that he serve in the social and cultural dimension would not be successful in the kriyā path unless he enacts such service. But all the same, there is a risk that such socializing might cause him to give up the path, hence the need for guidance by a kriyā master.

द्रुपदो द्रौपदेयाश्च
सर्वशः पृथिवीपते ।
सौभद्रश्च महाबाहुः
शङ्खान्दध्मुः पृथक्पृथक् ॥ १.१८॥
drupado draupadeyāśca
sarvaśaḥ pṛthivīpate
saubhadraśca mahābāhuḥ
śaṅkhāndadhmuḥ pṛthakpṛthak (1.18)

drupado — Drupada; draupadeyāś — sons of Draupadi; ca — and; sarvaśaḥ — all together, being grouped together; pṛthivī pate — O King of the province; saubhadraś — son of Subhadra; ca — and; mahābāhuḥ — strong—armed; śaṅkhān — conchshells; dadhmuḥ — blew; pṛthak pṛthak — one by one

...O king of the province, Drupada and the sons of Draupadi, being grouped together, and the strong—armed son of Subhadra, blew conchshells in series. (1.18)

Commentary:

It is no understatement that King Dhṛtarāṣṭra was the ruler of a major part of India at the time but to call him pṛthivī pate and to imply ruler of the earth, is flattery. Even though the Kurus had wide sovereignty beyond India, they did not rule every nook and cranny of the earth. After all, a man is limited even if he has wide sovereignty. Thus such titles are flattery. As a person using a blind body, we can know for sure that there was a limit to Dhṛtarāṣṭra's ruling capacity.

Here is mentioned an ally of the Pandavas, King Drupada, another person who was familiar with kriyā yoga. It was a common practice in their time. Draupadī is the daughter of King Drupada. She was the wife of all five Pandavas, a very unusual marital arrangement, which was approved by none other than the writer of the *Bhagavad Gītā*, Śrīla Vyāsadeva. Her sons were present on the battlefield, five total, one by each of the Pandavas brothers.

स घोषो धार्तराष्ट्राणां
हृदयानि व्यदारयत् ।
नभश्च पृथिवीं चैव
तुमुलो व्यनुनादयन् ॥ १.१९॥

sa ghoṣo dhārtarāṣṭrāṇāṁ
hṛdayāni vyadārayat
nabhaśca pṛthivīṁ caiva
tumulo vyanunādayan (1.19)

sa — the; ghoṣo (ghoṣaḥ) — noise; dhārtarāṣṭrāṇāṁ — the men of Dhṛtarāṣṭra; hṛdayāni — emotions; vyadārayat — disrupted; nabhaś — the sky; ca — and; pṛthivīṁ — the earth; caiva — and indeed; tumulo — vibrating sound; vyanunādayan — cause to resonate

The noise disrupted the emotions of the sons of Dhṛtarāṣṭra, and the vibrating sound caused the sky and earth to resonate. (1.19)

Commentary:

Whatever elation the Kuru people felt, after hearing Bhīṣma with his lionine—sounding conchshell, was dissipated by the responding vibration sounded from the conches of their opponents. It so affected the Kurus that it seemed to them that the sky and earth resonated when the Pandavas sounded their instruments.

अथ व्यवस्थितान्दृष्ट्वा
धार्तराष्ट्रान्कपिध्वजः ।
प्रवृत्ते शस्त्रसंपाते
धनुरुद्यम्य पाण्डवः ॥ १.२०॥

atha — then; vyavasthitān — in battle formation; dṛṣṭvā — after observing; dhārtarāṣṭrān — the sons of Dhṛtarāṣṭra; kapidhvajaḥ — the man with a monkey

atha vyavasthitāndṛṣṭvā
dhārtarāṣṭrānkapidhvajaḥ
pravṛtte śastrasaṁpāte
dhanurudyamya pāṇḍavaḥ (1.20)

insignia; pravṛtte — in the challenge; śastrasaṁpāte — in the clash of weapons; dhanur — bow; udyamya — raising; pāṇḍavaḥ — son of Pāṇḍu

Then after observing the sons of Dhṛtarāṣṭra in battle formation, the man with a monkey insignia, that son of Pandu, raised his bow in the challenge of the clash of weapons. (1.20)

Commentary:

It is interesting that while King Duryodhana, the actual contender on the Kuru side, came forward and observed his opponents, on the Pandavas side, the contender did not come forward. Instead his brother did. This brother was Arjuna, the man with the monkey insignia. Arjuna used the drawing of Hanumān for his pennant. Incidentally, Hanumān was a master kriyā yogi from the time of Śrī Rāma of Rāmāyaṇa. Hanumān also engaged in social and cultural activities and was the one who found Śrī Rāma's wife in Śrī Lankā, where she was held captive by the demon King Rāvaṇa.

The value of Arjuna's example as a kriyā yogi who now takes the forefront in defense of his brother, is that a kriyā yogi who is involved in social and cultural activities, is duty—bound to defend righteous persons. He is duty-bound to oppose those who are unrighteous.

Arjuna raised his bow to the challenge of the clash of weapons. Taking the forefront he wants everyone to know that he is empowered to enforce law and order. One way or the other, he will not tolerate injustice on the social and cultural scene. So long as he has to function there, he will use force if necessary to establish order for the sake of facilitating righteousness in the form of responsible living.

Many people who want to study kriyā do not fully understand the idea of responsible living. They feel that kriyā yoga might ease their hassles. Many are not skilled enough to defend responsibility in a world that is mostly inclined to irresponsibility. Such persons should note that to be a successful kriyā yogi, one must first follow in the footsteps of Arjuna. A neophyte may practice kriyā yoga, but that does not mean that he will complete the practice. He will not. It will not be possible because kriyā yoga requires expertise all around, both materially as well as spiritually.

हृषीकेशं तदा वाक्यम्
इदमाह महीपते ।
सेनयोरुभयोर्मध्ये
रथं स्थापय मेऽच्युत ॥१.२१॥
hṛṣīkeśaṁ tadā vākyam
idamāha mahīpate
senayorubhayormadhye
rathaṁ sthāpaya me'cyuta (1.21)

hṛṣīkeśaṁ — Hṛṣīkeśa, Krishna; tadā — then; vākyam — request; idam — this; āha — he spoke; mahīpate — O Lord of the earth; senayoḥ — of the two armies; ubhayoḥ — of the two; madhye — in the midst; rathaṁ — chariot; sthāpaya — cause to be parked; me — my; 'cyuta = acyuta — unaffected

Then he spoke this request to Hṛṣīkeśa, Krishna: O Lord of the earth, cause my chariot to be parked in the midst of the two armies, O unaffected one, (1.21)

Commentary:

Here another person is being addressed as Lord of the earth. This is a pattern in Vedic literatures, where there is glorification to the extent that in some readings one searches for clarity, trying to find the truth of the situation. Who indeed is the Lord of the earth? Sanjaya addressed Dhṛtarāṣṭra as ruler of the earth and now he stated that Arjuna addressed Śrī Krishna as Lord of the earth.

Arjuna also addresses Śrī Krishna as the unaffected one, a very significant title and one of interest to kriyā yogis. *Cyuta* means one who is affected, especially a person who is emotionally affected but *'cyuta* which is an abbreviation for acyuta means one who is not affected, who is spiritually situated to such an extent that he is unaffected by subtle or gross material shiftings.

In kriyā yoga we admit that we are affected at the moment. We strive to become unaffected in the near future by the transformation brought on in our psyche by the disciplines.

यावदेतान्निरीक्षेऽहं
योद्धुकामानवस्थितान् ।
कैर्मया सह योद्धव्यम्
अस्मिन्रणसमुद्यमे ॥ १.२२ ॥
yāvadetānnirīkṣe'haṁ
yoddhukāmānavasthitān
kairmayā saha yoddhavyam
asminraṇasamudyame (1.22)

yāvad — so that; etān — these; nirīkṣe — I can see; 'haṁ = a haṁ — I; yoddhu—kāmān — battle-hungry; avasthitān — armed warriors; kair — with whom; mayā — with myself; saha — with; yoddhavyam — should be fought; asmin — in this; raṇasamudyame — in the battle engagement

...so that I can see these battle—hungry, armed warriors, with whom I should fight in this battle engagement. (1.22)

__Commentary:__

Just as Duryodhana wanted to assess his opponents, Arjuna takes a stance to observe the persons whom he considers as opponents. Actually this mood of Arjuna shows that Arjuna forgot himself and is no longer acting as a kriyā student. Arjuna subjects himself to emotional fatigue. He takes the situation personally and does not see that he should fight on someone else's behalf. It is Yudhiṣṭhira who is contending for the throne not Arjuna.

When a kriyā student acts in the social and cultural setting and loses perspective and misunderstands his role, taking himself seriously as the primary agent, he is apt to make mistakes. He will, by the nature of action, fall under the sway of emotions and thus prove himself as being affected (cyuta). He will be in the opposite position to Śrī Krishna who is unaffected (acutya).

योत्स्यमानानवेक्षेऽहं
य एतेऽत्र समागताः ।
धार्तराष्ट्रस्य दुर्बुद्धेर्
युद्धे प्रियचिकीर्षवः ॥ १.२३ ॥
yotsyamānānavekṣe'haṁ
ya ete'tra samāgatāḥ
dhārtarāṣṭrasya durbuddher
yuddhe priyacikīrṣavaḥ (1.23)

yotsyamānān — those who are about to fight; avekṣe — I wish to observe; 'haṁ = a haṁ — I; ya — who; ete — these; 'tra = atra — here; samāgatāḥ — assembled together; dhārtarāṣṭrasya — of the son of Dhṛtarāṣṭra; durbuddher — of the evil—minded; yuddhe — in battle; priyacikīrṣavaḥ — desiring to please

I wish to observe those who are to fight, who assembled here desiring to please the evil-minded son of King Dhṛtarāṣṭra, in battle. (1.23)

Commentary:

The desire for such a view of the battle hungry men, who wanted to please Duryodhana, is not needed for a kriyā yogi. Arjuna is a kriyā yogi but he departed from the kriyā perspective at this stage. Arjuna slipped out from under the interest of kriyā yoga at this time. Thus he fell under the influence of social and cultural forces which are resistant to and which take a kriyā yogi away from the craft.

Arjuna has Śrī Krishna at his side but generally a practicing yogi does not have such a person sitting beside him in such situations. Instead one may be graced by the presence of a great yogi who might give one association from the astral world. Such association, however, may be ineffective if one lacks a keen psychic awareness and if one is not responsive.

We really do not wish to see those who are assembled to fight on behalf of evil kings or their sons. That has little to do with our personal development in spiritual life. Such affairs are continuous in the material world. We can always find such situations. We can easily observe, ponder, analyse and react to them for good or bad.

Such situations recur frequently in the material world. If one craves perplexity, he came to the right place in the material world. Here, there is perplexity in every direction. A kriyā yogi is not interested in the complications. At least he should not be because he has his own psychological maze to sort out. He really does not have the time or energy to be involved in social and cultural hassles.

In every home, in every village, in every town, in every thriving city, in every capital, in every country, on this planet internationally, there is perplexity. If that is what we seek, we will find it wherever we may roam. It is nothing special. What we really need to do is to turn inwards to look within our psyche and solve the perplexity that transpires there. That is kriyā yoga.

Avekṣe means I wish to observe. A kriyā yogi wishes to observe the operations in the psyche. That is the 1st stage of higher yoga. After making such observations and seeing that chaos and rampant disorder exist internally, he begins the stage called sensual withdrawal, which is pratyāhāra.

According to the tradition and according to Śrī Patañjali in his *Yoga Sūtras*, there are eight stages for yoga practice. These are the avoidance of prohibited activities (yama), the performance of approved conduct (niyama), the practice of postures (āsanas), the scientific operation of the breath mechanism (prāṇāyāma), sensual restraint and withdrawal (pratyāhāra), concentration or deliberate focusing of the intellect (dhāraṇa), contemplation (dhyāna) and trance states (samādhi).

The stage of observing the inner psyche begins somewhere between the scientific operation of the breath mechanism and the sensual restraint stages, between prāṇāyāma and pratyāhāra.

संजय उवाच
एवमुक्तो हृषीकेशो
गुडाकेशेन भारत ।
सेनयोरुभयोर्मध्ये
स्थापयित्वा रथोत्तमम् ॥१.२४॥

saṁjaya – Sanjaya; uvāca — said; evam — thus; ukto — being addressed; hṛṣīkeśo — Hrisikesa; guḍākeśena — by the thick—haired baron; bhārata — O descendant of Bharata; senayor — of the two armies; ubhayor — of the two; madhye — in the

saṁjaya uvāca
evamukto hṛṣīkeśo
guḍākeśena bhārata
senayorubhayormadhye
sthāpayitvā rathottamam (1.24)

middle; sthāpayitvā — caused to be positioned; rathottamam — best of the chariots

Sanjaya said: O descendant of Bharata, thus being addressed by Arjuna, the thick—haired baron, Krishna, who is known as Hṛṣīkeśa, caused the best of the chariots to be positioned in the midst of the two armies. (1.24)

Commentary:

Using a blind body, Dhṛtarāṣṭra fell into a fix and was unable to control his desire for physical vision. The lack of physical vision is not a handicap for the performance of kriyā yoga. Kriyā yoga has very little to do with physical vision, which is the operation of psychic vision being channeled through the optic nerves of the physical body.

In kriyā yoga, physical vision is a distraction. In some cases it causes the failure of the aspiring person, whereby his addiction to physical vision causes him not to have psychic insight. The eyes of jñāna, or knowledge, are regarded as intuitive perception by some. Others see it as a higher, more accurate sense of understanding. They do not acknowledge it as an actual vision in the visual sense. In reality, it is. It is an organ in the subtle body, just as these physical eyes are organs in this physical form.

Coming under the influence of Dhṛtarāṣṭra, and as the physical eyes of the King, Sanjaya got a psychic power whereby he could see physically anything that might occur far away. Of course, he did witness some of the battle scene but he also reviewed it, just as one would look at a film of something that transpired previously, except that Sanjaya is using mystic filming and mystic replay of the filming.

This was authorized by Sanjaya's kriyā yoga teacher, the writer of the *Bhagavad Gītā*, Śrī Krishna Dvaipāyana Vyāsadeva. Still, this is strictly speaking, a misuse of mystic power (siddhi). One should not use a siddhi just to please a blind man, especially one who was introduced to kriyā yoga, and who stubbornly neglected to practice and who persisted in the social and cultural ways of this world.

Because he fell under the influence of Dhṛtarāṣṭra, Sanjaya had to abuse his kriyā skill. He also had to open up his third eye for social and cultural purposes thus using a kriyā power to look for physical details with the organ of psychic vision (jñāna dipa).

Arjuna had the best of the chariots on the warfield but that does not mean that Sanjaya's observation of that would help his kriyā practice. After all, a person might have the best of chariots, the best automobile, and not be at all interested in kriyā yoga. Too close of an observation of any type of material phenomena causes the shutdown of psychic vision and forestalls our advancement in kriyā yoga. This is being viewed by Sanjaya, not because Śrī Krishna is a master of kriyā yoga or because Arjuna is a student of the science, but rather because Arjuna is a competitor to Dhṛtarāṣṭra's son, Prince Duryodhana, and also because Śrī Krishna had the physical power to disrupt the plans of Duryodhana and Dhṛtarāṣṭra. We must be clear about this. The motivation behind this vision, sought after by the blind king, was to use Sanjaya's kriyā skills to advance social and cultural affairs. That is not the purpose of associating with kriyā yogis. We should not allow others, be they fellow—students or non-interested parties, to use our kriyā progress for such matters.

Sometimes however, by the force of destiny one may be compelled to do this. As soon as possible, one should escape from such a fix and discipline oneself in such a way as to never be in a position to be used again.

Providence will not facilitate our kriyā advancement if we continually remain at its disposal for such usages. It is up to us, individually, to side—step such occurrences.

भीष्मद्रोणप्रमुखतः
सर्वेषां च महीक्षिताम् ।
उवाच पार्थ पश्यैतान्
समवेतान्कुरूनिति ॥ १.२५ ॥
bhīṣmadroṇapramukhataḥ
sarveṣāṁ ca mahīkṣitām
uvāca pārtha paśyaitān
samavetānkurūniti (1.25)

bhīṣma droṇa pramukhataḥ — in the presence of Bhisma, Droṇa; sarveṣām — of all these; ca — and; mahīkṣitām — rulers of the earth; uvāca — (Krishna) said; pārtha — O son of Pṛthā; paśyai 'etān — behold them; samavetān — are assembled together; kurūn — Kurus; iti — thus

In the presence of Bhishma, Droṇa and all those rulers of the earth, Krishna said: O son of Pṛthā, behold these Kurus who are assembled here together. (1.25)

Commentary:

In this verse Sanjaya assumes his own demeanor and resisted Dhṛtarāṣṭra's influence for a bit. This is because Sanjaya shifted his gaze from Arjuna to Śrī Krishna. Arjuna, as a student of kriyā yoga, fell under the socio—cultural forces. Śrī Krishna, a master kriyā yogi, does at all times, even when socially and culturally involved, transcend that influence. Therefore when Sanjaya shifted from Arjuna to Krishna, Sanjaya experienced an upliftment, a resituating on the kriyā yoga path.

Basically Śrī Krishna said that Arjuna could look at the Kurus as he wished. It was up to Arjuna, if he wanted, to subject himself to the socio—cultural scene and be situated in its influence. However, this is not such a good idea for a kriyā yogi student to put himself into such a position or to ask his teacher to position himself where he could view the world from an emotional perspective. This is not something we should do. We should not follow this particular example of Arjuna. Arjuna is a senior student of the kriyā path and in that sense he is our teacher, because he is further along the path than we are, but still we must discern which actions of his to follow. We must respect Arjuna always but we must also discern between Arjuna's treading of the kriyā path and Arjuna's departure from it.

Bhīṣma, Droṇa and all those rulers of the earth (mahikṣitam) had their political interest. This is why they were on the battlefield. These persons meant business, as Arjuna realized, and as Arjuna would further learn from Śrī Krishna. These people had no qualms about their social and cultural involvement. They staked political claims and were not at all shy about it. Such a timid kriyā student as Arjuna, should not allow himself to be subjected to the social and cultural influences, since he does not have a corresponding political interest which would motivate him to be aggressive.

तत्रापश्यत्स्थितान्पार्थः
पितॄनथ पितामहान् ।
आचार्यान्मातुलान्भ्रातॄन्
पुत्रान्पौत्रान्सखींस्तथा ।
श्वशुरान्सुहृदश्चैव
सेनयोरुभयोरपि ॥ १.२६ ॥

tatra apaśyat — there he saw; sthitān — standing; pārthaḥ — the son of Pṛthā; pitṝn — fathers; atha — then; pitāmahān — grandfathers; ācāryān — revered teachers; mātulān — maternal uncles; bhrātṝn — brothers; putrān — sons; pautrān — grandsons; sakhīṁs — friends; tathā — as well as; śvaśurān — fathers—in—law;

tatrāpaśyatsthitānpārthaḥ
pitṝnatha pitāmahān
ācāryānmātulānbhrātṝn
putrānpautrānsakhīṁstathā
śvaśurānsuhṛdaścaiva
senayorubhayorapi (1.26)

suhṛdaś = suhṛdaḥ — well-wishing men; caiva — and indeed; senayoḥ — in the two armies; ubhayoḥ — in the both; api — also

The son of Pṛthā saw men who were fathers, grandfathers, revered teachers, maternal uncles, brothers, sons, grandsons, as well as friends, fathers—in—law and well—wishing friends, standing there in both armies. (1.26)

Commentary:

When Arjuna was jarred loose from his kriyā yoga perspective, he was immediately put on the social and cultural plane, in terms of considering his bodily relations as the predominant reality. This is natural on that level.

Thus a kriyā yogi must try not to be shifted from the kriyā yoga view of seeing all living entities as relations on a similar footing. All the same, a kriyā yogi even though he sees all the living entities as being related to himself in some way or the other, does not move away from the primal task of self—purification. If somehow he does, as Arjuna did, he will definitely lose his foothold on the kriyā path.

As a matter of routine, even a kriyā yogi must conform to social and cultural expectations, in terms of seeing his father, mother, uncles, aunts, grandparents, teachers, siblings, dependents, as well as in—laws and friends, as being specially related to him and being worthy of special care and attention, but the kriyā yogi should know clearly that this is just formality and nothing more. One should not take this too seriously, because some who are not related might be in fact be dearer to a spirit than those who are related. Thus even though a kriyā yogi must to a degree conform to worldly dealings, he should not lose sight of the fact that it is mostly custom.

In this regard, Śrī Bābāji Mahasaya of a kriyā lineage, who serves as one of my spiritual masters, instructed me to expedite. I was once very distant from social and cultural ways, but Śrī Bābāji, a mahāyogī, using a sunlight yoga siddhi body, instructed me that I would advance much more rapidly if I would expedite these social customs whenever I encountered them in the material world. This advice of his was given in another way, long, long ago by Śrī Krishna to Arjuna, as we will hear in this *Gītā*.

तान्समीक्ष्य स कौन्तेयः
सर्वान्बन्धूनवस्थितान् ।
कृपया परयाविष्टो
विषीदन्निदमब्रवीत् ॥ १.२७ ॥
tānsamīkṣya sa kaunteyaḥ
sarvānbandhūnavasthitān
kṛpayā parayāviṣṭo
viṣīdannidamabravīt (1.27)

tān — them; samīkṣya — observing; sa — he; kaunteyaḥ — son of Kuntī; sarvān — all; bandhūn — relatives; avasthitān — armored; kṛpayā — with compassion; parayāviṣṭaḥ — overwhelmed by deep; viṣīdann — feeling discouraged; idam — this; abravīt — he said

Observing all his relatives in the armored state, that son of Kuntī was overwhelmed by deep compassion. Feeling discouraged, he spoke this: (1.27)

Commentary:

Because Arjuna was somehow jarred loose from the kriyā yoga perspective, he automatically defaulted to the customary way of viewing circumstances, in terms of always being partial to one's relatives, seeing everything in terms of this one lifetime and trying to facilitate one's family over others. Thus Arjuna became overwhelmed with emotions of compassion. His psychological energy broke down into compassionate feelings. He could no longer go through with the task of just doing his duty as a soldier for King Yudhiṣṭhira. His purpose at Kurukṣetra, which was to fight injustice and to bring on a state of just law and adequate order, was lost to his view at the time.

To a person in such a state, an armoured condition portends danger. Arjuna became thoroughly discouraged. On that level, one thinks and perceives the body of the spirit as the spirit itself. Thus any threat to the body appears to be a substantial risk to the very spirit. One then acts impulsively to save the body from doom, feeling that by doing so, one would save the dear spirit. Such is the materialistic demeanor adopted naturally on the social and cultural plane.

दृष्ट्वेमान्स्वजनान्कृष्ण
युयुत्सून्समवस्थितान् ।
सीदन्ति मम गात्राणि
मुखं च परिशुष्यति ॥ १.२८ ॥
dṛṣṭvemānsvajanānkṛṣṇa
yuyutsūnsamavasthitān
sīdanti mama gātrāṇi
mukhaṁ ca pariśuṣyati (1.28)

dṛṣṭvemaṁ — having seen this; svajanān — my people; kṛṣṇa — Krishna; yuyutsuṁ — eager for combat; samavasthitān— standing near; sīdanti — collapse; mama — my; gātrāṇi — legs; mukhaṁ — mouth; ca — and; pariśuṣyati — dries up

Having seen this situation of my own people, standing near, eager for combat, my legs collapse and my mouth dries up. (1.28)

Commentary:

It is interesting that Arjuna then addressed Śrī Krishna, who functioned as his charioteer. By the rule of military formation, Arjuna should have addressed his brother, King Yudhiṣṭhira, but Arjuna has a special confidential relationship with Śrī Krishna. That is the fortune of Arjuna. Not every kriyā yogi might be that lucky to have a kriyā teacher who is so cool—headed, and so devoid of the need to be worshipped and recognized by others, that he does not mind being treated as a friend.

However if one is sincere in kriyā practice, he could take recourse to mystic association in order to be near a kriyā teacher. The true kriyā teacher is similar in nature to Śrī Krishna, in the sense that he is not attached to being a spiritual master. He maintains ordinary friendly relations with students of the craft.

Arjuna experienced the social and cultural energy on a lower plane of existence. Subsequently his whole psyche broke down. How can this happen? This is the question. It happens by being shifted out of the stronger more clarifying energy to a weaker confusing force. One then perceives the world through that lower power and acts or refuses to act accordingly.

The whole science of kriyā yoga is meant to, gradually but surely, remove all the lower energy, permanently replacing it with the higher power, so that we can consistently and effortlessly function on the higher level. This is the long—term goal.

वेपथुश्च शरीरे मे
रोमहर्षश्च जायते ।
गाण्डीवं स्रंसते हस्तात्
त्वक् चैव परिदह्यते ॥ १.२९॥
vepathuśca śarīre me
romaharṣaśca jāyate
gāṇḍīvaṁ sraṁsate hastāt
tvak caiva paridahyate (1.29)

vepathuś — trembling; ca — and; śarīre — in the body; me — my; romaharṣaś — bristling of hair; ca — and; jāyate — takes place; gāṇḍīvaṁ — Gāṇḍīva bow; sraṁsate — falls; hastāt — from the hand; tvak — skin; caiva — and indeed; paridahyate — burns

A trembling is in my body and a bristling of my hairs takes place. The Gāṇḍīva bow falls from my hand. Indeed, my skin burns. (1.29)

Commentary:

Here Arjuna experienced further weakening due to a shift from the higher nature to a lower type of energy which weakens the psyche and activates the materialistic vision. When the spirit looks at the world through this energy, he perceives life in such a way that he becomes a wimp on the social and cultural plane. Of course many persons exist here, as wimps in their normal behavior, but a kriyā yogi is different. For him to be in such a position is quite abnormal.

न च शक्नोम्यवस्थातुं
भ्रमतीव च मे मनः ।
निमित्तानि च पश्यामि
विपरीतानि केशव ॥ १.३०॥
na ca śaknomyavasthātuṁ
bhramatīva ca me manaḥ
nimittāni ca paśyāmi
viparītāni keśava (1.30)

na — not; ca — and; śaknomy — I can; avasthātuṁ — to remain standing; bhramatīva — as if it wanders; ca — and; me — my; manaḥ — the mind; nimittāni — indications; ca — and; paśyāmi — I perceive; viparītāni — bad; keśava — beautiful—haired one

I cannot remain standing. My mind feels as if it wavers. I perceive bad indications, O beautiful—haired one. (1.30)

Commentary:

Even though Arjuna sunk low in terms of energy, he still perceives a friendly comforting relationship with Śrī Krishna. Now this relationship is a bit changed in the sense that he does not really see Śrī Krishna as a kriyā master. Instead he sees Krishna as an endearing friend, as someone who can comfort and give shelter in time of crisis. This is an underestimation of the value of Śrī Krishna. It is dictated by the same weakening energy.

We find that in kriyā yoga, when a student enters this weakening mood which is displayed by Arjuna, he regards the kriyā yoga teacher in exactly the same way and wants the teacher to serve his emotional needs. He desires that the teacher make things right for his emotional outlook in terms of stopping all things that hurt his feelings. That sort of attitude is not part of the scope of kriyā yoga.

न च श्रेयोऽनुपश्यामि
हत्वा स्वजनमाहवे ।
न काङ्क्षे विजयं कृष्ण
न च राज्यं सुखानि च ॥१.३१॥
na ca śreyo'nupaśyāmi
hatvā svajanamāhave
na kāṅkṣe vijayaṁ kṛṣṇa
na ca rājyaṁ sukhāni ca (1.31)

na — no; ca — and; śreyaḥ — benefit; 'nupaśyāmi = anupaśyāmi — I can imagine; hatvā — killing; svajanam — my folks; āhave — in battle; na — nor; kāṅkṣe — desired; vijayaṁ — victory; kṛṣṇa — O Krishna; na — nor; ca — and; rājyaṁ — political power; sukhāni — good feelings; ca — and

And I can imagine no benefit in killing off my kinfolk in battle. I do not desire victory, O Krishna, or political power, or good feelings. (1.31)

Commentary:

The intellect of Arjuna was also diminished by the energy that brought Arjuna down into the social and cultural plane. The energy now causes Arjuna's intellect to support it by justifying its behavior. It tries to enlist the services of Śrī Krishna by making absurd proposals.

Arjuna, as the spokesman for the weakening emotional force, states that there is no desire to kill kinsmen, or attain victory, or political power, or the resulting elation. But that is not the point at all. In fact Arjuna's personal feelings are irrelevant, for at Kurukṣetra, his duty was to fight for a just cause on behalf of his brother.

The weakening power presents these factors in a very misleading way by using the intellect to proposition Śrī Krishna to attempt to stop the upcoming battle. There was no benefit for Arjuna anyway. Thus the idea that he even sought a benefit is totally inappropriate. If a policeman is sent to recover stolen property from a thief, the policeman has nothing to gain by executing the instruction, since he will not be entitled to any of the stolen goods, which he confiscates.

किं नो राज्येन गोविन्द
किं भोगैर्जीवितेन वा ।
येषामर्थे काङ्क्षितं नो
राज्यं भोगाः सुखानि च ॥१.३२॥
kiṁ no rājyena govinda
kiṁ bhogairjīvitena vā
yeṣāmarthe kāṅkṣitaṁ no
rājyaṁ bhogāḥ sukhāni ca (1.32)

kiṁ — what value would there be; no — to us; rājyena — with political control of a nation; govinda — Chief of the cowherds; kiṁ — what use would there be?; bhogair — with enjoyments; jīvitena — with life; vā — or; yeṣām — whose; arthe — in the interest; kāṅkṣitaṁ — was desired; no — of us; rājyaṁ — political control; bhogāḥ — enjoyable aspects; sukhāni — pleasures; ca — and

What value to us would there be with political control of a nation, O Chief of the cowherds? What use would there be with the enjoyable aspects or with life? Those in whose interest, the political control, the enjoyments and pleasures, were desired by us, (1.32)

त इमेऽवस्थिता युद्धे
प्राणांस्त्यक्त्वा धनानि च ।
आचार्याः पितरः पुत्रास्
तथैव च पितामहाः ॥१.३३॥

ta — they; ime — these; 'vasthitā = avasthitā — are armored; yuddhe — in battle formation; prāṇāṁs — lives; tyaktvā — having left aside; dhanāni — financial assets; ca — and; ācāryāḥ — revered teachers;

ta ime'vasthitā yuddhe
prāṇāṁstyaktvā dhanāni ca
ācāryāḥ pitaraḥ putrās
tathaiva ca pitāmahāḥ (1.33)

pitaraḥ — fathers; putrās — sons; tathaiva — also; ca — and; pitāmahāḥ — grandfathers

...(they) are armed in battle formation, having left aside their lives and financial assets. These are revered teachers, fathers, sons and also grandfathers, (1.33)

मातुलाः श्वशुराः पौत्राः
स्यालाः संबन्धिनस्तथा ।
एतान्न हन्तुमिच्छामि
घ्नतोऽपि मधुसूदन ॥ १.३४ ॥
mātulāḥ śvaśurāḥ pautrāḥ
syālāḥ saṁbandhinastathā
etānna hantumicchāmi
ghnato'pi madhusūdana (1.34)

mātulāḥ — brothers of mothers; śvaśurāḥ — fathers of wives; pautrāḥ — grandsons; śyālāḥ — brothers—in—law; saṁbandhinas — relatives; tathā — also; etān — them; na — not; hantum — to kill; icchāmi — I desire; ghnato — those who are intent on killing; 'pi = api — even though; madhusūdana — slayer of Madhu

...brothers of our mothers, fathers of our wives, grandsons, brothers—in—law, and also their relatives. O slayer of Madhu, I do not desire to slay them even though they are intent on killing, (1.34)

अपि त्रैलोक्यराज्यस्य
हेतोः किं नु महीकृते ।
निहत्य धार्तराष्ट्रान्नः
का प्रीतिः स्याज्जनार्दन ॥ १.३५ ॥
api trailokyarājyasya
hetoḥ kiṁ nu mahīkṛte
nihatya dhārtarāṣṭrānnaḥ
kā prītiḥ syājjanārdana (1.35)

api — even; trailokya — of the three sectors, of the universe; rājyasya — political control; hetoḥ — on account of; kiṁ — what; nu — then; mahīkṛte — for the sake of the earth; nihatya — killing; dhārtarāṣṭrān — the sons of Dhṛtarāṣṭra; naḥ — to us; kā — what; prītiḥ — joy; syāj — might it be; janārdana — O motivator of people

...even for political control of the three sectors of the universe, how then for the earth? O motivator of people, what joy should be had by killing the sons of Dhṛtarāṣṭra? (1.35)

Commentary:

Arjuna addressed Śrī Krishna as Govinda, Chief of the cowherds. Krishna grew up as a cowherd boy in the countryside in a situation that had little to do with state politics. Thus Arjuna appeals to Krishna's humble background, in asking of the value of political control of a nation. Arjuna himself, as well as his four brothers, grew up in infancy in the forest with brahmin ascetics. Later they were taken to their ancestral capital city, where they entered into government responsibilities. Arjuna, therefore, could relate to Krishna's humble beginnings which were without political overtones.

Arjuna also asked in a challenging way and with due reason about the sanity of fighting a civil war. Victory is supposed to be enjoyed with family and friends but how can one enjoy it, if one kills off the very same relatives.

Arjuna was unwilling to use heroism for the sake of taking control of the universe according to his cosmological views at the time. He did not think it was worth it for him to kill relatives for the sake of gaining kingship even over the universe. He asked Śrī Krishna to describe the joy that could be derived from killing sons of Dhṛtarāṣṭra.

All these arguments are outside of the kriyā vision. This concerns the ordinary social and cultural considerations of a sympathetic compassionate human being, whose focus is social welfare on the material plane.

पापमेवाश्रयेदस्मान्
हत्वैतानाततायिनः ।
तस्मान्नार्हा वयं हन्तुं
धार्तराष्ट्रान्स्वबान्धवान् ।
स्वजनं हि कथं हत्वा
सुखिनः स्याम माधव ॥ १.३६ ॥
pāpamevāśrayedasmān
hatvaitānātatāyinaḥ
tasmānnārhā vayaṁ hantuṁ
dhārtarāṣṭrānsvabāndhavān
svajanaṁ hi kathaṁ hatvā
sukhinaḥ syāma mādhava (1.36)

pāpam — sin; evāśrayed = eva — even + āśrayed — should take hold; asmān — to us; hatvaitān = hatvā — having killed + etān — these; ātatāyinaḥ — offenders; tasmān — therefore; nārhā — unjustified; vayaṁ — we; hantuṁ — to kill; dhārtarāṣṭrān — sons of Dhṛtarāṣṭra; svabāndhavān — our relatives; svajanaṁ — our own people; hi — indeed; kathaṁ — how; hatvā — having killed; sukhinaḥ — happiness; syāma — should be; mādhava — descendant of Madhu

Having killed the offenders, sin will take hold of us. Therefore we are not justified to kill the sons of Dhṛtarāṣṭra, our relatives. Having killed our own people, how should we be happy, O descendent of Madhu? (1.36)

Commentary:

Happiness (sukhinah) is never the objective of a kriyā yogi, rather it might be clarity of vision and soberness. Happiness is a leading objective that causes the focus to be shifty. In this case, Arjuna speaks of happiness in association with family and friends, as he described, but that is not the objective of kriyā yoga, which concerns itself with individual practice for individual purification and psychic clarification. In fact, family and friends regularly form the basis for a failure in a yogi's endeavors. Usually relatives stress their bodily connection and make demands on the yogi on the basis of emotional energies which promote only social and cultural welfare at the expense of spiritual clarification.

Arjuna gives here a flattened analysis of the situation, citing that if the offenders were killed, sin would take hold of the Pandavas army, particularly Arjuna himself, Krishna who supported him, and the four brothers of Arjuna. However, this analysis is very shallow and ignores righteous duty or responsibility to oppose injustices.

It is not a kriyā yogi's business to go around righting wrongs even in terms of a person's past lives but it is also not his business to avoid duty or to come up with various excuses for why he should not serve society. It is not a kriyā yogi's business to take a non-violent stance to avoid completion of duties that involve chastising or even doing judicial violence to offenders. A yogi is not attached either way. Like Arjuna, who is a kriyā yogi, but who for the time being, stepped away from the kriyā practice, a kriyā yogi who functions in clarity, prefers not to be involved in any worldly affairs. If he has to participate, he takes the side of responsibility. He has no partiality. If any of his friends take to irresponsibility, the kriyā yogi will, for the time being, neglect such friends and side with those who exhibit righteous living.

यद्यप्येते न पश्यन्ति
लोभोपहतचेतसः ।
कुलक्षयकृतं दोषं
मित्रद्रोहे च पातकम् ॥ १.३७॥
yadyapyete na paśyanti
lobhopahatacetasaḥ
kulakṣayakṛtaṁ doṣaṁ
mitradrohe ca pātakam (1.37)

yadyapyete = yadi — if + api — even + ete — these; na — not; paśyanti — see; lobhopahata cetasaḥ = lobha — greed + upahata — possessed by + cetasaḥ — thoughts; kulakṣayakṛtaṁ = kula – clan + ksaya — destruction + kṛtaṁ — caused; doṣaṁ — fault; mitradrohe = mitra – friend + drohe — harm; ca — and; pātakam — crime

Even if these persons, their minds being possessed by greed, do not see the fault caused by the destruction of the clan and the crime of hurting a friend, (1.37)

कथं न ज्ञेयमस्माभिः
पापादस्मान्निवर्तितुम् ।
कुलक्षयकृतं दोषं
प्रपश्यद्भिर्जनार्दन ॥ १.३८॥

kathaṁ na jñeyamasmābhiḥ
pāpādasmānnivartitum
kulakṣayakṛtaṁ doṣaṁ
prapaśyadbhirjanārdana (1.38)

kathaṁ — how; na — not; jñeyam — to be understood; asmābhiḥ — by us; pāpād — from sin; asmān — from this; nivartitum — turn away; kulakṣaya = kula — clan + kṣaya — destruction; kṛtaṁ — caused; doṣaṁ — crime; prapaśyadbhiḥ — by due reason; janārdana — O motivator of human beings

...O motivator of human beings, why, by due reason, should we not understand that we should turn away from this sin, the crime caused by the destruction of the clan? (1.38)

Commentary:

The argument raised here by Arjuna is without substance. It is simply a display of weak emotions. It shows that Arjuna shifted from the kriyā vision into a justifying mood of avoiding duties that would irritate anyone.

If a person persists in actions that displace the rights of others he should be stopped by responsible members of society, whose duty is to correct injustices. Arjuna, under the influence of a weakened state of emotions, presents a false argument only considering what would happen if the civil war occurred. Really, the civil war was developed from Prince Duryodhana's usurpation of Yudhiṣṭhira's rights. That had to be rectified. Duryodhana stubbornly persisted in doing what was wrong and the war became necessary to stop him.

If Arjuna was shifted back into the kriyā yoga clarified view, he would have considered instead, that since these persons, their minds possessed by greed, did not see fault in depriving Yudhiṣṭhira of his share of the kingdom, then, by due reason, and as duty-bound, Arjuna and Śrī Krishna should challenge them.

Basically speaking, as kriyā yogis, we are not interested in these matters of the ancient family traditions (kuladharmah) or in the mere traditional values at large for society's sake (dharma). This is not our primary concern in kriyā yoga. This is only our secondary and subsidiary interest.

Since he was removed from the kriyā yoga perspective, Arjuna seized on the next best thing, our subsidiary concern, that of family values and national culture. That is not kriyā yoga. In kriyā yoga, these aspects take secondary importance in terms of obtaining material bodies using such bodies to acquire purification. The same family traditions and national culture through which we took such bodies, create impediments to the effectiveness of kriyā practice. Thus in the advanced stages, we carefully put aside such things as culture, the very thing which gave us shelter when we were in the world hereafter and needed human forms.

कुलक्षये प्रणश्यन्ति
कुलधर्माः सनातनाः ।
धर्मे नष्टे कुलं कृत्स्नम्
अधर्मोऽभिभवत्युत ॥ १.३९ ॥
kulakṣaye praṇaśyanti
kuladharmāḥ sanātanāḥ
dharme naṣṭe kulaṁ kṛtsnam
adharmo'bhibhavatyuta (1.39)

kulakṣaye — in destruction of the family clan; praṇaśyanti — vanish; kuladharmāḥ — family traditions; sanātanāḥ — ancient; dharme — in the traditional values; naṣṭe — in the removal; kulaṁ — clan; kṛtsnam — whole; adharmo — lawlessness; 'bhibhavatyuta = abhibhavati — it overpowers + uta — even

In the destruction of the clan, the ancient family traditions vanish. In the removal of the traditional values, the entire clan is overpowered by lawlessness. (1.39)

Commentary:

What Arjuna said is true, for after all, when the elderly relatives are killed in an untimely manner before they impart their learned experiences to the younger generation, then the youngsters suffer ignorance of certain basic skills, which are required for advancement of human civilization. If the youngsters are killed, the elderly people are checkmated in their efforts to transmit time-cultured values. However this does not mean, as Arjuna implied, that this is the highest objective for human life.

An advanced kriyā yogi understands the importance of family traditions and national culture. He does not discard it as useless for he knows very well, that if he does not become liberated, he will need such things for getting another form fit for continuation of kriyā practice. Nevertheless, the kriyā yogi is not like others who mostly feel that family tradition and national culture is the ultimate aim.

As Arjuna described, in the removal of traditional values, the family is overpowered by lawlessness. This will be explained in detail in subsequent verses. While true, it does not mean as he suggested that we should allow ourselves to drift from the kriyā yoga vision.

Arjuna made certain persons happy by feeling this way and by declaring these things. He acted as a spokesman for others and for other energies which detract from the serious advancement of any kriyā yogi. Admitedly those persons are the majority of the people using human bodies, being mostly materialistic entities. What Arjuna says here does not satisfy the rightly-situated kriyā yogi, but it shows that any of us who are not anchored in the kriyā view can, at any time betray ourselves by being shifted off to these cultural perceptions.

अधर्माभिभवात्कृष्ण
प्रदुष्यन्ति कुलस्त्रियः ।
स्त्रीषु दुष्टासु वार्ष्णेय
जायते वर्णसंकरः ॥ १.४० ॥

adharmābhibhavāt = adharma — lawlessness + abhibhavāt — from predominant; kṛṣṇa — O Krishna; praduṣyanti — are degraded; kulastriyaḥ — the women of the clan; strīṣu — in women; duṣṭāsu — degraded; vārṣṇeya — O clansman of

adharmābhibhavātkṛṣṇa
praduṣyanti kulastriyaḥ
strīṣu duṣṭāsu vārṣṇeya
jāyate varṇasaṁkaraḥ (1.40)

the Vṛṣṇis; jāyate — there arises; varṇasaṁkaraḥ — sexual intermixture of the classes

Due to the predominance of lawlessness, the women of the clan are degraded. In such women, O clansman of the Vṛṣṇis, there arises the sexual intermixture of the classes. (1.40)

<u>*Commentary:*</u>

Under the pressure of traditional energies, Arjuna presented his case for a class—laden society in which there is no intermarriage between the various segments of mankind. In that ideal view, a man with a priestly nature marries a woman who can complement his vocation. Another man with an administrative skill marries a woman of similar demeanor. A mercantile man marries a woman who is compatible with that occupation. And another man, who is fit to serve others, marries a maid. In other words, in such a society, all marriages are based on occupational similarity. This is called the varṇaśrām system, which means essentially that your life style or ashram is tied to your occupational capacity or varṇa. This all sounds good but in kriyā yoga, we are not as interested in ironing out the wrinkles in human society as we are in purifying our psyches.

As Arjuna was shifted from the kriyā yoga perspective, he moved under the banner of the vulgar consideration which deals with regulating sexual intercourse. In this view, a ruler and his officials, like Arjuna, lay out a government that regulates which woman will have intercourse with which man, thereby creating the institution of lineage marriage and prohibiting divorces and unregistered cohabitation. This is all well and good. Somebody ought to be concerned about such matters, which attempt to restrain the impulsions of the gross senses in their quest for vulgar satisfactions. However even though somebody should do this, it should not be the kriyā yogis. Someone near to a kriyā yogi may do this but not the kriyā yogi himself.

We must all realize that if per chance there is a war, even a civil war, and if many of the husbands die in that war, then the widowed women would try to remarry or be unified informally with other men. We should not assume that all of those women would be suffering. Some might even take boys of the age of their sons or men as old as their fathers and would still find this fulfilling.

संकरो नरकायैव
कुलघ्नानां कुलस्य च ।
पतन्ति पितरो ह्येषां
लुप्तपिण्डोदकक्रियाः ॥ १.४१ ॥
saṁkaro narakāyaiva
kulaghnānāṁ kulasya ca
patanti pitaro hyeṣāṁ
luptapiṇḍodakakriyāḥ (1.41)

saṁkaraḥ — sexual intermixture; narakāyaiva = narakāya — to hell + eva — indeed; kulaghnānāṁ = kula — clan + ghnānāṁ — destroyers; kulasya — of the clan; ca — and; patanti — are degraded; pitaro — the departed ancestors; hyeṣāṁ = hi — indeed + eṣām — of these; luptapiṇḍodakakriyāḥ = lupta — deprived of + piṇḍa — psychic cakes + udaka — psychic water + kriyāḥ — ceremonial rites

Indeed, the sexual intermixture causes the destroyers of the clan and the clan itself to go to hell. The departed ancestors of those clansmen, being deprived of the psychic cakes and water which are offered ceremonially, are degraded. (1.41)

Commentary:

Arjuna makes an astute observation here but, still, he presents these truths in support of the family tradition and national culture, contrary to the view of kriyā yoga. Certainly, if sexual intermixture occurs due to careless social relations, the person who causes the intermixture, as well as the victimized families, will see hell, not only on this level, but in the hereafter.

As Arjuna states, the departed ancestors become deprived of the psychic cakes, water, and the other subtle foodstuffs, so they beg elsewhere and become hungry and wretched on the astral plane. They take bodies in families where they have lodged little piety in their immediate past lives. Due to unconscious resentment, they suffer in infancy and they rebel as much as they can in their teenage years.

Every society has its system of offering subtle food, but not everyone does that formally as East Indians do. All of us are forced by pressure from the ancestors to give them food. And we do it by eating for ourselves and by eating for them as well, through our gross bodies. In a step further, the East Indians ritualize and formalize the process.

It is not that they have a monopoly. When a woman becomes pregnant and begins eating unusual foods, she is in fact, feeding subtle foods to the ancestors. When someone departs and the relatives affected by sorrow stop eating for a day or two, they are in fact, experiencing the starvation of the departed souls who long for physical food but who have no physical form to ingest it. However under the direction of their pandits and gurus, the East Indians make this into a religious ceremony. Supposedly their pandits and gurus are mystics who see the distressed spirits on the astral planes.

In kriyā yoga, this is not such a big deal. The kriyā yogi who has a foothold on the practice understands this, but he does not make the offering of psychic cakes his priority. We will not save anybody by doing a religious ceremony after he departs his body. We may do a ceremony as a matter of routine but we are not going to believe all that huff and puff of pandits and gurus who try to suggest that such a ceremony will bring the departed souls to heaven, or to the kingdom of God, or to birth in the respective family from which they just departed. That is not necessarily true.

दोषैरेतैः कुलघ्नानां
वर्णसंकरकारकैः ।
उत्साद्यन्ते जातिधर्माः
कुलधर्माश्च शाश्वताः ॥१.४२॥
doṣairetaiḥ kulaghnānāṁ
varṇasaṁkarakārakaiḥ
utsādyante jātidharmāḥ
kuladharmāśca śāśvatāḥ (1.42)

doṣair — with sins; etaiḥ — by these; kulaghnānāṁ — of the family destroyers; varṇasaṁkarakārakaiḥ = varṇasaṁkara — sexual intermixture of classes + kārakaiḥ — by producing; utsādyante — disappeared; jātidharmāḥ — individual skills; kuladharmāś — family duties; ca — and; śāśvatāḥ — long—standing, traditional

By the sins of the family destroyers and by the sexual intermixture of the classes, individual skills and traditional family duties disappear. (1.42)

Commentary:

It is definitely correct that individual skills and family duties disappear as a result of class mixture, but as kriyā yogis we are not interested to the extent that Arjuna extolled. Certainly, as a householder kriyā yogi, I myself, tried my best to institute individual skills and to foster family duties but that does not mean this is my main objective. In fact many of the very same children to whom I gave these, in the end rejected me, just because I am a kriyā yogi. We participate in the system but we do not like it all, because it is by nature, contrary. Somebody must establish these individual skills and family duties. We will hear from Śrī Krishna that ultimately He is the initiator of these, but that does not mean that this system of cultural advancement is kriyā yoga. Even though our supreme teacher, Śrī Krishna, is the master teacher of the upliftment, it is not kriyā yoga. That is the paradox. On one hand, we support cultural upliftment and on the other hand, we remain very callous to it. One should only be involved in cultural activities to the extent that it becomes mandatory to free oneself from material existence.

उत्सन्नकुलधर्माणां
मनुष्याणां जनार्दन ।
नरके ऽनियतं वासो
भवतीत्यनुशुश्रुम ॥ १.४३ ॥
utsannakuladharmāṇāṁ
manuṣyāṇāṁ janārdana
narake 'niyataṁ vāso
bhavatītyanuśuśruma (1.43)

utsanna kula dharmāṇāṁ = utsanna — destroyed + kuladharmāṇāṁ — of family customs; manuṣyāṇām — of men; janārdana — O Kṛṣṇa; narake — in hell; 'niyataṁ = aniyatam — indefinitely; vāso — dwelling; bhavatītyanuśuśruma = bhavati — it is + iti — was developed + anuśuśruma — we heard repeatedly

O Krishna, those who destroy the family customs dwell in hell indefinitely. This was declared repeatedly. (1.43)

Commentary:

Undoubtedly those who destroy the family dwell in hell indefinitely, but conversely those who support the family do not necessarily dwell in heaven. All the same, as kriyā yogis we are not interested in destroying the family but we will not maintain it any more than necessary. We do not have time for either activity. Our primary interest is kriyā practice. Those who upset moral values will definitely see hell but as kriyā yogis we cannot make cultural upliftment the priority. At the same time, we do not object to others who protect the culture. Let them complete with the task.

अहो बत महत्पापं
कर्तुं व्यवसिता वयम् ।
यद्राज्यसुखलोभेन
हन्तुं स्वजनमुद्यताः ॥ १.४४ ॥
aho bata mahatpāpaṁ
kartuṁ vyavasitā vayam
yadrājyasukhalobhena
hantuṁ svajanamudyatāḥ (1.44)

aho — O!; bata — what a wonder!; mahat — great; pāpaṁ — sin; kartuṁ — to perform; vyavasitā — committed to; vayam — we; yad — which; rājyasukhalobhena = rājya — aristocratic + sukha — pleasure + lobhena — with greed; hantuṁ — to kill; svajanam — own folks; udyatāḥ — eager for

O! What a wonder! We are committed to perform a great sin, being eager to kill our kinfolk, through greed for aristocratic pleasures. (1.44)

Commentary:

This is a tactful insult to Lord Krishna who is a supreme teacher of the kriyā craft. Persons like Lord Krishna, Lord Balarāma and Lord Shiva are masters of the craft. If they do not know what they are doing, then we as their students, are ignorant as well. Hence to insult any of them like this, would be a roundabout way of condemning ourselves. Admittedly, due to cultural complications, it seems that we are never able to complete the path. Still the course is there. Some rare yogis completed it successfully. Persons like Śrī Agastya Muni, Śrī Hanumānji and Śrī Matanga Rishi, did so, as well as Śrī Nārada and Śrī Shuka.

Arjuna wonders how Śrī Krishna, as well as his brothers and their friends, would perform a great sin in being eager to kill kinsmen through greed for the pleasures of aristocratic living. In fact, they are not going to kill the wayward kinfolk for that reason. Killing would take place in a civil war but the underlying reason for it in this case, is not what Arjuna perceives it to be. He sees in this way because he wavered from the kriyā yoga perspective.

यदि मामप्रतीकारम्
अशस्त्रं शस्त्रपाणयः ।
धार्तराष्ट्रा रणे हन्युस्
तन्मे क्षेमतरं भवेत् ॥१.४५॥
yadi māmapratīkāram
aśastraṁ śastrapāṇayaḥ
dhārtarāṣṭrā raṇe hanyus
tanme kṣemataraṁ bhavet (1.45)

yadi — if; mām — me; apratīkāram — unresisting; aśastraṁ — without weapons, unarmed; śastrapāṇayaḥ — those bearing weapons; dhārtarāṣṭrā — sons of Dhṛtarāṣṭra; raṇe — in battle; hanyuḥ — they may kill; tan — this; me — to me; kṣemataraṁ — greater happiness; bhavet — would be

If the weapon—bearing sons of Dhṛtarāṣṭra should kill me in battle, while I was unresisting, and unarmed, this to me would be greater pleasure. (1.45)

Commentary:

Here again we see evidence of Arjuna's reversion from the kriyā yoga perspective to the normal emotional plane. He says that if killed by the opposing Kurus while unarmed, then to him that would be a greater pleasure. In other words, Arjuna prefers to be a martyr, something that is contrary to the kriyā yoga course. It is part of the emotional way of acting for a famous position later on. Mahatma Gandhi, a famous politician in India, followed this course and was killed by an assassin. He was martyred and idolized by the East Indians. Recently another person who followed the same course and adopted many of Gandhi's tactics, was the Rev. Dr. Martin Luther King. Such great social liberators, however, are not kriyā yogis.

एवमुक्त्वार्जुनः संख्ये
रथोपस्थ उपाविशत् ।
विसृज्य सशरं चापं
शोकसंविग्नमानसः ॥१.४६॥
evamuktvārjunaḥ saṁkhye
rathopastha upāviśat
visṛjya saśaraṁ cāpaṁ
śokasaṁvignamānasaḥ (1.46)

evam — thus; uktvā — having spoken; arjunaḥ — Arjuna; saṁkhye — in the conflict; rathopastha = ratha — chariot + upastha — seat; upāviśat — sat down; visṛjya — casting aside; saśaraṁ — together with arrow; cāpaṁ — bow; śokasaṁvignamānasaḥ = śoka — sorrow + saṁvigna — overwhelmed + mānasaḥ — heart

Having spoken, Arjuna, who was in the midst of the conflict, sat down on his chariot. Casting aside his arrow and bow, he was overwhelmed with sorrow. (1.46)

Commentary:

This is the result of the sort of mood Arjuna displayed. In short, the result is emotional depression. If one does not succeed in the quest for martyrdom, one becomes saddened and depressed.

CHAPTER 2

Divine State*

संजय उवाच
तं तथा कृपयाविष्टम्
अश्रुपूर्णाकुलेक्षणम् ।
विषीदन्तमिदं वाक्यम्
उवाच मधुसूदनः ॥२.१॥
saṁjaya uvāca
taṁ tathā kṛpayāviṣṭam
aśrupūrṇākulekṣaṇam
viṣīdantamidaṁ vākyam
uvāca madhusūdanaḥ (2.1)

saṁjaya — Sanjaya; uvāca — said; taṁ — to him; tathā — in this way; kṛpayāviṣṭam — overcome with pity; aśrupūrṇākulekṣaṇam = aśru — tear + pūrṇa — filled + ākula — perplexed + īkṣaṇam — eyes; viṣīdantam — saddened with hopelessness; idaṁ — this; vākyam — response; uvāca — spoke; madhusūdanaḥ — killer of Madhu

Sanjaya said: To him who was overcome with pity, whose eyes were filled with tears, who was perplexed and saddened with hopelessness, the killer of Madhu spoke this response: (2.1)

Commentary:

Pity, though an admirable quality on the social and cultural planes, is not useful on the path of kriyā yoga. Neither is cruelty. Duty, however, is relevant either to assist someone dispassionately or to introduce a discipline to help someone solve a complication of destiny. Otherwise a kriyā yogi refrains from social and cultural affairs.

Sanjaya aptly addressed Śrī Krishna as Madhusūdana, the killer of Madhu, indicating that Śrī Krishna was a person who would never slip from the kriyā yoga stance. Krishna was known as the infallible one, as we hear later on.

श्रीभगवानुवाच
कुतस्त्वा कश्मलमिदं
विषमे समुपस्थितम् ।
अनार्यजुष्टमस्वर्ग्यम्
अकीर्तिकरमर्जुन ॥२.२॥
śrībhagavānuvāca
kutastvā kaśmalamidaṁ
viṣame samupasthitam
anāryajuṣṭamasvargyam
akīrtikaramarjuna (2.2)

śrī bhagavān — the Blessed Lord; uvāca — said; kutastvā = kutas — how + tvā — to you; kaśmalam — sickly emotion; idaṁ — this; viṣame — at a crucial time; samupasthitam — come; anāryajuṣṭam — not suitable for a cultured man; asvargyam — not facilitating heaven in the hereafter; akīrtikaram — causing disgrace; arjuna — O Arjuna

**The Mahābhārata contains no chapter headings. This title was assigned by the translator on the basis of verse 72 of this chapter.*

The Blessed Lord said: How has this sickly emotion come to you at a crucial time? It is not suitable for a cultured man. It does not facilitate heaven in the hereafter. It causes disgrace, O Arjuna. (2.2)

Commentary:

The sickly emotion, kaśmalam, the mood assumed by a kriyā yogi when he is shifted from the kriyā stance, is detrimental to a well—trained kriyā yogi like Arjuna. Still, it possessed him and presented itself as his identity. Such an emotion, according to Śrī Krishna, is not even desireable in the cultural sense if a man wants to achieved the heavenly world in the hereafter. He would be denied such a promotion if he succumbed to and acted under this emotion. Exactly how did that sickly emotion take over Arjuna? How was it possible for this emotion to control Arjuna from within his psyche even in the presence of Śrī Krishna?

Obviously that energy can take over any of us at any time. It has a back door into our psyche from the inner dimensions. It is so near that it compromises our resolution even when we stand beside a teacher like Śrī Krishna.

क्लैब्यं मा स्म गमः पार्थ
नैतत्त्वय्युपपद्यते ।
क्षुद्रं हृदयदौर्बल्यं
त्यक्त्वोत्तिष्ठ परंतप ॥२.३॥

klaibyaṁ mā sma gamaḥ pārtha
naitattvayyupapadyate
kṣudraṁ hṛdayadaurbalyaṁ
tyaktvottiṣṭha paraṁtapa (2.3)

klaibyaṁ — cowardly behavior; mā — not; sma — in fact; gamaḥ — should entertain; pārtha — O son of Patha; naitat — not this; tvayyupapadyate = tvayi — in your + upapadyate — is suitable; kṣudraṁ — degrading; hṛdayadaurbalyaṁ — emotional weakness; tyaktvottiṣṭha = tyaktva — give up + uttiṣṭha — stand up; paraṁtapa — scorcher of the enemy

O son of Pṛthā, you should not entertain cowardly behavior. This is not suitable for you. Give up this degrading emotional weakness. Stand, O scorcher of the enemy. (2.3)

Commentary:

Śrī Krishna addresses Arjuna here as the son of Pṛthā, Arjuna's mother. He could have addressed him as the son of Pāndu, Arjuna's departed father. This indicated that Arjuna was, at the time, more inclined to feminine behavior. In fact, kriyā yoga is not a favorite discipline of women. Kriyā yoga is threatening to the social and cultural organization. It threatens the security of human civilization. Therefore it is not favored by females.

This does not mean that Arjuna's mother was not a kriyā student. She was. She encouraged her sons in heroic acts but generally, women as a class are not inclined to kriyā yoga.

Arjuna's mother, Pṛthā, took up kriyā lessons earlier in her life but near the end, in old age, she adopted it more seriously as the story is told in *Mahābhārata* literature. This lady and women like Dhṛtarāṣṭra's wife, Gāndhārī, had some knowledge of the practice. These were exceptional women.

Śrī Krishna ordered Arjuna to abandon the degrading emotional weakness and to resume his normal self as a kriyā yogi who could apply physical disciplines to social circumstances and rise above material nature; but could Arjuna do this, so abruptly? As we will observe, it will take Arjuna some time before he fully recovers from the depression.

Śrī Krishna addressed Arjuna as scorcher of the enemy, a name Arjuna earned by his social and cultural actions which reflected his kriyā practice and military training. This was done to cause Arjuna to recover himself and shift back to his normal mood.

अर्जुन उवाच
कथं भीष्ममहं संख्ये
द्रोणं च मधुसूदन ।
इषुभिः प्रतियोत्स्यामि
पूजार्हावरिसूदन ॥ २.४॥
arjuna uvāca
kathaṁ bhīṣmamahaṁ saṁkhye
droṇaṁ ca madhusūdana
iṣubhiḥ pratiyotsyāmi
pūjārhāvarisūdana (2.4)

arjuna — Arjuna; uvāca — said; kathaṁ — how; bhīṣmam — Bhisma; ahaṁ — I; saṁkhye — in battle; droṇaṁ — Droṇa; ca — and; madhusūdana — O killer of Madhu; iṣubhiḥ — with arrows; pratiyotsyāmi — I will attack; pūjārhāv arisūdana = pūjārhāu — worthy of reverence + arisūdana — killer of the enemy, Krishna

Arjuna said: How will I attack in battle, Bhishma and Droṇa, who are worthy of reverence, O Krishna? (2.4)

Commentary:

In all cases, in kriyā yoga as well as in social and cultural life, it is questionable if one should attack those worthy of reverence. Arjuna now begins to tone down. His emotional sickness begins to subside.

Normally there is no reason to attack those who are revered. These include parents, school teachers and religious ministers. For his own sake, a kriyā yogi should never attack them. However in this existence one has to live beyond his own sake. He must also live as a matter of duty to ancestors, family, community, government and supernatural force. All these must be satisfied at one time or another. Thus a kriyā yogi might have to attack those who are worthy of reverence, but he should never do it for his own sake because he has nothing to gain from such acts. In all cases, if he attacks as a matter of duty, still he has nothing to gain by it. We must now look to the supreme teacher of kriyā yoga in action, to find out how and why we may attack such persons. I inform readers that the *Bhagavad Gītā,* which is famous as a philosophical discourse and a guideline for devotion to Krishna, is actually a course in how to apply kriyā yoga to worldly affairs. Further evidence will be provided in this commentary.

गुरूनहत्वा हि महानुभावान्
श्रेयो भोक्तुं भैक्ष्यमपीह लोके
हत्वार्थकामांस्तु गुरूनिहैव
भुञ्जीय भोगान्रुधिरप्रदिग्धान् ॥ २.५॥
gurūnahatvā hi mahānubhāvān
śreyo bhoktuṁ bhaikṣyam
apīha loke
hatvārthakāmāṁstu gurūn
ihaiva
bhuñjīya bhogān rudhira—
pradigdhān (2.5)

gurūn — the revered teachers; ahatvā — not killing; hi — in fact; mahānubhāvān — great—natured; śreyo — better; bhoktuṁ — to eat; bhaikṣyamapīha = bhaikṣyam — begging + api — also + iha — here; loke — on earth; hatvārthakāmāṅs = hatvā — having killed + artha — on the basis of + kāmān — impulsive desires; tu — but; gurūn — revered teachers; ihaiva = iha — here + eva — indeed; bhuñjīya — I would enjoy; bhogān — luxuries; rudhirapradigdhān = rudhira — bloody + pradigdhān — stained

In fact, it is better to eat by begging in this world than by killing the revered teachers who are great—natured. But having slain the venerable teachers on the basis of impulsive desires, I would enjoy blood—stained luxuries here on earth. (2.5)

Commentary:

For a kriyā yogi it is better to live by begging than to kill the revered teachers, especially those great—natured ones (mahā—anubhāvān). That is the preference. Still a kriyā yogi should never let his preference override his duty or prevent him from doing what is necessary.

A kriyā yogi, if he slays such venerable teachers as a matter of righted duty, should also not do it on the basis of impulsive desires. He should not after having slain them enjoy any bloodstained luxuries which they left behind. A kriyā yogi must remain detached in performance of his duty even in the aftermath, of a victory. In that way he remains emotionally clean and is saved from circumstancial reaction. Everyone, kriyā yogis and the rest, must at one time or another, serve as an agent of nature but in so doing, the kriyā yogi should not be enthralled by the outcome. Whatever nature motivates, nature will later renounce. One must understand this. One should not always rely on nature for support merely because she has used one as an agent for some act. This is part of the Samkhya philosophy, mentioned by Lord Krishna in verses 2.39, 5.4 and 13.27.

न चैतद्विद्मः कतरन्नो गरीयो
यद्वा जयेम यदि वा नो जयेयुः ।
यानेव हत्वा न जिजीविषामस्
तेऽवस्थिताः प्रमुखे धार्तराष्ट्राः ॥२.६॥
na caitadvidmaḥ kataranno garīyo
yadvā jayema yadi vā no jayeyuḥ
yāneva hatvā na jijīviṣāmas
te'vasthitāḥ pramukhe
dhārtarāṣṭrāḥ (2.6)

na — not; caitad — and this; vidmaḥ — we know; kataran — which of the alternatives; no = nah — for us; garīyo — is better; yad – which; vā — other; jayema — we should conquer; yadi — if; vā — or; no = naḥ — to us; jayeyuḥ — they should triumph over; yān — who; eva — indeed; hatvā — having killed; na — us; jijīviṣāmas — we desire to outlive; te — they; 'vasthitāḥ = avasthitāḥ — stand armed; pramukhe — before us; dhārtarāṣṭrāḥ — the sons of Dhṛtarāṣṭra

And this we do not know, which of the alternatives is better; whether we should conquer or if they should triumph over us. It concerns these sons of Dhṛtarāṣṭra who stand armed before us, and whom we would not desire to outlive, if they are killed. (2.6)

Commentary:

Actually we know very little about the intricacies of action. In this particular verse, Arjuna regained the track of a kriyā yogi. Since we do not know, because we cannot see past lives, we have to find out from someone who perceives, from a kriyā master, preferably from a senior master like Śrī Krishna. That person could tell us which is better in any given circumstance, whether to participate aggressively or to refrain completely.

As Arjuna states, a kriyā yogi is not too particular about his own body's survival. He has a sense of values which do not permit him to live at the expense of others. We should notice here how Arjuna is being shifted back into kriyā vision. Of greater note, it appears that Arjuna remained unaware of how he was shifted into the social and cultural perspective and how he was shifted back into the kriyā view.

Even though mentioned above that we should find out from someone who knows the appropriate action, still, that is easier said than done. We do not have Śrī Krishna before us as Arjuna did. The teachers available to us may not be as knowledgeable as Śrī Krishna. They may not see past lives which formed the foundation for present circumstances. This means that they may give faulty advice.

कार्पण्यदोषोपहतस्वभावः
पृच्छामि त्वां धर्मसंमूढचेताः
यच्छ्रेयः स्यान्निश्चितं ब्रूहि तन्मे
शिष्यस्तेऽहं शाधि मां त्वां प्रपन्नम्
॥२.७॥

kārpaṇyadoṣopahata—
svabhāvaḥ
pṛcchāmi tvāṁ dharma—
saṁmūḍhacetāḥ
yacchreyaḥ syānniścitaṁ
brūhi tanme
śiṣyaste'haṁ śādhi māṁ
tvāṁ prapannam (2.7)

kārpaṇyadoṣopahatasvabhāvaḥ = kārpaṇya — mercy—prone + doṣa — faulty weakness + upahata — overcome + svabhāvaḥ — my feelings (a person being afflicted with inappropriate mercy, a compulsive mercy—prone man); pṛcchāmi — I ask; tvāṁ — you; dharmasaṁmūḍhacetāḥ = dharma — sense of duty + saṁmūḍha — clouded by confusion + cetāḥ — mind (one whose sense of duty is clouded by confusion of mind); yacchreyaḥ = yac (yad) — which + chreyaḥ (śreyaḥ) — is better; syān — it should be; niścitaṁ — for certain; brūhi — tell; tan — this; me — to me; śiṣyas — student; te — of yours; 'haṁ = ahaṁ — I; śādhi — instruct; mām — me; tvāṁ — you; prapannam — submission

As a mercy-prone man, overcome by these feelings of pity, with my sense of duty clouded by mental confusion, I ask You to tell me with certainty, what is preferable. I am a student of Yours. Instruct me, who am submitted to You. (2.7)

Commentary:

From his admittance here, we can see that Arjuna did not have a set way of getting himself back on to the kriyā yoga perspective. By nature, he was a mercy-prone man (kārpanya). Thus if one has this type of nature, one can learn from studying its actions in the life of Arjuna. Arjuna however was perceptive enough in his psychology to know that his sense of duty was clouded by mental confusion. Thus a kriyā yogi must be able to recognize his mental condition.

Arjuna now presents himself to Śrī Krishna as a student (śiṣya). Arjuna certainly was Krishna's student for learning the application of kriyā yoga. Śrī Krishna was not Arjuna's sole teacher. Arjuna had others. In kriyā yoga, he even took lessons from his elder brother Yudhiṣṭhira who was now contesting the reign of the opposing Kurus. In kriyā yoga, we have many teachers. We do not accept only one teacher, because kriyā yoga is a complex science. Usually we learn its various skills from masters of the particular techniques. Śrī Krishna was Arjuna's teacher for the application of kriyā yoga to social and cultural affairs.

Unknown to many readers of the *Bhagavad Gītā,* including some famous teachers and devotees, Arjuna was already a successful student of kriyā yoga before he came to Kurukṣetra to stand before the opposing Kurus. The question is: If he was indeed a successful student, why did he suffer depression seeing the opposing army? Why did he request to be taught by Śrī Krishna? Simply put even though Arjuna was a successful student, he was not learned in the application of kriyā yoga to social and cultural affairs. That is an entirely different science. Kriyā yoga is not really meant for that application. It is basically a science of purifying the individual psyche for spiritual clarity, for leaving behind the social and cultural setting. Thus, it takes special techniques when in a worldly setting as Arjuna faced at Kurukṣetra.

Bhīṣma, the senior in the Kuru dynasty, Arjuna's great uncle, would have been the person to teach Arjuna the application of kriyā yoga to social and worldly affairs, but providence did not allow Bhīṣma the honor. Rather, we see here that Śrī Krishna, the supreme teacher of the science, taught Arjuna. Fortunately for us, we will learn of it from Krishna's instruction to Arjuna.

From many thousands of years later in posterity, we take the position as students of Śrī Krishna, and we ask Him as Arjuna did, to inspire us, as we submit ourselves to Him.

न हि प्रपश्यामि ममापनुद्याद्
यच्छोकमुच्छोषणमिन्द्रियाणाम् ।
अवाप्य भूमावसपत्नमृद्धं
राज्यं सुराणामपि चाधिपत्यम् ॥२.८॥
na hi prapaśyāmi mamāpanudyād
yacchokamucchoṣaṇam indriyāṇām
avāpya bhūmāvasapatnam ṛddhaṁ
rājyaṁ surāṇāmapi cādhipatyam (2.8)

na— not; hi— in fact; prapaśyāmi— I see; mamāpanudyād = mama— of me + apanudyāt —should remove; yac (yad) — which; chokam (śokam) — sadness; ucchoṣaṇam — absorbs; indriyāṇām — sensual enthusiasm; avāpya — acquiring; bhūmāvasapatnam = bhūmau — on earth + asapatnam — unrivaled; ṛddhaṁ — prosperity; rājyaṁ — rulership; surāṇām — of the angelic kingdom; api — also; cādhipatyam = ca — and + adhipatyam — sovereignty

In fact, I do not see, what would remove the sadness that absorbs my enthusiasm, even unrivaled rulership and prosperity on earth or sovereignty over the angelic kingdom. (2.8)

Commentary:

Some persons can be satisfied at least for the time being with unrivaled rulership and prosperity or even with sovereignty over the angelic world, but a person who has the kriyā yoga tendency cannot aspire in that way. Many devotees of Śrī Krishna exist and they are all great souls, special people, merely by the virtue of their devotional attraction to Him, but the kriyā yogi cannot be satisfied by leadership, prosperity and supernatural glory over others, even if these are administered in a devotional setting. This is how we can recognize a kriyā yogi. It is not that a kriyā yogi stands apart from the other devotees or that he is special in comparison with others. That is not it. By nature the kriyā yogi is just not satisfied being a leader of devotees or having prosperity in a devotional setting or ruling angelic beings.

संजय उवाच
एवमुक्त्वा हृषीकेशं
गुडाकेशः परंतप ।
न योत्स्य इति गोविन्दम्
उक्त्वा तूष्णीं बभूव ह ॥२.९॥
saṁjaya uvāca
evamuktvā hṛṣīkeśaṁ
guḍākeśaḥ paraṁtapa
na yotsya iti govindam
uktvā tūṣṇīṁ babhūva ha (2.9)

saṁjaya — Sanjaya; uvāca — said; evam — thus; uktvā — having appealed to; hṛṣīkeśaṁ — Kṛṣṇa; guḍākeśaḥ — Arjuna; paraṁtapa — scorcher of enemies; na — not; yotsya — I will fight; iti — thus; govindam — chief of the cowherds; uktvā — having spoken; tūṣṇīṁ — silently; babhūva — became; ha — indeed

Sanjaya said: O Dhṛtarāṣṭra, scorcher of enemies, after appealing to Krishna, Arjuna said to Govinda, the chief of cowherds, "I will not fight." Having said this, he became silent. (2.9)

Commentary:

Sanjaya now addressed King *Dhṛtarāṣṭra* as the scorcher of enemies. This was to offer respect to the blind King for listening attentively and for not becoming as emotional as Arjuna.

To illustrate the superiority of a kriyā yoga master, especially a supreme master as Lord Krishna, Sanjaya addressed Śrī Krishna, merely as Govinda, the chief of cowherds. A kriyā master does not require status. Kriyā yoga is such that it frees even ordinary beings from insecurity. Śrī Krishna had no such insecurities but since Dhṛtarāṣṭra was observing everything only by hearing and by mystic transference of visions, Sanjaya wanted to emphasize that a kriyā yoga master taps energy from a source completely removed from rulership and prosperity.

Sometimes established dynasties like the Kurus would berate Śrī Krishna or Śrī Balarāma as being country boys, merely cowherders and farmers. Here Sanjaya also addressed Śrī Krishna as a cowherd, but only to show that Arjuna, who was a prince from a prestigious dynasty, appealed to that country boy. Why was Arjuna doing that? Arjuna declared that he would not fight but he did so in resignation as a student who was willing to act once the teacher established a preference. The teacher did not have to be a ruler or a man of wealth.

Krishna will show powerful visions later on but that is not the reason Arjuna surrendered to Him. A person may have political leadership but he may not be a kriyā master. Another may be very wealthy and know nothing about kriyā. And yet another may have charisma and still be ignorant of how to shift somebody from depression to the kriyā vision.

तमुवाच हृषीकेशः
प्रहसन्निव भारत ।
सेनयोरुभयोर्मध्ये
विषीदन्तमिदं वचः ॥२.१०॥
tamuvāca hṛṣīkeśaḥ
prahasanniva bhārata
senayorubhayormadhye
viṣīdantamidaṁ vacaḥ (2.10)

tam — to him; uvāca — spoke; hṛṣīkeśaḥ — Kṛṣṇa; prahasan — smiling; iva — like; bhārata — O descendant of Bharata; senayoḥ — of the two armies; ubhayoḥ — of both; madhye — in the middle; viṣīdantam — dejected; idaṁ — this; vacaḥ — speech

Then, in the middle of both armies, Krishna, who was smiling, spoke this speech to the dejected Arjuna. (2.10)

Commentary:

As the supreme master of kriyā yoga, Śrī Krishna was smiling in a situation that Arjuna found to be distressing. However, the supreme kriyā teacher was not alone in standing before such a situation undisturbed. Others like Bhīṣma and Droṇa, who mastered sufficient kriyā practice and who were to some degree expert at applying it to social and cultural affairs, were also undisturbed. Both Arjuna and Duryodhana are shown here to be upset, as a result of drifting from the kriyā stance. Duryodhana spoke to his military instructor but he spoke in such a way as to disrespect the teacher. Therefore he was shifted into a position of arrogance. Arjuna was in a position to listen but he had lost the kriyā stance. This difference in their attitudes sets Arjuna apart from Duryodhana. Arjuna, though diverted, retained protection from a humility energy. Duryodhana was covered by an arrogant force which would lead him to ruination.

श्रीभगवानुवाच
अशोच्यानन्वशोचस्त्वं
प्रज्ञावादांश्च भाषसे ।
गतासूनगतासूंश्च
नानुशोचन्ति पण्डिताः ॥२.११॥
śrībhagavānuvāca
aśocyānanvaśocastvaṁ
prajñāvādāṁśca bhāṣase
gatāsūnagatāsūṁśca
nānuśocanti paṇḍitāḥ (2.11)

śrī—bhagavān – the Blessed Lord; uvāca — said; aśocyān — that which should be regretted; anvaśocas — mourned; tvaṁ — you; prajñāvādāṁś — intelligent statements; ca — and; bhāṣase — you express; gatāsūn — departed souls; agatāsūṁś — those not departed; ca — and; nānuśocanti = na — not + anuśocanti — mourn; paṇḍitāḥ — educated persons

The Blessed Lord said: You mourned for that which should not be regretted. And you expressed intelligent statements, but the educated persons mourn neither for the embodied or departed souls.(2.11)

Commentary:

By mourning for that which should not be regretted, Arjuna exposed himself as being removed from the kriyā vision. He now lacked the two preliminary perceptions of a kriyā yogi. The first one is perception of the spirit as an eternal reality, distinct and different from the material body. The second is that one should not cringe from compulsions of destiny, even if such occupations are unpalatable. These two perceptions link to a third perception, that of the Supreme Lord Whose approval is necessary for a prolonged favorable existence. If one acts in such a way as to draw His disapproval, one's temporary happiness will soon become a distressful situation.

Arjuna did express intelligent statements, but since he was shifted off from the kriyā perspective, his statements were being misused by the emotional energies. Such energies used true statements to add credence to their wishes. We will get some insight from Śrī Krishna as to how the emotional nature uses the intellect to support its views.

न त्वेवाहं जातु नासं
न त्वं नेमे जनाधिपाः ।
न चैव न भविष्यामः
सर्वे वयमतः परम् ॥२.१२॥
na tvevāhaṁ jātu nāsaṁ
na tvaṁ neme janādhipāḥ
na caiva na bhaviṣyāmaḥ
sarve vayamataḥ param (2.12)

na — no; tvevāhaṁ = tv (tu) — in fact + eva — alone + ahaṁ — I; jātu — ever; nāsaṁ = na — not + āsaṁ — I did exist; na — nor; tvaṁ — you; neme = na — nor + ime — these; jana—adhipāḥ — rulers of the people; na — not; caiva — and indeed; na — nor; bhaviṣyāmaḥ — we will exist; sarve – all; vayam — we; ataḥ — from now; param — onwards

There was never a time when I did not exist, nor you nor these rulers of the people. Nor will we cease to exist from now onwards. (2.12)

Commentary:

This is the first perception in kriyā yoga. One does not have to be a devotee of Śrī Krishna to experience this perception. Alternately, one can be a devotee and not experience this view. Some devotees of Krishna inherently believe this, even though they have no conscious recall being separate from their material bodies.

This perception is dependent on spiritual clarity and vision. It can also be dependent just on experiencing the separation of the gross and subtle body. By becoming conscious in dreams, one can experience the subtle body's separation from the physical form. This is not dependent on devotion to Lord Krishna. In addition in many other societies both inside and outside of India, the facts stated in the verse were discovered and introduced by persons who somehow realized that the spirit is not the same as the body. A human being does not have to be a follower of Śrī Krishna to understand this fact. The *Upanishads* attest Yama as the first human being to find out definitely that the body and soul were different. He then instructed Nachiketa. Elsewhere in other places like China, we have heard of completely independent discoveries by mystic perception of this truth.

Here in this verse, Śrī Krishna dismissed Arjuna's fear about killing the bodies of the opposing army. In effect Śrī Krishna informed Arjuna, that since Krishna, Himself, Arjuna and the rulers assembled there, existed always in the past and would exist onwards in the future for eternity, their bodies were as valueable as Arjuna suggested. The commodity of value was the spirits using such bodies, and that could not be interfered with by Arjuna.

This one statement of Śrī Krishna completely nullifies Arjuna's excuse about being sympathetic to the bodies of the opposing Kurus. Still, even though Śrī Krishna established this, Arjuna did not at the time, shift back to the kriyā vision. To him the emotional views were still reality.

देहिनोऽस्मिन्यथा देहे
कौमारं यौवनं जरा ।
तथा देहान्तरप्राप्तिर्
धीरस्तत्र न मुह्यति ॥२.१३॥
dehino'sminyathā dehe
kaumāraṁ yauvanaṁ jarā
tathā dehāntaraprāptir
dhīrastatra na muhyati (2.13)

dehinaḥ — of the embodied soul; 'smin = asmin — in this; yathā — as; dehe — in the body; kaumāraṁ — in childhood; yauvanam — in youth; jarā — in old age; tathā — so in sequence; dehāntaraprāptir = deha — body + antara — another + prāptiḥ — acquirement; dhīraḥ — wise person; tatra — on this topic; na — not; muhyati — is confused

As the embodied soul endures childhood, youth and old age, so another body is acquired in sequence. The wise person is not confused on this topic. (2.13)

Commentary:

Śrī Krishna now continues to address Arjuna's reasonings which were supportive of Arjuna's vision on the emotional plane. Arjuna might think, that even if the spirit was eternal, the current body is valuable because one would not get another body. As such, Śrī Krishna stated in advance, that one gets bodies one after another as one transmigrates.

On the basis of the life in the physical body, the embodied soul endures childhood, youth and old age, without having to worry about those changes. He gets those opportunities as a matter of course without even endeavoring for them. Similarly, on the basis of the subtle body, he will get another physical form. This is done in sequence (tatra). This happens naturally. It is inevitable. The soldiers will not have to work to achieve it. It is a part of nature and even without human endeavor it will take place.

मात्रास्पर्शास्तु कौन्तेय
शीतोष्णसुखदुःखदाः ।
आगमापायिनोऽनित्यास्
तांस्तितिक्षस्व भारत ॥२.१४॥
mātrāsparśāstu kaunteya
śītoṣṇasukhaduḥkhadāḥ
āgamāpāyino'nityās
tāṁstitikṣasva bhārata (2.14)

mātrāsparśāḥ — mundane sensations; tu — but; kaunteya — O son of Kuntī; śītoṣṇasukhaduḥkhadāḥ = śīta — cold + usna — heat + sukha — pleasure + duḥkha — pain + dāḥ — causing; āgamāpāyino = āgama — coming + apāyinaḥ — going; 'nityās = anityāḥ — not manifested continually; tāṁs — them; titikṣasva — you should cope; bhārata — O man of the Bharata family

O son of Kuntī, mundane sensations which cause cold and heat, pleasure and pain, do come and go. Cope with them, O man of the Bharata family. (2.14)

Commentary:

Somehow or the other, a man should overlook the mundane sensations (mātrāsparśās). These feelings exist in the emotional nature. Even though they are impressionable, they should not be used as a guideline for action in the material world. In the kriyā vision, one also perceives these feelings but one does so within his psyche from a lesser or greater distance according to how one mastered the practice.

यं हि न व्यथयन्त्येते
पुरुषं पुरुषर्षभ ।
समदुःखसुखं धीरं
सोऽमृतत्वाय कल्पते ॥२.१५॥
yaṁ hi na vyathayantyete
puruṣaṁ puruṣarṣabha
samaduḥkhasukhaṁ dhīraṁ
so'mṛtatvāya kalpate (2.15)

yaṁ — whosoever; hi — indeed; na — not; vyathayantyete = vyathayanti — afflict + ete — these mundane sensations; puruṣaṁ — that person; puruṣarṣabha — O bull among men; samaduḥkhasukhaṁ — steady in miserable and enjoyable conditions; dhīraṁ — wise man; so — he; 'mṛta tvāya = amṛtatvāya — to immortality; kalpate — is fit

O bull among men, these mundane sensations do not afflict the wise man who is steady in miserable or enjoyable conditions. That person is fit for immortality. (2.15)

Commentary:

In a very tactful way, Arjuna presented his case for not participating on the battlefield. Likewise, Śrī Krishna engages in tact, saying in a roundabout way, that even though Arjuna spoke some wise words, he could not be rated as a wise man steady in miserable and enjoyable conditions. Arjuna was unfit for the vision of a person who was in touch with the spirit's immortality. Here Śrī Krishna addresses the superior person as a *dhira*. He does not define that person as his devotee, for as I said before, a person can be perceptive of spiritual existence and not be a devotee of Śrī Krishna. And conversely a person may be a staunch devotee of Śrī Krishna and like Arjuna, lose the spiritual view.

नासतो विद्यते भावो
नाभावो विद्यते सतः ।
उभयोरपि दृष्टोऽन्तस्
त्वनयोस्तत्त्वदर्शिभिः ॥२.१६॥

nāsato = na— no + asatas — of the non—substantial things; vidyate— there is; bhāvo—enduring existence; nābhāvo = na — no + abhāvaḥ — lack of existence; vidyate — there is; sataḥ — substantial things; ubhayoḥ — of the two; api —

nāsato vidyate bhāvo
nābhāvo vidyate sataḥ
ubhayorapi dṛṣṭo'ntas
tvanayostattvadarśibhiḥ (2.16)

also; dṛṣṭaḥ — perceived; 'ntas = antaḥ — certainty; tvanayos = tu — but + anayoḥ — of these two; tattvadarśibhiḥ = tattva — reality + darśibhiḥ — by mystic powers

Of the non—substantial things, there is no enduring existence. Of the substantial things, there is no lack of existence. These two truths were perceived with certainty by the mystic seers of reality. (2.16)

Commentary:

Just before the time of Śrī Krishna, the sages who wrote the Upanishad, understood these truths by direct mystic perception that was gained by virtue of austerities in yoga practice. They came to certain conclusions and recorded their views. This verse is a statement of their opinions.

Basically this means that if something has eternal worth, its existence is assured. And if something has temporary value, it will not endure. The point however is that a limited being does not determine what is absolute and what is relative. That is determined by the layout of existence. If one cannot see this layout, then he will give value the temporary and underrate the eternal, as Arjuna did in overvaluing the material bodies of his relatives. The Supreme Being knows intimately what is absolute and what is relative but the limited beings in this world have the vision now and again.

अविनाशि तु तद्विद्धि
येन सर्वमिदं ततम् ।
विनाशमव्ययस्यास्य
न कश्चित्कर्तुमर्हति ॥२.१७॥
avināśi tu tadviddhi
yena sarvamidaṁ tatam
vināśamavyayasyāsya
na kaścitkartumarhati (2.17)

avināśi — indestructible; tu — indeed; tad — that factor; viddhi — know; yena — by which; sarvam — all; idaṁ — this world; tatam — is pervaded; vināśam — destructible; avyayasyāsya — of the everlasting principle; na — no; kaścit — anyone; kartum — to accomplish; arhati — can

Know that indestructible factor by which all this world is pervaded. No one can accomplish the destruction of that everlasting principle. (2.17)

Commentary:

This is the vision of the kriyā yogi — that he sees or tracks that indestructible factor by which this world is pervaded. Everywhere he goes, and in everything he does he should perceive that factor, for if he does so, he would not fall into the same fix Arjuna. That said, it is not an easy accomplishment to be always fixed in the higher view.

In as much as no one can destroy the everlasting principle which underlies this creation, so no one can accomplish the permanence of the material situation. This is due to natural causes which are themselves eternal principles.

अन्तवन्त इमे देहा
नित्यस्योक्ताः शरीरिणः ।
अनाशिनोऽप्रमेयस्य
तस्माद्युध्यस्व भारत ॥२.१८॥

antavanta — terminal; ime — these; dehā — bodies; nityasyoktāḥ = nityasya — of the eternal + uktāḥ — it is declared; śarīriṇaḥ — of the embodied soul; anāśinaḥ — of the indestructible; 'prameyasya = aprameyasya — of the

antavanta ime dehā
nityasyoktāḥ śarīriṇaḥ
anāśino'prameyasya
tasmādyudhyasva bhārata (2.18)

immeasurable; tasmāt — therefore; yudhyasva — fight; bhārata — O descendant of Bharata

It is declared that the bodies of the eternal, indestructible and immeasurable embodied soul are terminal. Therefore fight, descendent of the Bharatas. (2.18)

Commentary:

This was declared by the sages from the Upanishadic period. Śrī Krishṇa merely reminds Arjuna that such ideas were already established. Arjuna should make a decision on that basis.

य एनं वेत्ति हन्तारं
यश्चैनं मन्यते हतम् ।
उभौ तौ न विजानीतो
नायं हन्ति न हन्यते ॥२.१९॥
ya enaṁ vetti hantāraṁ
yaścainaṁ manyate hatam
ubhau tau na vijānīto
nāyaṁ hanti na hanyate (2.19)

ya — who; enaṁ — this embodied soul; vetti — concludes; hantāraṁ — the killer; yaścainaṁ = yas — who + ca — and + inam — this embodied soul; manyate — thinks; hatam — is killed; ubhau — both; tau — two viewers; na— not; vijānītaḥ— understood; nāyaṁ = na — not + ayam — this embodied soul; hanti — kill; na — nor; hanyate — can be killed

Both viewers do not understand, namely: He who concludes that the embodied soul is the killer and he who thinks that the embodied soul is killed. The embodied soul does not kill nor can he be killed. (2.19)

Commentary:

The mystic seers of reality perceive this existence in one way. Those without that view see this existence from another angle. A person without mystic perception sees the material body as the whole person. Thus if one body strikes another, it is said that the offender perpetrated a violence and that the offended was thereby victimized thereby. This is for social and cultural purposes but it is erroneous in pure spiritual terms.

Apart from the mystic seers of reality and those without mystic vision, there is a group of persons in between. They normally perceive everything in terms of actions of bodies. They believe that besides the body there is the spirit. They do not see the spirit but they believe in it, either by having an experience of it or becoming convinced by due reason. When Arjuna was shifted from the kriyā vision, he fell into the status of those who are in—between, who believe in the spirit or who experienced it previously, but who do not normally perceive it.

In the material world, a person is discouraged from perceiving spiritual existence. Thus it is natural that people would regard everything in terms of bodily actions, pegging the body as the person himself.

Here Śrī Krishna says that the embodied soul neither kills nor can he be killed, but the implications are not explained yet by Śrī Krishna. Before we can understand that statement, we must hear of the implications. The responsibility for killing a body must go somewhere. A man who murdered cannot be excused merely because he killed the body and not the soul. After all, he deprived a certain soul of its body.

न जायते म्रियते वा कदा चिन्
नायं भूत्वा भविता वा न भूयः ।
अजो नित्यः शाश्वतोऽयं पुराणो
न हन्यते हन्यमाने शरीरे ॥२.२०
na jāyate mriyate vā kadā cin
nāyaṁ bhūtvā bhavitā vā na bhūyaḥ
ajo nityaḥ śāśvato'yaṁ purāṇo
na hanyate hanyamāne śarīre (2.20)

na — not; jāyate — is born; mriyate — dies; vā — either; kadācin — at any time; nāyaṁ = na — nor + ayaṁ — this embodied soul; bhūtvā — having been; bhavitā — will be; vā — or; na — not; bhūyaḥ — again; ajo — birthless; nityaḥ — perpetual; śāśvataḥ — eternal; 'yaṁ = ayaṁ— this; purāṇaḥ — primeval; na— not; hanyate — is killed; hanyamāne — in the act of killing; śarīre — in the body

This embodied soul is not born, nor does it die at any time, nor having existed will it not be. Being birthless, eternal, perpetual and primeval, it is not slain in the act of killing the body. (2.20)

<u>Commentary:</u>

The embodied soul forms the core around which the various births and deaths take place, but the soul itself is neither coming into being nor going out of existence. Unfortunately, not every spirit understands this about itself and not every spirit experiences itself as an eternal principle. Due to a lack of long-range memory, as well as a lack of piercing insight, many spirits take themselves for granted as being material bodies. Knowing oneself to be eternal depends on being able to remember past lives. Thus the eternality of the spirit may not be understood or experienced by the spirit itself. It is difficult for the spirit to understand its own nature.

Śrī Krishna tactfully informed Arjuna that since the relatives and friends were all birthless, eternal, perpetual and primeval, none of them would be slain in the act of killing any of their bodies. In this way, Śrī Krishna incites Arjuna to fight regardless.

वेदाविनाशिनं नित्यं
य एनमजमव्ययम् ।
कथं स पुरुषः पार्थ
कं घातयति हन्ति कम् ॥२.२१॥
vedāvināśinaṁ nityaṁ
ya enamajamavyayam
kathaṁ sa puruṣaḥ pārtha
kaṁ ghātayati hanti kam (2.21)

vedāvināśinaṁ = veda — knows + avināśinaṁ — indestructible; nityaṁ — eternal; ya = yaḥ — who; enam — this; ajam — not born, birthless; avyayam — imperishable; kathaṁ — how; sa = saḥ — he; puruṣaḥ — person; pārtha — O son of Partha; kaṁ — whom; ghātayati — causes to kill; hanti — kills (directly); kam — whom

O son of Pṛthā, how can the person who knows this indestructible, eternal, birthless and imperishable principle, cause someone to be killed or even kill someone directly? (2.21)

<u>Commentary:</u>

This is an interesting question asked to Arjuna by Śrī Krishna. It applies to each of us as well. Obviously if one has the kriyā vision to see a spirit as distinct from its body, one knows that one cannot kill a spirit or cause spirits to be killed. All the same, one must also see in that vision that one could use a body to kill another body and thus deprive another spirit of its material body. Considering this, one would have to view life in an entirely different way but with a sense of responsibility.

वासांसि जीर्णानि यथा विहाय
नवानि गृह्णाति नरोऽपराणि ।
तथा शरीराणि विहाय जीर्णा;न्य्
अन्यानि संयाति नवानि देही ॥२.२२॥
vāsāṁsi jīrṇāni yathā vihāya
navāni gṛhṇāti naro'parāṇi
tathā śarīrāṇi vihāya jīrṇāny
anyāni saṁyāti navāni dehī (2.22)

vāsāṁsi — clothing; jīrṇāni — worn out; yathā — as when; vihāya — discarded; navāni — new; gṛhṇāti — takes; naro = naraḥ — person; 'parāṇi = aparāṇi — others; tathā — so; śarīrāṇi — bodies; vihāya — abandoned; jirṇāny — worn—out; anyāni— others; saṁyāti — encounters; navāni — new; dehī — the embodied soul

As when discarding old clothing, a person takes new garments, so the embodied soul abandons old bodies taking new ones. (2.22)

Commentary:

To further incite Arjuna, Śrī Krishna explained that the changing of bodies may be compared to the changing of garments. To Śrī Krishna it is that simple. However to us, what are the implications? From the perspective of the subtle body, taking on a new physical form equates to changing clothes. The subtle body provides the foundation for the various physical forms, just as the physical body is the foundation for various garments.

नैनं छिन्दन्ति शस्त्राणि
नैनं दहति पावकः ।
न चैनं क्लेदयन्त्यापो
न शोषयति मारुतः ॥२.२३॥

nainaṁ chindanti śastrāṇi
nainaṁ dahati pāvakaḥ
na cainaṁ kledayantyāpo
na śoṣayati mārutaḥ (2.23)

nainaṁ = na — not + enaṁ — this; chindanti — pierce; śastrāṇi — weapons; nainaṁ = na — not + enaṁ — this; dahati — burns; pāvakaḥ — fire; na — not; cainaṁ = ca — and + enaṁ — this; kledayantyāpo = kledayanti — soak + āpo = āpaḥ — water; na — nor; śoṣayati — dry out; mārutaḥ — the wind

Weapons do not pierce, fire does not burn, and water does not wet, nor does the wind dry that embodied soul. (2.23)

Commentary:

What endangers and what threatens the very existence of a living body poses no real threat to the spirit who uses or loses that body. The soul must certainly endure the ailments of a living body but ultimately, the spirit is only connected to those ailments in a superficial way.

अच्छेद्योऽयमदाह्योऽयम्
अक्लेद्योऽशोष्य एव च ।
नित्यः सर्वगतः स्थाणुर्
अचलोऽयं सनातनः ॥२.२४॥
acchedyo'yamadāhyo'yam
akledyo'śoṣya eva ca
nityaḥ sarvagataḥ sthāṇur
acalo'yaṁ sanātanaḥ (2.24)

acchedyaḥ — not to be pierced; 'yam = ayam — this; adāhyo = adāhyaḥ — not to be burnt; 'yam = ayam — this; akledyo = akledyaḥ — not to be moistened; 'śoṣya = aśoṣya — not to be dried; eva — indeed; ca — and; nityaḥ — eternal; sarvagataḥ — penetrant of all things; sthāṇuḥ — a permanent principle; acalo = acalaḥ — unmoving; 'yaṁ = ayaṁ — this; sanātanaḥ — primeval

This embodied soul cannot be pierced, cannot be burnt, cannot be moistened, cannot be dried. And indeed, this soul is eternal. It can penetrate all things. It is a permanent principle and is stable and primeval. (2.24)

Commentary:

The soul as Śrī Krishna described here needs no sympathy, regarding its appearance and disappearance. Something that can penetrate all things, which is a permanent principle, stable and primeval, which cannot be pierced, burnt, moistened or dried, requires no assistance at any time for its survival. In fact, no one can this soul a sense of security in terms of its ongoing existence.

Therefore, Arjuna was not crying for the souls which powered the bodies of his relatives and friends present on the battlefield. In verse 13, Śrī Krishna first began to describe this embodied soul (dehino/dehinah) in detail. Now the question remains as to why the embodied soul is harnessed to a material body in the first place.

अव्यक्तोऽयमचिन्त्योऽयम्
अविकार्योऽयमुच्यते ।
तस्मादेवं विदित्वैनं
नानुशोचितुमर्हसि ॥ २.२५ ॥
avyakto'yamacintyo'yam
avikāryo'yamucyate
tasmādevaṁ viditvainaṁ
nānuśocitumarhasi (2.25)

avyakto = avyaktaḥ — undisplayed; 'yam = ayam — this; acintyo = acintyah — unimaginable; 'yam = ayam — this; avikāryo = avikāryaḥ — unchanging; 'yam = ayam — this; ucyate — it is declared; tasmāt — therefore; evaṁ — thus; viditvainaṁ = viditva — knowing + enam — this; nānuśocitum = na — not + anuśocitum — to lament; arhasi — you should

This embodied soul is undisplayed, unimaginable, and unchanging. Therefore knowing this, you should not lament. (2.25)

Commentary:

As the background for these temporarily displayed bodies, the embodied soul is itself undisplayed and cannot be perceived usually. It is unchanging according to statements of the Upanishadic sages, statements now repeated and substantiated by Śrī Krishna. How is it then that this embodied soul becomes so involved with his body, that he thinks himself to be the body and the psychological energy which operates it? Arjuna, after he detoured from the kriyā yoga perspective, served as an example of a person whose spirit forgot itself and identified itself with the body and its psychological energies.

अथ चैनं नित्यजातं
नित्यं वा मन्यसे मृतम् ।
तथापि त्वं महाबाहो
नैनं शोचितुमर्हसि ॥ २.२६ ॥
atha cainaṁ nityajātaṁ
nityaṁ vā manyase mṛtam
tathāpi tvaṁ mahābāho
nainaṁ śocitumarhasi (2.26)

atha — furthermore; cainaṁ = ca — and + enaṁ — this; nityajātaṁ = nitya — continually + jātaṁ — being born; nityam — continually; vā — or; manyase — you think; mṛtam — dying; tathā 'pi = tathā – so + api — also; tvaṁ — you; mahābāho — strong—armed man; nainaṁ = na — not + enam — this; śocitum arhasi = śocitum — to mourn + arhasi — you can

And furthermore if you think that this embodied soul is continually being born or continually dying, even so, O strong—armed man, you should not lament. (2.26)

Commentary:

Śrī Krishna digressed, saying that even if the strong—armed Arjuna considered that the soul reincarnates repeatedly, born now and again, and dying in turn, only to be reborn, still there was no reason to think that the soul could be killed. Śrī Krishna addressed Arjuna as one of the persons who do not see mystic reality but who believe in it. They heard that the soul transmigrates and in their view it must be that the soul dies or becomes dormant and then returns afresh to begin a new existence.

Such a belief is not without its foundation in reality, in the sense that if the soul completely forgets his former births it is as if it died and was reborn afresh. When it takes the new birth it acts as if that was its first and last existence.

A person who does not recall any of his past lives, can only believe that he had previous existences. Consciously he relies on what he experiences in the present life, and he is driven from within by tendencies and instincts. Such a person, under the guidance of a mystic seer, might change perspective if he gains some mystic vision. Otherwise, he is left only with beliefs.

जातस्य हि ध्रुवो मृत्युर्
ध्रुवं जन्म मृतस्य च ।
तस्मादपरिहार्येऽर्थे
न त्वं शोचितुमर्हसि ॥२.२७॥

jātasya hi dhruvo mṛtyur
dhruvaṁ janma mṛtasya ca
tasmādaparihārye'rthe
na tvaṁ śocitumarhasi (2.27)

jātasya — of that which is born; hi — in fact; dhruvo = dhruvaḥ — certain; mṛtyur = mṛtyuḥ — death; dhruvaṁ — certain; janma — birth; mṛtasya — of that which is dead; ca — and; tasmādaparihārye = tasmāt — therefore + aparihārye — in what is unavoidable; 'rthe = arthe — in the assessment; na — not; tvaṁ — you; śocitum — to lament + arhasi — you should

In fact, of that which is born, death is certain; of that which is dead, birth is certain. Therefore in assessing what is unavoidable, you should not lament. (2.27)

Commentary:

Śrī Krishna explained a law of reality, which is that whatever appeared somewhere, will in time disappear from that place, and whatever disappeared from some place will appear somewhere else sooner or later. Therefore one should understand that the psychology which supports any living body, will go on to exist somewhere else after the body dies. This is certain. One should toughen emotionally and not lament.

Sometimes in religion, preachers try to establish that Śrī Krishna is different and that His body displayed before Arjuna was not subject to this rule of appearance and disappearance. However we cannot accept that proposal. Even a body displayed by Śrī Krishna as part of this material world will have to disappear by the very law of reality cited in this verse.

अव्यक्तादीनि भूतानि
व्यक्तमध्यानि भारत ।
अव्यक्तनिधनान्येव
तत्र का परिदेवना ॥२.२८॥

avyaktādīni = avyakta – undetected + ādīni— beginnings of a manifestation; bhūtāni — living beings; vyakta madhyāni = vyakta — visible + madhyāni — interim states; bhārata — O descendant

avyaktādīni bhūtāni
vyaktamadhyāni bhārata
avyaktanidhanānyeva
tatra kā paridevanā (2.28)

of Bharata; avyakta nidhanāny eva = avyakta — undetected + nidhanāni — ends of a manifestation + eva — again; tatra — there; kā — what; paridevanā — complaint

The living beings are undetected in the beginning of a manifestation, visible in the interim stages, and are again undetected at the end of a manifestation. What is the complaint? (2.28)

Commentary:

This detection and lack of detection applies to the gross senses. The subtle senses can detect the living being at all stages, but, since most human beings focus through gross senses, they interpret life in a gross way. All living entities in gross life forms have subtle senses. When, however, the psyche serves as a power supply for the gross body, the subtle senses cannot operate independently, and often become reliant on information from the gross form.

The example of a flashlight can show this. In a flashlight, a battery provides power. Therefore the battery is the main part of the apparatus. Still the battery cannot shine by itself. A bulb to produce illumination. Similarly in a gross body there is a power for operating the senses of smelling, tasting, seeing, touching and hearing.

As a battery does not understand itself or how it is being utilized for providing light, a spirit may not understand how its power activates the senses of the gross body. The battery of a flashlight is hardly noticed by users preoccupied with the shining light. Thus a living being is undetected at the beginning of a manifestation while in its father's or mother's body waiting to develop a baby form. It becomes visible after its form develops as a protruding embryo in the mother's form. Later on when its form dies, it becomes undetected again.

In yoga practice, one opens up the mystic perception and perceives these adjustments directly. The subtle senses are there. In kriyā yoga, we take up disciplines which free our spirit's energy from the hynotic pull of the gross senses. By the practice of pratyāhār in the 5th stage of yoga, a sensual energy restraint is achieved. This enables perception through the subtle senses.

आश्चर्यवत्पश्यति कश्चिदेनम्
आश्चर्यवद्वदति तथैव चान्यः ।
आश्चर्यवच्चैनमन्यः शृणोति
श्रुत्वाप्येनं वेद न चैव कश्चित् ॥२.२९॥
āścaryavatpaśyati kaścidenam
āścaryavadvadati tathaiva
cānyaḥ
āścaryavaccainamanyaḥ śṛṇoti
śrutvāpyenaṁ veda na caiva
kaścit (2.29)

āścaryavat — wonderful; paśyati — perceives; kaścidenam = kaścid — someone + enam — this; āścaryavad — fantastic; vadati — describes; tathai 'va = tathā — so + eva — indeed; cānyaḥ = ca — and + anyah — another person; āścaryavaccainam = āścaryavat — amazing + ca — and + enam — this; anyaḥ — another; śṛṇoti — hears; śrutvāpyenaṁ = srutva — having heard + api — also + enaṁ — this; veda — knows; na — not; caiva = ca — and + eva — in fact; kaścit — anyone

Someone perceives this embodied soul as being wonderful. Another person describes it as amazing. Another hears of it as being fantastic. And even after hearing this, no one knows this embodied soul in fact. (2.29)

Commentary:

The spirit is difficult to track and understand. Some human beings, who perceive it by direct mystic vision, regard it as a wonder. This means that even the spirit regards itself as a wonder. It is fascinated by its own existence. Some human beings may describe the spirit in writing after hearing of it from someone else, or after reading of it in books like the *Bhagavad Gītā*. Such a person may describe it as being amazing. Another person may hear of it as being fantastic.

However Śrī Krishna states that even after hearing, a person does not know the spirit in fact. This is because hearing, in this case, is not a direct perception. Merely hearing of spiritual objects does not give sufficient experience of such things. One must perceive directly to really understand it.

देही नित्यमवध्योऽयं
देहे सर्वस्य भारत ।
तस्मात्सर्वाणि भूतानि
न त्वं शोचितुमर्हसि ॥२.३०॥
dehī nityamavadhyo'yaṁ
dehe sarvasya bhārata
tasmātsarvāṇi bhūtāni
na tvaṁ śocitumarhasi (2.30)

dehī — embodied soul; nityam — eternally; avadhyo = avadhyaḥ — non—killable; 'yaṁ = ayaṁ — this; dehe — in the body; sarvasya — of all, in all cases; bhārata — O descendant of Bharata; tasmāt — therefore; sarvāṇi — all; bhūtāni — beings; na — no; tvaṁ — you; śocitumarhasi = śocitum — to mourn + arhasi — should

In the body, in all cases, this embodied soul is always non—killable, O descendant of Bharata. Therefore you should not mourn for any of these beings. (2.30)

Commentary:

Since a human being cannot understand the full significance of the spirit simply by hearing, those who lack experience but who accept the authority of persons like Śrī Krishna, must for the time being, take instructions from such authorities or from Śrī Krishna Himself as Arjuna did. The first instruction in this case is not to mourn for any of these living beings. This is the first adjustment that one makes on the path of kriyā yoga. However this is easier said that done, since the mourning tendency is embedded in the psyche of a human being.

स्वधर्ममपि चावेक्ष्य
न विकम्पितुमर्हसि ।
धर्म्याद्धि युद्धाच्छ्रेयोऽन्यत्
क्षत्रियस्य न विद्यते ॥२.३१॥
svadharmamapi cāvekṣya
na vikampitumarhasi
dharmyāddhi
yuddhācchreyo'nyat
kṣatriyasya na vidyate (2.31)

svadharmam — your assigned duty; api — also; cāvekṣya = ca — and + avekṣya — looking, mentally considering; na — no; vikampitum — to consider alternatives; arhasi — you should; dharmyād = dharmyāt — from righteousness; dhi = hi — indeed; yuddhācchreyo = yuddhāt — from battle + chreyo = śreyas — better; 'nyat = anyat — other; kṣatriyasya — of the son of a king; na — no; vidyate — there is

And considering your assigned duty, you should not look for alternatives. In fact, for the son of a king, there is no other duty which is better than a righteous battle. (2.31)

Commentary:

This is a technical piece of advice for kriyā yogis. If we analyze this in detail, Śrī Krishna said that Arjuna should accept his particular duty (svadharman). Śrī Krishna does not talk about devotion to Himself here but only about responsible actions (dharma) in terms of social and cultural birth circumstances. These circumstances involved with Arjuna's body as the son of a king (kṣatriya).

If Arjuna wanted a better alternative such as acting as the son of a brahmin or acting as a priest, teacher or ascetic, then Śrī Krishna rejected that desire. This is a very tough verse if we look squarely. It means that as kriyā yogis, we can become perfected even if we function responsibly in terms of the type of body we took in the present lifetime. We are not required to procure a higher status but should determine our assigned destiny in terms of this birth oppurtunity.

यदृच्छया चोपपन्नं
स्वर्गद्वारमपावृतम् ।
सुखिनः क्षत्रियाः पार्थ
लभन्ते युद्धमीदृशम् ॥ २.३२ ॥
yadṛcchayā copapannaṁ
svargadvāramapāvṛtam
sukhinaḥ kṣatriyāḥ pārtha
labhante yuddhamīdṛśam (2.32)

yadṛcchayā — by a stroke of luck; copapannaṁ = ca — and + upapannaṁ — made available; svargadvāram = svarga — heaven + dvāram — gate; apāvṛtam — is open; sukhinaḥ — thrilled, happy; kṣatriyāḥ — warriors; pārtha — O son of Pṛthā; labhante — get; yuddham — battle opportunity; īdṛśam — such

And by a stroke of luck, the gate of heaven is opened. Thrilled are the warriors who get such a battle opportunity, O son of Pṛthā. (2.32)

Commentary:

Śrī Krishna encouraged Arjuna to fight on the basis of showing that the opportunity for battle was a stroke of good luck (yadṛcchayā). Śrī Krishna indicated that other warriors would usually be thrilled, not saddened by the circumstance.

As kriyā yogis, it is found sometimes that when we get a chance to be householders, we lament or try to avoid it, thinking that its undesirable, and not recognizing the chance from destiny for us to perform righteous duty (svadharman).

Sometimes a kriyā yogi gains an opportunity to serve society in some functional way that hardly relates to his ascetic practice and he whimsically turns away from it, feeling it would detract from spiritual endeavors. Unfortunately for us, we do not have Śrī Krishna standing physically before us as did Arjuna and we may not be sensitive enough to Śrī Krishna or another master of kriyā yoga to be inspired by them and take such glorious opportunities. However here in this *Gītā*, Śrī Krishna explained in detail why we should seize the opportunity.

अथ चेत्त्वमिमं धर्म्यं
संग्रामं न करिष्यसि ।
ततः स्वधर्मं कीर्तिं च
हित्वा पापमवाप्स्यसि ॥ २.३३ ॥
atha cettvamimaṁ dharmyaṁ
saṁgrāmaṁ na kariṣyasi
tataḥ svadharmaṁ kīrtiṁ ca
hitvā pāpamavāpsyasi (2.33)

atha — now; cet — if; tvam — you; imaṁ — this; dharmyaṁ — appropriate duty; saṁgrāmaṁ — warfare; na — not; kariṣyasi — will conduct; tataḥ — then; svadharmaṁ — own duty; kīrtiṁca = kīrtiṁ — reputation + ca — and; hitvā — having neglected; pāpam — sin, fault; avāpsyasi — will acquire

Now if you do not conduct this righteous war, then, by neglecting your duty and reputation, you will acquire a fault. (2.33)

Commentary:

If a human being neglects his or her appropriate duty (dharman), there will be reactions. It does not matter if such a human being is a devotee of Krishna, a kriyā yogi, or an atheist. In fact, the overall reality will certainly overtake a person who cannot figure out what he ought to do or must do as necessity. This, of course, does not compensate for the ignorance of the average human being. Those who are truly ignorant, who have no training and understanding, are cushioned by their lack of awareness when the reaction falls, while the others who have some sense suffer terribly.

Arjuna had a reputation to maintain. Śrī Krishna, who elsewhere in the *Gītā* portrayed Himself as the Supreme God, reminds Arjuna of this now. One may asks, what does an ordinary human being, or a simple devotee of Krishna, or a kriyā yogi devotee of Śrī Krishna, have to do with reputation? Unavoidably even the most insignificant human being has some small circle of influence in which he or she operates. Thus the small reputation in that circle would suffer if one neglects duty.

Reputation loses its importance when a person makes the effort for spiritual life, but since it is an eternal aspect of the spirit, it cannot be fully abandoned. Thus Śrī Krishna spiced no words when He drew this to Arjuna's attention. Śrī Krishna stated a very subtle truth, namely, that if one neglects duty (svadharman) and reputation (kirtim), one automatically acquires a fault (pāpam).

अकीर्तिं चापि भूतानि
कथयिष्यन्ति तेऽव्ययाम् ।
संभावितस्य चाकीर्तिर्
मरणादतिरिच्यते ॥२.३४॥
akīrtiṁ cāpi bhūtāni
kathayiṣyanti te'vyayām
saṁbhāvitasya cākīrtir
maraṇādatiricyate (2.34)

akīrtiṁ — downfall; cāpi = ca — and + api — also; bhūtāni — the people; kathayiṣyanti — will speak; te — of you; 'vyayām = avyayām — continually; saṁbhāvitasya — for an honored man; cākīrtir = ca — and + akīrtiḥ — loss of reputation; maraṇād = maraṇāt — than the loss of body; atiricyate — is harder to bear

The people will speak of your downfall continually. And for an honored man, the loss of reputation is harder to bear than the loss of his body. (2.34)

Commentary:

Śrī Krishna cited the possibility of Arjuna's downfall (akirtim), stating that the people will speak of it continually. Such condemnation would bear negative consequences for Arjuna. Further, Śrī Krishna explained that in the long run, Arjuna would regret the loss of reputation, since from history we understand that for an honored man, condemnation is harder to bear than the loss of his body.

Being a kriyā yogi takes courage. Still one should not miscalculate or underestimate the emotional component of one's nature. One should know the hazards of carelessness and not act foolishly in a way that gives a show of courage now and much regret later. Even so this does not mean that a kriyā yogi should accept the entire range of opportunities presented by the social and cultural display. We must participate only in our assigned duty and should never take an iota more.

भयाद्रणादुपरतं
मंस्यन्ते त्वां महारथाः ।
येषां च त्वं बहुमतो
भूत्वा यास्यसि लाघवम् ॥२.३५॥
bhayādraṇāduparataṁ
maṁsyante tvāṁ mahārathāḥ
yeṣāṁ ca tvaṁ bahumato
bhūtvā yāsyasi lāghavam (2.35)

bhayād = bhayāt — because of fear; raṇād = raṇāt — from the excitement of battle; uparataṁ — withdraw from; maṁsyante — they think; tvāṁ — you; mahārathāḥ — great warriors; yeṣāṁ — of whom; ca — and; tvaṁ — you; bahumato = bahumataḥ — high opinion; bhūtvā — had; yāsyasi — you will come; lāghavam — insignificance

The great warriors will think that because of fear, you withdrew from battle. And to those who held a big opinion, you will appear to be insignificant. (2.35)

Commentary:

It may be counter-stated that a kriyā yogi should not be concerned about the opinions of others but such a proposal is unrealistic, because even a kriyā yogi is not absolute. He must stay in perspective. In so far as the opinions of others are relevant, he cannot afford to neglect their views.

We observe, sometimes, that persons who are devotees of Krishna take on from their spiritual master, a view that they are not at all responsible to anyone but their guru and Śrī Krishna. And of course, in a practical sense, this suggestion alludes that they are only responsible to their guru because Śrī Krishna is not physically present. They follow the complete or incomplete, partial or full understanding of the *Gītā* given by their guru. Such persons then look at the world in a very impractical way, neglecting all other people but their guru. This inevitably leads to a crisis. This happens because they have not applied this verse and others which are supplemental to it.

As soon as one takes a human body he becomes responsible to many human beings in the social and cultural environment. Even though he is responsible to God and to religious teachers, here Śrī Krishna insists on the obligation to social and cultural leaders.

It may be asked: Who cared what the great warriors thought, especially since they sided with the enemy? The answer is here before us, in that Śrī Krishna Himself cared.

In kriyā yoga, we understand that we should be very mindful of resentments. Bad feelings find a person wherever he or she may go. One cannot hide from resentment unless one becomes fully liberated or unless the bad feelings go into dormancy. Arjuna might have thought that he could leave the battlefield and live peacefully with ascetics at forest retreats but Śrī Krishna alerted him that certain resentments from both the common people and the great warriors would find Arjuna wherever he went In Arjuna's case, some of his friends would think that he was fearful and ran away. He would then be blamed for military failure if they fought and were defeated. Then from the opponents, there would be ridicule since Arjuna had deprived them of an opportunity for competitive fighting.

These energies of reciprocation would have to be faced by Arjuna. They would disrupt his peace of mind.

अवाच्यवादांश्च बहून्
वदिष्यन्ति तवाहिताः ।
निन्दन्तस्तव सामर्थ्यं
ततो दुःखतरं नु किम् ॥२.३६॥

avācyavādāṁśca = avācya — not to be said, slurred + vādān — words, saying + ca — and; bahūn — many; vadiṣyanti — will speak; tavāhitāḥ = tava — about you + ahitāḥ — enemies; nindantas — laughed at; tava — of

avācyavādāṁśca bahūn
vadiṣyanti tavāhitāḥ
nindantastava sāmarthyaṁ
tato duḥkhataraṁ nu kim (2.36)

you; sāmarthyaṁ — capability; tato = tataḥ — from that; duḥkhataraṁ — greater grief; nu — but; kim — what

The enemies will say many slurs about you, thus laughing at your capability. But, what would be a greater grief than this? (2.36)

Commentary:

The enemy will laugh saying that Arjuna had martial skill but not the courage to use it. Śrī Krishna asked Arjuna to regard that upcoming assault of criticism and ridicule. Actually a kriyā yogi cannot continue his meditations successfully if he remains under such psychological bombardment. Somehow he has release from it and he will not escape it by avoiding duty. Only the completion of destined activity frees a man from such resentments.

It may be asked: What does it matter if others laughs? The answer is that it matters only if destiny is supportive and reinforces their derision. As kriyā yogis we should be careful with destiny. When someone's opinion is an echo of destiny's view, a kriyā yogi should heed.

हतो वा प्राप्स्यसि स्वर्गं
जित्वा वा भोक्ष्यसे महीम् ।
तस्मादुत्तिष्ठ कौन्तेय
युद्धाय कृतनिश्चयः ॥२.३७॥
hato vā prāpsyasi svargaṁ
jitvā vā bhokṣyase mahīm
tasmāduttiṣṭha kaunteya
yuddhāya kṛtaniścayaḥ (2.37)

hato = hataḥ — be killed; vā — either; prāpsyasi — you will achieve; svargaṁ — angelic world; jitvā — having conquered; vā — or; bhokṣyase — you will enjoy; mahīm — the nation; tasmād = tasmāt — therefore; uttiṣṭha — stand up; kaunteya — O son of Kuntī; yuddhāya — to battle; kṛtaniścayaḥ — be decisive

Either be killed and achieve the angelic world or having conquered, enjoy the nation. Therefore stand up and be decisive, O son of Kunti. (2.37)

Commentary:

Śrī Krishna addressed Arjuna as the son of Kunti, because Kunti, the mother of the Pandavas, had once berated the five heroes, her sons, for not retaliating when Duryodhana and his company unfairly deprived them of their share of the Kuru sovereignty.

Śrī Krishna presented to Arjuna the alternatives; which were to participate and lose in this world while gaining in the angelic realm for bravery and compliance with destiny or to participate, be victorious and, as a consequence, take part in ruling the country.

At this point, if Arjuna had done what Śrī Krishna told him, about standing and being decisive in battle then the *Gītā* would be completed here. Instead the *Gītā* continues because Arjuna was not convinced. Arjuna was still incapacitated. Śrī Krishna as the master kriyā teacher had not done enough to dislodge the emotionsof Arjuna.

सुखदुःखे समे कृत्वा
लाभालाभौ जयाजयौ ।
ततो युद्धाय युज्यस्व
नैवं पापमवाप्स्यसि ॥२.३८॥

sukhaduḥkhe = sukha — happiness + duḥkhe — in distress; same — in the same emotions; kṛtvā — having regard; lābhālābhau — gains or losses; jayājayau — victory or defeat; tato = tataḥ — them; yuddhāya — to

sukhaduḥkhe same kṛtvā
lābhālābhau jayājayau
tato yuddhāya yujyasva
naivaṁ pāpamavāpsyasi (2.38)

battle; yujyasva — apply yourself; naivaṁ = na — not + evaṁ — thus; pāpam — sin,demerit; avāpsyasi — you will get

Having regarded happiness, distress, gains, losses, victory and defeat, as the same emotions, apply yourself to battle. Thus you will get no demerit. (2.38)

Commentary:

The underlying attitude of a kriyā yogi is described in very simple terms. Simple as it may seem, it requires much practice under superior guidance for a student of kriyā to attain it unless such a student was born with natural kriyā instincts. A psychology which regards happiness, distress, gains, losses, victory and defeat as one and the same emotion, is usually odd. The human psyche operates on the very principle of diverse emotions. Most human beings live on excitement and depression which reflect different responses to social and cultural life.

In Chapter One, Arjuna was mired in depression. He was not dhira (steady), as Lord Krishna indicated in verse 15, as aforementioned:

yaṁ hi na vyathayantyete puruṣaṁ puruṣarṣabha
samaduḥkhasukhaṁ dhīraṁ so'mṛtatvāya kalpate (2.15)

O bull amongst men, these mundane sensations do not afflict the wise man who is steady in miserable and enjoyable conditions. That person is fit for immortality. (2.15)

Śrī Krishna wanted Arjuna to make a marked change of attitude to a wise man steady in miserable and enjoyable conditions and not afflicted by mundane sensations. He wanted Arjuna to remain anchored in this state as a permanent psychology.

Thus Śrī Krishna told Arjuna to resign himself to the role of warrior, either to be killed or achieve the angelic world, or having conquered the opponents, live in this world for the time being and supervise the nation as a brother of the ruler. Arjuna had to dismiss fear and emotional consideration in order to stand up and be decisive.

Śrī Krishna then surprisingly said that if Arjuna maintained a mood of indifference to emotional overtones and still executed his duty as warrior, then Arjuna would get no fault.

This is a potentially controversial statement. We need to hear more from Śrī Krishna before we can understand it. For one, suppose Arjuna or any other kriyā yogi made a mistake, while remaining emotionally detached in the performance of duty. What would happen to the consequences of that error? Would there be no repercussion? Śrī Krishna will further clarify this in Chapter 4, Verses 16 and 21, and then definitely in Verse 4.41.

Merely because a kriyā yogi is detached, does not mean that he will not make mistakes. Besides, he may again slip into the emotional state, by falling from the kriyā stance, for whatever happened before can certainly occur again. Arjuna can again succumb to a weakened psychological state. Even in the presence of Śrī Krishna, Arjuna can again think in a way that is inconsistent with the kriyā views. We will read more from Śrī Krishna, before we become convinced.

एषा तेऽभिहिता सांख्ये
बुद्धिर्योगे त्विमां शृणु ।
बुद्ध्या युक्तो यया पार्थ
कर्मबन्धं प्रहास्यसि ॥ २.३९ ॥
eṣā te'bhihitā sāṁkhye
buddhiryoge tvimāṁ śṛṇu
buddhyā yukto yayā pārtha
karmabandhaṁ prahāsyasi (2.39)

eṣā — this; te — to you; bhihitā = abhihitā — stated; sāṁkhye — in Sāṁkhya philosophy; buddhir = buddhiḥ — insight; yoge — in yoga discipline; tvimāṁ = tu — but + imāṁ — this; śṛṇu — hear; buddhyā — with the insight; yukto = yuktaḥ — yoked; yayā — by which; pārtha — O son of Pṛthā; karmabandhaṁ — complication of action; prahāsyasi — you will avoid

As explained in the Sāṁkhya philosophy, this vision is the insight, but hear of its application in yoga practice. Yoked with this insight, O son of Pṛthā, you will avoid the complication of action. (2.39)

Commentary:

This verse is a synopsis of what Śrī Krishna taught Arjuna. Śrī Krishna gave Arjuna a crash course in the application of yogic insight to worldly life. This is called karma yoga. As will be explained in Chapter Four, Śrī Krishna claimed that He formerly taught this to certain legendary kings and that He would introduce Arjuna to the practice.

I want to point out to readers that this is the main idea of the *Gītā*. Its main idea is not bhakti (devotion) but rather the application of an existing yoga practice to worldly life. From this verse we can infer that the objective of yoga when applying it to worldly life is to avoid the implications of action. A kriyā yogi should participate in social and cultural affairs in such a way as to not be degraded by the involvement.

Śrī Krishna stated that the tenets of the Samkhya philosophy are perceived by insight through yoga practice but still anyone who was not gifted in the skill of sinless participation, required preliminary traning. Such a person must be trained by a kriyā master, someone like Śrī Krishna.

This means that once we master yoga and gain insight into whatever the Samkhya advocates, the next effort is to apply ourselves sinlessly in the social and cultural setting. We should not switch back to normal vision when we encounter baffling circumstances but should keep the yogic insight and make decisions from that stance. In this way we avoid complications and do not attract sinful reactions.

The big fear for a person who performed yoga and gained the Samkhya insight, is that if he again returns to the social and cultural setting, he will become implicated and suffer reactions. Here Śrī Krishna gave the key to avoiding all that, which is to remain in the Samkhya insight while functioning in worldly life.

I must emphasize now that a philosophical study of Samkhya does not give one the insight of Samkhya . One gets it by the performance of yoga, so that one's psyche changes and one's subtle senses are shifted away from the gross body. One cannot fully develop the insight by merely hearing from a teacher, even by only hearing from Śrī Krishna. Arjuna not only heard, but he performed the yoga completely. In addition, Śrī Krishna gave Arjuna divine revelations later on. Thus there is no possibility of developing the full insight by hearing only.

नेहाभिक्रमनाशोऽस्ति
प्रत्यवायो न विद्यते ।
स्वल्पमप्यस्य धर्मस्य
त्रायते महतो भयात् ॥२.४०॥
nehābhikramanāśo'sti
pratyavāyo na vidyate
svalpamapyasya dharmasya
trāyate mahato bhayāt (2.40)

nehābhikramanāśo = na — not + iha — in this insight + abhikrama — endeavor + nāśo (nāśaḥ) — loss; asti — it is; pratyavāyo = pratyavāyaḥ — reversal; na — not; vidyate — there is; svalpam — a little; apy = api — even; asya — of this; dharmasya — of righteous practice; trāyate — protects; mahato = mahataḥ — from the great; bhayāt — from danger

In this insight, no endeavor is lost nor is there any reversal. Even a little of this righteous practice protects from the great danger. (2.40)

Commentary:

Śrī Krishna assured that if one acts in the world in a way consistent with yogic insight, no loss or reversal will occur. Even a little of such righteous action, would protect the person from the great danger which follows if he neglected his appropriate duty (dharmyam, B.G. 2.33) or performed such duty with emotional regard for happiness and distress, gains or losses and victory or defeat. In fact a little of this practice would strengthen the performer so that in the future, his reinforced habit of acting with the yogic insight would be more instilled in his nature.

व्यवसायात्मिका बुद्धिर्
एकेह कुरुनन्दन ।
बहुशाखा ह्यनन्ताश्च
बुद्धयोऽव्यवसायिनाम् ॥२.४१॥
vyavasāyātmikā buddhir
ekeha kurunandana
bahuśākhā hyanantāśca
buddhayo'vyavasāyinām (2.41)

vyavasāyātmikā — intentional determination; buddhir = buddhih — technical insight; ekeha = eka — one view + iha — in this instance; kurunandana — O dear man of the Kuru family; bahuśākhā — many offshoots; hyanantāś = hi — in fact + anantāḥ — endless; ca — and; buddhayo = buddhayaḥ — views; 'vyavasāyinām = avyavasāyinām — of the person with many hopes

When a person's intentional determination is guided by technical insight, he experiences one view, O dear man of the Kuru family. But the views of a person with many hopes are diverse and endless. (2.41)

Commentary:

Śrī Krishna said that when we have that technical insight and allow it to guide our intentions then we have only one view; but if we have many hopes, our views become diversified and we become indecisive. Arjuna developed that technical insight, for he was a kriyā yogi of accomplishment. Somehow he was shifted from it and did not, on this occasion, allow it to guide his intentions. Instead his emotions took control and managed his psyche, showing him many excuses for not doing his duty.

यामिमां पुष्पितां वाचं
प्रवदन्त्यविपश्चितः ।
वेदवादरताः पार्थ
नान्यदस्तीति वादिनः ॥२.४२॥

yām — which; imām — this; puṣpitāṁ — poetic; vācaṁ — quotation; pravadantyavipaścitaḥ = pravadanti — they proclaim + avipaścitaḥ — ignorant reciters; vedavādaratāḥ — enjoying Vedic Sanskrit

yāmimāṁ puṣpitāṁ vācaṁ
pravadantyavipaścitaḥ
vedavādaratāḥ pārtha
nānyadastīti vādinaḥ (2.42)

poetry; pārtha — O son of Pṛthā; nānyad = na — not + anyat — anything; astīti = asti — it is + iti — thus; vādinaḥ — saying

This is poetic quotation which the ignorant reciters proclaim, O son of Pṛthā. Enjoying the Vedic verses, they say there is no other written authority. (2.42)

Commentary:

Śrī Krishna informed Arjuna, that whatever Arjuna said previously which was quoted from the *Vedas*, the ultimate scriptures in the time of Arjuna, were verses which ignorant reciters proclaim. Arjuna followed their example, but only because he shifted away from the insight of kriyā yoga. Śrī Krishna openly criticizes the Vedic reciters and the *Vedas* itself. Śrī Krishna suggests that there were other authoritative writings besides the *Vedas*.

In this verse Śrī Krishna releases Arjuna from certain insecurities, which cause Arjuna to lean on the Vedic reciters for support in the effort to turn away from his battlefield duties, obligations which were unpalatable.

कामात्मानः स्वर्गपरा
जन्मकर्मफलप्रदाम् ।
क्रियाविशेषबहुलां
भोगैश्वर्यगतिं प्रति ॥२.४३॥
kāmātmānaḥ svargaparā
janmakarmaphalapradām
kriyāviśeṣabahulāṁ
bhogaiśvaryagatiṁ prati (2.43)

kāmātmānaḥ — people of a sensuous nature; svargaparā — people intent on going to the swarga (angelic) world; janmakarmaphalapradām = janma – rebirth + karma – cultural act + phala – pay—off + pradām — offering; kriyāviśeṣabahulāṁ = kriyā – ceremonial rites + viśeṣa — specific + bahulāṁ — various; bhogaiśvaryagatiṁ = bhoga — enjoyment + aiśvarya — political power + gatiṁ — aim; prati — toward

Those reciters, being people of a sensuous nature, being intent on going to the Svarga angelic world, offering such rebirth as payoff for cultural activities, make themselves busy in various specific ceremonial rites, and focus on enjoyment and political power. (2.43)

Commentary:

In order to make a livelihood through the performance of rituals, the Vedic priests sell their ceremonial expertise to wealthy patrons. They promise the patrons heaven by explaining that if they subscribe to the ceremonies and willingly pay the stipulated fees, while supporting beneficial cultural activities which improve human society, they would surely go to the Svārga angelic world after the death of their bodies, thus avoiding having to take rebirth on earth immediately after this life is finished.

Śrī Krishna indicated that this was a farce and that Vedic priests could not possibly substantiate such a guarantee, because as He stated, their actual focus is enjoyment and political power (bhogaiśvaryagatim).

This can be explained simply as follows. Vedic priests who have little or no mystic insight usually abhor yoga practice. By constant repetition in ceremonial rites, they specialize in the procedures and perform these with more expertise than the mystics. Their expertise however does not guarantee the results advocated. Since in their process they do not require any harsh austerities like those practiced in haţha yoga and prāṇāyāma, they attract more common people than do the mystics. They especially attract the ruling classes and mercantile community.

Since they do not have reliable insight and cannot see directly into the Svārga angelic world or any other dimension, they have only a belief in such subtle territory. Sharing this belief with their congregations, they promise that if one would do ceremonies and follow their advice for piety, one would definitely go to the Svārga angelic world.

Absent the mystic focus which transcends this physical dimension, such Vedic priests instead focus into this world for the enjoyment and status which can be procured here. These people are of a sensual nature (kāmātmānah). That is indicated by their lack of interest in yoga austerities and their natural attraction for social and cultural affairs which have religious over—coating (kriyāviśeṣabahulām). They are involved in kriyā but not in kriyā yoga or not in yoga as it is applied in kriyā or ceremonial rites.

Not all patrons of these Vedic priests are fooled. Now and again, one or two such people do reach the Swārga angelic world, to enjoy life in that paradise for a time, but most supporters are merely reborn in this world in some human or animal body. Obviously Śrī Krishna disliked the Vedic priests who operated such religious farces.

भोगैश्वर्यप्रसक्तानां
तयापहृतचेतसाम् ।
व्यवसायात्मिका बुद्धिः
समाधौ न विधीयते ॥२.४४॥
bhogaiśvaryaprasaktānāṁ
tayāpahṛtacetasām
vyavasāyātmikā buddhiḥ
samādhau na vidhīyate (2.44)

bhogaiśvaryaprasaktānāṁ = bhoga — pleasure + aiśvarya — power + prasaktānāṁ — of the attached, of the prone; tayāpahṛtacetasām = tayā — by this + apahṛta — captivated + cetasām — idea; vyavasāyātmikā = vyavasāya — focused determination + ātmikā — self; buddhiḥ — intellect; samādhau — in meditation; na — not; vidhīyate — is experienced

Being absorbed by this way of life, pleasure—prone and power-seeking people, are captivated by this idea. Thus in meditation, the self—focused intellect is not experienced by them. (2.44)

<u>*Commentary:*</u>

Being captivated by this sort of life, whereby in this world one sanctifies his business and leisure with a religious overcoating, as authorized by Vedic priests or by others like them, one is unable to focus on the spiritual reality during meditation.

But it is not only the non—yogis who experience this. We too, as neophyte kriyā yogis are unable to experience the self—focused intellect in meditation. This self—focused intellect called by Śrī Krishna vyavasāyātmikā buddhim, is developed in deep meditation, but only after one turns away from the physical senses objects, conserves sensual power, contains it and then refocus it as directed by the kriyā yoga teachers like Śrī Krishna. This is a mystic skill developed after long practice.

त्रैगुण्यविषया वेदा
निस्त्रैगुण्यो भवार्जुन ।
निर्द्वंद्वो नित्यसत्त्वस्थो
निर्योगक्षेम आत्मवान् ॥२.४५॥

traiguṇya — three moods; viṣayā — phases; vedā — Vedas; nistraiguṇyo = nistraiguṇyaḥ — without the three moody phases; bhavārjuna = bhava — be + arjuna — Arjuna; nirdvandvo = nirdvandvaḥ — without fluctuation; nityasattvastho = nityasattvasthaḥ = nitya – always + sattva —

traiguṇyaviṣayā vedā
nistraiguṇyo bhavārjuna
nirdvaṁdvo nityasattvastho
niryogakṣema ātmavān (2.45)

reality + sthaḥ — fixed; niryogakṣema — without grasping and possessiveness; ātmavān — soul—situated

Three moody phases are offered by the Vedas. Be without the three moods, O Arjuna. Be without the moody fluctuations. Be always anchored to reality. Be free from grasping and possessiveness. (2.45)

Commentary:

Generally speaking, the scope of the *Vedas* has to do with using and operating the three moody phases of material nature. The *Vedas* have transcendental objectives but that is not the general instruction there. The Veda is, more or less a manual for mundane living for the time of the Vedic period which was before the advancement of Upanishadic sages who developed what Śrī Krishna called the self—focused meditative intellect. Śrī Krishna wanted Arjuna to apply kriyā yoga expertise in being anchored in reality (nityasattvastah).

यावानर्थ उदपाने
सर्वतः संप्लुतोदके ।
तावान्सर्वेषु वेदेषु
ब्राह्मणस्य विजानतः ॥२.४६॥
yāvānartha udapāne
sarvataḥ saṁplutodake
tāvānsarveṣu vedeṣu
brāhmaṇasya vijānataḥ (2.46)

yāvān — as much; artha — importance; udapāne — in a well; sarvataḥ — in all directions; saṁplutodake = saṁpluta — flowing + udake — in water; tāvān — so much; sarveṣu — in the entire; vedeṣu — in the Vedas; brāhmaṇasya — of a brahmin; vijānataḥ — perceptive

For as much importance as there is in a well when suitable water flows in all directions, so much worth is in the entire Vedas for a perceptive brahmin. (2.46)

Commentary:

The *Vedas* are supposed to be the property of the brahmins, who traditionally are said to be the only ones who understand those texts. The question is: Who is a brahmin? Śrī Krishna seemed to distinguish between a non—perceptive brahmin and a perceptive one. He added the word vijānatah, indicating that there are grades of brahmins. Previously he called such a person a tattvadarśih. This means that a Brahmin, according to Śrī Krishna's standard, must have mystic insight.

In the time of Śrī Krishna, a brahmin was someone born from a man who was already a brahmin. Those people specialized in religious rites and various mystic insights, since such religions dealth with invoking supernatural persons from the unseen world. If however, the brahmin is not perceptive, he would speculate on the outcome of a ceremony since he could not see directly into the subtle world. He would have to assure his congregation even though he lacked supernatural vision. He would indulge in pretences.

Śrī Krishna explained that a truly perceptive Brahmin, even though he may use the procedures outlined in the *Vedas*, would not depend fully on the literature since he would see directly into the subtle world.

कर्मण्येवाधिकारस्ते
मा फलेषु कदाचन ।
मा कर्मफलहेतुर्भूर्
मा ते सङ्गोऽस्त्वकर्मणि ॥ २.४७ ॥
karmaṇyevādhikāraste
mā phaleṣu kadācana
mā karmaphalaheturbhūr
mā te saṅgo'stvakarmaṇi (2.47)

karmaṇyevādhikāraste = karmaṇi — in performance + eva — alone + adhikāraḥ — command, privilege + te — your; mā — not; phaleṣu — in the aftermath of consequences; kadācana — at any time; mā — not; karmaphalahetur = karmaphala — a result + hetur (hetuh) — motivation; bhūr = bhūḥ — be; mā — not; te — your; saṅgo = sangah — attachment; 'stv = astu — should be; akarmaṇi — non—action, idleness

The command is yours while performing, but not at any time in the aftermath of consequences. Do not be motivated by a result, nor harbor an attachment to idleness. (2.47)

Commentary:

This is a crucial instruction for all kriyā yogis, in terms of what attitude they should assume while performing in the social and cultural environments. We can perform. That is our privilege but it is not our opportunity to seek the results of activity, nor should we remain idle if destiny pressures us to perform.

Most people act on the expecion of a favorable or unfavorable result or they remain indifferent if they perceive no gain in acting but a kriyā yogi should act when pressed by destiny regardless of the expected result. Rather than foreseeing the results and then deciding to act, one becomes disciplined in not seeing the results at all. When one initially comes to kriyā yoga one may habitually check for favorable results but gradually one should change this psychology so that one does not waste any energy on this. Rather, one becomes supersensitive to the demands of providence and puts all energy into completing duties.

The self needs to understand and accept pleasantly, what Śrī Krishna told Arjuna: that the privilege is to perform duties only. It should not be to hunt for consequences or try to calculate the outcomes.

In social and cultural existence, this is what happens: The self perceives a future that is partially true and partially false. Then it might act. If the self perceives a future wherein there is no benefit, it tries to cease action. It assumes reluctance. The reluctance is addressed in this verse as idleness or non—action (akarmaṇi). Many prospective kriyā yogis take the single lifestyle as monks or bachelors because they see no advantage in being householders or grihastas. They become reluctant to act. Many others like them find no reason also to take a job or to earn a livelihood because they feel they would not benefit from earning money. On that basis they refuse to act or become reluctant to participate.

Worldly people usually act after they see a benefit but since their intellects are defective, what they perceive before hand as a result, is usually a false perception. Providence is so complicated that it is impossible for their intellects to perfectly prefigure what destiny will do. Since their vision of the future is only partially true at best, their actions on the basis of such mistaken insight bring disappointment and pain.

Despite repeated frustration, worldly people keep on following the lead of their intellects in making decisions. They are frustrated repeatedly. It is not their fault either. They can only follow the intellect and life energy indications, because that is the way the spirits are connected within the psyche. In kriyā yoga, until a yogi becomes advanced, he also falls victim to the faulty intellect except that when he is occasionally inspired with a clear view of reality and can bypass the normal way of faulty decision-making. Since the kriyā yogi sees that it is possible to get out, he strives for improvement by adopting the kriyā disciplines which cause changes in the psyche, life energy and intellect.

It is not easy to escape the calculative powers of the intellect. For kriyā yogis it is possible only after much practice. To keep working and working on and on in the material world, while not anticipating the good or bad consequences, was difficult for Arjuna even while standing next to Śrī Krishna.

When Śrī Krishna instructed that we act in an unprejudiced way in relation to the results of our actions, and that we not harbor attachment to idleness, it means that we have to stop our nature from doing this. That is not easy. These are psychological traits, not gross physical things. It is difficult to even perceive how these traits motivate us, much less stopping them. Still, let us proceed in this *Gītā* to get more hints of how we can put this advice into practice.

These basic instructions of kriyā yoga are very important. Some kriyā yogis, who have not completed the practice but who followed leaders of devotion to Krishna, concluded that they can attain these aspects without practicing kriyā yoga. Thus they do not feel it is necessary to work internally to change their psychology. However, I do not ascribe to their belief about devotion to Krishna. I feel that if a yogi has devotion or learned it from those who stress devotion, then the yogi should strive achieve changes in his psyche by more consistent endeavor in kriya yoga so that his devotion to Krishna would be purified further. In my view, finding devotion to Krishna or realizing its importance only increases the need to intensify kriyā yoga practice. I do not agree with the teachers who suggest that devotion itself will bring on the required purity of love for Krishna. I feel that the love of Krishna should be purified further by earnest use of kriyā yoga.

योगस्थः कुरु कर्माणि
सङ्गं त्यक्त्वा धनंजय ।
सिद्ध्यसिद्ध्योः समो भूत्वा
समत्वं योग उच्यते ॥२.४८॥
yogasthaḥ kuru karmāṇi
saṅgaṁ tyaktvā dhanaṁjaya
siddhyasiddhyoḥ samo bhūtvā
samatvaṁ yoga ucyate (2.48)

yogasthaḥ— in yoga attitude; kuru — do perform; karmāṇi — actions; saṅgaṁ — attachment to crippling emotions; tyaktvā — having abandoned; dhanaṁjaya — conqueror of wealthy countries; siddhyasiddhyoḥ — to success or failure; samo = samaḥ — attitude of indifference; bhūtvā — be; samatvaṁ — indifference; yoga — yogic practice; ucyate — it is said

So perform actions in the yoga mood. Attachment to crippling emotions should be abandoned, O conqueror of wealthy countries. Be indifferent to success or failure. It is said that indifference denotes yoga. (2.48)

Commentary:

Yogasthah means in the yogic mood, in the position of practicing yoga and keeping the psychological vision and feeling developed through its techniques. Here Śrī Krishna teaches Arjuna to maintain the yoga stance while performing acts in the social and cultural fields of life. This is the application to worldly life. This is yoga as it is applied to karma. Śrī Krishna instructed Arjuna to abandon attachment to crippling emotions, but that which can be easily said by a kriyā teacher is difficult to implement by the kriyā student who is not proficient. The crippling emotions are the ones which overcame Arjuna when he sat down on the chariot and refused to fight. These emotions rise within the psyche when it ranges over the projected or actual results of an action. The problem is that the psyche does this automatically and continually. The will power does not have to operate for this to occur, because the psyche has an automatic mechanism which causes it to range over projected or actual results.

This is why one has to practice mystic techniques to change the psyche. The mechanisms within the psyche move very fast in analyzing results. It is so fast that usually the spirit does not see the calculations but is only perceptive of the conclusions of the intellect. The spirit then approves or disapproves of an action suggested by the intellect in a biased way. This brings on excitement to act, crippling emotions not to act, or precautions which develop into indifference.

In kriyā yoga, one should be indifferent not to actions, but rather to the mind's analysis of projected success or failure of an action, particularly if that action is a duty presented before one by providence. This, Śrī Krishna said, is the evidence of yoga practice in the life of a student who acts in a social and cultural setting.

The above two verses, text 47 and 48, are the essence of kriyā yoga in its application to social and cultural life. These two verses should be remembered at all times. What they advocate, should be instituted firmly in a kriyā yogi's life. We cannot fail in our bid for perfection if we master what is discussed in the verses. If one acts in the world with the mastership defined in those verses, then one will complete terminal actions which will cause the release or curtailment of one's material existence.

If a kriyā yogi cannot finish his material existence without a certain amount of social and cultural interaction, then that interaction will be counterproductive for him if he does not first act with the mastership defined here. On one hand, such a kriyā student will not be successful in his advanced kriyā practice, if he cannot act in the world. On the other hand he will become more implicated in the world if he acts without the mastership. Hence the mastership is most important. He must receive training from a kriyā teacher in how to change his nature, so that he can act in the ways prescribed by Śrī Krishna in verses 47 and 48.

दूरेण ह्यवरं कर्म
बुद्धियोगाद्धनंजय।
बुद्धौ शरणमन्विच्छ
कृपणाः फलहेतवः ॥२.४९॥
dūreṇa hyavaraṁ karma
buddhiyogāddhanaṁjaya
buddhau śaraṇamanviccha
kṛpaṇāḥ phalahetavaḥ (2.49)

dūreṇa — by far; hyavaraṁ = hi — surely + avaraṁ — inferior + karma — cultural action; buddhiyogād = buddhiyogāt — intellectual discipline through yoga; dhanaṁjaya — victor of wealthy countries; buddhau — mystic insight; śaraṇam — location of confidence; anviccha — put; kṛpaṇāḥ — low and pathetic; phalahetavaḥ — people motivated for a result

Surely, cultural action is by far inferior to intellectual discipline through yoga, O victor of wealthy countries. One should take shelter in mystic insight, for how pathetic are those who are motivated by the promise of results. (2.49)

Commentary:

Buddhi yoga is buddhi yoga, which means it is yoga discipline through which a spirit gains control of the functions of the buddhi organ in the subtle body. He gains control in such a way as to stop its automatic operations. These automatic operations cause the spirit to follow the false conceptions of the buddhi and thereby lead the spirit endlessly down the social and cultural path.

Buddhi yoga is attained by pratyāhār sensual withdrawal and by concentration, the 5th and 6th stages of yoga. This, as Śrī Krishna states, is far better than mere cultural activity in the material world.

Even though cultural actions are put down by Śrī Krishna, still we see that Śrī Krishna insisted that Arjuna should be culturally involved. While inferior, the kriyā yogi cannot avoid cultural actions all together because they are his duty. Thus, he must act on them in a way that breaks off or terminates his material existence.

To do that he must master buddhi yoga, the control of his intellect, so that when he performs duty, the intellect does not misguide him. That is the technicality of this verse.

At this point I must as the commentator thank Śrī Krishna and Śrī Balarāma, His brother, as well as Lord Shiva and numerous kriyā yoga teachers of mine who brought me to the level of being able to represent Śrī Krishna here by this commentary, in which Śrī Krishna's words are echoed again across the centuries with this light of understanding. When I felt I should do this commentary, I had no idea that Śrī Krishna would stand over my shoulder and dictate so much to me about what He explained to Arjuna.

I wanted to do a commentary for the instructions that He gave to Uddhava in Canto Eleven of Śrīmad Bhāgavatam Purāṇa. I had already began that but I felt that my previous commentary of the Gītā, is published as Bhagavad Gītā Explained, was all I would do on the Gītā. However I was mistaken. I see now, as I am shown by Śrī Krishna, that the Gītā is a precise document of kriyā yoga.

बुद्धियुक्तो जहातीह
उभे सुकृतदुष्कृते ।
तस्माद्योगाय युज्यस्व
योगः कर्मसु कौशलम् ॥२.५०॥
buddhiyukto jahātīha
ubhe sukṛtaduṣkṛte
tasmādyogāya yujyasva
yogaḥ karmasu kauśalam (2.50)

buddhiyukto = buddhiyuktaḥ — a person disciplined by the reality—piercing insight; jahātīha = jahāti — he discards + iha — here; ubhe — both; sukṛtaduṣkṛte — pleasant and unpleasant work; tasmād = tasmāt — therefore; yogāya — to yoga; yujyasva — take yourself to; yogaḥ — yogic mood; karmasu — in performance; kauśalam — skill

A person who is disciplined by the reality—piercing insight discards in each life both pleasant and unpleasant work. Therefore take to the yogic mood. Yoga gives skill in performance. (2.50)

Commentary:

Here we are told about the advanced kriyā yogis. They are reliant on the reality—piercing insight which supports them on the psychological plane, in such a way that they do not falter or get excited on the basis of their projected, actual, imagined or real perceptions of the results of action.

The advanced yogi takes care of all the pleasant and unpleasant work which is thrown before him by providence and which providence indicates as his duty. In so doing he cleans up his participation in the material world and satisfies the sum total energy as well as the supernatural and natural people who required services.

Śrī Krishna advised that we take to the yogic mood since it gives skill in cultural performance. Of course taking to the yogic mood like this requires training and practice.

कर्मजं बुद्धियुक्ता हि
फलं त्यक्त्वा मनीषिणः।
जन्मबन्धविनिर्मुक्ताः
पदं गच्छन्त्यनामयम् ॥२.५१॥
karmajaṁ buddhiyuktā hi
phalaṁ tyaktvā manīṣiṇaḥ
janmabandhavinirmuktāḥ
padaṁ gacchantyanāmayam (2.51)

karmajaṁ — produced by actions; buddhiyuktā — disciplined mystic seers; hi — indeed; phalaṁ — result; tyaktvā — having abandoned; manīṣiṇaḥ — wise people; janmabandhavinirmuktāḥ = janma — rebirth + bandha — bondage + vinirmuktāḥ — freed from; padaṁ — place; gacchanty = gacchanti — go; anāmayam — misery—free

Having abandoned the results which are produced by actions, and being freed from the bondage of rebirth, those wise people, the disciplined mystic seers, go to the misery—free place. (2.51)

Commentary:

The secret to ending material existence is described in this verse as having abandoned the results, which are produced by actions. Note that this is not leaving aside the actions themselves but only the results produced from them. The actions go on in the life of an advanced yogi, unless he was permitted by providence to step aside and focus only on the misery—free places (padam anāmayam).

The actions are usually required, because in the gross and subtle material existence, the presence of a spirit continually attracts and activates energies based on the spirit's interactions in the said world for millions of years prior. It is only when and if the spirit can exit from these places, that the energies are not activated in relation to him.

Now, if the actions are performed in a yogic mood, there would be no complications. Instead the interaction would solve puzzles and loosen entanglements. Thus eventually by more mastership and by getting a waiver from providence, the kriyā yogi gets more time for practice. He reaches a stage of retirement from those types of duties which were imposed by providence. Then, even if he still has a material body or still has a subtle material form, he begins to experience the misery—free places continually and he goes there as soon as his gross body disintegrates by the time factor.

यदा ते मोहकलिलं
बुद्धिर्व्यतितरिष्यति ।
तदा गन्तासि निर्वेदं
श्रोतव्यस्य श्रुतस्य च ॥२.५२॥
yadā te mohakalilaṁ
buddhirvyatitariṣyati
tadā gantāsi nirvedaṁ
śrotavyasya śrutasya ca (2.52)

yadā — when; te — you; mohakalilaṁ — delusion—saturated mind; buddhir (buddhiḥ) — discrimination; vyatitariṣyati — departs; tadā — then; gantāsi — you will become; nirvedaṁ — disgusted; śrotavyasya — with what is to be heard; śrutasya — what was heard; ca — and

When from your delusion—saturated mind, your discrimination departs, you will become disgusted with what is to be heard and what was heard. (2.52)

Commentary:

This verse described a technique which is mastered at a median stage of practice. In that procedure, one trains his buddhi organ to not focus itself within the imagination. When the buddhi organ focuses within the imagination, all sorts of visions and sounds are created in the mind. One then follows these as a person follows a film show to a glorious or tragic ending. One then acts in the social and cultural setting according to what was seen in the imagination. Invariably such actions are faulty because the mental conception usually does not match reality.

It is a fact, however, that this focusing in the imagination is a natural faculty of the buddhi organ. To stop it, is most difficult. Most people cannot even imagine how they could control such a subtle process within their psyche. In kriyā yoga we control this after long detailed practice being supervised by a kriyā master. If we read this verse, we can see that to Śrī Krishna, this process is very easy. To Him it is merely a mystic move made by a kriyā yogi. For Arjuna it will be just that, once he becomes convinced by Śrī Krishna, but for us it is not easy.

A kriyā student becomes disgusted with people who are not kriyā yoga masters and who try to hold his attention to preach what they think should be heard. One becomes disgusted because these people waste time getting nowhere, and they desire to waste the time of others, especially the aspiring yogis. One becomes disgusted with them as soon as one experiences the intellect as an organ in the subtle body, as a subtle object, not as a feeling of understanding, and as soon as one stops that organ's impulsive imaginations. When one harnesses tightly his intellect so that it stops all these thinkings and picturizations, then one avoids the association of spiritual masters who are not kriyā teachers, even those who are devotees of Krishna but who abhor and avoid the kriyā method.

श्रुतिविप्रतिपन्ना ते
यदा स्थास्यति निश्चला ।
समाधावचला बुद्धिस्
तदा योगमवाप्स्यसि ॥२.५३॥
śrutivipratipannā te
yadā sthāsyati niścalā
samādhāvacalā buddhis
tadā yogamavāpsyasi (2.53)

śrutivipratipannā = śruti — scriptural information + vipratipannā —false, misleading; te — you; yadā — when; sthāsyati — will remain; niścalā — unmoving, steady; samādhāvacalābuddhis = samādhau — in deep meditation; acalā — without moving, stable; buddhis (buddhiḥ) — intelligence; tadā — then; yogam — yoga discipline; avāpsyasi — will master

When, rejecting misleading scriptural information, your intelligence remains steady without moody variation, being situated in deep meditation, you will master the yoga disciplines. (2.53)

Commentary:

The misleading scriptural information is the incentive type of scriptural statements which occur in scriptures anywhere. Such incentive information stimulates the non—kriyā yogis who are looking for an easy way out, something suitable to the mind in its present condition. Śrī Krishna already described some of these projected fantasies in verse 43 where he spoke of hoping for the Svārga angelic world and for enjoyment and political power on this plane.

Once the kriyā yogi is free from the sensual excitements invoked by incentive statements in the scriptures, he can move on to a steady practice through which he develops deep meditation (samādhav/samādau) with a stable (acalā) intelligence which does not imagine impulsively. This is the most advanced stage of kriyā yoga called samādhi. This is the complicated high level of yoga practice. Śrī Krishna has already gone very far, way beyond our level of accomplishment. He will, however, backtrack as Arjuna raises questions.

अर्जुन उवाच
स्थितप्रज्ञस्य का भाषा
समाधिस्थस्य केशव ।
स्थितधीः किं प्रभाषेत
किमासीत व्रजेत किम् ॥२.५४॥
arjuna uvāca
sthitaprajñasya kā bhāṣā
samādhisthasya keśava
sthitadhīḥ kiṁ prabhāṣeta
kimāsīta vrajeta kim (2.54)

arjuna – Arjuna; uvāca — said; sthitaprajñasya — of the person who is situated in clear penetrating insight; kā — what; bhāṣā — description; samādhisthasya — one who is anchored in deep meditation; keśava — Keśava, Kṛṣṇa; sthitadhīḥ — one who is steady in objectives; kiṁ — whom; prabhāṣeta — should speak; kim — how; āsīta — should sit; vrajeta — move; kim — how

Arjuna said: In regards to the person who is situated in clear, penetrating insight, would you please describe him? Speak of the person who is anchored in deep meditation, O Keśava Krishna. As for the man who is steady in objectives, how would he speak? How would he sit? How would he act? (2.54)

Commentary:

Śrī Krishna, Keshava, described a person expert at remaining steady in spiritual perception and never shifting from it. Now Arjuna wants more details of such a person. Arjuna also wants to know how such a person can be recognized physically. Thus far Śrī Krishna gave the description of the psychology of such a person, but if a person cannot see inside the mind and psyche, he can only gage by what he sees physically. Thus Arjuna asks for outward indications of such a person regarding how he might speak, sit and act.

श्रीभगवानुवाच
प्रजहाति यदा कामान्
सर्वान्पार्थ मनोगतान् ।
आत्मन्येवात्मना तुष्टः
स्थितप्रज्ञस्तदोच्यते ॥२.५५॥
śrībhagavānuvāca
prajahāti yadā kāmān
sarvānpārtha manogatān
ātmanyevātmanā tuṣṭaḥ
sthitaprajñastadocyate (2.55)

śrī bhagavān — the Blessed Lord; uvāca — said; prajahāti — abandons; yadā — when; kāmān — cravings; sarvān — all; pārtha — O son of Pṛthā; manogatān — escapes from mental dominance; ātmanyevātmanā = ātmani — in the spirit + eva — only + ātmanā — by the spirit; tuṣṭaḥ — being self—content; sthitaprajñastadocyate = sthitaprajñaḥ — one whose insight is steady + tadā — then + ucyate — is identified

The Blessed Lord said: When someone abandons all cravings, O son of Pṛthā, and escapes from mental dominance, being self content, then that person is identified as one with steady insight. (2.55)

Commentary:

Sanjaya addressed Śrī Krishna here as Bhagavan which means the Blessed Lord. Sometimes the term is used as a formality or annotation for respect. Sometimes it is flattery. We will see that Krishna is proved to be the Blessed Lord. Later on, when Śrī Krishna shows Arjuna the Universal Form.

Now we get a description of the person with the clear penetrating insight. This description is not a physical one. Unless we have some mystic vision and unless that vision is clear and free from prejudices, we would not be able to find such a person. Some regard their spiritual teacher as such a person and by the prejudice of wanting to glorify that person, the followers fail to develop mystic insight in order to actually see if their authority fits the description.

This verse is definitive for us as kriyā yogis, in terms of what we wish for ourselves. We want to reach a stage whereby we consistently abandon cravings and escape from the mental dominance of the buddhi organ which impulsively and automatically plans and causes the body to execute activities which cause us further implications in material existence. If we desire to remain in the spiritual self—identity as spiritual selves, we must develop the steady spiritual insight.

For us as kriyā yogis, we are not very interested in glorifying a guru. We honestly want to get a technique from the guru through which we can alter the flaws in our psyche, so that changes are made in our interaction with our life force, intellect and causal bodies, changes which would free us from lower dominance.

दुःखेष्वनुद्विग्नमनाः
सुखेषु विगतस्पृहः ।
वीतरागभयक्रोधः
स्थितधीर्मुनिरुच्यते ॥२.५६ ॥
duḥkheṣvanudvignamanāḥ
sukheṣu vigataspṛhaḥ
vītarāgabhayakrodhaḥ
sthitadhīrmunirucyate (2.56)

duḥkheṣvanudvignamanāḥ = duḥkheṣv (duḥkheṣu) — in miserable conditions + anudvigna — free from worries + manāḥ — mind; sukheṣu — in good conditions; vigataspṛhaḥ — free from excitement; vītarāgabhayakrodhaḥ = vīta — steps aside + rāga — passion + bhaya — fear + krodhaḥ — anger; sthitadhīr = sthitadhīḥ — steady in meditation; munir = muniḥ — wise man; ucyate — is said to be

Furthermore, someone who in miserable conditions remains free from worries, and who in good conditions remains free from excitement, who steps aside from passion, fear and anger, and who is steady in meditation is considered to be a wise man. (2.56)

Commentary:

Here is another abstract description which does not give us physical hints. Someone might fake these by showing physically that he is happy and calm even in miserable circumstances, that he is not excited when there is sufficient cause for elation and that he is not passionate, fearful and angry. All of this can be feigned.

In kriyā yoga however we are not really looking for anyone to show us these things in themselves but rather to show techniques by which we can acquire these traits in our psyche. To remain free from worries in miserable conditions, we have to free the buddhi from its natural habits of contemplating and analyzing such conditions. The buddhi would like very much to eliminate miserable conditions. We have to alter it, so that it gives up its need to eliminate the misery conditions of the world. Freedom from excitement is gained by controlling the intake of the senses and the subsequent reactions felt within the buddhi and the life force energy.

यः सर्वत्रानभिस्नेहस्
तत्तत्प्राप्य शुभाशुभम् ।
नाभिनन्दति न द्वेष्टि
तस्य प्रज्ञा प्रतिष्ठिता ॥२.५७॥
yaḥ sarvatrānabhisnehas
tattatprāpya śubhāśubham
nābhinandati na dveṣṭi
tasya prajñā pratiṣṭhitā (2.57)

yaḥ— who; sarvatrā — in all circumstances; anabhisnehaḥ — without crippling affections; tattat = tad tad—this or that; prāpya— meeting; śubhāśubham — enjoyable and disturbing factors; nābhinandati = na — not + abhinandati — excited; na — nor; dveṣṭi — distressed; tasya — his; prajñā — reality—piercing consciousness; pratiṣṭhitā — is established

A person who, in all circumstances, is without crippling affections, who, when meeting enjoyable or disturbing factors, does not get excited nor distressed, his reality—piercing consciousness is established. (2.57)

Commentary:

Here a key term is given, sarvatrā, meaning in all circumstances, everywhere. If we can find a person who in all circumstances, not just some, remains without crippling affections and who, when meeting enjoying or disturbing factors, does not get excited, nor depressed, then we know that such a person has the reality—piercing consciousness. The next step then is to ask such a person for instructions whereby we can work with ourselves to develop these attributes.

It is obvious that as great as Arjuna was, as the dear friend and associate of Śrī Krishna and as a successful kriyā student, still he was not such a person, since from time to time, he was shifted back out of reality—piercing consciousness. The question is: What is it that makes a person become established permanently in the reality—piercing consciousness? Is it his category, as a certain type of spiritual being? Is it his special relationship with Śrī Krishna? What is it?

यदा संहरते चायं
कूर्मोऽङ्गानीव सर्वशः ।
इन्द्रियाणीन्द्रियार्थेभ्यस्
तस्य प्रज्ञा प्रतिष्ठिता ॥२.५८॥
yadā saṁharate cāyaṁ
kūrmo'ṅgānīva sarvaśaḥ
indriyāṇīndriyārthebhyas
tasya prajñā pratiṣṭhitā (2.58)

yadā — when; saṁharate — pulls; cāyaṁ = ca — and + ayam — this; kūrmo = kūrmaḥ — tortoise; 'ṅgānīva = aṅgānīva = aṅgāni — limbs + iva — like, compared to; sarvaśaḥ — fully; indriyāṇīndriyārthebhyas = indriyani — senses + indriyarthebhyaḥ — attractive things; tasya — his; prajñā — reality—piercing vision; pratiṣṭhitā — is established

When such a person pulls fully out of moods, he or she may be compared to the tortoise with its limbs retracted. The senses are withdrawn from the attractive things in the case of a person whose reality—piercing vision is established. (2.58)

Commentary:

Unless the self enters into samādhi, it remains somewhat involved in moods. When it is exempt from moods, it may be compared to a tortoise with limbs retracted. This is a complete pratyāhār sensual withdrawal technique when the various sensual orbs of the buddhi organ are drawn in and the sensual pursuits cease for the time being. Then the yogi might be in a trance of stilled consciousness or he might be focused elsewhere into the spiritual environment in which the subtle and gross material phenomena are non—existent.

By constant practice, the yogi guarantees that he will not relapse into sensuality when he leaves his present body. He does not rely on the assurances given in the incentive parts of scripture because his discrimination is lifted from the habit of focusing into the imaginative compartment of the intellect. He endeavors with mystic disciplines to withdraw the senses from the attractive objects. After repeatedly doing this, his nature is transformed. This is described in the next verse:

विषया विनिवर्तन्ते
निराहारस्य देहिनः।
रसवर्जं रसोऽप्यस्य
परं दृष्ट्वा निवर्तते॥ २.५९॥
viṣayā vinivartante
nirāhārasya dehinaḥ
rasavarjaṁ raso'pyasya
paraṁ dṛṣṭvā nivartate (2.59)

viṣayā = viṣayāḥ — temptations; vinivartante — turn away; nirāhārasya — from (without) indulgence; dehinaḥ — of the embodied soul; rasavarjaṁ = rasa — memory or mental flavor of past indulgences + varjaṁ — except for, besides; raso = rasah — memories (mental flavors); 'pyasya = apyasya = apy (api) — even + asya — of him; paraṁ — higher stage; dṛṣṭvā — having experienced; nivartate — leaves

The temptations themselves turn away from the disciplinary attitude of an ascetic, but the memory of previous indulgences remain with him. When he experiences higher stages, those memories leave him. (2.59)

Commentary:

Eventually, after doing many austerities the temptations of the sense objects seem as if they become discouraged in trying to lure the yogi into sensual life. The sensual life is merely an opening to the life of responsibilities. And the yogi sees that. It is an enticement to get the yogi to link himself into the world of responsible living (dharma). It becomes attractive through the offer of vices like sexual indulgence and manipulation. If the yogi accepts such offers, then he signs a subtle contract to take up responsibilities in the future life.

Seeing these enticements for what they are, the yogi repeatedly turns away from them and tries to alert neophytes about the nature of the temptations. At last he sees that it is not really his duty to signal others about it, and he increases his efforts for self—reform. Then he has a chance of being successful, since it requires his full endeavor to become freed. It is not that he should not help others but rather, that he cannot free himself by partial reform. He has to use all the energy to free himself. Realizing this he turns away from trying to convince others.

At that point the temptations turn away from him. He sees, within his psyche, memories of previous indulgence rising one after the other. These include some from the subtle world and some from previous lives. Many of these memories haunt him when he tries to meditate. He goes through a period of abject remorse over the fact that he subjected himself or was exposed to sense objects. He vows to avoid such environments in the future. Of course he cannot avoid environments that are imposed because he is not absolute but he can avoid whatever environment he may willfully pursue.

At that point the yogi considers the supernatural beings, the departed ancestors, those who now use material bodies, the Supreme God and His parallel divinities and the overall sum total energies, since any of these can apply pressure that is beyond his control. Simultaneously, he realizes that he is responsible for whatever he willfully imposed on himself.

Gradually and painstakingly, taking help from the mahāyogīs especially from Mahādeva Lord Shiva and those great sages who accompany Mahādeva, he experiences higher states (param) and the lower memories leave him, fading as he becomes unresponsive to those impressions. He becomes increasingly resistant to them as he practices the appropriate mystic kriyās.

Being occupied with this purification, he is no longer distracted. He is reduced to being a student of the mahāyogīs. His ambition for other things fades away.

यततो ह्यपि कौन्तेय
पुरुषस्य विपश्चितः।
इन्द्रियाणि प्रमाथीनि
हरन्ति प्रसभं मनः ॥२.६०॥
yatato hyapi kaunteya
puruṣasya vipaścitaḥ
indriyāṇi pramāthīni
haranti prasabhaṁ manaḥ (2.60)

yatato = yatataḥ — concerning an aspiring seeker; hyapi = hi — indeed + api — also; kaunteya — son of Kuntī; puruṣasya — of the person; vipaścitaḥ — of the discerning educated; indriyāṇi — the senses; pramāthīni — tormenting; haranti — seize, adjust; prasabhaṁ — impulsively, by impulse; manaḥ — mentally

Concerning an aspiring seeker, O son of Kuntī , concerning a discerned educated person, the senses do torment him. By impulses, the senses do adjust his mentality. (2.60)

Commentary:

This is what happens when one first comes to kriyā yoga practice. At that stage the impulsions, the senses, do torment the seeker. By impulsions in the psyche, the sense objects adjust the mentality, regardless of what process one uses. It is at this stage that one realizes that one is being fooled by religious teachers who give so many methods which simply do not adjust the psyche. As a last resort, because everything else failed for conquest of one's nature, one takes to kriyā yoga.

Some impulsions are pushed into the buddhi by the life force. Others are injected from the causal cavity. Once they enter the buddhi, this subtle sensual mechanism tries to ease itself by fulfillments. When the impulsions enter the buddhi, they inject themselves into the senses. The senses, in turn, motivate the physical and subtle bodies for manifesting appropriate fulfillments. Then the buddhi organ forms justifications to support the actions.

These actions comprise various vulgar and not—so—vulgar vices which ruin the psyche. Thus when the ascetic understands this, he realizes that he has an internal war on his hands. He has destructive forces in him. At that point he loses interest in religions which offer cheap salvation. Śrī Krishna gave a summary description of the process of kriyā yoga in no uncertain terms. Let us listen as He charts it out:

तानि सर्वाणि संयम्य
युक्त आसीत मत्परः।
वशे हि यस्येन्द्रियाणि
तस्य प्रज्ञा प्रतिष्ठिता ॥२.६१॥

tāni — these; sarvāṇi — all (senses); saṁyamya — restraining; yukta — yogically disciplined; āsīta — should sit; matparaḥ — focused on Me, on My interest; vaśe — in control; hi — indeed; yasyendriyāṇi = yasya

tāni sarvāṇi saṁyamya
yukta āsīta matparaḥ
vaśe hi yasyendriyāṇi
tasya prajñā pratiṣṭhitā (2.61)

— of whom + indriyāṇi — of the sensuality; tasya — of him; prajñā — vision; pratiṣṭhitā — anchored

Restraining all these senses, being disciplined in yoga practice, an ascetic should sit, being focused on Me. The vision of a person whose sensuality is controlled, remains anchored in reality. (2.61)

Commentary:

This is the 6th and 7th stages of yoga practice which consist of focusing the buddhi organ on a particular object within or outside the psyche. It is interesting that Śrī Krishna began with this instruction which is a description of the 6th stage of yoga practice called dhāraṇa (concentration). What has happened to the five prior stages? Does Śrī Krishna regard those as elementary? Some commentators summarized this verse as being a piece of bhakti (devotion) and others say it is bhakti yoga not just bhakti. This is because here for the first time in the *Bhagavad Gītā*, Śrī Krishna uses the pronoun, mat, which means "on me". There can be no doubt that Śrī Krishna is talking about Himself personally.

The process of samyama is the process of advanced pratyāhāra which is the 5th stage of yoga practice. Accordingly then, for a person to apply this advice, he must have already mastered the 5th stage of yoga practice. Some religious teachers say that one does not have to sit as Krishna says here (āsīta) but rather one can just love Krishna and by devotion to Krishna, one can focus on Krishna.

For kriyā yoga however, we know that one must master all stages of yoga up to the 5th stage, before one can focus on Krishna as described, and one does have to sit in posture to do this.

This focus on Śrī Krishna means focusing on the spiritual body of Śrī Krishna. It does not mean looking at the Krishna Mūrti, the Krishna form, in the temple. That is a different type of focus. This is the focusing of the sensually-withdrawn shutdown buddhi organ into the spiritual environment.

It can only be done if the yogi closes his access to all objects on the physical side. These include the object of the Krishna Form which is established in the temple.

Śrī Krishna claims, in this verse, that a person who can focus on Him as He exists on the spiritual side would remain anchored in reality, when he returns to this side of existence and acts here. The fact is that Śrī Krishna's material body was present before Arjuna. Even though Arjuna viewed and focused on it, he could not remain anchored in reality. Standing side-by-side that physical form used by Śrī Krishna at the time, Arjuna could not keep himself in the spiritual perspective. Later in the *Gītā*, Arjuna will focus into the supernatural world to see the Universal Form, after which he will remain anchored in the kriyā view.

ध्यायतो विषयान्पुंसः
सङ्गस्तेषूपजायते ।
सङ्गात्संजायते कामः
कामात्क्रोधोऽभिजायते ॥२.६२॥
dhyāyato viṣayānpuṁsaḥ
saṅgasteṣūpajāyate
saṅgātsaṁjāyate kāmaḥ
kāmātkrodho'bhijāyate (2.62)

dhyāyato = dhyāyataḥ — considering; viṣayān — sensual objects; puṁsaḥ — a person; saṅgas — attachment; teṣupajāyate = teṣu — in them + upajāyate — is born, is created; saṅgāt — from attachment; saṁjāyate — is born; kāmaḥ — craving; kāmāt – from craving; krodho = krodhah — anger; 'bhijāyate = abhijāyate — is derived

The act of considering sensual objects, creates in a person, an attachment to them. From attachment comes craving. From this craving, anger is derived. (2.62)

क्रोधाद्भवति संमोहः
संमोहात्स्मृतिविभ्रमः ।
स्मृतिभ्रंशाद्बुद्धिनाशो
बुद्धिनाशात्प्रणश्यति ॥ २.६३ ॥
krodhādbhavati saṁmohaḥ
saṁmohātsmṛtivibhramaḥ
smṛtibhraṁśādbuddhināśo
buddhināśātpraṇaśyati (2.63)

krodhād = krodhāt — from anger; bhavati — becomes (comes); saṁmohaḥ — delusion; saṁmohāt — from delusion; smṛti — conscience + vibhramaḥ — vanish; smṛtibhraṁśād = smṛtibhraṁśāt = smṛti — memory, judgement + bhraṁśāt — from fading away; buddhināśo = buddhināśaḥ = buddhi –discerning power + nāśaḥ — lose, affected; buddhināśāt = buddhi — discernment + nāśāt — from loss, from being affected; praṇaśyati — is ruined

From anger, comes delusion. From this delusion, the conscience vanishes. When he loses judgment, his discerning power fades away. Once the discernment is affected, he is ruined. (2.63)

Commentary:

After describing the 6th stage of yoga, that of dhāraṇa, concentration on spiritual objects, Śrī Krishna now describes how the sensuality works when it focuses on the physical side.

This explanation by Śrī Krishna is fine, except that the act of considering sensual objects is for the most part non-deliberate or non-willful. The mind's acceptance of sensual objects and their impressions occurs involuntarily for the most part. It is not that in all cases we deliberately consider the sense objects. In most cases, the mind finds these objects regardless of our interest or lack of interest in them.

The psyche operates in such a way that the spirit's approval or disapproval is not necessary for the enactment of any considerations of sense objects. Automatically an attachment develops even for objects which are pursued non-willfully. From that attachment, craving is felt. If the craving is not fulfilled, then frustration or anger develops. And from that, a delusion and depression is felt. Then one loses any sense of conscience and acts irrationally.

The key to understanding this syndrome is to realize that the spirit is not in control of the psyche. The psyche has its automatic mode of operation which transpires even without the approval of the spirit.

This means that once a person decides to make the effort for self reform and self realization, he must put himself or be put into an environment where sensual cravings and repulsions are discontinued. Such an environment is called an ashram, a place especially created to tone down the excitement which the senses crave.

It used to be that an ashram hardly had any facility for sexual mixing, since in the time of the *Upanishads*, the time just before the advent of Śrī Krishna, ashrams were supervised by married men, sages, who tutored boys for training in yoga practice. Nowadays, however, this changed. The word ashram nowadays could mean anything. In some ashrams there might be males and females who mix under supervision but it is not the same as the ashram in the time of Śrī Krishna. We must keep this in mind, since whatever Śrī Krishna says, bears meaning in the past cultural setting.

As another example, today in some ashrams there are colorfully dressed Mūrtis. These are sacred images of Deities. Previously in the forest retreats, the Mūrtis were not so colorfully displayed. Those Mūrtis, which were colorful, were formerly in the houses of kings and wealthy merchants only. Nowadays, however, we find colorful displays in the ashrams of sannyasis or gurus. Times changed. We must keep this in mind while reading the *Gītā*, so that we do not superimpose present adjustments upon the times of the *Gītā* and then believe or be led to believe that our contemporary scene applies directly.

रागद्वेषवियुक्तैस्तु
विषयानिन्द्रियैश्चरन् ।
आत्मवश्यैर्विधेयात्मा
प्रसादमधिगच्छति ॥२.६४॥
rāgadveṣaviyuktaistu
viṣayānindriyaiścaran
ātmavaśyairvidheyātmā
prasādamadhigacchati (2.64)

rāgadveṣaviyuktais = rāga — cravings + dveṣa — disliking + viyuktaiḥ — discontinued; tu — if, however; viṣayān — attractive objects; indriyaiścaran = indriyaiḥ — by the senses + caran — interacting; ātmavaśyair = ātmavaśyaiḥ — disciplined person; vidheyātmā — a well—behaved person; prasādam — grace of providence; adhigacchati — gets

If, on the other hand, cravings and dislikings are continued and the attractive objects and senses continue interaction, a disciplined person who is usually well—behaved, gets the grace of providence. (2.64)

Commentary:

Once a person gets into the ashram or hermitage environment and once his cravings and repulsions are discontinued, then the attractive objects and the senses will continue to interact, but to a much lesser degree. This is provided the ashram life effectively reduces the cravings and repulsions and does not restrict them in one area. while causing them to be excited in another.

Any time they meet, the sense objects and the pursuing senses will continue interaction no matter what. If there is a slight memory, the mind which was barred from excitements externally, will delve deeply inside itself and indulge through the facility of imagination. This is quite automatic.

However as Śrī Krishna informs us, a disciplined person who is usually well—behaved will get the grace of providence, the result of which, Śrī Krishna will describe in the next verse. The indication here is if one assumes the ashram life even in a setting similar to the Upanishadic period and dissimilar to what passes today for ashram life, then still, if he is not disciplined and well-behaved, he will not get the grace of providence. He will soon become disgruntled or dissatisfied with the ashram routine and its lack of excitement, and he will return to worldly life.

Many people go to an ashram and then discover that it is not to their liking because of its bland, plain and simple lifestyle. Because of the lack of excitement, they find it boring. Others enter a modern type of ashram in which excitements are provided by super—smart sannyasis. Such situations however do not fall under the category of this verse.

प्रसादे सर्वदुःखानां
हानिरस्योपजायते ।
प्रसन्नचेतसो ह्याशु
बुद्धिः पर्यवतिष्ठते ॥२.६५॥

prasāde — the grace of providence producing spiritual peace of mind; sarvaduḥkhānāṁ = sarva — all + duḥkhāṇāṁ — of the emotional distresses; hānir = hāniḥ — cessation, end; asyopajāyate = asya — of him + upajāyate — is produced; prasannacetaso = prasannacetasaḥ = prasanna — peaceful + cetasaḥ— of mind; hyāśu = hy (hi) — indeed + āśu — at once;

prasāde sarvaduḥkhānāṁ
hānirasyopajāyate
prasannacetaso hyāśu
buddhiḥ paryavatiṣṭhate (2.65)

buddhiḥ — intelligence; paryavatiṣṭhate — becomes stable

By the grace of providence, all the emotional distresses cease for him. Being of a pacified mind, his intelligence at once, becomes stable. (2.65)

Commentary:

We have to remember that in the Upanishadic period, boys went to teachers to learn the yoga discipline, very early on in life. Some stayed and completed austerities to perfection, while others returned home, married, settled down as householders and then in elderly years, returned to the forest reserves to complete the austerities. This is the history. Therefore we must try to understand the *Gītā* in that context and not project it into the modern era with the fancy ashrams being created by smart sannyasis.

For a boy the emotional distresses would cease quickly because such distresses from his current life would pertain mostly to attachment for his mother and a dislike of the disciplinary tone of his father and other authoritive figures.

As long as his temperament was naturally disciplined and well-behaved, rather than own-way and mischievous, then the grace of providence would work wonders on him in the ashram environment supervised by seasoned reality—piercing mystic sages. Being of a pacified mind because of the simple environment and the orderliness of his daily activities, his intelligence would become stable in a short time. He would not have to struggle for this.

However in our case, where we looked at television, grew up under the subjugation of radio, and went to schools where we mixed with children from various backgrounds, participated in vices like cigarette smoking, drinking of alcohol, taking of intoxicants, having sexual intercourse and reading all sorts of contrary literature, it cannot be expected that we would absorb the same grace of providence. Hence we should not apply this verse to ourselves. Certainly, the grace of Providence is as active and available now, as in the time of Śrī Krishna, but our condition puts a damper on it. We cannot assimilate it as boys did in those ancient times, even though many sannyasis and spiritual leaders would lead us to believe otherwise.

नास्ति बुद्धिरयुक्तस्य
न चायुक्तस्य भावना ।
न चाभावयतः शान्तिर्
अशान्तस्य कुतः सुखम् ॥२.६६॥
nāsti buddhirayuktasya
na cāyuktasya bhāvanā
na cābhāvayataḥ śāntir
aśāntasya kutaḥ sukham (2.66)

nāsti = na — no + asti — is; buddhir = buddhiḥ — proper discernment; ayuktasya — of the uncontrolled person; na — not; cāyuktasya = ca — and + ayuktasya — of the uncontrolled person; bhāvanā — concentration; na — not; cābhāvayataḥ = ca — and + abhāvayataḥ — a person lacking concentration; śāntir = śāntiḥ — peace; aśāntasya — lacking emotional stability; kutaḥ — how is it to be achieved; sukham — happiness

In comparison, never is there proper discernment in an uncontrolled person. He is not capable of concentration. One who lacks concentration cannot get inner peace. For one who lacks emotional stability, how will happiness be achieved? (2.66)

Commentary:

Reading this in the context of the last two verses is very important. That context is the ashram environment, where a person goes, and either settles down or does not, depending on his good or bad nature from before. This is a description of persons who are in the ashram setting, but who are discovered to be unsettled even there. Even in that ideal setting where there is no agitation, where no excitements are created just to pacify the followers, even there, a person might remain as an uncontrolled individual, being incapable of concentration and thus lacking inner peace, emotional stability and the resultant happiness.

The issue here is the past life of the person concerned. If in the past life, the person was not following such a peaceful, nonsensational life, then it is unlikely his psyche will tolerate such a bland and plain environment. He will have to leave such a place and go where excitements are easily procured.

These aspects like natural self control, capacity for deep concentration, emotional stability and self satisfaction, are not stressed in many modern ashrams. Instead, they define self control as the ability to do what one is told. Concentration for them is to view a colorfully—decorated Deity. Emotional stability is to identify with group security. Self satisfaction is the fulfillment of the senses in a setting where fragrance is smelled, pleasing or stimulating music is heard and food sanctified in ceremonies is superfluously appreciated. Such a life, though serviceable in its own way, is not what is discussed in these *Gītā* verses.

इन्द्रियाणां हि चरतां
यन्मनोऽनुविधीयते ।
तदस्य हरति प्रज्ञां
वायुर्नावमिवाम्भसि ॥२.६७॥
indriyāṇāṁ hi caratāṁ
yanmano'nuvidhīyate
tadasya harati prajñāṁ
vāyurnāvamivāmbhasi (2.67)

indriyāṇāṁ — of the senses; hi — indeed; caratāṁ — wandering; yan = yad — when; mano = manaḥ — the mind; 'nuvidhīyate = anuvidhīyate — is prompted; tadasya = tad — that + asya — of it; harati — it utilizes; prajñāṁ — of the discernment; vāyur = vāyuḥ — the wind; nāvam — a ship; ivāmbhasi = iva — like + ambhasi — in the water

When the mind is prompted by the wandering senses, it utilizes the discernment, just as in water, the wind handles a ship. (2.67)

Commentary:

The discernment is the decisive part of the buddhi organ which resides in the head of the subtle body. The wandering senses are the edge—lights of that buddhi. The senses or subtle sensors constantly seek out objects by ranging over whatever is available in any given environment. As soon as a particular sense detects anything that is desirable, it prompts the mind to open itself for information about the said object. In the meantime, the discernment becomes engaged in judging the usefulness or uselessness of the object in terms of its enjoyment content. This happens effortlessly with or without the spirit's approval.

As Śrī Krishna informed us, we may compare the operation of the senses, mind and discernment to that of the wind handling a ship. Even if a ship is anchored, it is affected by wind. If it is not anchored then it is affected to a greater degree. The impressions detected by the senses serve like a wind force, sometimes a fury, to blow the entire mind mechanism here and there accordingly.

तस्माद्यस्य महाबाहो
निगृहीतानि सर्वशः ।
इन्द्रियाणीन्द्रियार्थेभ्यस्
तस्य प्रज्ञा प्रतिष्ठिता ॥२.६८॥
tasmādyasya mahābāho
nigṛhītāni sarvaśaḥ
indriyāṇīndriyārthebhyas
tasya prajñā pratiṣṭhitā (2.68)

tasmād — therefore; yasya — of the person who; mahābāho — O powerful Arjuna; nigṛhītāni — retracts; sarvaśaḥ — in every interaction; indriyāṇīndriyārthebhyas = indriyāṇi — sensual feelings + indriyārthebhyaḥ — of the attractive objects; tasya — his; prajñā — discernment; pratiṣṭhitā — remains constant

Thus, O Arjuna, concerning the person who, in every interaction retracts the sensual feelings from the attractive objects; his discernment remains constant. (2.68)

Commentary:

This type of person is the exception to the rule, because most of us as human beings are unable to do this in every interaction (sarvaśah). We do it in some but not in all. Thus we fall below the standard. Obviously then, our discernment is not constant. And neither was Arjuna's.

या निशा सर्वभूतानां
तस्यां जागर्ति संयमी ।
यस्यां जाग्रति भूतानि
सा निशा पश्यतो मुनेः ॥२.६९॥
yā niśā sarvabhūtānāṁ
tasyāṁ jāgarti saṁyamī
yasyāṁ jāgrati bhūtāni
sā niśā paśyato muneḥ (2.69)

yā — which; niśā — void; sarvabhūtānāṁ — all ordinary people; tasyāṁ — in this; jāgarti — is perceptive; saṁyamī — the sense—controlling person; yasyāṁ — in what; jāgrati — is exciting; bhūtāni — the masses of people; sā — that; niśā — is void; paśyato = paśyataḥ — of the perceptive; muneḥ — of the sage.

The sense—controlling person is perceptive of that which is void to the ordinary people. What is exciting to the masses of people is void to the perceptive sage. (2.69)

Commentary:

Śrī Krishna does not mention His devotee but rather the samyamī, the sense-controlling person, who does so by virtue of mastership of yoga practice, or samyama. Samyama is the concentration of mind which is practiced and achieved in the last three stages of yoga practice.

The sense-controlling person who mastered those last three stages of yoga is perceptive of things which appear dull to ordinary people. What is exciting to such persons is void to him. This is why he could live peacefully and with satisfaction in the plain and simple ashram environment created by sages during the Upanishadic period.

आपूर्यमाणमचलप्रतिष्ठं
समुद्रमापः प्रविशन्ति यद्वत् ।
तद्वत्कामा यं प्रविशन्ति सर्वे
स शान्तिमाप्नोति न कामकामी॥२.७०॥

āpūryamāṇam — becoming filled; acala – not moving about + pratiṣṭham — remaining stationary; samudram — the ocean; āpaḥ — the waters; praviśanti — they enter; yadvat — in which; tadvat — similarly; kāmā = kāmāḥ — cravings; yaṁ — whom; praviśanti — enter,

āpūryamāṇamacalapratiṣṭhaṁ
samudramāpaḥ praviśanti yadvat
tadvatkāmā yaṁ praviśanti sarve
sa śāntimāpnoti na kāmakāmī (2.70)

arise; sarve — all; sa — he; śāntim — true satisfaction; āpnoti — gets; na — not; kāmakāmī — one who craves for every desire

Becoming filled, not flowing about, remaining stationary, the ocean absorbs the waters that enter it. Similarly, a person who remains calm when cravings arise gets true satisfaction, but not the person who craves for every desire. (2.70)

Commentary:

Nowadays many spiritual masters dismiss this verse as unnecessary and no longer relevant. Citing recent incarnations of Godhead and citing statements from scripture which nullify this verse, they say that when cravings arise, one does not need to remain calm since one will get a transcendental or spiritual result if one craves God or something that pertains to God. But such a statement is not in this verse.

If we want to understand these verses, we should for the time being, put aside the modern practices. First of all, a person must have reached the ashram. He must have practiced sufficiently to calm himself to the point where his senses are completely restrained and filled with the conserved energies, the way the ocean is filled with water. Then as indicated in the previous verse he should have mastered samyama, the last three stages of the yoga practice of concentration, contemplation and samādhi. Then after such mastery, whenever cravings arise, he would remain calm and still feel the true satisfaction.

विहाय कामान्यः सर्वान्
पुमांश्चरति निःस्पृहः ।
निर्ममो निरहंकारः
स शान्तिमधिगच्छति ॥२.७१॥

vihāya kāmānyaḥ sarvān
pumāṁścarati niḥspṛhaḥ
nirmamo nirahaṁkāraḥ
sa śāntimadhigacchati (2.71)

vihāya — rejects; kāmān — cravings; yaḥ — who; sarvān — all; pumāṁścarati = pumān — person + carati — acts; niḥspṛhaḥ — free of lusty motivation; nirmamo = nirmamaḥ — indifferent to possessions; nirahaṁkāraḥ — free from impulsive assertion; sa — he; śāntim — contentment; adhigacchati — attains

The person who rejects all cravings, whose acts are free of lusty motivation, who is indifferent to possessions, who is free of impulsive assertion, attains contentment. (2.71)

Commentary:

The person who rejects all cravings differs from the person who takes his cravings and legitimizes them by using them to serve God as his guru stipulates. We are talking about the rejection of all cravings not the sanctification or conversion of cravings. Sarvam means all. Here again we discuss the person who is free of lusty motivation, not the person whose lust is being used to serve the guru and God.

We are talking about the person who is indifferent to possessions not the person who is indifferent only to possessions unrelate to the temple or deity or spiritual teacher.

We hear about the person who is free of impulsive assertion because in the time of the Upanishad, teachers specialized in giving up such assertion by abandoning support of the sense of initiative in order to realize the bare spirit all by itself without the mechanisms of the subtle body. Such a person, Śrī Krishna said, attains contentment (śāntim). This shantim is not love of God or happiness derived from seeing the Deity form of God.

एषा ब्राह्मी स्थितिः पार्थ
नैनां प्राप्य विमुह्यति ।
स्थित्वास्यामन्तकालेऽपि
ब्रह्मनिर्वाणमृच्छति ॥२.७२॥
eṣā brāhmī sthitiḥ pārtha
naināṁ prāpya vimuhyati
sthitvāsyāmantakāle'pi
brahmanirvāṇamṛcchati (2.72)

eṣā — this; brāhmī — divine; sthitiḥ — state; pārtha — son of Pṛthā; naināṁ = na — not + enām — this; prāpya — does have; vimuhyati — is stupefied; sthitvā — is fixed; 'syām = asyām — in this; antakāle — at the time of death; 'pi = api — also; brahma – divinity + nirvāṇam — full stoppage of mundane sensuality; ṛcchati — attains

This divine state is required, O son of Pṛthā. If a man does not have this, he is stupefied. At the time of death, the full stoppage of mundane sensuality and the attainment of divinity is attained by one who is fixed in this divine state. (2.72)

Commentary:

Śrī Krishna states here that this is a divine state (brāhmī stitih). It is not the only divine state but it is the one Śrī Krishna described in this verse. Accordingly, to this view, if a man does not achieve this inner peace which comes from mastery of the three highest stages of yoga practice (samyama), then he is stupefied and after leaving this body he attains neither divinity nor the full stoppage of mundane sensuality.

More or less, until this point, Śrī Krishna tactfully told Arjuna that all the compassion in the world, would not give a man the divine state, but the supreme dispassion which ignores excitements and which brings on self contentment, would take a man to the divine state known as brāhmī sthitih. Of final interest in this verse, is the term nirvāṇam which means the full stoppage of mundane sensuality. That is an objective on the kriyā yoga path.

CHAPTER 3

Cultural Activity and Renunciation*

अर्जुन उवाच
ज्यायसी चेत्कर्मणस्ते
मता बुद्धिर्जनार्दन ।
तत्किं कर्मणि घोरे मां
नियोजयसि केशव ॥ ३.१ ॥
arjuna uvāca
jyāyasī cetkarmaṇaste
matā buddhirjanārdana
tatkiṁ karmaṇi ghore māṁ
niyojayasi keśava (3.1)

arjuna — Arjuna; uvāca — contested; jyāyasī — is better; cet = ced — if; karmaṇaḥ — than physical action; te — your; matā — idea; buddhirjanārdana = buddhiḥ — mental action + janārdana — motivator of men; tatkiṁ = tat (tad) — them + kiṁ — why; karmaṇi — in action; ghore — in horrible; māṁ — me; niyojayasi — you urge; keśava — handsome—haired one

Arjuna contested: O motivator of men, if it is Your idea that the mental approach is better than the physically—active one, then why do You urge me to commit horrible action, O handsome—haired One? (3.1)

Commentary:

The mental approach seems to be contradictory to the physically-active one. Thus Arjuna asked for clarification. This is the problem with kriyā yoga and the application of it. On one hand kriyā yoga is presented as the termination of physical involvements (karmaṇas) and the adopting of subtle perception (buddhir). On the other hand, some kriyā yogis find that they must repeatedly become involved in social and cultural affairs.

Admittedly a few kriyā students did yoga and did not have to return to worldly life as householders and as people who earned a livelihood. All the others returned and became involved in worldly affairs. Some of these returnees lost the practice entirely, forgetting everything about yoga and merging in the crowd of worldly people who go on living as if they are their material bodies.

When one enters into kriyā practice and picks up the idea that he would be ending off his material existence by it (nirvāṇam), he becomes discouraged when he hears that he must again become socially involved.

A kriyā student, like Arjuna, may ask the teacher of the necessity to return to social life since it is counterproductive to kriyā practice. Arjuna asked about the horrors of warfare. For the kriyā student it might be a question of the spiritually-destructive effects of householder life.

**The Mahābhārata contains no chapter headings. This title was assigned by the translator on the basis of verse 4 of this chapter.*

As a kriyā teacher, I have the opportunity to advise many young men who aspire for kriyā skill. Usually I advise such youngsters to get a spouse, form a household and continue their practice in the meantime, so that when these responsibilities decrease, they may complete kriyā practice. Such students, usually look at me with surprise, being appalled at the recommendation. They wanted to avoid social responsibilities, and so they feel frustrated when I advise them to take up duties.

व्यामिश्रेणैव वाक्येन
बुद्धिं मोहयसीव मे ।
तदेकं वद निश्चित्य
येन श्रेयोऽहमाप्नुयाम् ॥ ३.२ ॥
vyāmiśreṇaiva vākyena
buddhiṁ mohayasīva me
tadekaṁ vada niścitya
yena śreyo'hamāpnuyām (3.2)

vyāmiśreṇaiva = vyāmiśreṇa — with this two—way + iva — like this; vākyena — with a proposal; buddhiṁ — intelligence; mohayasīva = mohayasi — you baffle + iva — like this; me — of me; tad — this; ekaṁ — one; vada — tell; niścitya — surely; yena — by which; śreyo = śreyaḥ — the best; 'ham = aham — I; āpnuyām — I should get

You baffle my intelligence with this two-way proposal. Mention one priority, by which I would surely get the best result. (3.2)

Commentary:

I had this experience with many prospective students of kriyā yoga, in that they desire just one priority to follow, a clear and direct instruction that involves only one system.

One will be baffled in trying to get out of this material existence, because the destinies are complicated and intertwining. It is not merely a matter of what a student thinks he should have; rather, he has to deal with the Supervising Universal Lord. That person will not allow any living being to leave the material existence, until certain duties are completed. A kriyā teacher, if perceptive, will know what is required of each student. He will not encourage anyone to avoid duties, because he knows very well that the Supervising Universal Lord cannot be superseded by any limited entity.

Arjuna thought of circumventing the social system completely but later on, when Śrī Krishna displayed the Universal Form, Arjuna realized that it was not possible to escape material existence conveniently except by the method approved by that Lord.

A kriyā teacher cannot protect his students from such a Lord but he can assist the student to acquire that Lord's approval. Therefore we must advise students to face their duties and perform them in a terminal way, by using the mastership that is gained in the practice of kriyā yoga. This is what the *Gītā* teaches. The *Gītā* is the guideline or curriculum of how to apply kriyā yoga to worldly life, in such a way as to end material existence by gaining the waiver of the Supervising Universal Lord.

A person may or may not believe in God when he comes to kriyā yoga. He may not be inclined to any particular religion. That is not the issue here. The factor here is practicality, in that whatever we are required to do to be successful, must be executed. If we have to recognize that Supervising Universal Lord, then we had better do it and achieve the objective. It is not a sentimental belief system. If there is Somebody who is God and if He presents requirements for freedom from these responsibilities, then the quicker we can appease Him, the better off we will be.

Generally people who are serious about kriyā yoga, are not inclined to chase after gurus and glorify them. We are more for a process of development which we can practice to achieve mastership. It is not our system to just have faith and to solely rely on grace. We want to work for and to earn our perfection as we proceed, but that does not mean that we are atheists.

Arjuna requests a priority so that his path of life would be straight forward and simple but actually, life is not that simply laid out. Therefore we will have to give up our need for such simplicity and live in the practical way. Since this existence is intertwining and complicated because of so many lives and so many involvements and mostly because there is supernatural supervision which crosses into the mundane world, we will have to agree to a complicated solution.

It is not just one priority as Arjuna suggests because there are so many varying factors and personalities who must be taken into account. An exit from material existence cannot be had that simply. Admittedly in some scriptures and even in some statements made in this *Gītā* by Śrī Krishna, there are suggestions that it might be a very simple event for a person to achieve salvation or spiritual perfection, but these statements, even those made by the Divinities, are usually an incentive only. Those proposals are in a sense, figurative, because the maze of material existence is very intertwining and our attachment to material nature is very compelling. It has a long, long history.

श्रीभगवानुवाच
लोकेऽस्मिन्द्विविधा निष्ठा
पुरा प्रोक्ता मयानघ ।
ज्ञानयोगेन सांख्यानां
कर्मयोगेन योगिनाम् ॥ ३.३ ॥
śrībhagavānuvāca
loke'smindvividhā niṣṭhā
purā proktā mayānagha
jñānayogena sāṁkhyānāṁ
karmayogena yoginām (3.3)

śrī bhagavān — the Blessed Lord; uvāca — said; loke — in this physical world; 'smin = asmin — in this; dvividhā — of the two—fold; niṣṭhā — standard; purā — previously; proktā — was taught; mayā — by me; 'nagha = anagha — O blameless one, good man; jñānayogena — mind regulations by yoga practice; sāṁkhyānāṁ — of the Sāṁkhya philosophical yogis; karmayogena — action regulation by yoga practice; yoginām — of the non—philosophical yogis

The Blessed Lord said: In the physical world, a two—fold standard was previously taught by Me, O Arjuna, my good man. This was mind regulation by the yoga practice of the Sāṁkhya philosophical yogis and the action regulation by the yoga practice of the non—philosophical yogis. (3.3)

Commentary:

This is a piece of history. If anyone studies the *Vedas* and then studies the *Upanishads* in that order, he will realize that the development of the spiritual course for human beings came about gradually. The stress on bhakti and on bhakti yoga came about later after the Upanishadic period. During the time of Śrī Rāma, the bhakti and the bhakti yoga systems began to pick up momentum because by then, cultured human beings were moving away from fire sacrifices and were gaining the upper hand over cave men, wild animals and hostile climates.

We have to understand that the creation of this planet, as we now know it, took billions of years. It is not that God or a Creative agent of God (Brahmā) created this planet as we find it today. At first this planet was a hot mass. And then gradually over millions of years it cooled down. The climate we experience today was not always manifested on this planet which in its past history was mostly hostile to human existence.

In the past, sometimes the aquatics thrived. Sometimes the big creatures like dinosaurs thrived. Sometimes crude human beings, the so—called cave men thrived. Periodically refined human bodies, like the ones we use, thrived. In the Vedic period which is recent in terms of astronomical time, some sages tried to get human beings to organize themselves as advised by Brahmā, a supernatural personality. Gradually when the Vedic sages like Agni and others were successful, the Upanishadic period came on. But the stress on bhakti and bhakti yoga came later. This is why here in the *Gītā*, Śrī Krishna admits only a two—fold standard.

Bhakti and bhakti yoga are vital but they were not the system of consideration initially, so they are not mentioned here by Śrī Krishna. If one reads the *Vedas* and the Upanishad, this point will become evident.

In the Vedic times, the sages had to deal with survival of their material bodies. Just by saying a wrong syllable in the rudimentary Sanskrit used at the time, they could destroy their own bodies or create things that were undesirable. Bhakti and bhakti yoga were not foremost on their minds. Later, in the Upanishadic period, we see bhakti and bhakti yoga coming into focus. Still, at the time, the psychological research into the Absolute Truth and the hunt for mystic experience was the priority. It is said that a sage by the name of Yama was the first of the people in the Upanishadic period, to consciously leave his material body and experience himself as being separate from it in a subtle form.

Two types of yogis are mentioned in this verse, as being oriented towards two systems of practice, which Śrī Krishna said He previously taught. Use of the word, *previously*, must mean in previous lives or in other dimensions through which inspirations and revelations filtered back into this world. In the current life of Himself and Arjuna, Śrī Krishna served as a student to some sages who explained to Him the yoga system afresh. In addition, Sri Krishna was instructed in the most advanced kriyā practices by Sage Upamanyu who instructed Him in how to practice, so that he could call Lord Shiva for an interview. This is described in the *Mahābhārata*.

The two types of yogis mentioned are Samkhya yogis and the haţha yogis who did not have a strong philosophical interest. Both of these yogis learned haţha yoga but only the Samkhyas progressed further to perfect jñāna yoga; the non—philosophically inclined persons went back to cultural life and tried to do karma yoga. Both were proficient in haţha yoga but one was inclined to mystic activities and the other to physical activities for social, cultural and political causes. Thus Śrī Krishna claims to have established a two—fold training process (dvidvidhā).

Śrī Krishna's yoga practice under the direction of the mahāyogīn Upamanyu is summarized as follows:

In the Anusasanika Parva of the *Mahābhārata*, Section 14, there is a narration of how Bhīṣma, the eldest of the Kurus, declined a request by Yudhiṣṭhira to describe the one thousand names of Lord Shiva, saying that he was quite incompetent to sing the glories of Maheshvara, Lord Shiva. Bhīṣma recommended that Lord Krishna give the one thousand names, Shiva Sahasranama, because he said that only Śrī Krishna could understand Shiva.

A great yogin sage named Tandi sung those one thousand names long, long ago. It was heard by Upamanyu, who lived in the time of Śrī Krishna. This Upamanyu, another great yogin told those one thousand names to Śrī Krishna, when Śrī Krishna lived at his hermitage and performed austerities under his direction.

Śrī Krishna agreed to tell those one thousand names to Yudhiṣṭhira and others, there at the place where Bhīṣma was to leave his body on the battlefield of Kurukṣetra. As the story goes, one of Śrī Krishna's wives, named Jāmbavatī, asked Śrī Krishna to beget sons who were comparable to those which He gave one of her co—wives named Rukmiṇī, and to follow the same course of austerities prior to begetting as he did in the case of the sons of Rukmiṇī.

This occurred some 12 years after Rukmiṇī's son, Pradyumna had killed the demon Sambara. Śrī Krishna took leave of Jāmbavatī, gained permission from his elders, and then said goodbye to Gada and Śrī Balarāma, his elder brother. He went to the Himalaya Mountains. There he found a nice place for practice but this location was the hermitage of the great yogin Upamanyu, the descendant of Vyaghrapāda. That area had many wonders of nature. Many wild animals roamed there but the predatory creatures did not attack the gentle ones in that vicinity. This was due to the over—riding holy atmosphere which charmed the ferocious creatures.

Śrī Krishna saw many ascetics who appeared like pillars of fire. Some lived on air only, some on water. Some did audible repetition of prayers. Others were engaged in inaudible repetition. Some were cleansing their psychologies by practicing compassion. Other yogins sat in trance meditation. Some lived on smoke only, some on fire, some on milk. Some drank and ate like the cows do, not using their hands nor cooking anything. Some kept two stones for husking grain. Some used their teeth only for the same. Some drank moon rays. Some drank froth only. Some were dressed in rags, some in animal skins, some in tree bark.

Entering that place, Śrī Krishna perceived all the supernatural rulers present there. He saw a great yogin sage with matted locks, who was dressed in rags. The person blazed with fire with his austerities and purifying energies. He was the Sage Upamanyu.

Śrī Krishna offered formal respects by bowing to this person who was the spiritual master of that place. Upamanyu, recognizing Śrī Krishna, said, "Welcome to You, whose eyes are shaped like lotus petals. Today, by Your visit, my penances resulted in the highest gain. You, who are worthy of my admiration, honor me here today. You, who are worthy of being seen, came to me today."

Śrī Krishna then discussed the purpose of His journey to the Himalayas to perform a penance for begetting sons for Jāmbavatī and to do this by invoking Lord Shiva. The mahāyogīn Upamanyu told Śrī Krishna that Mahādeva Shiva resided at that very place along with his wife, the goddess Umā.

Upamanyu then explained that in his boyhood, his mother advised him to worship Śrī Mahādeva Shiva, because he had a desire to drink nectarian milk which his parents could not provide because they were poor ascetics living in a remote forest. The mahāyogīn then did penance standing on his left toe for one thousand years, then for the same period each, he subsisted on fruits, then on fallen leaves, then on water and lastly he subsisted on air for 700 years. This added up to about one thousand years in the time of the celestial people. After this, disguised as Indra, the King of the angelic people, Lord Shiva came to Upamanyu. The yogin did not realize the disguise of Lord Shiva and merely stressed that he wanted to talk to Lord Shiva and not to Indra.

Then Śrī Mahādeva shed the disguise and with him appeared Lord Brahmā and Lord Nārāyaṇa who were on his left side. Close to Shiva was Umā, his wife, as well as Skanda, his son. In front of Shiva was Nandī, his associate servant.

Hearing this story of the accomplishment of the Spiritual Master of that place, Śrī Krishna asked the authority for a sight of Lord Shiva. The mahāyogīn Upamanyu said that in the sixth month, Śrī Krishna would see Lord Shiva and would get whatever was desired. They conversed for eight days which to Śrī Krishna seemed like one hour. Then Upamanyu gave Lord Krishna formal initiation as a disciple and described the penances for seeing Lord Shiva.

Lord Krishna, as the student of that great yogin, did the yoga austerities as He was shown. In the first month, He lived on fruits alone, in the second, on water, and in the third, fourth and fifth, he lived on air alone, standing on one foot with arms raised, without sleeping. Then suddenly He saw Lord Shiva with Umā, the goddess of the material nature. They were shining like a thousand suns combined. Lord Shiva said to Śrī Krishna, "Behold O Krishna, My form which You wish to see. Speak to Me as desired. You adored Me hundreds and thousands of times in the past in many of Your incarnations. No one in these three worlds is so dear to Me as You are."

Lord Krishna discussed with Lord Shiva and with Goddess Umā, the reason for the penance. Then Lord Shiva and the Goddess granted Krishna all that was requested.

न कर्मणामनारम्भान्
नैष्कर्म्यं पुरुषोऽश्नुते ।
न च संन्यसनादेव
सिद्धिं समधिगच्छति ॥३.४॥
na karmaṇāmanārambhān
naiṣkarmyaṁ puruṣo'śnute
na ca saṁnyasanādeva
siddhiṁ samadhigacchati (3.4)

na — not; karmaṇām — concerning cultural activity; anārambhān — not being involved; naiṣkarmyaṁ — freedom from cultural activity; puruṣo = puruṣaḥ — a person; 'śnute = aśnute — attains; na — not; ca — and; saṁnyasanādeva = saṁnyasanād (saṁnyasanāt) — from renunciation + eva — alone; siddhiṁ — spiritual perfection; samadhigacchati — achieves

A man does not attain freedom from cultural activity merely by not being involved in social affairs. And not by renunciation alone, does he achieve spiritual perfection. (3.4)

Commentary:

The technicality here for us as kriyā yogis is this: We will not become exempt from cultural activity merely by staying out of the cultural field. This is because there is a controller who is the Supervising Universal Lord. He will not permit us to escape responsibilities and liabilities from the past, merely by abstinence from cultural activities. This might be our plan of action but it will not work, because normally He does not approve of it.

In addition, the mundane energy itself will not agree to our proposal for a sudden stoppage of cultural activity. This is why we see that many monks who start spiritual missions, end up participating in cultural activities, even though they are witty enough to pass off their participation as seva (divine work) or as bhakti (devotional services). Some of them label it as selfless work. The truth is that they are forced back into the world by the Supervising Universal Lord and by material nature. They are not allowed to be completely exempt from cultural activities.

On the other hand, those who remain in isolation and who do not participate in any sort of cultural activities, are rarely able to achieve spiritual perfection (siddhim) by renunciation alone. Very few achieve this, since only a few are permitted that by the Supervising Universal Lord and by their very, very slim relationship to material nature. Only those who took a body after they fulfilled the obligations in the recent past life, can get the required exemptions, not others. Thus we see that some who were yogis in their past lives and who completed the obligations formerly, begin their practice early on in the new life and as if by some divine grace or special providence, they make the quantum leap and attain liberation.

All others must strike a balance between the performance of certain terminal cultural acts and the application of renunciation. The trick is to understand clearly what the demands of the Supervising Universal Lord are and to fulfill these as efficiently as possible. If one gains an exemption from Him, one is sure to be successful in yoga practice.

न हि कश्चित्क्षणमपि
जातु तिष्ठत्यकर्मकृत् ।
कार्यते ह्यवशः कर्म
सर्वः प्रकृतिजैर्गुणैः ॥३.५॥
na hi kaścitkṣaṇamapi
jātu tiṣṭhatyakarmakṛt
kāryate hyavaśaḥ karma
sarvaḥ prakṛtijairguṇaiḥ (3.5)

na — no; hi — indeed; kaścit — anyone; kṣaṇamapi = kṣaṇam — a moment + api — also; jātu — ever; tiṣṭhatyakarmakṛt = tiṣṭhati — exists + akarmakṛt — not acting; kāryate — caused to act; hyavaśaḥ = hi — indeed + avaśaḥ — against their wishes; karma — vibration; sarvaḥ — everyone; prakṛtijair = prakṛtijaiḥ — produced by material nature; guṇaiḥ — variations of mundane energy

No one, even momentarily, ever exists without vibration. By the variations of mundane energy in material nature, everyone, even against their wishes, is forced to perform. (3.5)

Commentary:

It is not just the Supervising Universal Lord who may upset the advancement of a yogi but also material nature itself, because as Śrī Krishna authoritatively stated, no one, even momentarily, ever exists without vibration. Every one of us is forced into activity even against our wish. This is reality. We must accept this. A kriyā yogi must be realistic if he wants to succeed. He should recognize the laws of nature and be coordinated with them.

कर्मेन्द्रियाणि संयम्य
य आस्ते मनसा स्मरन् ।
इन्द्रियार्थान्विमूढात्मा
मिथ्याचारः स उच्यते ॥३.६॥
karmendriyāṇi saṁyamya
ya āste manasā smaran
indriyārthānvimūḍhātmā
mithyācāraḥ sa ucyate (3.6)

karmendriyāṇi — bodily limbs; saṁyamya — restraining; ya = yaḥ — who; āste — sits; manasā — by the mind; smaran — remembering; indriyārthān — attractive objects; vimūḍhātmā = vimūḍha — deluded + ātmā — self; mithyācāraḥ — deceiver; sa — he; ucyate — it is declared

A person who while restraining his bodily limbs sits, with the mind remembering attractive objects, is a deceiver. So it is declared. (3.6)

Commentary:

If one sits to meditate and still remembers the attractive objects, either deliberately or impulsively as forced on by the mind and the emotional energy in it, then it is to be understood that one has not gained exemption from cultural activities. If however, one does not understand this and persists in the isolation, then one is declared to be a deceiver. This is because one gives people the impression that one has transcended the physical plane when, in fact, one is still tightly connected to it.

Śrī Krishna very tactfully informed that Arjuna would not be able to meditate since any effort to do so would result in Arjuna's compulsive thinking of opponents. Thus it was best for Arjuna to deal with the situation and to resolve that confrontation for the satisfaction of the Supervising Universal Lord.

Even though yoga involves the restraining of bodily limbs in āsana postures, still that is not the entire process. With the mind, the yogi is supposed to restrain his subtle brain or buddhi. That entails breath regulation and sensual energy retraction. Āsana postures are not the complete process. Even though it may give observers the impression that one is a yogi, it does not actually make one into a yogi unless one restrains the mind from remembering the attractive objects.

यस्त्विन्द्रियाणि मनसा
नियम्यारभतेऽर्जुन ।
कर्मेन्द्रियैः कर्मयोगम्
असक्तः स विशिष्यते ॥३.७॥
yastvindriyāṇi manasā
niyamyārabhate'rjuna
karmendriyaiḥ karmayogam
asaktaḥ sa viśiṣyate (3.7)

Yas (yaḥ)— whosoever; tvindriyāṇi = tv (tu) — however + indriyāṇi — the senses; manasā — by the mind; niyamyārabhate = niyamya — controlling + ārabhate — endeavors; 'rjuna— Arjuna; karmendriyaiḥ — by the limbs; karmayogam — regulating his work by yoga practice; asaktaḥ — without attachment; sa = saḥ — he; viśiṣyate — is superior

However, whosoever endeavors to control the senses by the mind, O Arjuna, and who restricts the limbs through regulating his work by yoga practice, without attachment, is superior. (3.7)

Commentary:

Some commentators feel that Śrī Krishna meant cultural work and religious work as yoga practice, but this assumption is misleading. We deny it. Karma yoga, in the *Gītā*, does not mean just social, cultural or political work or any other type of work, including religious work, which is performed without the application of yoga practice. For some people this is very difficult to accept because they want to use the *Gītā* to endorse such activities as karma yoga. However, there is no need to do this. There are verses in the *Gītā*, which approve such activities but those verses occur elsewhere with appropriate descriptions. We will point them out in this commentary.

Even though in modern times karma yoga has come to mean religious activities without yoga, that is not the meaning intended by Śrī Krishna in the *Bhagavad Gītā*. One should not be embarrassed or ashamed of the truth of the matter. In this verse, Śrī Krishna gave a description of the skill of karma yoga, which is yoga expertise applied to social, cultural and political life. Arjuna was in the political field as a prince. He had to apply what he already practiced and mastered in yoga to that sort of life. Thus he would mindfully control the senses through the yoga disciplines he had learned and practiced. He would restrict his limbs by regulating his activities through whatever bodily control he already mastered in haţha yoga practice. He could do so without attachment by the power of being emotionally hardened.

नियतं कुरु कर्म त्वं
कर्म ज्यायो ह्यकर्मणः ।
शरीरयात्रापि च ते
न प्रसिध्येदकर्मणः ॥३.८॥

niyataṁ — moral; kuru — do; karma — cultural duty; tvaṁ — you; karma — performance; jyāyo = jyāyaḥ — better; hy akarmaṇaḥ = hi — indeed + akarmaṇaḥ — than non—action; śarīrayātrāpi = śarīra — body + yātrā — maintenance + api

niyataṁ kuru karma tvaṁ
karma jyāyo hyakarmaṇaḥ
śarīrayātrāpi ca te
na prasidhyedakarmaṇaḥ (3.8)

— even; ca — and; te — your; na — not; prasidhyet — could be achieved; akarmaṇaḥ — without activity

Moral action should be done by you. Performance is better than non—performance. Even the maintenance of your body could not be achieved without activity. (3.8)

Commentary:

Niyama is the 2nd stage of yoga practice which consists of approved actions. These are mostly moral activities which are socially, culturally and politically beneficial to one and all. Śrī Krishna here tells Arjuna that the performance of moral activities is better than the lack of it. He cites the fact that activity is so essential that a person cannot maintain his body without it. In fact, even those who get the exemption from cultural acts, must maintain their bodies in some way or another. Those yogis who enter trance do so after performing many activities in haṭha yoga and prāṇāyāma. So in all respects some sort of activity is performed.

So long as one has to complete duties, as ordained by the Supervising Universal Lord, then it is best that one performs, since the refusal to do so, would draw the non—approval of the Supreme Personality, which would result in the failure of yoga practice.

यज्ञार्थात्कर्मणोऽन्यत्र
लोकोऽयं कर्मबन्धनः ।
तदर्थं कर्म कौन्तेय
मुक्तसङ्गः समाचर ॥३.९॥
yajñārthātkarmaṇo'nyatra
loko'yaṁ karmabandhanaḥ
tadarthaṁ karma kaunteya
muktasaṅgaḥ samācara (3.9)

yajñārthāt = yajña — religious fulfillment and ceremony + ārthāt — for the sake of; karmaṇo = karmaṇaḥ — from action; 'nyatra = anyatra — besides; loko = lokaḥ — world; 'yaṁ = ayaṁ — this; karmabandhanaḥ — something bound by action; tadartham = tad — this + arthaṁ — purpose, value; karma — cultural activity; kaunteya — son of Kuntī; muktasaṅgaḥ — freedom from attachment; samācara — act promptly

Besides action for religious fulfillment and ceremony, this world, is action—bound. Act for the sake of religious fulfillment and ceremony, O son of Kuntī. Be free from attachment. Act promptly. (3.9)

Commentary:

Yajnārtha is the religious fulfillment and ceremonies which were suggested and approved by the Supervising Universal Lord. These actions are not part of the regular social, cultural and political course of human civilization.

Śrī Krishna informed us that whatever is initiated by the Supervising Universal Lord is separate and distinct from the other actions which take place, but in any case a person must act. Sometimes he is compelled to perform for the sake of that Supreme Lord. Sometimes he acts for the satisfaction of others. In all cases a kriyā yogi should act without attachment. To do this he puts himself into a stage of detached consciousness as he practiced in the mystic kriyā techniques.

Arjuna, who was to represent that Supervising Universal Lord, had to squash the opposing Kurus because they acted irresponsibly in governing the country. If Arjuna left the battlefield he would have discarded yajñārtha, thereby rejecting the Divine Will and invoking Its disapproval.

The idea here is this: Even though one might be a kriyā yogi intending to end one's material existence, still one is duty bound to serve the Supervising Universal Lord. At no time does one become free from the jurisdiction of that Supreme Lord, even though He might give one a waiver from cultural actions, including the ones to be performed on His behalf.

A kriyā yogi should never get the idea that he is God or that there is no God or that he is completely exempt from the views of the God. At all times, in his conditioned or liberated states, he is under the jurisdiction of that Supreme Personality.

सहयज्ञाः प्रजाः सृष्ट्वा
पुरोवाच प्रजापतिः ।
अनेन प्रसविष्यध्वम्
एष वोऽस्त्विष्टकामधुक् ॥३.१०॥
sahayajñāḥ prajāḥ sṛṣṭvā
purovāca prajāpatiḥ
anena prasaviṣyadhvam
eṣa vo'stviṣṭakāmadhuk
(3.10)

sahayajñāḥ — along with religious fulfillment and ceremony; prajāḥ — first human beings; sṛṣṭvā — having created; purovāca = pura — long ago + uvāca — said; prajāpatiḥ — procreator Brahma; anena — by this; prasaviṣyadhvam — may you produce; eṣaḥ — this; vo = vaḥ — your; 'stviṣṭakāmadhuk = astviṣṭakāmadhuk = astu — may it be + iṣṭakāmadhuk — for granting desires

Long ago, having created the first human beings, along with religious fulfillment and ceremonies, the Procreator Brahmā said: By this worship procedure, you may be productive. May it cause the fulfillment of your desires. (3.10)

Commentary:

These supernatural authorities like Brahmā, the Procreator, have a monopoly on the creation. They spread out a franchise through which we operate later on in the creation. Even though such persons may not be physically present, still we have to understand that they wield supernatural power. That energy does affect the physical reality. We ourselves, the physical beings, must give up the physical forms and take on subtle bodies. This means that we cannot avoid the supernatural controllers indefinitely.

Śrī Krishna informs that Brahmā established the human species and set up certain worship procedures, which were mandatory. Because He created the environment and working conditions for the living beings who were produced after, Brahmā has the authority to give guidelines for living. Brahmā, by intuition, knew what his sons should do to live easily in this creation without much reaction from material nature and with the approval of the Supreme Lord. Thus as a good father, he gave his sons information which caused their success.

देवान्भावयतानेन
ते देवा भावयन्तु वः।
परस्परं भावयन्तः
श्रेयः परमवाप्स्यथ ॥३.११॥
devānbhāvayatānena
te devā bhāvayantu vaḥ
parasparaṁ bhāvayantaḥ
śreyaḥ paramavāpsyatha
(3.11)

devān — supernatural rulers; bhāvayatānena = bhāvayatā — may you cause to flourish + anena — by this procedure; te — they; devā — the supernatural rulers; bhāvayantu — may they bless you; vaḥ — you; parasparaṁ — each other; bhāvayantaḥ — favorably regarding one another; śreyaḥ — well—being; param — highest; avāpsyatha — you will achieve

By this procedure, you may cause the supernatural rulers to flourish. They, in turn, may bless you. In favorably regarding each other, the highest well—being will be achieved. (3.11)

Commentary:

Here we get more information as to why a kriyā yogi may not get out of the material world without first completing certain social, cultural and political duties. There are several reasons: There is the Supervising Universal Lord. There is also the Procreator Brahmā. There are the supernatural rulers (devān). Arjuna was in the same situation of having to satisfy these authorities.

Śrī Krishna gave a synopsis of what it takes to satisfy these personalities. It is not that a human being appeases each and every one of them, but he cannot attain liberation without getting a waiver from the Supervising Universal Lord. At the time of the battle, Arjuna did not have such an exemption. Thus for him, to turn away would have been a very foolish action.

We do not get a detailed description of the religious fulfillment and ceremony which was prescribed but this does confirm such activity. By following the worship procedures, the human beings would cause the supernatural rulers to flourish. And they in turn would bless the humans. In the favorable regard of each other, the highest well—being would be achieved for each. From the tone of this instruction of Brahmā, we get the feeling that he is not one of the supernatural rulers indicated. They are persons commissioned by him to supervise the creation.

इष्टान्भोगान्हि वो देवा
दास्यन्ते यज्ञभाविताः ।
तैर्दत्तानप्रदायैभ्यो
यो भुङ्क्ते स्तेन एव सः ॥३.१२॥
iṣṭānbhogānhi vo devā
dāsyante yajñabhāvitāḥ
tairdattānapradāyaibhyo
yo bhuṅkte stena eva saḥ
(3.12)

iṣṭān — most desired; bhogān — enjoyable people and things; hi — indeed; vo = vaḥ — to you; devā — supernatural rulers; dāsyante — they will give; yajñabhāvitāḥ — manifested through prescribed austerity and religious ceremony; tair = taiḥ — by those; dattān — given items; apradāyaibhyo = apradāya — not offering + ebhyaḥ — to them; yo = yaḥ — who; bhuṅkte — enjoys; stena — a thief; eva — only; saḥ — he

The supernatural rulers, being manifested through prescribed austerity and religious ceremony, will, indeed, give you the most desired people and things. Whosoever does not offer those given items to them, but who enjoys these, is certainly a thief. (3.12)

Commentary:

According to this, the supernatural rulers had no material bodies but were manifested to the human beings who cooperated with the stipulations of Brahmā. How they were manifested, is not stated. The process for bringing in such manifestation is given as prescribed austerity and religious ceremony. It may be said however, that such a procedure, even if it operated in the Vedic era, is irrelevant now, since today most human beings procure happiness without following such procedures.

This has some truth in it, but we must also understand that at this stage of the creative cycle, the stipulations of Brahmā only appear to be ineffective. As Śrī Krishna says in the last sentence, those who do not offer the given items to the supernatural rulers, but who enjoy nevertheless, are thieves. At least that is Śrī Krishna's view. That opinion carries some weight. This will be explained in the next verse.

यज्ञशिष्टाशिनः सन्तो
मुच्यन्ते सर्वकिल्बिषैः ।
भुञ्जते ते त्वघं पापा
ये पचन्त्यात्मकारणात् ॥३.१३॥
yajñaśiṣṭāśinaḥ santo
mucyante sarvakilbiṣaiḥ
bhuñjate te tvaghaṁ pāpā
ye pacantyātmakāraṇāt (3.13)

yajñaśiṣṭāśinaḥ = yajñaśiṣṭa — sanctified items used after a religious ceremony + āśinaḥ — utilizing; santo = santaḥ — virtuous souls; mucyante — they are released; sarvakilbiṣaiḥ — from all faults; bhuñjate — consume; te — they; tvaghaṁ = tv (tu) — but + aghaṁ — impurity; pāpā — wicked people; ye — who; pacantyātmakāraṇāt = pacanti — prepare + ātma — self + kāraṇāt — for the sake of

(Krishna continued): The virtuous people who utilize the items after they are sanctified by prescribed ceremony, are released from all faults. But the wicked ones who prepare for their own sake, consume their own impurity. (3.13)

Commentary:

This is not simply Krishna's opinion, for as He clarified in other parts of the *Gītā*, the living entity, the spirit, has more than one existence and the supernatural people can affect future births and express their disapproval in other settings. Even though modern people do not generally adhere to the stipulations of Brahmā, still they are under the gaze of the Supervising Universal Personality.

A kriyā yogi should note this and not act whimsically or refrain from action just by his own fancy.

अन्नाद्भवन्ति भूतानि
पर्जन्यादन्नसंभवः ।
यज्ञाद्भवति पर्जन्यो
यज्ञः कर्मसमुद्भवः ॥३.१४॥
annādbhavanti bhūtāni
parjanyādannasaṁbhavaḥ
yajñādbhavati parjanyo
yajñaḥ karmasamudbhavaḥ (3.14)

annād=annāt— from nourishment; bhavanti— are produced; bhūtāni — the creatures; parjanyād = parjanyāt — from rain clouds; anna — nourishment; saṁbhavaḥ — originated; yajñād = yajñāt — from prescribed austerity and religious ceremony; bhavati — exists; parjanyo = parjanyaḥ — rain; yajñaḥ — prescribed austerity and religious ceremony; karma — cultural action; samudbhavaḥ — is caused

The creatures are produced from nourishment. From rain clouds, nourishment originated. From prescribed austerity and religious ceremony, rain clouds are produced. And prescribed austerity and religious ceremony are caused by cultural activities. (3.14)

Commentary:

Śrī Krishna explained why the material existence is not irrelevant to spiritual communication and why a living being should adhere to Brahmā's stipulations. Beginning with the creature forms, especially in the human form, Śrī Krishna explains a simple truth, that these physical forms are produced from nourishment. Nourishment or food is caused by rainfall. The rainfall, Śrī Krishna states, is produced by prescribed austerity and religious ceremony. This is not just superstition. Modern astronomers use unmanned space probes to find water on nearby planets, since in their view, water preceeds physical life.

At this point we may or may not agree with Śrī Krishna. If what He says about rainfall is true, then that fact must be verified supernaturally. From the physical perspective it is accepted that rainfall is produced from the clouds which are caused by the sun's action of evaporating water from the land, rivers and seas.

For the sake of following the explanations, we will go along with Krishna's ideas. He claims that rain is produced from prescribed austerity and religious ceremony, which in turn is produced by cultural activities. This goes back to the human beings. This shows that the earthly environment is to a greater extent dependent on the cultural acts of human beings. Obviously, the connection must be supernatural, because from the geographic perspective, the human beings are not that significant even though their impact can negatively or positively affect the environment.

कर्म ब्रह्मोद्भवं विद्धि
ब्रह्माक्षरसमुद्भवम् ।
तस्मात्सर्वगतं ब्रह्म
नित्यं यज्ञे प्रतिष्ठितम् ॥३.१५॥
karma brahmodbhavaṁ viddhi
brahmākṣarasamudbhavam
tasmātsarvagataṁ brahma
nityaṁ yajñe pratiṣṭhitam (3.15)

karma — cultural activity; brahmodbhavaṁ = brahma — the Veda + udbhavaṁ — produced; viddhi — be aware; brahmākṣarasamudbhavam = brahma — Supreme Spirit + akṣara — the unaffected spiritual reality + samudbhavam — produced; tasmāt — hence; sarvagataṁ — all—pervading; brahma — spirit person; nityaṁ — always; yajñe — in prescribed austerity and religious ceremony; pratiṣṭhitam — is situated

Cultural activity is produced from the Personified Veda. The Personified Veda comes from the unaffected Supreme Spirit. Hence the all—pervading Supreme Spirit is always situated in prescribed austerity and religious ceremony. (3.15)

Commentary:

Cultural activity, though performed by human beings, does not originate with them. It seems as though it does come from their hearts and minds, but actually it does not. From this information, we hear that it originates from the Personified Veda, who is Brahmā, the Procreator. As stated Brahmā comes from the unaffected Supreme Spirit (brahmākṣara). Hence, according to this deduction, the all—pervading Supreme Spirit is always situated in prescribed austerities and religious ceremony, because He is the ultimate cause of the creation and of the inspirations and instructions which come through His agent, the Procreator Brahmā.

एवं प्रवर्तितं चक्रं
नानुवर्तयतीह यः ।
अघायुरिन्द्रियारामो
मोघं पार्थ स जीवति ॥३.१६॥
evaṁ pravartitaṁ cakraṁ
nānuvartayatīha yaḥ
aghāyurindriyārāmo
moghaṁ pārtha sa jīvati (3.16)

evaṁ — thus; pravartitaṁ — perpetuated; cakraṁ — circular process; nānuvartayatīha = na — not + anuvartayati — cause to be perpetuated + iha — on earth; yaḥ — who; aghāyurindriyārāmo = aghāyurindriyārāmaḥ = aghāyuḥ — malicious + indriyārāmaḥ — sensually—happy person; moghaṁ — worthless; pārtha — son of Pṛthā; sa = saḥ — he; jīvati — lives

O son of Pṛthā, a person who does not cause this circular process to be perpetuated here on earth, lives as a malicious, sensually—happy and worthless person. (3.16)

Commentary:

This blunt opinion of the all-pervading Supreme Spirit applies to Arjuna as well as to us. If we do not contribute to this circular process, then we are considered as malicious, sensually-happy and worthless. Then how could that apply to someone who took up austerities forsaking the sensual world, in an effort to fend off involvements? The answer is that such a person will not succeed and will, of necessity, be forced to think of sensual memories while he tries to meditate. Let us recall a verse spoken by Śrī Krishna already:

karmendriyāṇi saṁyamya ya āste manasā smaran
indriyārthānvimūḍhātmā mithyācāraḥ sa ucyate (3.6)

A person who, while restraining his bodily limbs, sits with mind remembering attractive objects, is a deceiver. So it is declared. (3.6)

The implication is that if one goes off to be a recluse and tries to meditate for spiritual emancipation, he will not be successful if the Supreme Lord did not give him an exemption from cultural activities. Without the waiver he will be left to his own devices. He will be under the spell of the various psychic energies which will ruin his meditation.

यस्त्वात्मरतिरेव स्याद्
आत्मतृप्तश्च मानवः ।
आत्मन्येव च संतुष्टस्
तस्य कार्यं न विद्यते ॥३.१७॥
yastvātmaratireva syād
ātmatṛptaśca mānavaḥ
ātmanyeva ca saṁtuṣṭas
tasya kāryaṁ na vidyate (3.17)

yastvātmaratireva = yas (yaḥ) — who + tv (tu) — but + ātma — spiritual self + ratir (ratiḥ) — pleased + eva — surely; syāt — should be; ātmatṛptaśca = ātma — self + tṛptaḥ — satisfied + ca — and; mānavaḥ — a human being; ātmanyeva = ātmany (ātmani) — in the self, internally + eva — only; ca — and; saṁtuṣṭaḥ — content; tasya — of him; kāryaṁ — cultural duty; na — no; vidyate — it is experienced

A person who is spiritually-pleased, self-satisfied and internally-content, has no cultural duties. (3.17)

Commentary:

As neophyte kriyā yogis who are longing for freedom from material existence, our concern is this: Such a person obtained an exemption from cultural duties. He has the waiver from the Supervising Universal Lord. How did he acquire it? This is not a sentimental matter, because we see that many who are devotees of Śrī Krishna do not get that exemption. Some of them go on year after year, month after month and in many cases, life after life, happily without it.

As scientifically-minded people who are not satisfied to remain as Śrī Krishna's devotees in the material world, we are honest with ourselves in knowing that we want to get out. Thus our interest focuses on how such a person who is spiritually-pleased, self-satisfied and spiritually-content got the waiver from cultural duties?

He could not have acquired the waiver after attaining the self—satisfied, spiritually—content state because we know that one gets this only after being relieved from the chores of material existence and after focusing on the samādhis and various psychic disciplines and clarifications which lead to that sort of complete self satisfaction.

We recognize that Arjuna was not in that condition when he broke down in tears on the chariot. How then can a kriyā yogi get the opportunity whereby he could be free to practice advanced kriyā yoga in order to reach this stage? He must be free to practice without pressures for cultural upliftment. He must be allowed the time to complete the disciplines uninterruptedly. At the time of battle, Arjuna did not have the waiver. Thus Śrī Krishna described a person who was far beyond Arjuna's stage.

नैव तस्य कृतेनार्थो
नाकृतेनेह कश्चन ।
न चास्य सर्वभूतेषु
कश्चिदर्थव्यपाश्रयः ॥३.१८॥
naiva tasya kṛtenārtho
nākṛteneha kaścana
na cāsya sarvabhūteṣu
kaścidarthavyapāśrayaḥ (3.18)

naiva = na — not + eva — indeed; tasya — regarding him; kṛtenārtho = kṛtena — with action + artho (arthaḥ) — gain; nākṛteneha = na — not + akṛtena — with non—action + iha — in this case; kaścana — anyone; na — not; cāsya = ca — and + asya — of him; sarvabhūteṣu — in all mundane creatures; kaścit — any; arthavyapāśrayaḥ = artha — purpose + vyapāśrayaḥ — depending

The person who does not aspire for gain in an action or in an inaction, is not reliant on any mundane creature. (3.18)

Commentary:

Now we get a technicality that is worth noting. In trying to get the waiver we have to qualify ourselves in certain ways, one of which is mentioned in this verse. As in every case of applying for some status, one has to meet certain requirements.

Some commentators, being all too eager to find a method of total exemption from reliance on anyone anywhere, have suggested the meaning of this verse as a total independence from any and everyone. In their view, one reaches what is called the stage of kevala or absoluteness. Sometimes this is presented as oneness with everything or becoming God. However, such an interpretation is not scientific.

What this verse really means hinges on the meaning of the word bhūta from which bhūteṣu is derived. The word sarva means all. The word bhūta limits the application of this verse to mundane creatures. It does not apply to supernatural people or divine personages.

This verse says that if by elementary practice, a kriyā yogi can develop the skill of not aspiring for gain or for elation and satisfaction, then he becomes non—reliant on mundane creations.

This will not develop by discernment alone, but by cultural involvements in which one practices how not to be reward—seeking and how not to enjoy legitimate exemptions from action. This instruction applies directly to Arjuna who was to practice this at Kurukṣetra. This is part of the karma yoga training, which is the skill of applying psychological detachment to social, cultural and political involvements.

In order to become free from mundane involvements entirely, we must first be involved, as Arjuna was told by Śrī Krishna. We must practice the detachment while acting as duty-bound and also whenever we get a waiver from such action.

तस्मादसक्तः सततं
कार्यं कर्म समाचर ।
असक्तो ह्याचरन्कर्म
परमाप्नोति पूरुषः ॥३.१९॥
tasmādasaktaḥ satataṁ
kāryaṁ karma samācara
asakto hyācarankarma
paramāpnoti pūruṣaḥ (3.19)

tasmād = tasmāt — therefore; asaktaḥ — unattached; satataṁ — always; kāryaṁ — duty, required tasks; karma — action; samācara — perform; asakto = asaktaḥ — unattached; hyācarankarma = hy (hi) — indeed + ācaran — executing + karma — action; param — the highest stage; āpnoti — gets; pūruṣaḥ — a person

Therefore, being always unattached, perform the action which is your duty. By being detached and executing the required tasks, a person gets the highest stage. (3.19)

Commentary:

As I stated, these particular verses have to do mostly with karma yoga which is karma with the application of yoga expertise. Verse 19 is a clear explanation of this. Please note it. Here Śrī Krishna speaks of performing the action which is the person's duty but being unattached while doing so. This non—attachment is what is developed while practicing the yoga disciplines through which one develops a psyche which is resistant to emotional and climatic diversities. That will be explained more in other verses. Śrī Krishna stated that by being detached while executing the required tasks, which are mandatory performances in the social, cultural and political areas, a person gets to the higher stages as described in verse 17.

Anyone who feels that karma yoga is seva (religious services) or bhakti (devotional services) or naiṣkarm (selfless services), please take note of these verses. Detach yourselves from your objectives for a moment. Study what Śrī Krishna suggested here. Note that Arjuna was not doing religious service, or temple service in devotion, or selfless service in printing religious books or serving the public. He was to engage in a ghastly civil war.

कर्मणैव हि संसिद्धिम्
आस्थिता जनकादयः ।
लोकसंग्रहमेवापि
संपश्यन्कर्तुमर्हसि ॥३.२०॥
karmaṇaiva hi saṁsiddhim
āsthitā janakādayaḥ
lokasaṁgrahamevāpi
saṁpaśyankartumarhasi (3.20)

karmaṇaiva = karmaṇa — by cultural activities + eva — alone; hi — indeed; saṁsiddhim — perfection; āsthitā — attained; janakādayaḥ = janaka – Janaka + ādayaḥ — beginning with; lokasaṁgrahamevāpi = loka — world + saṁgraham — maintenance + eva — only + api — only; saṁpaśyan — seeing mentally; kartum — to act; arhasi — you should

Beginning with Janaka, perfection was attained by cultural activities alone. Seeing the necessity for world maintenance, you should act. (3.20)

Commentary:

To our dismay, here Śrī Krishna tactfully dismissed Arjuna's personal needs as well as asserted what the Supervising Universal Lord desires, which is for Arjuna to forego his own priorities and serve for the benefit of the world by chastising the opposing Kurus.

Arjuna was to throw aside his own dear—felt desires and act for world maintenance (lokasamgraham). The Supervising Universal Lord, is more concerned with the overall situation than he is with the personal development of anyone, and to boot, He wants to enlist our services even if it means that we will be put into a state of anguish or even if we will be repulsed by the ghastly actions. That personality could care less if we desire to be exempt. Of course, in verse 18, Śrī Krishna gave an allowance for those who have conscientious objection, which is, that if in complying with the order for participation, we do not aspire for gain and if when given a holiday from action, we do not become elated, then we would be put into a condition where we become unreliant on any mundane creature. From there we could advance further until we reach the highest stage of being spiritually pleased, self satisfied and spiritually content, having no cultural duties to perform.

Śrī Krishna spoke of Arjuna seeing the necessity for world maintenance and then acting to suit. In reality, the person seeing is not Arjuna but rather the Supervising Universal Lord. Arjuna is seeing Him, viewing His vision. What Arjuna had to see what we should see is that we have no alternative but to comply with what the Supreme Person sees. We should act on behalf of the Supreme Person according to His will.

Śrī Krishna cites the example of Janaka, a king of antiquity who pioneered karma yoga and attained perfection by its performance. In the *Upanishads* also, rulers were proficient at this karma yoga. It is not in our interest as kriyā yogis to become rulers or to follow the path of Janaka but those persons who are like Janaka may take note of this verse.

Generally the kriyā yogi wants to attain perfection through jñāna yoga and not through karma yoga but both paths are available as taught by Śrī Krishna or by any other of the divine personages. The two paths are mentioned by Śrī Krishna as being the content of the *Gītā*. Let us review the verse:

śrībhagavānuvāca
loke'smindvividhā niṣṭhā purā proktā mayānagha
jñānayogena sāṁkhyānāṁ karmayogena yogināṁ (3.3)

The Blessed Lord said: In the physical world, a two—fold standard was previously taught by Me. O Arjuna, my good man. This was mind regulation by the yoga practice of the Sāṁkhya philosophical yogis and the action regulation by the yoga practice of the non-philosophical yogis. (3.3)

Despite this verse, it is clear that even though Arjuna wanted to take the jñāna yoga route, Śrī Krishna barred him and introduced karma yoga instead. Śrī Krishna explained that for Arjuna at that stage, karma yoga was necessary. It would contribute to later success in jñāna yoga, which is what Arjuna desired to do. Arjuna was fond of jñāna yoga not karma yoga but it appears that the Supervising Universal Lord objected to Arjuna's practice of the former due to the need for Arjuna's services on the battlefield and due also to the fact that Arjuna was not advanced enough to gain the waiver from cultural work. Arjuna was gain—seeking at the time. He was not detached. This disqualified him for exemption from cultural services.

यद्यदाचरति श्रेष्ठस्
तत्तदेवेतरो जनः ।
स यत्प्रमाणं कुरुते
लोकस्तदनुवर्तते ॥३.२१॥
yadyadācarati śreṣṭhas
tattadevetaro janaḥ
sa yatpramāṇaṁ kurute
lokastadanuvartate (3.21)

yadyad — whatever; ācarati — does; śreṣṭhaḥ — the greatest; tattad = tad tad — this and that; evetaro (evetaraḥ) = eva — only + itaraḥ — the others; janaḥ — perform; sa = saḥ — he; yat — what; pramāṇaṁ — trend; kurute — establishes; lokastadanuvartate = lokaḥ — the world + tad — that + anuvartate — pursues

Whatever a great person does, for that only, others aspire. Whatever trend he establishes, the world pursues. (3.21)

Commentary:

This is an incentive for us to do as we are told by the Supervising Universal Lord. It is a round—about way of saying that a great person will be held responsible for his own, and for his followers' mishaps, even when such followers imitate him without invitation.

Thus the Supreme Lord will book us for any liabilities incurred by followers who imitate or aspire to do whatever we enact, including actions of refusal to cooperate with Him. This is a statement about accountability. It is for this reason that a perceptive kriyā yogi shies away from fame. Through fame, one acquires a bloated lopsided reputation, which is enjoyed by naive leaders, but of which a kriyā yogi is fearful. Such a reputation causes many human beings to follow one's path to their doom, and one is held accountable by God.

By this verse, a law of charisma or an explanation of human psychology is given, whereby whatever a great person does, others take up as a matter of course due to the helplessness in attraction to great people. Whatever trend of action or inaction, that he establishes by behavior, almost every other human being pursues. The followers may be thwarted from their righted duties assigned by the Supervising Universal Lord. Obviously that Supreme Lord will not approve if a famous person diverts human beings away from divine influences.

Arjuna's idea for himself to be a jñāna yogi is great but considering that Arjuna is famous and that he was a role model and celebrity, this desire converts into danger, if it is not compliant to divine will. Hence Śrī Krishna warned that if Arjuna were to depart from the warfield, others might follow in imitation, and Arjuna would be liable for their rejection of righted duty, which was set before them circumstantially by the Supervising Universal Lord. Śrī Krishna brought this to Arjuna's attention in another way in the last verse:

karmaṇaiva hi saṁsiddhim āsthitā janakādayaḥ
lokasaṁgrahamevāpi saṁpaśyankartumarhasi (3.20)

Beginning with Janaka, perfection was attained by cultural activities alone. Seeing the necessity for world maintenance, you should act. (3.20)

There are many spiritual masters bask in the glory of having attracted many followers after such gurus advertised themselves through literature, radio and television. Many such spiritual masters do not comprehend these verses. They snatch many persons away from social, cultural and political involvements, feeling that these are inferior activities which should be given up for spiritual life. Here, however, we see that Śrī Krishna did not allow Arjuna to follow a strictly spiritual path. At the time, Arjuna was not permitted to go on pilgrimage to temples, nor to go and live in the ashram of a spiritual master. Arjuna had to stay and complete political duties. The spiritual masters are so interested in popularity, which is such a sweet delicacy, that they ignore the liabilities and fail to see that they might be irritating the Supervising Universal Personality.

न मे पार्थास्ति कर्तव्यं
त्रिषु लोकेषु किंचन ।
नानवाप्तमवाप्तव्यं
वर्त एव च कर्मणि ॥३.२२॥
na me pārthāsti kartavyaṁ
triṣu lokeṣu kiṁcana
nānavāptamavāptavyaṁ
varta eva ca karmaṇi (3.22)

na — not; me — of me; pārthāsti = pārtha — O son of Pṛthā + asti — is; kartavyaṁ — should be done; triṣu — in the three divisions; lokeṣu — in the universe; kiṁcana — anything specific; nānavāptamavāptavyaṁ = na — not + anavāptam — not attained + avāptavyaṁ — to be acquired; varta — I function; eva — yet; ca — and; karmaṇi — in cultural activities

For Me, O son of Pṛthā, there is nothing specific that must be done in the three divisions of the universe. And there is nothing that I have not attained nor should acquire, and yet I function in cultural activities. (3.22)

Commentary:

Śrī Krishna without declaring His stance in reference to the Supervising Universal Lord, now sets Himself apart from Arjuna and every other man on that battlefield. It sounds as though Śrī Krishna separates Himself from every limited being who must comply with the Supreme Lord or face consequences through divine disapproval. Who is Śrī Krishna that He should say this?

He saids that for Him there was nothing specific to be done but if Arjuna did not enact specific duties, he would face consequences which would disrupt and prevent any spiritual aspirations Arjuna might have. Actually, Śrī Krishna described Himself as being totally exempt from the stipulations of the Supervising Universal Lord which filter down into human society and manifest as mandatory cultural activities, according to the formula given by Śrī Krishna before:

annādbhavanti bhūtāni parjanyādannasaṁbhavaḥ
yajñādbhavati parjanyo yajñaḥ karmasamudbhavaḥ (3.14)
karma brahmodbhavaṁ viddhi brahmākṣarasamudbhavam
tasmātsarvagataṁ brahma nityaṁ yajñe pratiṣṭhitam (3.15)

The creatures are produced from nourishment. From rain clouds, nourishment originated. From prescribed austerity and religious ceremony, rain clouds are produced. And prescribed austerity and religious ceremony are caused by cultural activities. (3.14)

Cultural activity is produced from the Personified Veda. The Personified Veda comes from the unaffected Supreme Spirit. Hence the all—pervading Supreme Spirit is always situated in prescribed austerities and religious ceremony. (3.15)

Claiming complete exemption from the stipulations Brahmā placed on his mind—born sons, Śrī Krishna then stated that although He has an exemption, He still functions culturally. The idea is that Arjuna must do as he is told.

यदि ह्यहं न वर्तेयं
जातु कर्मण्यतन्द्रितः ।
मम वर्त्मानुवर्तन्ते
मनुष्याः पार्थ सर्वशः ॥३.२३॥
yadi hyahaṁ na varteyaṁ
jātu karmaṇyatandritaḥ
mama vartmānuvartante
manuṣyāḥ pārtha sarvaśaḥ (3.23)

yadi — if; hyahaṁ = hy (hi) — perchance + ahaṁ — I; na — not; varteyaṁ — should perform; jātu — ever; karmaṇyatandritaḥ = karmaṇy (karmaṇi) — in work + atandritaḥ — attentively; mama — of me, my; vartmānuvartante = vartma — pattern + anuvartante — they follow; manuṣyāḥ — human beings; pārtha — O son of Pṛthā; sarvaśaḥ — in all respects

If perchance, I did not perform attentively, then all human beings, O son of Pṛthā, would follow Me in all respects. (3.23)

Commentary:

Indirectly this statement puts Śrī Krishna in a centrally charismatic position relative to all human beings. Śrī Krishna thinks that if He did not perform culturally, people would follow Him in all respects. It implies that He would be liable for the ensuing chaos, even though He stated that He is not accountable to anyone as Arjuna and others are. This is indicated in the next verse.

उत्सीदेयुरिमे लोका
न कुर्यां कर्म चेदहम् ।
संकरस्य च कर्ता स्याम्
उपहन्यामिमाः प्रजाः ॥३.२४॥
utsīdeyurime lokā
na kuryāṁ karma cedaham
saṁkarasya ca kartā syām
upahanyāmimāḥ prajāḥ (3.24)

utsīdeyur = utsīdeyuh — would perish; ime — these; lokā — worlds; na — not; kuryāṁ — I should engage; karma — cultural activity; cedaham = cet — if + aham — I; saṁkarasya — of the social chaos; ca — and; kartā — producer; syām — I should be; upahanyām — I should destroy; imāḥ — these; prajāḥ — creature

If I should not engage in cultural activity, these worlds would perish. And I would be a producer of social chaos. I would have destroyed these creatures. (3.24)

Commentary:

Not just this natural world, but the celestial and supernatural ones as well, would be ruined by Krishna's avoidance of cultural activity. Such is the great claim that Śrī Krishna made for Himself.

सक्ताः कर्मण्यविद्वांसो
यथा कुर्वन्ति भारत ।
कुर्याद्विद्वांस्तथासक्तश्
चिकीर्षुर्लोकसंग्रहम् ॥३.२५॥
saktāḥ karmaṇyavidvāṁso
yathā kurvanti bhārata
kuryādvidvāṁstathāsaktaś
cikīrṣurlokasaṁgraham (3.25)

saktāḥ — attached; karmaṇyavidvāṁso = karmaṇyavidvāṁsaḥ = karmaṇi — in activities + avidvāṁsaḥ — unintelligent; yathā — as; kurvanti — they act; bhārata — O son of the Bharata family; kuryād = kuryāt — he should perform; vidvāṁs — the wise person; tathāsaktaś = tathā — so + asaktaḥ — detached; cikīrṣur = cikīrṣuḥ — intending to do; lokasaṁgraham = loka — society + saṁgraham — maintenance

As the unintelligent people perform with attachment to cultural activity, O son of the Bharata family, so the wise person should act, but in a detached manner, for the maintenance of society. (3.25)

Commentary:

After one has perfected some of the yoga disciplines to a degree, at least to the degree of detachment, one can safely perform in the cultural field and act as the worldly people do, but with detachment, doing good for society (lokasamgraham). Undoubtedly some are born with the required detachment but Śrī Krishna and Arjuna did practice the yoga disciplines nevertheless. By practicing the disciplines, whatever aptitude for detachment a person brought from a past life, he would reinforce in himself.

न बुद्धिभेदं जनयेद्
अज्ञानां कर्मसङ्गिनाम् ।
जोषयेत्सर्वकर्माणि
विद्वान्युक्तः समाचरन् ॥३.२६॥
na buddhibhedaṁ janayed
ajñānāṁ karmasaṅginām
joṣayetsarvakarmāṇi
vidvānyuktaḥ samācaran (3.26)

na — not; buddhibhedaṁ = buddhi – intelligence + bhedaṁ — breaking (broken intelligence, indetermination); janayet — should produce; ajñānāṁ — of the simpletons; karmasaṅginām — of those attached to action; joṣayet — should inspire to be satisfied; sarvakarmāṇi — all actions; vidvān — the wise person; yuktaḥ — disciplined; samācaran — performing

One should not produce indetermination in the minds of the simpletons. A wise person should inspire them to be satisfied by action. The wise one should be disciplined in behavior. (3.26)

Commentary:

This pertains to setting an example for simpleminded people who see cultural activities as the ultimate aim. In the presence of such persons, a yogi should inspire them by acting as if he is satisfied with moral performance and duty fulfillments. Actually the yogi would be happy. He would be relieved since he would appease the Supervising Universal Lord. Common people may think that his happiness is derived from cultural accomplishments.

Seeing this happiness and conceiving of it in their own way, they would be inspired to be productive. This would cause their promotion in the social field.

प्रकृतेः क्रियमाणानि
गुणैः कर्माणि सर्वशः ।
अहंकारविमूढात्मा
कर्ताहमिति मन्यते ॥३.२७॥
prakṛteḥ kriyamāṇāni
guṇaiḥ karmāṇi sarvaśaḥ
ahaṁkāravimūḍhātmā
kartāhamiti manyate (3.27)

prakṛteḥ — of the primal mundane energy; kriyamāṇāni — performed; guṇaiḥ — by the variations; karmāṇi — actions; sarvaśaḥ — in all cases; ahaṁkāravimūḍhātmā = ahaṁkāra – falsely-asserted identity + vimūḍha — confused + ātmā — self; kartāham = kartā — performer + aham — I; iti — thus; manyate — he thinks

In all cases, actions are performed by variations of the primal mundane energy. But the identity-confused person thinks: "I am the performer." (3.27)

Commentary:

Although the Supervising Universal Lord serves as the ultimate mover, He is more or less just a remote cause of mundane action. Śrī Krishna declared that in all cases (sarvaśah), the actions are performed by variations of the primal mundane energy (prakṛteh). However, being confused, we usually think we are the performers. The yogi also becomes confused in this matter but periodically he snaps out of it.

Vimūḍhātma means the confused spirit (ātma). Since he is harnessed to the gross and subtle bodies, he considers the reflection of his energy to be himself. He thinks that he is an actor in cultural affairs. Thus, he endures joys and sufferings, accomplishments and frustrations, until he is freed from the false view.

It is interesting that on one hand, Śrī Krishna advised Arjuna to act and Krishna said that He Himself, participated by self responsibility. Now the same Śrī Krishna denies that any of the spirits are acting in fact.

तत्त्ववित्तु महाबाहो
गुणकर्मविभागयोः।
गुणा गुणेषु वर्तन्त
इति मत्वा न सज्जते ॥३.२८॥
tattvavittu mahābāho
guṇakarmavibhāgayoḥ
guṇā guṇeṣu vartanta
iti matvā na sajjate (3.28)

tattvavit — reality—perceiving person; tu — but; mahābāho — O powerful man; guṇakarmavibhāgayoḥ = guṇa — moods of nature + karma — action + vibhāgayoḥ — in two—fold basis; guṇa — the variation of material nature; guṇeṣu — in the variations of material nature; vartanta — they interact; iti — thus; matvā — having thought; na — no; sajjate — is attached

But, O powerful man, having considered that variations of material nature interact with variations of material nature, the reality—perceiving person is not attached to action. (3.28)

Commentary:

The real reason, for being detached from the social and cultural scenes, is clearly stated by Śrī Krishna. This vision, however, is only possessed by the reality—perceiving personalities, the tattvavits, or those who know the tattvas by direct mystic perception. The rest of us see indirectly by what we were told or by what was written by a tattvavit. We are subjected to error in conception since our minds faultily conceive of the information.

This verse explains that the detachment exhibited by a reality-perceiving person, is done on the basis of his vision of things. It does not occur on the basis of a philosophical conception or on the basis of an assumption that the variations of material nature are interacting in all cases.

प्रकृतेर्गुणसंमूढाः
सज्जन्ते गुणकर्मसु।
तानकृत्स्नविदो मन्दात्
कृत्स्नविन्न विचालयेत् ॥ ३.२९ ॥

prakṛterguṇasaṁmūḍhāḥ
sajjante guṇakarmasu
tānakṛtsnavido mandāt
kṛtsnavinna vicālayet (3.29)

prakṛter = prakṛteḥ — of subtle material nature; guṇasaṁmūḍhāḥ = guṇa — variations of material nature + saṁmūḍhāḥ — deluded people; sajjante — they are attached; guṇakarmasu — in the mood—motivated activities; tān — them; akṛtsnavido = akṛtsnavidaḥ — partially—knowing; mandāt — foolish people; kṛtsnavin — the person who understands the whole reality; na — not; vicālayet — should unsettle

Those who are deluded by the variations of material nature are attached to mood—motivated activities. The person who understands the reality should not unsettle those foolish people who have partial insight. (3.29)

Commentary:

So far we have heard of two types of activities with variations of one type. The first type extolled, is the detached yogicly—produced regulated activities which Arjuna was supposed to perform. The second type is described in this verse as being mood-motivated (guṇakarmasu). However, Śrī Krishna also said in verse 27 that, in all cases, the activities are performed by material nature. Therefore the technicality is the type of motivation.

Either we are motivated by material nature directly or we are motivated by the Supervising Universal Lord, but in all cases, the action is performed by material nature.

Those who are deluded by the variations of material nature, who remain attached to the mood—motivated activities, do not exhibit detachment, except when they are discouraged by material nature for one reason or another, based on the sensual perception of their subtle bodies and the aggressive or passive mood of their life force. Those who are pushed by the Supervising Lord, apply detachment every step of the way in their activities.

It is not easy, however, to discern between the two types of personalities. This is why Arjuna asked this question in the previous chapter:

arjuna uvāca
sthitaprajñasya kā bhāṣā samādhisthasya keśava
sthitadhīḥ kiṁ prabhāṣeta kimāsīta vrajeta kim (2.54)

Arjuna said: In regards to the person who is situated in clear, penetration insight, would you please describe him: Speak of the person who is anchored in deep meditation, O Keśava, Krishna. As for the man who is steady in objectives, how would he speak? How would he sit? How would he act? (2.54)

Arjuna had to adopt the superior motivation which was coming from the Supervising Universal Spirit. Arjuna was to remain detached while acting culturally, but he was not to disrupt the productive activities of the ordinary people who are always mood—motivated. His plan to leave the battlefield would be disruptive to the ordinary soldiers. He would then be responsible for his refusal to fight and for the negative impact on other soldiers. Even though they have partial insight and even though their actions are motivated by whims, still they should not be unsettled by Arjuna or by any of us.

मयि सर्वाणि कर्माणि
संन्यस्याध्यात्मचेतसा ।
निराशीर्निर्ममो भूत्वा
युध्यस्व विगतज्वरः ॥३.३०॥
mayi sarvāṇi karmāṇi
saṁnyasyādhyātmacetasā
nirāśīrnirmamo bhūtvā
yudhyasva vigatajvaraḥ (3.30)

mayi — to me; sarvāṇi — all; karmāṇi — working power; saṁnyasyādhyātmacetasā = saṁnyasya — entrusting + adhyātmacetasā — by meditation on the Supreme Spirit; nirāśīr — from cravings; nirmamo = nirmamaḥ — indifferent to selfishness; bhūtvā — being; yudhyasva — do fight; vigatajvaraḥ = vigata — departed + jvaraḥ — feverish mood

All your working power should be entrusted to Me. On the Supreme Spirit, you should meditate. Being free from cravings, indifferent to selfishness, do fight. Be a man whose feverish mood has departed. (3.30)

Commentary:

Śrī Krishna now acclaims Himself as the adhyātma, the Foremost Spirit, the Supervising Universal Lord. He instructs that Arjuna entrust all working power to Him and disregard the cravings felt within his psyche, as well as remain indifferent to his own natural feelings of selfishness in terms of survival. The feverish mood about committing violence to relatives was to depart from him.

This statement by Śrī Krishna is easy for Arjuna to apply because Śrī Krishna stands next to him. What about those who do not have Śrī Krishna besides us? Some say that we should surrender to a teacher who is in disciplic succession from Śrī Krishna and who is an acclaimed pure devotee. What if such a person is pure only some of the time? What if he slips out of the proper motivation periodically, just as Arjuna did on that occasion?

ये मे मतमिदं नित्यम्
अनुतिष्ठन्ति मानवाः ।
श्रद्धावन्तोऽनसूयन्तो
मुच्यन्ते तेऽपि कर्मभिः ॥३.३१॥
ye me matamidaṁ nityam
anutiṣṭhanti mānavāḥ
śraddhāvanto'nasūyanto
mucyante te'pi karmabhiḥ (3.31)

ye — whosoever; me — My; matam — idea; idam — this; nityam — constantly; anutiṣṭhanti — they apply; mānavāḥ — human beings; śraddhāvanto = śraddhāvantaḥ — having faith; 'nasūyanto = anasūyantaḥ — not complaining; mucyante — are freed; te — they; 'pi = api — also; karmabhiḥ — from the consequences of action

Those human beings, who believe My idea, constantly applying it, having faith and not complaining, are freed from the consequences of action. (3.31)

Commentary:

Here Śrī Krishna does not interject any agent of His, someone to tell us what to do when Krishna is not present, rather He talks about directly believing His idea and constantly applying it without complaint while being inspired by the Supervising Universal Spirit, who Krishna now identifies as Himself.

ये त्वेतदभ्यसूयन्तो
नानुतिष्ठन्ति मे मतम् ।
सर्वज्ञानविमूढांस्तान्
विद्धि नष्टानचेतसः ॥३.३२॥
ye tvetadabhyasūyanto
nānutiṣṭhanti me matam
sarvajñānavimūḍhāṁstān
viddhi naṣṭānacetasaḥ (3.32)

ye — who; tvetad = tv (tu) — but + etad — this; abhyasūyanto = abhyasūyantaḥ — discrediting; nānutiṣṭhanti = na — not + anutiṣṭhanti — they practice; me — My; matam — idea; sarvajñānavimūḍhāṁs = sarva — all + jñāna — insight + vimūḍhāṁs — muddled; tān — them; viddhi — know; naṣṭān — jinxed; acetasaḥ — senseless

Know that those who discredit this instruction and do not practice My ideas, being of muddled insight, are jinxed and senseless. (3.32)

Commentary:

Śrī Krishna readily condemns anyone who does not practice His ideas. Here also we see that Śrī Krishna does not mention any agent who is to explain His ideas to us. Thus far in the *Gītā*, He has not stipulated that we have somebody explain these ideas and set themselves up as His spokesperson.

सदृशं चेष्टते स्वस्याः
प्रकृतेर्ज्ञानवानपि ।
प्रकृतिं यान्ति भूतानि
निग्रहः किं करिष्यति ॥३.३३॥
sadṛśaṁ ceṣṭate svasyāḥ
prakṛterjñānavānapi
prakṛtiṁ yānti bhūtāni
nigrahaḥ kiṁ kariṣyati (3.33)

sadṛśaṁ — according to; ceṣṭate — one acts; svasyāḥ — from one's own; prakṛter = prakṛteḥ — from material nature; jñānavān — wise man; api — also; prakṛtiṁ — material nature; yānti — they submit; bhūtāni — the creatures; nigrahaḥ — restraint; kiṁ — what; kariṣyati — will do

A human being, even a wise man, acts according to his material nature. The creatures submit to material nature. What will restraint do? (3.33)

Commentary:

Generally, in translations, svasyāh prakṛter is interpreted, as either His nature or His tendency. However that does not clarify what is said here by Śrī Krishna and what Śrī Krishna said earlier about material nature performing all activities.

The key word in this verse is svasyāh which means from one's own. This is important because it focuses on the individual's personal connection with and absorption of material nature. This applies even to a wise man who is consistently being motivated by the Supervising Universal Lord.

Some say that one changes completely and is not involved with the material energy once one surrenders to Śrī Krishna, but here that is not indicated. One still has to work with material nature, even after one becomes a wise man guided by Śrī Krishna as described and expert in the detachment recommended.

It is interesting that Śrī Krishna, Who identified Himself as the Supreme Spirit, the Foremost Personality (adhyātma 3.30), asked the question about restraint, regarding what it could or could not do?

It is not that restraint does nothing at all, otherwise there would be no value in Śrī Krishna's instruction for Arjuna to restrain himself emotionally. Exactly what does restraint accomplish?

इन्द्रियस्येन्द्रियस्यार्थे
रागद्वेषौ व्यवस्थितौ ।
तयोर्न वशमागच्छेत्
तौ ह्यस्य परिपन्थिनौ ॥३.३४॥
indriyasyendriyasyārthe
rāgadveṣau vyavasthitau
tayorna vaśamāgacchet
tau hyasya paripanthinau (3.34)

indriyasyendriyasyārthe = indriyasya — of a sense organ + indriyasya — of a sense organ + arthe — in an attractive object; rāgadveṣau = rāga — the response of liking + dveṣau — the response of disliking; vyavasthitau — deep—seated; tayor = tayoḥ — of these two; na — not; vaśam — power; āgacchet — should be influenced; tau — two; hyasya = hy (hi) — indeed + asya — of him; paripanthinau — two hindrances

The response of liking or disliking that is felt between a sense and an attractive object, is deep—seated. One should not be influenced by the power of these two moods. They are hindrances. (3.34)

Commentary:

This is important for us to understand. The liking and disliking responses will be felt even by wise men, even by those who follow the motivations of the Supervising Universal Lord. The difference is that the wise man is able to see these moods in his psyche and then ignore them, while others are forced by the impulsions.

श्रेयान्स्वधर्मो विगुणः
परधर्मात्स्वनुष्ठितात् ।
स्वधर्मे निधनं श्रेयः
परधर्मो भयावहः ॥३.३५॥
śreyānsvadharmo viguṇaḥ
paradharmātsvanuṣṭhitāt
svadharme nidhanaṁ śreyaḥ
paradharmo bhayāvahaḥ (3.35)

śreyān — better; svadharmo = svadharmaḥ — one's righteous duty; viguṇaḥ — imperfect; paradharmāt — than the righteous duty of another; svanuṣṭhitāt = sv (su) — good, great + anuṣṭhitāt — than done; svadharme — in one's righteous duty; nidhanaṁ — death; śreyaḥ — it is better; paradharmo = paradharmaḥ — righteous duty of another; bhayāvahaḥ = bhaya — risk + āvahaḥ — bringing on

Better to do one's righteous duty imperfectly, than to do the duty of another with great efficiency. Death is better in the course of one's duty but the task of another is risky. (3.35)

Commentary:

The risk here has to do with contravening the will of the Supervising Universal Lord, such that even if one does the duty of another person with great efficiency, one will still be held accountable for completing one's assigned duties. From the stern tone of Śrī Krishna, we get an indication that the Supervising Universal Lord would regard the completion of another's duty as an interference. Thus it is better to face one's duty, even if it is dangerous to one's material body, than to forego it and complete the duty of someone else safely.

For Arjuna the advice was direct: Better that he would face his duty in battle and die in its performance than to take up the task of the ascetics whose duty was to sit, contemplate and meditate.

अर्जुन उवाच
अथ केन प्रयुक्तोऽयं
पापं चरति पूरुषः ।
अनिच्छन्नपि वार्ष्णेय
बलादिव नियोजितः ॥३.३६॥
arjuna uvāca
atha kena prayukto'yaṁ
pāpaṁ carati pūruṣaḥ
anicchannapi vārṣṇeya
balādiva niyojitaḥ (3.36)

arjuna — Arjuna; uvāca — said; atha — then; kena — by what?; prayukto = prayuktaḥ — forced; 'yaṁ = ayam — this; pāpaṁ — evil; carati — commits; pūruṣaḥ — a person; anicchannapi = anicchan — unwilling + napi (api) — even; vārṣṇeya — family man of the Vṛṣṇis; balād = balāt — from force; iva — as if; niyojitaḥ — compelled

Arjuna said: Then explain, O family man of the Vṛṣṇis, by what is a person forced to commit an evil unwillingly, just as if he were compelled to do so? (3.36)

Commentary:

This is exactly what each of us wants to ask Śrī Krishna or another kriyā yoga teacher. We find that we are unwillingly compelled to commit evil actions. Even when we are reluctant to perform them and exert willpower against their promptings, still we are forced into such acts. What urges this?

श्रीभगवानुवाच
काम एष क्रोध एष
रजोगुणसमुद्भवः ।
महाशनो महापाप्मा
विद्ध्येनमिह वैरिणम् ॥३.३७॥
śrībhagavānuvāca
kāma eṣa krodha eṣa
rajoguṇasamudbhavaḥ
mahāśano mahāpāpmā
viddhyenamiha vairiṇam (3.37)

śri bhagavān — the Blessed Lord; uvāca — said; kāma — craving; eṣa — this; krodha — anger; eṣa — this; rajoguṇasamudbhavaḥ = rajo (rajaḥ) — passion + guṇa — emotion + samudbhavaḥ — source; mahāśano (mahāśanaḥ) = mahā — great + aśana — consuming power; mahāpāpmā = mahā — much + pāpmā — damage; viddhyenam = viddhi — recognize + enam — this; iha — in this case; vairiṇam — enemy

The Blessed Lord said: This force is craving. This power is anger. The passionate emotion is the source. It has a great consuming power and does much damage. Recognize it as the enemy in this case. (3.37)

Commentary:

The force manifests in our psyche as anger and craving but the root of it is passionate emotional energy. It has great consuming power, says Śrī Krishna. It does much damage; it diverts us from sensible actions which promote long-range benefits.

धूमेनाव्रियते वह्निर्
यथादर्शो मलेन च ।
यथोल्बेनावृतो गर्भस्
तथा तेनेदमावृतम् ॥ ३.३८ ॥
dhūmenāvriyate vahnir
yathādarśo malena ca
yatholbenāvṛto garbhas
tathā tenedamāvṛtam (3.38)

dhūmenāvriyate = dhūmena — by smoke + āvriyate — is obscured; vahnir = vahniḥ — the sacrificial fire; yathā — similarly; 'darśo = ādarśaḥ — mirror; malena — with dust; ca — and; yatholbenāvṛto = yatholbenāvṛtaḥ = yatho (yatha) — similarly + ulbena — by skin + āvṛtaḥ — is covered; garbhaḥ — embryo; tathā — so; tenedam = tena — by this + idam — this; āvṛtam — is blocked

As the sacrificial fire is obscured by smoke, and similarly as a mirror is shrouded by dust or as an embryo is covered by skin, so a man's insight is blocked by the passionate energy. (3.38)

Commentary:

Unless the passionate energy is dissipated or unless it is pierced or parted away, one cannot have the spiritual insight. One can still reason out the difference between the body and the soul and the difference between the gross body and the intermeshed subtle one, but reasoning is different to direct subtle perception.

The passionate energy (rajoguṇa 3.37) is removed by special disciplines. When one completes these, his psychic insight develops from within the psyche and the covering which shrouds the buddhi organ is parted. This happens from within. The passionate energy surrounds the buddhi on all sides and prohibits the light of it from spreading to higher zones.

आवृतं ज्ञानमेतेन
ज्ञानिनो नित्यवैरिणा ।
कामरूपेण कौन्तेय
दुष्पूरेणानलेन च ॥ ३.३९ ॥
āvṛtaṁ jñānametena
jñānino nityavairiṇā
kāmarūpeṇa kaunteya
duṣpūreṇānalena ca (3.39)

āvṛtam — is adjusted; jñānam — discernment; etena — by this; jñānino = jñāninaḥ — educated people; nityavairiṇā = nitya — eternal + vairiṇā — by the enemy; kāmarūpeṇa = kāma — yearning for various things + rūpeṇa — by the sense or form of; kaunteya — son of Kuntī; duṣpūreṇānalena = duspūreṇa — is hard to satisfy + analena — by fire; ca — and

The discernment of educated people is adjusted by their eternal enemy which is the sense of yearning for various things. O son of Kuntī, the lusty power, is as hard to satisfy as it is to keep a fire burning. (3.39)

Commentary:

This discernment is the buddhi organ in the subtle body. The spirit takes help from this buddhi organ in determinations. Without that organ, the spirit would make no objective contact with the subtle and gross mundane objective world. As such being reliant on the buddhi, the spirit is misled when it is influenced and limited by the passionate energy. Śrī Krishna said that as the sense of yearning for things, it serves as an eternal enemy. This is because the passionate force is reflected in the buddhi organ as desires for various things.

Such yearnings influence the buddhi to plan for fulfillments. This uses up the psychological energies to procure costly experiences. However, the nature of the lusty energy is that it creates fresh desires as soon as the older ones are fulfilled or frustrated. Śrī

Krishna says that it is as hard to satisfy as it is to keep a fire burning. Keeping the spirit bound in the syndrome of aspiring for fulfillment, the passionate energy effectively blocks the spirit's use of psychological insight. This energy is used by the passionate force to imagine fulfillments and then procure them by various endeavors that lead to fulfillment or frustration according to how those plans are accepted or rejected by providence.

इन्द्रियाणि मनो बुद्धिर्
अस्याधिष्ठानमुच्यते ।
एतैर्विमोहयत्येष
ज्ञानमावृत्य देहिनम् ॥ ३.४० ॥
indriyāṇi mano buddhir
asyādhiṣṭhānamucyate
etairvimohayatyeṣa
jñānamāvṛtya dehinam (3.40)

indriyāṇi — the senses; mano = manaḥ — the mind; buddhir = buddhiḥ — the intelligence; asyādhiṣṭhānam = asya — if this + adhiṣṭhānam — warehouse; ucyate — it is authoritatively stated; etair = etaiḥ — with these; vimohayatyeṣa = vimohayaty (vimohayati) — confuses + eṣa — this; jñānam — insight; āvṛtya — is shrouded; dehinam — embodied soul

It is authoritatively stated that the senses, the mind and the intelligence are the combined warehouse of the passionate enemy. By these faculties, the lusty power confuses the embodied soul, shrouding his insight. (3.40)

Commentary:

This is important information for us as kriyā yogis. If we know where the enemy resides, we have a far better chance of defeating it. Here we are informed that it lives and stays in the senses, the mind and the intelligence. The next step is to find out where these three aspects are located. This is an internal battle for the procurement of insight. The struggle is with the passionate force, the lusty power in the psyche. The intelligence is the calculative perceiving organ in the head of the subtle body. The mind is the compartment in which the intellect is housed. The senses are offshoots of the buddhi organ. They spread their sensing powers in all directions through hearing, touching, seeing, tasting and smelling. The sensual power is expressed inside the body through subtle nerves in the subtle form and gross nerves in the gross body. The senses include the various gross and subtle sense organs as well as the survival sense or life force.

By inhabiting and limiting the senses, mind and intellect, the lusty power consumes psychological power and shrouds potential insights.

तस्मात्त्वमिन्द्रियाण्यादौ
नियम्य भरतर्षभ ।
पाप्मानं प्रजहिह्येनं
ज्ञानविज्ञाननाशनम् ॥ ३.४१ ॥
tasmāttvamindriyāṇyādau
niyamya bharatarṣabha
pāpmānaṁ prajahihyenaṁ
jñānavijñānanāśanam(3.41)

tasmāt — thus; tvam — you; indriyāṇyādau = indriyāṇi — senses + ādau — initially; niyamya — regulating; bharatarṣabha — powerful man of the Bharata family; pāpmānaṁ — degrading power; prajahi — squelch, destroy; hyenaṁ = hy (hi) — certainly + enaṁ — this; jñānavijñānanāśanam = jñāna — knowledge + vijñāna — discernment + nāśanam — ruining

Thus regulating the senses initially, you should, O powerful man of the Bharata family, squelch this degrading power which ruins knowledge and discernment. (3.41)

Commentary:

Niyama is the 2nd stage of yoga practice when one is advised by a teacher on what to do in the cultural field and in personal relations. However, in the 5th stage, one is again given certain approved conducts for the psychology. These concern regulation of the senses (indriyāṇi). The 1st stage of yoga practice is yama which provides rules prohibiting certain psychological conduct. These are continued in the 5th stage of pratyāhār, restraint of the sensual energies.

Arjuna is addressed by Śrī Krishna as a powerful man, one compared to a bull (ṛṣabha), but that bullish power was to be applied psychologically in this case to make Arjuna move away from the cow-like feminine emotional energies which weakened him. This again shows what karma yoga really is, as the application of psychological strength developed in yoga practice, being applied to life in the social, cultural and political fields.

Arjuna was to compress or squelch the degrading power of the passionate force, which developed into lusty power (kāma), and which ruined his knowledge and discernment, barring him from compliance with the Supervising Universal Lord, the Person whom Śrī Krishna identified Himself as in verse 30:

mayi sarvāṇi karmāṇi saṁnyasyādhyātmacetasā
nirāśīrnirmamo bhūtvā yudhyasva vigatajvaraḥ (3.30)

All your working power should be entrusted to Me. On the Supreme Spirit, you should meditate. Being free from cravings, indifferent to selfishness, do fight. Be a man whose feverish mood has departed. (3.30)

इन्द्रियाणि पराण्याहुर्
इन्द्रियेभ्यः परं मनः ।
मनसस्तु परा बुद्धिर्
यो बुद्धेः परतस्तु सः ॥३.४२॥
indriyāṇi parāṇyāhur
indriyebhyaḥ paraṁ manaḥ
manasastu parā buddhir
yo buddheḥ paratastu saḥ (3.42)

indriyāṇi — the senses; parāṇyāhur = parāṇi — are energetic; āhur (āhuḥ) — the ancient psychologists say; indriyebhyaḥ — the senses; paraṁ — more energetic; manaḥ — the mind; manasas — in contrast to the mind; tu — but; parā — more sensitive; buddhir = buddhiḥ — the intelligence; yo = yaḥ — which; buddheḥ — in reference to the intelligence; paratas — most sensitive; tu — but; saḥ — he, the spirit

The ancient psychologists say that the senses are energetic, but in comparison to the senses, the mind is more energetic. In contrast to the mind, the intelligence is even more sensitive. But in reference, the spirit is most elevated. (3.42)

Commentary:

Even though the spirit is more elevated than the intelligence, the mind and the senses, a particular spirit may not realize his superiority. This is due to his lack of objectivity and his proneness to being utilized by the psychological mechanism which he mistakenly considers to be himself. The psyche of the spirit is not the spirit itself, but the spirit must acquire detachment to understand this.

As a human being relies on his eyes to see into the physical world and as the human being hardly observes how his eyes operates and hardly examines the visual organ in detail, so the spirit hardly looks into the discriminative faculty, which is the buddhi organ in the subtle body. The embodied spirits hardly understand their relationship to the senses, the mind and intelligence, but the ancient psychologists, the sages of the Upanishadic period, took note and developed a course for humans to realize themselves as being distinct from the subtle organs in the psyche.

एवं बुद्धेः परं बुद्ध्वा
संस्तभ्यात्मानमात्मना ।
जहि शत्रुं महाबाहो
कामरूपं दुरासदम् ॥ ३.४३ ॥
evaṁ buddheḥ paraṁ buddhvā
saṁstabhyātmānamātmanā
jahi śatruṁ mahābāho
kāmarūpaṁ durāsadam (3.43)

evaṁ — thus; buddheḥ — than the intelligence; paraṁ — higher; buddhvā — having understood; saṁstabhyātmānamātmanā = saṁstabhya — keeping together + ātmānam — the personal energies + ātmanā — by the spirit; jahi — uproot; śatruṁ — enemy; mahābāho — O powerful man; kāmarūpaṁ — form of passionate desire; durāsadam — difficult to grasp

Thus having understood what is higher than intelligence, keeping the personal energies under control of the spirit, uproot, O powerful man, the enemy, the form of passionate desire which is difficult to grasp. (3.43)

Commentary:

I understand from a careful study of the Upanishads, that there are the senses, mind, intelligence, the sense of initiative, and the chitta (super-subtle pranic energy). Then there is the spirit. The psyche which the spirit inhabits also houses the senses, mind, intelligence, initiative for action, and super-subtle motivating force. These are called the personal energies (ātmānam) in this verse.

We should note also that even though, initially, Śrī Krishna named the passionate energy as the great consuming power, He now stresses its form of lust (kāmarūpam). By itself the passionate energy does not have as much force as in its developed form which we experience as lust. Once it develops, it is almost impossible to restrain. It expends itself for procuring fulfillment and then converts that into disappointment and exhaustion. Thus in the previous verse, Śrī Krishna said that at the moment when the passionate force is about to develop one should squelch it.

At first one has to understand the theory of this philosophy, which is the Samkhya analysis. Having understood that and knowing that the spirit is the highest, one should keep the personal energies under control by practicing gross and subtle yoga in the eightfold process of yama, niyama, āsana, prāṇāyāma, pratyāhār, dhāraṇa, dhyāna, and samādhi. By psychological strength developed from that practice, one may apply himself as advised by Śrī Krishna.

Śrī Krishna flatly states that the lusty power, which is the developed form of the passionate energy, is difficult to grasp. This is mental grasping, not the application of physical gripping. This is a mystic activity. Persons who are not expert at kriyā yoga can only pretend to control the lusty power because the acts for curbing it are psychic and mystic only. Physical actions do not effectively curb it. Physical morality is preliminary only. Subtle morality is the real accomplishment but that is an entirely different affair. Persons who are preoccupied with physical morality are not on the path of kriyā yoga, nor are those who join a religious society preoccupied with its status and image. We are to root out the lusty power which is the developed form of the passionate energy but that can only be done on the psychological plane. Hence there exists the need for meditation in which we squelch and finally get rid of that power altogether. It is a mystic process achieved through mastery of psychological control and psychic energy intake through advanced yoga practice, which begins with pratyāhār and continues in the advanced stages with dhāraṇa (concentration), dhyāna (contemplation) and samādhi (absorption trance states). All of these are based on elementary yoga practice of yama (prohibition), niyama (approved activities), āsana (haţha yoga postures) and prāṇāyāma (breath practices).

CHAPTER 4

Disciplines of Accomplishment*

श्रीभगवानुवाच
इमं विवस्वते योगं
प्रोक्तवानहमव्ययम् ।
विवस्वान्मनवे प्राह
मनुरिक्ष्वाकवेऽब्रवीत् ॥४.१॥
śrībhagavānuvāca
imaṁ vivasvate yogaṁ
proktavānahamavyayam
vivasvānmanave prāha
manurikṣvākave'bravīt (4.1)

śrī bhagavān — the Blessed Lord; uvāca — said; imaṁ — this; vivasvate — to Vivasvat; yogaṁ — yogic skill of controlling personal energies; proktavān — having explained; aham — I; avyayam — perpetual; vivasvān — Vivasvat; manave — to Manu; prāha — explained; manur = manuḥ — Manu; ikṣvākave — to Ikṣvāku; 'bravīt = abravīt — imparted.

The Blessed Lord said: I explained to Vivasvat, this perpetual teaching of controlling the personal energies through yoga. Vivasvat explained it to Manu. Manu imparted it to Ikṣvāku. (4.1)

Commentary:

Here yoga is given and nothing else. Thus we should be confident of the practice of yoga and not allow anyone to dislodge us from it. It is okay to add something to yoga but it is not good to reject the entire practice for something else.

Vivasvāt, Manu and Ikṣvāku were kings. They had the technique of karma yoga, the skill of applying their yogicly—hardened psychology to political affairs. Śrī Krishna claims here to have taught Vivasvāt. He mentions the karma yoga process as a perpetual teaching course taught again and again to generation after generation. The focus is the teaching as it was transferred from one king to his successor. Arjuna is a prince. It is required for him. Those of us who are not in the political field and who are kriyā yogis must also do karma yoga on a smaller scale when we manage households and businesses or whenever we interact in society.

एवं परंपराप्राप्तम्
इमं राजर्षयो विदुः ।
स कालेनेह महता
योगो नष्टः परंतप ॥४.२॥
evaṁ paraṁparāprāptam
imaṁ rājarṣayo viduḥ
sa kāleneha mahatā
yogo naṣṭaḥ paraṁtapa (4.2)

evaṁ — thus; paraṁ parāprāptam = paraṁ parā — a series of teachers + prāptam — received; imaṁ — this; rājarṣayo = rājarṣayaḥ — yogi kings; viduḥ — they knew; sa = saḥ — it; kāleneha = kālena — in time + iha — here on earth; mahatā — long; yogo = yogaḥ — yogic discipline; naṣṭaḥ — was lost; paraṁtapa — O burner of enemy forces

**The Mahābhārata contains no chapter headings. This title was assigned by the translator on the basis of verse 32 of this.chapter.*

Thus, received through a series of teachers, the yogi kings knew this skill of controlling the personal energies. After a long time, here on earth, this yoga application was lost, O burner of enemy forces. (4.2)

Commentary:

The yogi kings (rājarṣayo) were rulers who were adept at yoga practice and who learned from their fathers how to apply the psychological strengths they developed in yoga to political administration. This is exactly what Śrī Krishna taught Arjuna in the *Bhagavad Gītā*. In modern times, *Bhagavad Gītā* is portrayed as a book for missionaries but readers should specifically note that it was taught to rulers, Arjuna himself being the brother of a contending ruler. Again and again we see the word yoga. Śrī Krishna stressed it repeatedly.

Śrī Krishna states that after a long time, the application of yoga skills to political administration was lost. Please note that Śrī Krishna has not mentioned bhakti yoga or devotion to Himself. He speaks of the skill of applying a yogicly—disciplined psychology to the political administration performed by rulers. This is not missionary activity. It is important for us to free ourselves from the idea spread by the missionaries, that the *Gītā* is their exclusive property and that Śrī Krishna meant this lecture for them. Certain parts of the *Gītā* do apply directly to temple activities, but the *Gītā* as a whole is targeted to rulers who were skilled in yoga and who wanted to learn how to apply their yoga skills to political life. We may also apply it to ourselves as householder kriyā yogis or even as bachelor kriyā yogis but we must still keep in mind that it was taught to rulers.

The disciplic succession mentioned here is one from Śrī Krishna to other rulers only. This is not a succession from a temple sannyasi to his disciples who are not ruling society. This is a succession passing through martially—inclined students like Arjuna, persons who will use weapons if necessary, persons who were duty bound as soldiers and policemen of society. This is the *Gītā* for the most part.

Śrī Krishna claims here to have reinstated that training from one ruler to another. In the cases mentioned it was from a king to his son. Now at the time of the *Gītā* speech it was between Śrī Krishna and His cousin Arjuna. Śrī Krishna claimed Himself as the original teacher.

स एवायं मया तेऽद्य
योगः प्रोक्तः पुरातनः ।
भक्तोऽसि मे सखा चेति
रहस्यं ह्येतदुत्तमम् ॥४.३॥

sa evāyaṁ mayā te'dya
yogaḥ proktaḥ purātanaḥ
bhakto'si me sakhā ceti
rahasyaṁ hyetaduttamam (4.3)

sa = saḥ — it; evāyaṁ = eva — indeed + ayaṁ — this; mayā — by me; te — to you; 'dya = adya — today; yogaḥ — yoga technique; proktaḥ — is explained; purātanaḥ — ancient; bhakto = bhaktaḥ — devoted; 'si = asi — you are; me — of me; sakhā — friend; ceti = ca — and + iti — thus; rahasyaṁ — confidential teaching; hyetad = hi — truly + etad — this; uttamam — best

Today, this ancient yoga technique is explained to you by Me, since you are devoted to Me and are My friend. Indeed, this is confidential and is the best teaching. (4.3)

Commentary:

Now definitely for the first time in the *Gītā*, devotion (bhakti) is included. It is interesting, because in the first verse of this chapter, the succession from Vivasvāt is from a king to his son. Now however, Śrī Krishna stated that His reason for teaching Arjuna was Arjuna's devotional loyalty and dear friendship (sakhā).

Some commentators, being anxious to give bhakti a prominent place in the *Gītā*, magnify its significance by stating that the only reason for Śrī Krishna to speak the *Gītā* to Arjuna was Arjuna's devotion to Śrī Krishna. However we must also note that in the first verse of this chapter, devotion is not indicated, since the succession passed through rulers to their sons, who were successors to the throne.

Certainly, Arjuna was not the son of Śrī Krishna. Śrī Krishna, in that time, had sons who were not present at the Battle of Kurukṣetra. Since Arjuna was not the son of Śrī Krishna, and since Arjuna was not in succession from Śrī Krishna, then Śrī Krishna's teaching of the skill to Arjuna was somewhat inconsistent with the tradition of passing the skill from a ruler to his son. Why has Śrī Krishna deviated from this system? The reasons are now revealed as bhakto and sakho, the devoted loyalty and dear friendship of Arjuna. Those rulers of antiquity considered the teaching to be confidential and to be the best education they could get, because by it, their governing actions did not bring spiritually-damaging reactions or sins.

अर्जुन उवाच
अपरं भवतो जन्म
परं जन्म विवस्वतः ।
कथमेतद्विजानीयां
त्वमादौ प्रोक्तवानिति ॥४.४॥
arjuna uvāca
aparaṁ bhavato janma
paraṁ janma vivasvataḥ
kathametadvijānīyāṁ
tvamādau proktavāniti (4.4)

arjuna — Arjuna; uvāca — said; aparaṁ — later; bhavato = bhavataḥ — Your Lordship; janma — birth; paraṁ — earlier; janma — birth; vivasvataḥ — Vivasvat; katham — how; etad — this; vijānīyāṁ — I should understand; tvam — you; ādau — in the beginning, before; proktavān — having explained; iti — thus

Arjuna said: Your Lordship's birth was later. The birth of Vivasvat was earlier. How should I understand that You explained this before? (4.4)

Commentary:

From the information Arjuna had, Vivasvāt was born long, long before Śrī Krishna, thousands of years before. Hence how could Arjuna take what Krishna said at face value? Even if Arjuna trusted Śrī Krishna to that extent, he could not verify that information because he had no means at his disposal to check on Śrī Krishna's previous appearances or previous births.

Convention dictates that we accept a person as being born for the first time. Even if we suspect that a person might be an incarnation of someone from the past, still by convention, we regard the person's present body as his first. Thus Arjuna followed the convention. These pressing influences caused him to shift from the kriyā vision. Still, a limited spirit using kriyā vision cannot see unlimitedly but he may have revelations and true visions of certain phases of the past from time to time.

श्रीभगवानुवाच
बहूनि मे व्यतीतानि
जन्मानि तव चार्जुन ।
तान्यहं वेद सर्वाणि
न त्वं वेत्थ परंतप ॥४.५॥

śrī bhagavān — the Blessed Lord; uvāca — said; bahūni — many; me — of Me; vyatītāni — transpired; janmāni — births; tava — your; cārjuna = ca — and + arjuna — Arjuna; tānyahaṁ = tāny (tāni) — them + ahaṁ — I; veda — I recall; sarvāṇi — all;

śrībhagavānuvāca
bahūni me vyatītāni
janmāni tava cārjuna
tānyahaṁ veda sarvāṇi
na tvaṁ vettha paraṁtapa (4.5)

na — not; tvaṁ — you; vettha — you remember; paraṁtapa — O scorcher of the enemies

The Blessed Lord said: Many of My births transpired, and yours, Arjuna. I recall them all. You do not remember, O scorcher of the enemies. (4.5)

Commentary:

As a scorcher of the enemies (paramtapa), Arjuna had grasp on some of the situations encountered in his life. That was his history from the past, to always have a footing in the particular life he lived, but he did not have a grasp on the memory of past lives. Śrī Krishna however described Himself as having perpetual grasp on history.

This verse reveals the perpetual association of Śrī Krishna and Arjuna in the same type of devotional loyalty and friendship of Arjuna to Śrī Krishna, with Arjuna consistently having a grasp on whatever conditions his body was born into, but consistently forgetting his past life, and with Śrī Krishna being detached from new bodily conditions and always being aware of their past.

As kriyā yogis, we get a lesson from Śrī Krishna. Our natural and strong focus on present conditions reinforces our forgetfulness of the past. Hence the need for the practice of detachment and the refocusing of ourselves on long—range objectives while loosening grip of the short-range aspects. This requires psychological disciplinary practices in kriyā yoga.

अजोऽपि सन्नव्ययात्मा
भूतानामीश्वरोऽपि सन् ।
प्रकृतिं स्वामधिष्ठाय
संभवाम्यात्ममायया ॥४.६॥
ajo'pi sannavyayātmā
bhūtānāmīśvaro'pi san
prakṛtiṁ svāmadhiṣṭhāya
saṁbhavāmyātmamāyayā (4.6)

ajo = ajaḥ — birthless; 'pi = api — even though; sann = san — being; avyayātmā = avyaya — imperishable + ātmā — person; bhūtānām — of the creatures; īśvaro = īśvaraḥ — Lord; 'pi = api — even; san — being; prakṛtiṁ — material energies; svām — my own; adhiṣṭhāya — controlling; saṁbhavāmyātmamāyayā = sambhavāmy (saṁbhavāmi) — I become visible + ātma — self + māyayā — by supernatural power

Even though I am birthless and My person is imperishable, and even though I am the Lord of the creatures, by controlling My material energies, I become visible by My supernatural power. (4.6)

Commentary:

Here for the first time in the *Gītā*, Śrī Krishna makes a bold declaration of Himself as the Lord of the creatures (bhūtānām īśvaro). There is a technicality in that the limited spirits are also birthless. There are also imperishable if we regard them as only their spirits and not as the psyche which houses or harnesses the spirit. The big difference between them and Śrī Krishna is that He controls His material energies and effectively wields supernatural power.

Śrī Krishna is not the only one with supernatural energy. The limited spirits have that too. Śrī Krishna is not the only one with mundane energy at His disposal. The limited entities have some tiny bit of it in their possession, but they only have partial control over their supernatural being, while the rest of it, is impulsively operated. Their material energy stays in touch with them psychically but most of it lies beyond the control of their will power.

In kriyā yoga we study these aspects, as they pertain to ourselves in relationship to material nature and our mystic expressions and impulsions. We aspire for more directive control, so that we can be less manipulated by material nature and so that more supernatural power can be exhibited.

It is important to understand the distinction and similarities between us and Śrī Krishna, the Lord of the creatures. Once we know our scope and that of Krishna, we can begin working to improve our condition. We can take help from Śrī Krishna and other superior beings for an upgrade. The *Gītā* itself is an effort by Śrī Krishna to elevate Arjuna. It teaches a great deal about self improvement.

As the Supreme Lord, Śrī Krishna does not have to endeavor, but as limited spirits, we must endeavor to upgrade ourselves and to maintain the improvements. As Arjuna was unable to maintain himself and would have to endeavor repeatedly, not only while the *Gītā* was spoken, but also later on in his life, so we must strive to keep ourselves elevated.

यदा यदा हि धर्मस्य
ग्लानिर्भवति भारत ।
अभ्युत्थानमधर्मस्य
तदात्मानं सृजाम्यहम् ॥४.७॥
yadā yadā hi dharmasya
glānirbhavati bhārata
abhyutthānamadharmasya
tadātmānaṁ sṛjāmyaham (4.7)

yadā yadā — whenever; hi — indeed; dharmasya — of righteousness; glānir = glāniḥ — decrease; bhavati — it is; bhārata — O son of the Bharata family; abhyutthānam — increasing; adharmasya — of unrighteousness, of wickedness; tadā — then; 'tmānaṁ = ātmānaṁ — My self; sṛjāmyaham = sṛjāmy (sṛjāmi) — show + aham — I

Whenever there is a decrease of righteousness, O son of the Bharata family, and when there is an increase of wickedness, then I show Myself. (4.7)

Commentary:

As the Supervising Universal Lord, Śrī Krishna shows Himself to the world whenever there is a decrease in righteousness and an increase in wickedness, but this does not mean that His showing brings about an immediate adjustment. As we see here, Śrī Krishna showed Himself physically at Kurukṣetra and wanted Arjuna enact out the divine disapproval, but still it was not immediate. It took time. There was a power struggle between the disciplinary opinions of Śrī Krishna and the views of the others which was sorted out gradually.

Some have criticized this verse, indicating that Śrī Krishna told an untruth here, since Śrī Krishna has not recently appeared with the same body as He did in the time of Arjuna. He has not shown Himself in every instance of a decrease in righteousness or an increase in wickedness. This criticism is based on a misunderstanding.

The key to understanding this verse is to know that even though Śrī Krishna shows Himself in each instance of moral degression and decadent expansion, still He may not act immediately. It takes time. As the Supervising Universal Lord, He is aware of the degrading conditions as they transpire from moment to moment. He does react in one way or the other, but those reactions, on the supernatural plane, take time to manifest subtly and physically.

परित्राणाय साधूनां
विनाशाय च दुष्कृताम् ।
धर्मसंस्थापनार्थाय
संभवामि युगे युगे ॥४.८॥

paritrāṇāya sādhūnāṁ
vināśāya ca duṣkṛtām
dharmasaṁsthāpanārthāya
saṁbhavāmi yuge yuge (4.8)

paritrāṇāya — to protect; sādhūnāṁ — of the saintly persons; vināśāya — to destruction; ca — and; duṣkṛtām — of the wicked people; dharmasaṁsthāpanārthāya = dharma — righteousness + saṁsthāpana — the establishing of + arthāya — for the sake of; saṁbhavāmi — I come into visible existence; yuge yuge — from era to era

To protect the saintly people, to destroy the wicked ones, and to establish righteousness, I come into the visible existence from era to era. (4.8)

Commentary:

This coming into visible existence means into physical or into subtle existence from time to time, at His discretion, all depending on the inability of the saintly people to protect themselves from the onslaught of criminal elements. The value of the saintly persons is that they establish and maintain righteousness. If they are unable to do so or if their efforts are thwarted, blocked or prevented, Śrī Krishna appears directly or sends an agent.

An example is before us in the *Bhagavad Gītā*, where Śrī Krishna incited Arjuna to chastise the wicked ones for the sake of establishing and maintaining righteousness. Instead of acting directly, Śrī Krishna incited Arjuna to be the agent. He instructed that all of Arjuna's working power (karmaṇi) be entrusted to Him, to Krishna. That was in verse 30 of Chapter Three:

mayi sarvāṇi karmāṇi saṁnyasyādhyātmacetasā
nirāśīrnirmamo bhūtvā yudhyasva vigatajvaraḥ (3.30)

All your working power should be entrusted to Me. On the Supreme Spirit, you should meditate. Being free from cravings, indifferent to selfishness, do fight. Be a man whose feverish mood has departed. (3.30)

This is of interest to us as kriyā yogis, since it means that in times of increased wickedness, we might be asked to act in the social, cultural or political arenas. Being asked to participate by the Supervising Universal Lord, we would be unable to refuse without invoking His disapproval, something which would affect our spiritual progression. Thus we must be willing and able to assist Him, at least until we could get a waiver from such activity.

We should note also that those who claim that merely by the commission of Śrī Krishna, we can act without incurring sinful reactions, are surely mistaken. Here in the *Gītā*, Arjuna had to be trained in karma yoga or the application of psychological yoga skills to political life. Arjuna could not execute the instruction immediately after receiving an order, even from Śrī Krishna Himself. Arjuna had to be trained. Thus a kriyā yogi must be prepared to honor the request of the Supervising Universal Lord and he must be pre-trained otherwise he will not be able to represent that Lord without making mistakes.

This explains clearly the disgraces suffered by many disciples of the spiritual masters who came advocating themselves as empowered and bonafide representatives of Śrī Krishna, and who gave orders which were followed but which led many of their disciples into dire straits.

Some of these spiritual masters were only partially empowered but they presented themselves as fully empowered. Others were empowered and disempowered on occasion, but they pretended to be empowered all the time. Some were simply over-confident, popularity-crazed teachers. In any case, we should take care to be pre-trained if we are to represent the Supervising Universal Lord upon His request. As we see here with Śrī Krishna, Arjuna was providentially, by virtue of his birth as son of a king, placed in a position to properly represent the Supreme Lord, Who is usually unseen on the physical plane but Who possesses on—going supernatural forms which empower personalities. It so happened that Arjuna had Śrī Krishna there on the chariot to give training. We are not in such a position. Arjuna's birth as the son of a king, was cited by Śrī Krishna:

svadharmamapi cāvekṣya na vikampitumarhasi
dharmyāddhi yuddhācchreyo'nyat kṣatriyasya na vidyate (2.31)
yadṛcchayā copapannaṁ svargadvāramapāvṛtam
sukhinaḥ kṣatriyāḥ pārtha labhante yuddhamīdṛśam (2.32)
atha cettvamimaṁ dharmyaṁ saṁgrāmaṁ na kariṣyasi
tataḥ svadharmaṁ kīrtiṁ ca hitvā pāpamavāpsyasi (2.33)

And considering your assigned duty, you should not look for alternatives. In fact, for the son of a king, there is no other duty which is better than a righteous battle. (2.31)

And by a stroke of luck, the gate of heaven is opened. Thrilled are the warriors who get such a battle opportunity, O son of Pṛthā. (2.32)

Now if you do not conduct this righteous war, then, by neglecting your duty and reputation, you will acquire a sin. (2.33)

In these verses, Śrī Krishna indicated that the Supervising Universal Lord and Material Nature gave Arjuna a valuable opportunity to affect the situation. If Arjuna rejected the chance, then he would incur the disapproval of the Supreme Lord, Who was, at the time, Śrī Krishna Himself existing both on the supernatural and physical planes. In addition, Śrī Krishna indicated that even if one does not have the karma yoga training which was given to the yogi kings like Janaka, then one should still try to act as instructed despite the chance that one's actions would be imperfect. Śrī Krishna said:

śreyānsvadharmo viguṇaḥ paradharmātsvanuṣṭhitāt
svadharme nidhanaṁ śreyaḥ paradharmo bhayāvahaḥ (3.35)

Better to do one's righteous duty imperfectly, than to do the duty of another with great efficiency. Death is better in the course of one's duty but the task of another is risky. (3.35)

Thus even if we are not pre-trained it is better that we attempt whatever we are instructed by the Supreme Lord or by His empowered agent. We should be sure that the agent actually reflects His wishes at the time and is not pretending to be inspired.

जन्म कर्म च मे दिव्यम्
एवं यो वेत्ति तत्त्वतः ।
त्यक्त्वा देहं पुनर्जन्म
नैति मामेति सोऽर्जुन ॥४.९॥
janma karma ca me divyam
evaṁ yo vetti tattvataḥ
tyaktvā dehaṁ punarjanma
naiti māmeti so'rjuna (4.9)

janma — visitation; karma — deed; ca — and; me — of me; divyam — supernatural; evaṁ — thus; yo = yaḥ — who; vetti — realizes; tattvataḥ — in truth; tyaktvā — abandoning; dehaṁ — body; punarjanma = rebirth; naiti = na — not + eti — goes; mām — to Me; eti — goes; so = saḥ — he; 'rjuna = arjuna — Arjuna

One who knows My supernatural visitation and deeds, who truly realizes this while abandoning his body, does not seek rebirth. He goes to Me, O Arjuna. (4.9)

Commentary:

This discusses a very strong attraction for the Supreme Lord Śrī Krishna. It is the attraction to His super-excellent way of interfacing with the material world. The crux of the matter, as explained previously regards Śrī Krishna having no obligations in this world and not being attracted to any accomplishments here:

na me pārthāsti kartavyaṁ triṣu lokeṣu kiṁcana
nānavāptamavāptavyaṁ varta eva ca karmaṇi (3.22)

For Me, O son of Pṛthā, there is nothing specific that must be done in the three divisions of the universe. And there is nothing that I have not attained nor should acquire, and yet I function in cultural activities. (3.22)

If one becomes attracted to Śrī Krishna as described above, then one will, by force of that attraction, work in a way that gains Krishna's approval. Ideally, one would undertake a social, cultural or political mission of Śrī Krishna, a mission which ideally is performed in the attitude of karma yoga as described by the Lord and as prescribed for Arjuna. Thus one would follow the trend-setting pattern established by Śrī Krishna and would not enact bothersome activities which draw His disapproval.

yadyadācarati śreṣṭhas tattadevetaro janaḥ
sa yatpramāṇaṁ kurute lokastadanuvartate (3.21)

Whatever a great person does, for that only, others aspire. Whatever trend he establishes, the world pursues. (3.21)

In cooperating like this with Śrī Krishna, one would cause a decrease in social disorder as more of the living beings would follow the plan of Śrī Krishna, one that He impresses upon them through their cooperation with Him. Let us review two more verses:

yadi hyahaṁ na varteyaṁ jātu karmaṇyatandritaḥ
mama vartmānuvartante manuṣyāḥ pārtha sarvaśaḥ (3.23)
utsīdeyurime lokā na kuryāṁ karma cedaham
saṁkarasya ca kartā syām upahanyāmimāḥ prajāḥ (3.24)

If perchance, I did not perform attentively, then all human beings, O son of Pṛthā, would follow Me in all respects. (3.23)

If I should not engage in cultural activity, these worlds would perish. And I would be a producer of social chaos. I would have destroyed these creatures. (3.24)

Duryodhana was one such leader of men who did not cooperate with Krishna. The trend which Duryodhana set was followed by other leaders and by ordinary men. Obviously, there is by necessity, an allowance for deviation from the Supreme Will. That privilege comes with certain liabilities which cause bad reactions involving those wayward leaders.

Understanding the supernatural visitation and deeds of Śrī Krishna involves more than just mental realization or attractive fascination with Krishna. The main part is one's ability to perform karma yoga as described in the *Gītā*. One who knows this would not go for rebirth and would appear elsewhere as referred by the Supreme Being. Due to strong reliance on Śrī Krishna and by the magnetic pull of His glory, such a person would become resistant to other types of attraction which normally cause haphazard rebirths or appearances in other places.

As neophyte kriyā yogis, such a proposition of Śrī Krishna draws our attention. We are attracted to it, but we lack sufficiently purity to hold the pull of Śrī Krishna. At present we wave back and forth between the attraction to Krishna and the competing attraction to other entities. In a sense we are a bit like Duryodhana, and a bit like Arjuna too. Thus we will have to listen keenly for the methods of purification which would remove from our nature, those energies which cause our attraction to the competing people, places and things.

वीतरागभयक्रोधा
मन्मया मामुपाश्रिताः ।
बहवो ज्ञानतपसा
पूता मद्भावमागताः ॥४.१०॥
vītarāgabhayakrodhā
manmayā māmupāśritāḥ
bahavo jñānatapasā
pūtā madbhāvamāgatāḥ (4.10)

vītarāgabhayakrodhā = vīta — gone + rāga — craving + bhaya — fear + krodhā — anger; manmayā — think of Me; mām — Me; upāśritāḥ — rely on; bahavo = bahavaḥ — many; jñānatapasā — by austerity/education; pūtā — purified; madbhāvam — my level of existence; āgatāḥ — attained

Many, whose cravings, fear and anger are gone, who are totally focused on Me, who are purified by austerity and education, attained My level of existence. (4.10)

Commentary:

Now the advanced kriyā yogis are mentioned. They alone attain Śrī Krishna's level of existence, existing side by side with Him, the Supreme Being. Their craving, fear and anger no longer exist. Their attention is totally focused on what Śrī Krishna desires for them. They are purified beforehand by austerity and spiritual education. This is an individual development not a group effort. Each yogi devotee must endeavor to reach the required purity.

ये यथा मां प्रपद्यन्ते
तांस्तथैव भजाम्यहम् ।
मम वर्त्मानुवर्तन्ते
मनुष्याः पार्थ सर्वशः ॥४.११॥
ye yathā māṁ prapadyante
tāṁstathaiva bhajāmyaham
mama vartmānuvartante
manuṣyāḥ pārtha sarvaśaḥ (4.11)

ye — who; yathā — as; māṁ — me; prapadyante — they rely; tāṁs = tan — them; tathaiva = tathā — so + eva — indeed; bhajāmyaham = bhajāmy (bhajāmi) — relate to + aham — I; mama — my; vartmānuvartante = vartma — course of action + anuvartante — are affected; manuṣyāḥ — human beings; pārtha — son of Pṛthā; sarvaśaḥ — everywhere

As they rely on Me, so I relate to them, O son of Pṛthā. All human beings, everywhere, are affected by My course of action. (4.11)

Commentary:

The relationship hinges on how the devotee relates to Śrī Krishna. It is not a mental decision or even an emotional one. It forms according to actions which confirm or oppose the Supreme Will. In so far as our mentality causes us to confirm and our emotions push us to act as required by Him, we **will** get positive feedback from Him.

As the Supervising Universal Lord, His course of action affects all human beings everywhere, causing them to either assist Him and manifest His designs or to resist Him and counteract His plans.

As kriyā yogis, we know that we may rely on others besides Krishna. We can rely on other powerful beings and on lesser persons who do not care at all about Śrī Krishna and His views. We can even rely on material nature. Even if we claim ourselves as devotees of Krishna, we still have to respond to urges within our psyche, motivations which may put us at odds with Krishna's views. It happens repeatedly. Arjuna, the dear friend and loyal devotee of Krishna, was himself put at odds with Śrī Krishna.

काङ्क्षन्तः कर्मणां सिद्धिं
यजन्त इह देवताः ।
क्षिप्रं हि मानुषे लोके
सिद्धिर्भवति कर्मजा ॥४.१२॥
kāṅkṣantaḥ karmaṇāṁ siddhiṁ
yajanta iha devatāḥ
kṣipraṁ hi mānuṣe loke
siddhirbhavati karmajā (4.12)

kāṅkṣantaḥ — wanting; karmaṇāṁ — of ritual action; siddhiṁ — success; yajanta — they worship; iha — here on earth; devatāḥ — supernatural authorities; kṣipraṁ — quickly; hi — indeed; mānuṣe — in the humans; loke — in the world; siddhir = siddhiḥ — fulfillment; bhavati — there is, comes to be; karmajā — produced of ritual action

Wanting their ritual action to succeed, people in the world, worship the supernatural authorities. Quickly in this human world, there is fulfillment which comes from ritual action. (4.12)

Commentary:

Ritual is not the same as ritual action, for the ritual is the formality and the ritual action is the actual process of attainment. The formality serves three purposes, namely: public acknowledgement of supernatural agency, public declaration of intentions, and lastly reinforcement of the confidence. Both the ritual and the ritual action might be seen by others but, in each, some techniques remain secret from the public view.

It is interesting that Śrī Krishna, who acknowledged Himself as the Supreme Lord, showed distaste for the ritual and ritual actions which acknowledge the existence of His supernatural agents regulating this world. He does not, it seems, approve of the separate worship of His agents but only wants their recognition to occur in relation to Him as their Manager.

Śrī Krishna however, being quite realistic, frankly admits the individuality of both the worshippers and the supernatural agents who ideally, should represent His views alone. He suggests that fulfillments will quickly come to those who worship these supernatural people.

चातुर्वर्ण्यं मया सृष्टं
गुणकर्मविभागशः ।
तस्य कर्तारमपि मां
विद्ध्यकर्तारमव्ययम् ॥४.१३॥

cāturvarṇyaṁ mayā sṛṣṭaṁ
guṇakarmavibhāgaśaḥ
tasya kartāramapi māṁ
viddhyakartāramavyayam (4.13)

cāturvarṇyaṁ — the four career categories; mayā — by me; sṛṣṭaṁ — instituted; guṇa — habit; karma — work tendency; vibhāga – distribution; śaḥ — by; tasya — of it; kartāram — creator; api — also; māṁ — me; viddhyakartāram = viddhy (viddhi) — know + akartāram — one not required to act; avyayam — eternal

According to the distribution of habits and work tendencies, the four career categories were instituted by Me. Know that I am never required to participate. (4.13)

Commentary:

Arjuna fit into the second category, that of government administration. As the Supervising Universal Lord, Śrī Krishna stated that serving under an assigned career is not a waste of time. It all depends on the Supreme Lord's intentions for a particular human being.

Since this career posting is divinely ordained, it cannot be abolished or ignored without consequences. Thus a human being should perform his divinely-ordained duty and not be diverted to something else. A kriyā yogi, in so far as he lacks an exemption from the divine people, must stick to his category in terms of a career as a priestly man, an administrator, a businessman or a laborer.

A status—conscious person might find it suitable to move up the social scale but if his promotion is not approved by the Divine Supervisor, it will result in a demotion later on.

न मां कर्माणि लिम्पन्ति
न मे कर्मफले स्पृहा ।
इति मां योऽभिजानाति
कर्मभिर्न स बध्यते ॥४.१४॥
na māṁ karmāṇi limpanti
na me karmaphale spṛhā
iti māṁ yo'bhijānāti
karmabhirna sa badhyate (4.14)

na — not; māṁ — me; karmāṇi — actions; limpanti — they entrap; na — not; me — of me; karmaphale — in a pay—off; spṛhā — desire; iti — thus; māṁ — me; yo = yaḥ — who; 'bhijānāti = abhijānāti — understands; karmabhir = karmabhiḥ — by actions; na — not; sa = saḥ — he; badhyate — is entrapped

Actions do not entrap Me. The desire for payoff is not in Me. The person who understands this is not entrapped by action. (4.14)

Commentary:

A person who understands that Krishna is not entrapped by actions and that Krishna has no desire for a payoff becomes so attracted to Śrī Krishna, that he abandons mundane pursuits and adheres to the request of Krishna. Adherence to Krishna's request causes this person not to be entrapped by actions.

That person is shielded by the same supernatural buffer which Krishna radiates and which prevents Krishna from succumbing to the influence of material nature and its reactions brought on by material nature. The reactions may still come to such a person, but nevertheless he would be psychologically impervious to them.

एवं ज्ञात्वा कृतं कर्म
पूर्वैरपि मुमुक्षुभिः ।
कुरु कर्मैव तस्मात्त्वं
पूर्वैः पूर्वतरं कृतम् ॥४.१५॥
evaṁ jñātvā kṛtaṁ karma
pūrvairapi mumukṣubhiḥ
kuru karmaiva tasmāttvaṁ
pūrvaiḥ pūrvataraṁ kṛtam (4.15)

evaṁ — thus; jñātvā — having understood; kṛtaṁ — done; karma — functional work; pūrvair = pūrvaih — by the ancient rulers like Janaka; api — even; mumukṣubhiḥ — by those who desire liberation; kuru — perform; karmaiva = karma — cultural acts + eva — indeed; tasmāt — therefore; tvaṁ — you; pūrvaiḥ — by the yogi kings like Janaka; pūrvataraṁ — before; kṛtam — performed

Having understood this conclusion, functional work was done, even by the yogi kings who desired liberation. Therefore you should perform cultural acts, just as it was done before. (4.15)

Commentary:

Śrī Krishna encouraged Arjuna to fight the battle just as the ancient yogi kings participated in cultural and political affairs for the establishment of righteousness in human society. Arjuna needed to relinquish his fear of participation and take the commission from Śrī Krishna to fight no matter what. Śrī Krishna did not see that Arjuna had any other alternative.

किं कर्म किमकर्मेति
कवयोऽप्यत्र मोहिताः ।
तत्ते कर्म प्रवक्ष्यामि
यज्ज्ञात्वा मोक्ष्यसेऽशुभात् ॥४.१६॥
kiṁ karma kimakarmeti
kavayo'pyatra mohitāḥ
tatte karma pravakṣyāmi
yajjñātvā mokṣyase'śubhāt (4.16)

kiṁ — what; karma — action; kiṁ — what; akarmeti = akarma — no action + iti — thus; kavayo = kavayaḥ — eloquent philosophers; 'py = api — even; atra — in this matter; mohitāḥ — confused; tat — this; te — to you; karma — action; pravakṣyāmi — I will discuss; yaj = yad — which; jñātvā — knowing; mokṣyase — you will be freed; 'śubhāt = aśubhāt — from undesirable circumstances

What is action? What is not an action? Even eloquent philosophers are confused on this subject. I will discuss the subject of action with you. Knowing this, you will be freed from undesirable circumstances. (4.16)

Commentary:

From the indications given so far, Śrī Krishna defines actions as those acts which are reflective of the divine will. For example, in Arjuna's case, staying on the battlefield to act as Śrī Krishna's agent would be an action. If however, Arjuna dismounted the chariot and renounced his affiliation with the Kurus, that would be an inaction or a refusal to comply with the divine will.

On the other hand, from the spiritual view, Arjuna's compliance with divinity would be an inaction, since according to Śrī Krishna, those actions bear no reaction on the performer due to his acquired immunity which is borrowed from Śrī Krishna's infallible radiance. Arjuna's non—compliance would be an action since it would be without immunity and would incur the disapproval of the Supervising Universal Lord.

कर्मणो ह्यपि बोद्धव्यं
बोद्धव्यं च विकर्मणः ।
अकर्मणश्च बोद्धव्यं
गहना कर्मणो गतिः ॥४.१७॥
karmaṇo hyapi boddhavyaṁ
boddhavyaṁ ca vikarmaṇaḥ
akarmaṇaśca boddhavyaṁ
gahanā karmaṇo gatiḥ (4.17)

karmaṇo = karmaṇaḥ — of action; hyapi = hy (hi) — indeed + api — also; boddhavyaṁ — should be known; boddhavyaṁ — should be recognized; ca — and; vikarmaṇaḥ — inappropriate action; akarmaṇaś = akarmaṇaḥ — no action + ca — and; boddhavyaṁ — should be understood; gahanā — difficult to comprehend; karmaṇo = karmaṇaḥ — of action; gatiḥ — the course

Indeed, appropriate action should be known and one should also recognize the inappropriate type. The effect of no action should be understood. The course of action is difficult to comprehend. (4.17)

Commentary:

The course of action is indeed difficult to comprehend, since it involves pleasing the Supreme Lord and since a human being, even one on par with Arjuna, might be baffled when his psychology shifts away from the kriyā view and he loses track of the divine prerogatives.

As Śrī Krishna pointed out, the effect of taking no action at all, should be understood, for that is also a kind of action. Appropriate actions should be defined as that which is approved. Inappropriate action is that to which Śrī Krishna is opposed to.

कर्मण्यकर्म यः पश्येद्
अकर्मणि च कर्म यः ।
स बुद्धिमान्मनुष्येषु
स युक्तः कृत्स्नकर्मकृत् ॥४.१८॥
karmaṇyakarma yaḥ paśyed
akarmaṇi ca karma yaḥ
sa buddhimānmanuṣyeṣu
sa yuktaḥ kṛtsnakarmakṛt (4.18)

karmaṇyakarma = karmaṇy (karmaṇi) — in performance + akarma — non—action; yaḥ — who; paśyed = paśyet — he should see; akarmaṇi — in non—action; ca — and; karma — action; yaḥ — who; sa = saḥ — he; buddhimān — wise person; manuṣyeṣu — of human beings; sa = saḥ — he; yuktaḥ — skilled in yoga; kṛtsnakarmakṛt = kṛtsna – all + karmakṛt — action performance

He who perceives the non—acting factor in a performance and sees an acting factor when there is no action, is the wise person among human beings. He is skilled in yoga and can perform all actions. (4.18)

Commentary:

When there is no action, there is the action of restraint. When the said restraint is applied, there is no external action but an internal force comes on. All the same when the yogi acts in compliance to the divine will, it is a kind of nonaction, since he functions only as a reflective agent of the divine, and since he is shielded by divine radiance. Such a person, who is skilled in yoga application, can do almost anything without danger of contamination, as long as his actions reflect the divine. If he misjudges, however, he will undoubtedly incur a reaction.

यस्य सर्वे समारम्भाः
कामसंकल्पवर्जिताः ।
ज्ञानाग्निदग्धकर्माणं
तमाहुः पण्डितं बुधाः ॥४.१९
yasya sarve samārambhāḥ
kāmasaṁkalpavarjitāḥ
jñānāgnidagdhakarmāṇaṁ
tamāhuḥ paṇḍitaṁ budhāḥ (4.19)

yasya — one whom; sarve — all; samārambhāḥ — endeavors; kāmasaṁkalpa varjitāḥ = kāma — desire + saṁkalpa — intention + varjitāḥ — not mixed into; jñānāgni dagdha karmāṇaṁ = jñāna — knowledge + āgni — fiery force + dagdha — burnt, destroyed + karmāṇaṁ — action, reactionary work; tam — him; āhuḥ — call; paṇḍitaṁ — learned man; budhāḥ — wise man

He for whom desires and intentions are not mixed into his endeavors, who destroyed reactionary work by the fiery force of his knowledge, he, the wise men call a pandit or learned man. (4.19)

Commentary:

This person must be already free from personal motivations, such that his own desires and intentions are not mixed in when he acts for the divine. Such a person deserves the title of pandit or learned man.

This person is not bogged down in material existence by the cultural activities which usually keep a spirit time-bound in haphazard transmigrations. This person's reactionary work is destroyed by the fiery force of his knowledge about Śrī Krishna and about how to accurately reflect Him.

त्यक्त्वा कर्मफलासङ्गं
नित्यतृप्तो निराश्रयः ।
कर्मण्यभिप्रवृत्तोऽपि
नैव किंचित्करोति सः ॥४.२०॥
tyaktvā karmaphalāsaṅgaṁ
nityatṛpto nirāśrayaḥ
karmaṇyabhipravṛtto'pi
naiva kiṁcitkaroti saḥ (4.20)

tyaktvā — given up; karmaphalāsaṅgaṁ = karma — action + phala — pay—off + āsaṅgaṁ — attachment, quest; nityatṛpto (nityatṛptaḥ) = nityaḥ — always + tṛptaḥ — satisfied; nirāśrayaḥ — not dependent; karmaṇy = karmaṇi — in performance; abhipravṛtto = abhipravṛttaḥ — proceeding, functioning; 'pi = api — even; naiva = na — not + eva — indeed; kiṁcit — anything; karoti — does; saḥ — he

Giving up the quest for a payoff from actions, being always satisfied, not depending on anything, he does nothing at all even while performing. (4.20)

Commentary:

This person, even while performing, relinquishes his personal interest in worldly life and remains attuned to the divine will. Losing interest in a payoff from actions, being always satisfied and not depending on anyone for mundane fulfillment, he does not attract reactions.

निराशीर्यतचित्तात्मा
त्यक्तसर्वपरिग्रहः ।
शारीरं केवलं कर्म
कुर्वन्नाप्नोति किल्बिषम् ॥४.२१॥
nirāśīryatacittātmā
tyaktasarvaparigrahaḥ
śārīraṁ kevalaṁ karma
kurvannāpnoti kilbiṣam (4.21)

nirāśīr — without hoping; yatacittātmā = yata — reserved + citta — thought + ātmā — spirit; tyaktasarvaparigrahaḥ = tyakta — giving up + sarva — all + parigrahaḥ — tendency for grasping; śārīraṁ — body; kevalaṁ — alone; karma — action; kurvan — functioning; nāpnoti = na — not + āpnoti — acquire; kilbiṣam — fault

Without hoping, being reserved in thought and spirit, giving up all tendency for grasping, using the body effectively for action, he does not acquire a fault. (4.21)

Commentary:

This person has transcended the human tendency to aspire for hope. With a mind blank of expectations, having no particular interest besides being sensitive to and compliant with the divine will, he does not acquire a fault. Those actions of his which reflect divine will, carry liability for the Supreme Person, and not for him. Any corresponding reactions that reach him, are retransmitted to the Supreme Being.

This person's nature is transformed in such a way that the natural tendency for grasping is neither felt internally nor exhibited externally, except in the instances when the Supervising Universal Lord uses his psyche for a specific purpose.

यदृच्छालाभसंतुष्टो
द्वंद्वातीतो विमत्सरः ।
समः सिद्धावसिद्धौ च
कृत्वापि न निबध्यते ॥४.२२॥
yadṛcchālābhasaṁtuṣṭo
dvaṁdvātīto vimatsaraḥ
samaḥ siddhāvasiddhau ca
kṛtvāpi na nibadhyate (4.22)

yadṛcchā — by chance; lābha — benefit; saṁtuṣṭaḥ — satisfied; dvandvātīto (dvandvātītaḥ) = dvandva — likes and dislikes + atītaḥ — ignoring; vimatsaraḥ — free from envy; samaḥ — even—minded; siddhāv = siddhau — in success; asiddhau — in failure; ca — and; kṛtvā — having performed; 'pi = api — also; na — no; nibadhyate — is implicated

Being satisfied by benefit which comes by chance, ignoring likes and dislikes, being free from envy, even—minded in success and failure, and having performed, a man is still not implicated. (4.22)

Commentary:

Benefits which come by chance, manifest as a result of past endeavors of various persons and forces. Usually a human being interprets such benefits within the scope of what he can remember in his present life. This is of course an error in judgment since whatever happens today is based on numerous factors from the unknown past. It is a certain arrogance that causes a human being to fit circumstances into the present memory. In kriyā yoga we seek to remove this presumption by various austerities which make us free beings and which open the door of subconscious memories.

The benefits which come by chance, should only be used as advised by the Supreme Lord; otherwise they should not be touched by a living being, even if he perceives them and even if he feels tempted to exploit them. Basically speaking, the enjoying propensity fades proportionately as one advances kriyā practice.

If the yogi can remain in an even—minded state even in success of endeavors or in failures, he does not become implicated. The evenness of mind allows him to hear the Supreme Lord and make the necessary adjustments as dictated by the Divinity.

गतसङ्गस्य मुक्तस्य
ज्ञानावस्थितचेतसः ।
यज्ञायाचरतः कर्म
समग्रं प्रविलीयते ॥४.२३॥
gatasaṅgasya muktasya
jñānāvasthitacetasaḥ
yajñāyācarataḥ karma
samagraṁ pravilīyate (4.23)

gatasaṅgasya = gata — gone + saṅgasya — of attachment; muktasya — of the liberated person; jñānāvasthitacetasaḥ = jñāna — knowledge + avasthita — established + cetasaḥ — of an idea; yajñāyācarataḥ = yajñāya — for austerity and religion + ācarataḥ — doing; karma — action; samagraṁ — completely; pravilīyate — cancels

Concerning a person whose attachment is finished, who is liberated, whose idea is established in knowledge, any of his action which is done solely for austerity and religion, does cancel completely. (4.23)

Commentary:

A living being has is always to something. He cannot be totally detached. If he becomes detached from one reality, he becomes attached to another one simultaneously. Thus to accommodate that tendency, one has to lean in one direction to disengage from another position. However to lean in the higher direction, one has to be purified; otherwise, one will return to the lower plane. It is simply a matter of preferred reliance. One must lean while performing purificatory austerities of kriyā yoga, and then gradually one is purified. As the purifications take effect permanently, one can move to the higher plane and associate with higher persons like Lord Krishna and Lord Shiva.

When the lower attachments are finished, one is liberated from the lower interactions which spur painful reactions. Thereafter one's actions are cancelled out. They do not bring about new lower obligations. At that stage, such actions are done either as austerity for further purification or for religion while acting under the supervision of the Supreme Lord. There is no need, however, to make disciples and to cause them to worship one's person merely because one acts as an agent of the Supreme. This is hardly necessary. In fact it is a great distraction for the yogi and also thoroughly misleading for the said followers.

ब्रह्मार्पणं ब्रह्महविर्
ब्रह्माग्नौ ब्रह्मणा हुतम् ।
ब्रह्मैव तेन गन्तव्यं
ब्रह्मकर्मसमाधिना ॥४.२४॥

brahmārpaṇaṁ brahmahavir
brahmāgnau brahmaṇā hutam
brahmaiva tena gantavyaṁ
brahmakarmasamādhinā (4.24)

brahmārpaṇaṁ = brahma — spiritual existence + arpaṇam — ceremonial articles; brahma — spiritual existence; havir = haviḥ — sacrificial ingredients, ghee; brahmāgnau = brahma — spiritual existence + agnau — in fire; brahmaṇā — by the qualified brahmin priest; hutam — offering oblations; brahmaiva = brahma — spiritual existence + eva — indeed; tena — by him; gantavyaṁ — to be attained; brahmakarmasamādhinā = brahma — spiritual existence + karma — activity + samādhinā — by meditative contact

Spiritual existence is the basis of his ceremonial articles. It is the foundation of sacrificial ingredients. The perceptive priest pours the stipulated items into the fiery splendor of spiritual existence. It is the spiritual existence which is attained by a person who keeps contact with the spiritual level while acting. (4.24)

Commentary:

This is mystic jargon, pertaining to a time when the perceptive priest (brahmaṇā) performed physical rituals which reflected events on the mystic plane. Nowadays the priests do not have mystic insights. Most of them are fraudulent. They pay service to the traditional ceremonies but they lack the corresponding insight. Besides, the environment is not responsive to their Sanskrit invocations. In the *Mahābhārata* of which the *Bhagavad Gītā* is a part, we hear of warriors who invoked explosives and other armaments merely by Sanskrit sounds. That is no longer possible. Brahmin priests today speak the Sanskrit language but are unable to produce anything by their sounding of it. Some say the fault lies in incorrect pronunciation but this is just an excuse. Formerly if there was an incorrect pronunciation something to the contrary occurred, but now nothing happens. It is not the pronunciation but rather the unresponsive environment which nolonger vibrates to the resonance of Sanskrit.

By kriyā yoga, we maintain in contact with the spiritual level while acting just as the ancient perceptive brahmins did but we do not act on a large scale as some of them did. In the following verses, our processes are described. These verses from 25 through 30 of this chapter are very important in defining what a kriyā teacher should be versed in. These definitions free us from deception by those who say they are representatives of Śrī Krishna or the Absolute Truth, but who actually exploit the ignorance of seekers. In these verses, Śrī Krishna defines clearly who is to be a teacher for the kriyā yogis. He also describes the various disciplines of kriyā yoga, for it has more than one course to it.

दैवमेवापरे यज्ञं
योगिनः पर्युपासते ।
ब्रह्माग्नावपरे यज्ञं
यज्ञेनैवोपजुह्वति ॥४.२५॥
daivamevāpare yajñaṁ
yoginaḥ paryupāsate
brahmāgnāvapare yajñaṁ
yajñenaivopajuhvati (4.25)

daivam — to a supernatural authority; evāpare = eva — indeed + apare — some; yajñaṁ — austerity and religious ceremony; yoginaḥ — yogis; paryupāsate — practice; brahmāgnāv = brahmāgnau — in the fiery brilliance of spiritual existence; apare — others; yajñaṁ — austerity and religious ceremony; yajñenaivopajuhvati = yajñena — by austerity and religious ceremony; eva — indeed + upajuhvati — they offer

Some yogis perform austerity and religious ceremony in relation to a supernatural authority. Others offer austerity and religious ceremony as the sacrifice into the fiery brilliance of spiritual existence. (4.25)

Commentary:

These procedures related to yogins (yoginah), some of whom are devotees and others who are non-devotees. The point is that we cannot say this verse refers to devotees alone or that Śrī Krishna was using the term yoginah to mean devotees or bhaktas.

We have to understand that previously in the time of Śrī Krishna, yoga was such a basic discipline and an educational requirement that all the ascetics, monks and religious people were required to be qualified with it. It is different nowadays but still we cannot update the *Gītā* by stating that yoginah means devotees of Krishna who chant holy names, attend temple functions and offer worshipful ceremonies to a spiritual master in succession from Śrī Krishna.

Yoginah is a plural term. In verse 34 the term jñāninah is also as a plural term meaning perceptive teachers. We cannot say that jñāninah means one teacher. It is a plural term. In addition, we should not smartly use jñāninah as our teacher in one place and then elsewhere condemn the term as being a description of monist philosophers. These terms have consistent meanings in the *Gītā*. If we distort that, we indirectly ridicule Śrī Krishna, just for the sake of putting ourselves forward as absolute authorities under His name.

From text 25 through text 30, there is a list of teachers and their qualifications. These are the spiritual masters (jñāninah) recognized by Śrī Krishna. These are all yogis or people who practiced the eightfold process of yoga beforehand. In Chapter Six, Śrī Krishna will describe the yoga process from its elementary stage upwards.

This text 25 lists two of those teachers as follows:

1). Those who are expert in worshipping a deity, a supernatural authority (daivam). *They do so by performing austerity and religious ceremony which is requested of them by that authority. In other words, they pick up information from scriptures, from their predecessors and from direct revelation in how to satisfy and how to communicate with the said supernatural figure. Their austerities and* *ceremonies are not described by Śrī Krishna because it would depend on the particular deity.*

Śrī Krishna is one such supernatural person, even though He does not mention Himself specifically. The value of being a yogi beforehand is this: The worshipper gains mystic insight which allows him to actually communicate with the said authority who is on another plane of existence. The person may or may not use a Deity form, an Image which is inhabited by the supernatural figure, but even so, some mystic perception is required for accurate communication. Thus the requirements for the worshipper to be a yogi is tantamount.

2). Those who worship spiritual energy (brahmāgnau). *These persons also must be yogis beforehand, otherwise they would not have perception of the spiritual energy and would be left with their mental concepts. These persons are usually regarded as impersonalists because they avoid worshipping a supernatural personality (daivam). Their tendency is to accept the Absolute Truth as a spiritual power only.*

These persons, though regarded as impersonalists and though they naturally avoid personal worship, are not imagining spiritual energy. They were supposed to be expert in yoga austerities beforehand, and by that mystic perception, they see spiritual energy and offer their austerity and religious ceremony in relation to it.

It may be contested that if the energy worshippers are correct then the personalist yogis are incorrect or or one may propose the converse. However, that is not in contention here. Śrī Krishna does not raise the issue. Here He recognized both types of yogis as having valid processes, as we shall read in verses 31 and 32.

Both the personalist and impersonalist worshippers are ritualistic yogis as described in this verse. Thus Śrī Krishna has rated both as following courses which will lead to spiritual advancement. Human beings who have the tendency for ritual are of two types, those having a personalist bent and those having an impersonalist one.

As kriyā yogis, we adopt the mood of Śrī Krishna of not condemning either of these yogi ritualists. We do not want to form a bias against either of them, regardless of our particular tendency for personal or impersonal worship.

श्रोत्रादीनीन्द्रियाण्यन्ये
संयमाग्निषु जुह्वति ।
शब्दादीन्विषयानन्ये
इन्द्रियाग्निषु जुह्वति ॥४.२६॥
śrotrādīnīndriyāṇyanye
saṁyamāgniṣu juhvati
śabdādīnviṣayānanye
indriyāgniṣu juhvati (4.26)

śrotrādīnīndriyāṇy = śrotrādīnīndriyāṇi = śrotra — hearing + ādīni — and related aspects + indriyāṇi — senses; anye — others; saṁyamāgniṣu = saṁyama — restraint + agniṣu — in the fiery power; juhvati — they offer; śabdādīn = śabda — sound + ādīn — and so on; viṣayān — sensual pursuits; anye — others; indriyāgniṣu — in the fiery energy of sensuality; juhvati — they offer

Other yogis offer hearing and other sensual powers into the fiery power of restraint. Some offer sound and other sensual pursuits into the fiery sensual power. (4.26)

Commentary:

This refers to other yogis who have also mastered yoga and who apply the psychological expertise and emotional hardening of their nature, as well as their super-concentration abilities, to various disciplines. Here in verse 26, two types of pratyāhār yogis are mentioned. These are:

1) Those who restrain their sensual outputs by pulling in and stopping the out-pouring of their hearing ability and any of the other senses like touching, seeing, tasting and smelling. *These yogis first control one of those senses. Thereafter, they work on restraining the others, one by one.*

Eventually, they restrain the entire sensual mechanism which is an offshoot of the buddhi organ in the brain of the subtle body. By pulling in the subtle sensual mechanism, these yogis effectively control their relationship with the external world. They greatly reduce its effects on them. The restraint of the senses also gives them increased mystic perception and causes supernatural abilities to be realized.

2) Those yogis who vibrated sound into the sense of hearing and who direct other sense objects into the appropriate matching senses. *They use sounds like* ***Om****. In modern times they also use sounds like* ***Hare Krishna*** *and direct such sound into the appropriate sense organs. Those who specialize in sounds like* ***Om****, practice subtle meditation. Those who use sounds like Hare Krishna work mostly with their physical tongue to vibrate the sound, while using the physical ear to hear it. The mystic yogis may vibrate* ***Om*** *within their heads audibly or inaudibly. They hear it within their heads. Other sense objects like surfaces for touching, forms for seeing, flavors for tasting and aromas for smelling are used in the same way either as gross or subtle objects and are pegged to the appropriate senses. This is a type of pratyāhār where the sensuality ends its pursuits.*

When done from a personalist stance, the offering of sound and other sensual pursuits into the sensual power is licensed as Deity worship in terms of chanting the Holy Name of the Deity, touching the Deity form, seeing the Deity's features, tasting the

foods offered to the Deity and smelling scents given to the Deity. When it is done without a Deity it is considered as an impersonalist practice.

सर्वाणीन्द्रियकर्माणि
प्राणकर्माणि चापरे ।
आत्मसंयमयोगाग्नौ
जुह्वति ज्ञानदीपिते ॥४.२७॥
sarvāṇīndriyakarmāṇi
prāṇakarmāṇi cāpare
ātmasaṁyamayogāgnau
juhvati jñānadīpite (4.27)

sarvāṇīndriyakarmāṇi = sarvāṇi — all + indriyakarmāṇi — sensual actions; prāṇakarmāṇi = prāṇa — breath function + karmāṇi — activities; cāpare = ca — and + apare — some; ātmasaṁyamayogāgnau = ātmasaṁyama — self—restraint + yogāgnau — in fiery yoga austerities; juhvati — they offer; jñānadīpite = jñāna — experience + dīpite — illuminated

Some ascetics subject the sensual actions and the breath function to self—restraint by fiery yoga austerities, which are illuminated by experience. (4.27)

Commentary:

These are the yogis who perform mystic kriyās. They specialize in haţha yoga and prāṇāyāma. Through advanced prāṇāyāma techniques which are mentioned in text 29, and advanced haţha yoga which is mentioned in 30, they develop the ability to see on the subtle and supersubtle planes by third eye vision, buddhi vision and prāṇa vision. They develop the mastership of suppression of sensual action. They rid themselves of lower energy intake. These persons are expert kriyā yogis. They consider the practice of yoga to be the ways and means of perfection. Śrī Krishna accredited yoga practice as their objective (yogāgnau).

द्रव्ययज्ञास्तपोयज्ञा
योगयज्ञास्तथापरे ।
स्वाध्यायज्ञानयज्ञाश्च
यतयः संशितव्रताः ॥४.२८॥
dravyayajñāstapoyajñā
yogayajñāstathāpare
svādhyāyajñānayajñāśca
yatayaḥ saṁśitavratāḥ (4.28)

dravya — property + yajñās — austerity and religious ceremony; tapo (tapaḥ) — self denial + yajñā — austerity and religious ceremony; yoga —eight—part yoga process + yajñāḥ — austerity and religious ceremony; tathāpare = tathā — as well as + apare — some others; svādhyāyajñānayajñāśca = svādhyāya — study of the Veda + jñāna — knowledge + yajñāḥ — austerity and religious ceremony + ca — and; yatayaḥ — ascetics; saṁśitavratāḥ = saṁśita — strict + vratāḥ — vows

Persons whose austerity and religious ceremony involve the control of material possession, those whose austerity and religious life involve some self—denial, as well as some others whose penance and religious procedure is the eight—part yoga discipline, and those whose austerity and religious ceremony is the study of the Veda and the acquirement of knowledge, all these are regarded as ascetics with strict vows. (4.28)

Commentary:

Some yogis focus on controlling property and money. There are many ways of doing this all depending on the nature of the yogi. Others use self denial and austerity, barring themselves from one thing or the other. Some just stick to the eightfold yoga process and steadfastly maintaining their practice, seeing yoga as the means and the end. Some others take up study of the *Vedas* and other related scriptures. They consider their theoretical views as the objective. All these are regarded as ascetics with strict vows.

अपाने जुह्वति प्राणं
प्राणेऽपानं तथापरे ।
प्राणापानगती रुद्ध्वा
प्राणायामपरायणाः ॥४.२९॥
apāne juhvati prāṇaṁ
prāṇe'pānaṁ tathāpare
prāṇāpānagatī ruddhvā
prāṇāyāmaparāyaṇāḥ (4.29)

apāne — in exhalation; juhvati — they offer; prāṇam — inhalation; prāṇe — in inhalation; 'pānaṁ = apāṇaṁ — in exhalation; tathāpare = tathā — similarly + apare — others; prāṇāpāna gatī = prāṇa — energizing air + apāna — de—energizing air + gatī — channel; ruddhvā — restraining; prāṇāyāmaparāyaṇāḥ = prāṇa — inhaling + āyāma — regulate + parāyaṇāḥ — intent

Some offer inhalation into the exhalation channels; similarly others offer the exhalation into the inhalation channels, thus being determined to restrain the channels of the energizing and de-energizing airs. (4.29)

Commentary:

Some yogis stick to prāṇāyāma. By it they progress through the four higher stages of yoga, namely pratyāhār sensual restraint and conservation, dhāraṇa concentration of psychic attention, dhyāna contemplation on higher levels of reality, and samādhi absorption in spiritual nature.

अपरे नियताहाराः
प्राणान्प्राणेषु जुह्वति ।
सर्वेऽप्येते यज्ञविदो
यज्ञक्षपितकल्मषाः ॥४.३०॥
apare niyatāhārāḥ
prāṇānprāṇeṣu juhvati
sarve'pyete yajñavido
yajñakṣapitakalmaṣāḥ (4.30)

apare — others; niyatāhārāḥ — persons restrained in diet; prāṇān — fresh air; prāṇeṣu — into the previous inhalations; juhvati — impel; sarve — all; 'pyete (apyete) = apy (api) — also + ete — these; yajñavido = yajñavidaḥ — those who know the value of an act of sacrifice; yajñakṣapitakalmaṣāḥ = yajña — austerity and religious ceremony + kṣapita — destroyed, removed + kalmaṣāḥ — impurities

Others who were restrained in diet, impel fresh air into the previously inhaled air. All these ascetics whose impurities were removed by austerity and religious ceremony understand the value of an act of sacrifice. (4.30)

Commentary:

Some who master haṭha yoga and who practice prāṇāyāma, are inspired to become completely restrained in diet for further progression. They control their psychic energies by doing bhastrika (rapid breathing) and its related breath exercises and sensual control techniques in kriyā yoga. Śrī Krishna appraises these ascetics (yatayah 4.28) as comprehending the value of an act of sacrifice. As I stated earlier some of these may or may not be devotees. Still, Śrī Krishna does not issue a bias. He rates not their affiliation with Him but rather, their practice.

यज्ञशिष्टामृतभुजो
यान्ति ब्रह्म सनातनम्।
नायं लोकोऽस्त्ययज्ञस्य
कुतोऽन्यः कुरुसत्तम ॥४.३१॥
yajñaśiṣṭāmṛtabhujo
yānti brahma sanātanam
nāyaṁ loko'styayajñasya
kuto'nyaḥ kurusattama (4.31)

yajñaśiṣṭāmṛtabhujo = yajñaśiṣṭāmṛtabhujaḥ = yajñaśiṣṭa — the physical result of a sacrifice + amṛta — the psychological enjoyment + bhujaḥ — enjoying; yānti — they go; brahma — to the spiritual region; sanātanam — primeval; nāyaṁ = na — not + ayaṁ — this; loko = lokaḥ — world; 'sty = asty (asti) — is (properly utilized); ayajñasya — of a person who performs no austerity or religious ceremony; kuto = kutaḥ — how can it be?; 'nyaḥ = anyaḥ — other; kurusattama — best of the Kurus

Those who enjoy the physical and psychological results of a sacrifice, go to the primeval spiritual region. This world is not properly utilized by those who do not perform austerity or religious ceremony. How then can the other world be, O best of the Kurus? (4.31)

Commentary:

Those ascetics who enjoy by actual experience, the physical as well as the psychological results of their sacrifice, go to the primeval spiritual region, on the condition that their efforts were complete. The physical enjoyment may be there but the psychological one must be present for the effects to extend to the spiritual region.

Śrī Krishna gave His opinion that this physical world is properly utilized only when one performs austerity and religious ceremonies which match the descriptions given by Him in the *Gītā*. He suggests to Arjuna that a person cannot enjoy the hereafter without performing such austerity and religious ceremony. The conclusion is that the world was created for that particular purpose. The methods are definitely not stereotyped, since Śrī Krishna named so many alternative processes as being valid. He did not give just one procedure nor did He state that one method was the only way.

एवं बहुविधा यज्ञा
वितता ब्रह्मणो मुखे ।
कर्मजान्विद्धि तान्सर्वान्
एवं ज्ञात्वा विमोक्ष्यसे ॥४.३२॥
evaṁ bahuvidhā yajñā
vitatā brahmaṇo mukhe
karmajānviddhi tānsarvān
evaṁ jñātvā vimokṣyase (4.32)

evaṁ — thus; bahuvidhā — many types; yajñā — disciplines of accomplishment; vitatā — expounded; brahmaṇo = brahmaṇaḥ — of spiritual existence; mukhe — in the mouth; karmajān — action—produced; viddhi — know; tān — them; sarvān — all; evaṁ — thus; jñātvā — having realized; vimokṣyase — you will be freed

Many types of disciplines of accomplishment were expounded in the mouth of the spiritual existence. Know them all to be produced from action. Realizing this, O Arjuna, you will be freed. (4.32)

Commentary:

Śrī Krishna again acknowledged the various disciplines which were expounded from time to time by great human personages as they were inspired or as these were revealed to them by divine people who used human forms and acted as the Mouth of the Supreme Itself.

The point, however, is that these valid procedures required action on the physical and psychological levels. Arjuna needed to realize this and become freed from hesitation. The recommendation for Arjuna was martial action done with the detachment developed in advanced yoga practice.

श्रेयान्द्रव्यमयाद्यज्ञाज्
ज्ञानयज्ञः परंतप ।
सर्वं कर्माखिलं पार्थ
ज्ञाने परिसमाप्यते ॥४.३३॥
śreyāndravyamayādyajñāj
jñānayajñaḥ paraṁtapa
sarvaṁ karmākhilaṁ pārtha
jñāne parisamāpyate (4.33)

śreyān — better; dravyamayād = dravyamayāt — than property; yajñāj = yajñāt — than control and ritual regulation; jñānayajñaḥ = jñāna — theoretical knowledge and primitive practical knowledge + yajñaḥ — control and ritual regulation; paraṁtapa — scorcher of the enemy; sarvaṁ — all; karmākhilaṁ = karma — activity + akhilaṁ — without exception; pārtha — son of Pṛthā; jñāne — as conclusion; parisamāpyate — is realized completely

Better than property control and its ritual regulation is knowledge control and its ritual regulation, O scorcher of the enemy. Every activity without exception, O son of Pṛthā, is realized as a conclusion in the final analysis. (4.33)

Commentary:

Śrī Krishna gave the idea that some of the methods are inferior to others. Methods that involve the sacrifice of material possessions (dravya) are definitely inferior to those which involve the control of theoretical knowledge and of primitive techniques. In any case, every activity without exception is to be evaluated to form a conclusion. The person should assess the worth of each process by evaluating its result.

Property control and its ritual regulation are an elementary method. Once mastered, one should evolve to knowledge control and its ritual regulation. This is a comprehensive process and thus one cannot abandon property control while in pursuit of knowledge control. They exist side by side at the advanced level. Property control is the initial process and knowledge control completes it. Ultimately, all activity has a conclusion or leads to a specific result.

तद्विद्धि प्रणिपातेन
परिप्रश्नेन सेवया ।
उपदेक्ष्यन्ति ते ज्ञानं
ज्ञानिनस्तत्त्वदर्शिनः ॥४.३४॥
tadviddhi praṇipātena
paripraśnena sevayā
upadekṣyanti te jñānaṁ
jñāninastattvadarśinaḥ (4.34)

tad — this; viddhi — know; praṇipātena — by submitting as a student; paripraśnena — by asking questions; sevayā — by serving as requested; upadekṣyanti — they will teach; te — you; jñānaṁ — knowledge; jñāninas = jñāninaḥ — those who know; tattvadarśinaḥ — perceptive reality—conversant sages

This you ought to know. By submitting yourself as a student, by asking questions and by serving as requested, the perceptive reality—conversant teachers will teach you the knowledge. (4.34)

Commentary:

Every method described in verses 25 through 30 can be learned from any adept teacher who has developed mystic sensual perception to pierce the hidden aspects of reality. To be a student one should submit oneself for learning, ask questions and serve as requested. There is no stipulation here about honored worship of a guru or treating him as if he were God. The submission is one as a student approaching respectfully for an education and a practical technique.

यज्ज्ञात्वा न पुनर्मोहम्
एवं यास्यसि पाण्डव ।
येन भूतान्यशेषेण
द्रक्ष्यस्यात्मन्यथो मयि ॥४.३५॥
yajjñātvā na punarmoham
evaṁ yāsyasi pāṇḍava
yena bhūtānyaśeṣeṇa
drakṣyasyātmanyatho mayi (4.35)

yaj = yad — which; jñātvā — having known; na — not; punar — again; moham — delusion; evaṁ — thus; yāsyasi — you succumb; pāṇḍava — O son of Pāndu; yena — by which; bhūtāny = bhūtāni — living beings; aśeṣeṇa — without exception, all; drakṣyasy = drakṣyasi — you will perceive; ātmany = ātmani — in the self; atho — then; mayi — in me

Having known that experience, you will never again succumb to delusion, O son of Pāndu. By that experience, you will perceive all beings in relation to yourself and then in relation to Me. (4.35)

Commentary:

The experience is the direct perception of reality either as the Supreme Being or as the Supreme Energy, according to the seeker's tendency for personal or impersonal worship. In both cases, the seeker will reach a state of perceiving all beings in relation to himself and then, in the more advanced stage in relation to Śrī Krishna or the Supreme Absolute, according to tendency.

अपि चेदसि पापेभ्यः
सर्वेभ्यः पापकृत्तमः ।
सर्वं ज्ञानप्लवेनैव
वृजिनं संतरिष्यसि ॥४.३६॥

api — even; ced — if; asi — you are; pāpebhyaḥ — of the culprits; sarvebhyaḥ — of all; pāpakṛttamaḥ — most wicked; sarvaṁ — all; jñānaplavenaiva = jñāna — experience + plavena — by conveyance + eva

api cedasi pāpebhyaḥ
sarvebhyaḥ pāpakṛttamaḥ
sarvaṁ jñānaplavenaiva
vṛjinaṁ saṁtariṣyasi (4.36)

— indeed; vṛjinaṁ — bad tendencies; saṁtariṣyasi — you will overcome

Even if you were the most wicked of the culprits, you will overcome all bad tendencies by the conveyance of this experience. (4.36)

Commentary:

By that experience one overcomes bad tendencies. This applies to both the personalists and impersonalists. Both shed bad tendencies after experiencing the Supreme Person or the Supreme Cause. The experience frees a person from his limited identity and its faults. This is explained by an analogy in the next verse.

यथैधांसि समिद्धोऽग्निर्
भस्मसात्कुरुतेऽर्जुन ।
ज्ञानाग्निः सर्वकर्माणि
भस्मसात्कुरुते तथा ॥४.३७॥
yathaidhāṁsi samiddho'gnir
bhasmasātkurute'rjuna
jñānāgniḥ sarvakarmāṇi
bhasmasātkurute tathā (4.37)

yathaidhāṁsi = yathā — as + idhāṁsi (edhāṁsi) — firewood; samiddho = samiddhaḥ — set on fire; 'gnir = agnir — fire; bhasmasāt kurute — it reduces to ashes; 'rjuna (arjuna) = Arjuna; jñānāgniḥ = jñāna — realize knowledge + agniḥ — fiery potency; sarvakarmāṇi = sarva — all + karmāṇi — actions; bhasmasāt kurute — it reduces to nothing; tathā — so

As when wood is set on fire, it is reduced to ashes, O Arjuna, so the fiery potency of realized knowledge reduces all actions to nothing. (4.37)

Commentary:

The experience of the Supreme Person or the Supreme Cause extinguishes the lower aspects of a person's nature, shifting the person to the higher level of the spirit, for both personalists or impersonalists. In either case the person gets a full waiver from lower existence.

न हि ज्ञानेन सदृशं
पवित्रमिह विद्यते ।
तत्स्वयं योगसंसिद्धः
कालेनात्मनि विन्दति ॥४.३८॥
na hi jñānena sadṛśaṁ
pavitramiha vidyate
tatsvayaṁ yogasaṁsiddhaḥ
kālenātmani vindati (4.38)

na — nothing; hi — indeed; jñānena — with direct experience; sadṛśaṁ — compared with; pavitram — purifier; iha — in this world; vidyate — is relevant; tat — that realization; svayaṁ — himself; yogasaṁsiddhaḥ = yoga — yoga practice + saṁsiddhaḥ — perfected; kālenātmani = kālena — in time + ātmani — in the self; vindati — he locates

Nothing, indeed, can be compared with direct experience. No other purifier is as relevant in this world. That man who himself is perfected in yoga practice, will in time, locate the realization in himself. (4.38)

Commentary:

In all cases, nothing compares with direct experience. Hearing from a self-realized teacher or from anybody who claims to know the truth, does not match direct experience. Ultimately it is direct experience which must be acquired.

No other purifier is as effective. Nothing else results in such a complete change in the nature and habits of the individual concerned. All should strive for direct experience, leaving aside other lesser means.

Yogasamsiddha is perfected yoga practice. Śrī Krishna's definition of yoga is given in Chapter Six. The value of yoga, given here, is that the man who perfects its practice locates the experience of the Supreme Person or the Supreme Cause, within his psyche. He no longer has to rely on divine or mundane hearsay. This is the purpose of kriyā yoga, for the person to acquire transcendental experience. Kriyā yoga is for those who, by nature, are not satisfied merely by hearing, conceptualizing and believing.

श्रद्धावाँल्लभते ज्ञानं
तत्परः संयतेन्द्रियः ।
ज्ञानं लब्ध्वा परां शान्तिम्
अचिरेणाधिगच्छति ॥४.३९॥
śraddhāvāṁllabhate jñānaṁ
tatparaḥ saṁyatendriyaḥ
jñānaṁ labdhvā parāṁ śāntim
acireṇādhigacchati (4.39)

śraddhāvān — one who has faith; labhate — he gets; jñānaṁ — the experience; tatparaḥ = tad — that + paraḥ — being devoted to; saṁyatendriyaḥ = saṁyata — restraining + indriyaḥ — sensual energy; jñānaṁ — experience; labdhvā — having acquired; parāṁ — supreme; śāntim — peace; acireṇādhigacchati = acireṇa — quickly + adhigacchati — goes

One who has faith, gets the experience. Being devoted to restraining the sensual energy, having acquired the experience, he goes quickly to the supreme peace. (4.39)

Commentary:

Faith here means faith in the yoga process which has sensual restraint as its 5th stage (pratyāhār). That 5th stage was described in verse 26 as samyama:

srotradini 'ndriyany anye samyamagnisu juhvati

Other yogis offer hearing and other sensual powers into the fiery power of restraint.

By completing the pratyāhār stage of yoga practice, one goes quickly to the supreme peace. By isolating the senses from their destructive yearnings, one allows higher perceptions to occur and one attains the supreme peace.

अज्ञश्चाश्रद्दधानश्च
संशयात्मा विनश्यति ।
नायं लोकोऽस्ति न परो
न सुखं संशयात्मनः ॥४.४०॥
ajñaścāśraddadhānaśca
saṁśayātmā vinaśyati
nāyaṁ loko'sti na paro
na sukhaṁ saṁśayātmanaḥ (4.40)

ajñaścāśraddadhānaśca = ajñaḥ — ignorant person + ca — and + aśraddadhānaḥ — faithless person + ca — and; saṁśayātmā = saṁśaya — doubtful + ātmā — self; vinaśyati — is degraded; nāyaṁ = na — not + ayaṁ — this; loko = lokaḥ — world; 'sti = asti — is; na — not; paro = paraḥ — beyond the physical world; na — not; sukhaṁ — in happiness; saṁśayātmanaḥ = saṁśaya — doubting + ātmanaḥ — for the self

The ignorant person, the faithless one who is doubtful, is degraded. Neither this physical world, nor the dimensions beyond this, nor happiness, is for the person who is doubtful. (4.40)

Commentary:

Here again faith deals with the yoga process indicated above and not with anything else. We have to stay in context and not divert these meanings to other ideas. The indication is that one who lacks faith in the pratyāhār sensual restraint endeavor, will become degraded. Neither this physical world, nor the dimensions beyond it, nor even genuine happiness is for the person who doubts the sensual restraint process. Indeed, he will be mesmerized by gross sensual perception and, in the course of time, will become ruined.

योगसंन्यस्तकर्माणं
ज्ञानसंछिन्नसंशयम् ।
आत्मवन्तं न कर्माणि
निबध्नन्ति धनंजय ॥४.४१॥
yogasaṁnyastakarmāṇaṁ
jñānasaṁchinnasaṁśayam
ātmavantaṁ na karmāṇi
nibadhnanti dhanaṁjaya (4.41)

yogasaṁnyastakarmāṇaṁ = yoga — yoga technique + saṁnyasta — renounced + karmāṇaṁ — action; jñānasaṁchinnasaṁśayam = jñāna — realized knowledge + saṁchinna — removed + saṁśayam — doubt; ātmavantaṁ — self—composed; na — no; karmāṇi — cultural activities; nibadhnanti — they bind; dhanaṁjaya — O conqueror of wealthy countries

Cultural activities do not implicate a person whose actions are renounced through techniques developed in yoga practice, whose doubt is removed by realized knowledge and who is self—composed, O conqueror of wealthy countries. (4.41)

Commentary:

Finally, Śrī Krishna definitely addresses karma yoga as the application of yogicly—produced psychological maturity to social, cultural and political affairs. Here Śrī Krishna clearly tells Arjuna that he should apply the sensual restraints on the battlefield and still fight as a matter of obligatory duty.

He states that activities do not implicate a person whose actions are renounced through yoga techniques and whose doubts were removed by mystic experience of the supernatural reality which overrides this physical plane. Arjuna was to perform his duty and not worry about consequences. Those reactions concerned only the Supreme Lord. Arjuna should be self-composed (ātmavantam), immune to all influences except those from the Supreme Lord, Whose will and energy superseded everyone.

तस्मादज्ञानसंभूतं
हृत्स्थं ज्ञानासिनात्मनः ।
छित्त्वैनं संशयं योगम्
आतिष्ठोत्तिष्ठ भारत ॥४.४२॥
tasmādajñānasaṁbhūtaṁ
hṛtsthaṁ jñānāsinātmanaḥ
chittvainaṁ saṁśayaṁ yogam
ātiṣṭhottiṣṭha bhārata (4.42)

tasmād = tasmāt — therefore; ajñānasaṁbhūtaṁ = ajñāna — ignorance + saṁbhūtaṁ — produced by; hṛtsthaṁ — lodged in your being; jñānāsinā = jñāna — realized knowledge + asinā — by the cutting effect; 'tmanaḥ = ātmanaḥ — of yourself; chittvainaṁ = chittva — having severed entirely + enaṁ — this; saṁśayam — doubt; yogaṁ — to yogic technique; ātiṣṭhottiṣṭha = ātiṣṭha — resort to + uttiṣṭha — make a stand; bhārata — man of the Bharata family

Therefore having severed entirely, with the cutting instrument of realized knowledge, this doubt that comes from the ignorance, lodged in your being, resort to yogic technique and make a stand, O man of the Bharata family! (4.42)

Commentary:

Śrī Krishna ordered Arjuna to participate in the battle. Arjuna must realize the Supreme Person and His overriding influences. He must identify himself as an agent of the Supreme, taking commission from Śrī Krishna to act on the battlefield, while resorting to the yogic techniques he formerly practiced.

Finally in this last verse of Chapter Four, Arjuna is ordered to make a stand as a divine agent.

It is interesting that there are more chapters to the *Bhagavad Gītā*, since at this point, if Arjuna was convinced, He could have repossessed his bow and arrow, straightened his posture and fought as directed by Śrī Krishna. Unfortunately, Arjuna was not yet convinced. He was not yet under the kriyā yoga vision as described by Śrī Krishna.

Author's Notation:

This Edition of Bhagavad Gītā which is a service to the kriyā yogis, is sponsored first of all by my Śrī Śrī Krishna and Balarāma Deities, as well as by Lord Shiva. There was an idea by Lord Shiva for me to compose a text on the complexities and haphazards of taking rebirth. So far, I was unable to compose that book but in this edition some of the information is included, since Lord Krishna touched on the matter repeatedly.

After I finished the previous commentary of Bhagavad Gītā which was entitled Bhagavad Gītā Explained, Lord Krishna felt that there was something more to be said and that some ideas should be polished. Some criticism came after certain people read the publication. Their critical views are regarded in this commentary. While the previous commentary was an open text, open to anyone, this one is closed to many and opened only to kriyā yogis.

When I finished the commentary to Chapter Four, Śrī Bābāji Mahasaya came on the morning of July 31, 2001. With him was the famous Śrī Paramahamsa Yogananda, the person who first popularized the kriyā path in the Western Countries. As I looked on, Śrī Bābāji instructed Śrī Paramhansaji to give me certain energies. Some of these were energies that were to be exposed in Śrī Paramahamsa's commentaries on Bhagavad Gītā but instead he hid them in that book in cryptic language. Some more of those energies pertained to practices Śrī Paramhamsa performed, but which he did not integrate sufficiently to comment upon during his lifetime.

After some association, I noticed that Śrī Bābāji Mahasaya signaled for Śrī Paramhamsaji to leave. Then Śrī Bābāji said to me, "He was distracted by his quest for wealthy followers. He allowed some desires from the chitta to influence him for fulfillments for an empire. I waited many years for someone to explain these ideas for kriyā yogis. Take my blessings."

With that he smiled broadly and then left. I then considered what transpired. I thought, "I will do the Gītā but there is no guarantee that it will be what Bābāji wanted. And besides, I have my own defects to eliminate. One agent has one defect and the other has a different blemish. That is how it is."

But as I thought of this, Śrī Bābāji sent a message through the atmosphere. It read, "You have got the critical energy. You understand its usage. What do I care about blemishes? Just you remember text 4.38. With Paramhamsaji, we waited and waited. But with you we have an agent who can bear weight of these blessings. We have no fear."

As the agent-writer, I must now tell the readers that Śrī Bābāji and one of his disciples, Śrīla Satyeshwarananda Swamiji, did years ago, give me some kriyās for using the critical energy. I began to use these after they trained me. Śrīla Satyeshwarananda has his own way of explaining the use of these energies but he did show me how to operate them. I have not seen him for some time. I am grateful for his showing the technique. It is my duty to try to explain these in this commentary. Readers should know that I never met Śrīla Satyeshwarananda physically. All communications took place on the subtle planes.

Yogi Madhvācārya

CHAPTER 5

Disciplined Use of Opportunities by a Yogi*

अर्जुन उवाच
संन्यासं कर्मणां कृष्ण
पुनर्योगं च शंससि ।
यच्छ्रेय एतयोरेकं
तन्मे ब्रूहि सुनिश्चितम् ॥५.१॥
arjuna uvāca
saṁnyāsaṁ karmaṇāṁ kṛṣṇa
punaryogaṁ ca śaṁsasi
yacchreya etayorekaṁ
tanme brūhi suniścitam (5.1)

arjuna – Arjuna; uvāca — said; saṁnyāsaṁ — renunciation of involvement; karmaṇām — of social activity; kṛṣṇa — Krishna; punar — again; yogaṁ — the application of yoga austerities to worldly life; ca — and; śaṁsasi — you approved; yacchreya = yad — which + chreya (śreyaḥ) — better; etayor = etayoḥ — of these two; ekaṁ — one; tan — this; me — to me; brūhi — tell; suniścitam — with certainty

Arjuna said: You approved renunciation of social activity and also mentioned the application of yoga to worldly life. Which one of these is better? Tell me this with certainty. (5.1)

Commentary:

The complication of kriyā yoga mentioned by Arjuna, is that it involves both the renunciation of social activities and the application of yoga austerities to the same social field. It is a seemingly paradoxical craft. The end goal is removal from social, cultural and political affairs but initially that requires involvement in the same affairs. As the saying goes, one must fight fire with fire or meet one danger with another.

Even Arjuna, a superior human being, wanted a clear-cut separation between renunciation of social activity and the application of yoga austerities. He could not see that one could safely mix yoga with worldly life. He thought there should be one or the other, either involvement in worldly life or isolation for yoga practice.

Arjuna saw no viable connection between the two, nor did he see how one could use the emotional maturity gained by yoga practice in the worldly field. Śrī Krishna's expertise in applying yoga skills to worldly life, comes to the forefront here, as He will school Arjuna in the skill of it. This same skill is being taught to us, the kriyā yogis, since we, like Arjuna, face a dilemma of wanting to renounce the social life of householders or avoid the danger of becoming monks who mix with the public.

**The Mahābhārata contains no chapter headings. This title was assigned by the translator on the basis of verse 2 of this chapter.*

Just as Arjuna cannot abandon his political duties without absorbing consequences, we cannot turn away from our domestic or monastic duties without reactions which would upset our spiritual path. Thus we have much to learn from Śrī Krishna in this *Bhagavad Gītā*. This discourse is perfect for people like us who must stay on in the worldly field but who want to surpass the dangers that come with more involvement. Śrī Krishna can teach us, as He taught Arjuna, how to act here without being involved, performing in a terminal way. This is the karma yoga of the *Gītā*, something we need to learn from Śrī Krishna.

श्रीभगवानुवाच
संन्यासः कर्मयोगश्च
निःश्रेयसकरावुभौ ।
तयोस्तु कर्मसंन्यासात्
कर्मयोगो विशिष्यते ॥५.२॥
śrībhagavānuvāca
saṁnyāsaḥ karmayogaśca
niḥśreyasakarāvubhau
tayostu karmasaṁnyāsāt
karmayogo viśiṣyate (5.2)

śrī—bhagavān – the Blessed Lord; uvāca — said; saṁnyāsaḥ — total renunciation of social opportunities; karmayogaśca = karmayogaḥ — disciplined use of social opportunities by a yogi + ca — and; niḥśreyasakarāv = niḥśreyasa – ultimate happiness + karāv (karau) — leading to; ubhau — both; tayos — of the two; tu — but; karmasaṁnyāsāt — than the renunciation of cultural activity; karmayogo = karmayogaḥ — disciplined use of social opportunities by a yogi; viśiṣyate — is better

The Blessed Lord said: Both methods, the total renunciation of social opportunities and the disciplined use of opportunities by a yogi, lead to ultimate happiness. But of the two aspects, the disciplined use of opportunities in a yogic mood is better than total renunciation of cultural activity. (5.2)

Commentary:

Here Śrī Krishna clarifies that for Arjuna, sannyasa is not as good as karma yoga. This is not a contrast between yoga and devotional service but rather between sannyasa and karma yoga. In this case, Śrī Krishna points Arjuna in the direction of karma yoga but this does not apply in all cases.

By stating that karma yoga is better for Arjuna, Śrī Krishna is not referring to all persons. When Śrī Krishna instructed Uddhava he did not say that karma yoga was better but rather he directed Uddhava on the path of jñāna yoga. Uddhava wanted to take the route of bhakti yoga but Śrī Krishna directed him to perform austerities in jñāna yoga. Some commentators claim that Uddhava was directed to bhakti yoga, but the Sanskrit is clear in the Eleventh Canto of Śrīmad Bhāgavatam.

For Arjuna, karma yoga is better and for any of us who are without a divine waiver from responsibilities, it is also better. If however we have not performed sufficient yoga austerities, we will falter in karma yoga, until we begin to learn austerities and apply them towards our advancement. Luckily for Arjuna he was already proficient, as we hear in the *Mahābhārata* literature.

Since we lack a waiver from cultural activities, sannyasa or the total abandonment of social, cultural and political involvement would be a ruinous path. We should therefore not follow any missionary who pushes us in that direction at this stage of our development. Later on, if we reach a more advanced stage and thereby acquire the waiver from the Lord, we can embrace that path, leaving aside cultural involvement.

Even though both methods, the total renunciation of social opportunities and the disciplined use of them by a yogi, lead to the ultimate happiness, neither of them is the final stage. Of the two, total renunciation is the more advanced level. We would have to practice yoga, gain proficiency and then seek the disciplined use of opportunities. Then again, when we get a waiver, we may take the path of total renunciation. Śrī Uddhava was pointed to this path by Śrī Krishna, in contrast to Arjuna who required the more elementary stage of having to take up the opportunities.

So long as we participate in the social, cultural and political world, social involvement in a disciplined yogic mood is best. So long as the Supervising Universal Lord requires our services, then it is certainly the best path, since Śrī Krishna would not approve of other activities.

ज्ञेयः स नित्यसंन्यासी
यो न द्वेष्टि न काङ्क्षति ।
निर्द्वंद्वो हि महाबाहो
सुखं बन्धात्प्रमुच्यते ॥५.३॥
jñeyaḥ sa nityasaṁnyāsī
yo na dveṣṭi na kāṅkṣati
nirdvaṁdvo hi mahābāho
sukhaṁ bandhāt pramucyate (5.3)

jñeyaḥ — to be known; sa = saḥ — he; nityasaṁnyāsī = nitya — consistent + saṁnyāsī — a renouncer of social opportunities; yo = yaḥ — who; na — not; dveṣṭi — dislikes; na — not; kāṅkṣati — craves; nirdvandvo = nirdvandvaḥ — indifferent to opposite features; hi — indeed; mahābāho — O strong—armed man; sukhaṁ — easily; bandhāt — from implication; pramucyate — is freed

Indeed, a person who neither dislikes nor craves, who is indifferent to opposite features, should be recognized as a consistent renouncer, O strong—armed man. He is easily freed from implication. (5.3)

Commentary:

Here Śrī Krishna encouraged Arjuna to face the battle, to perform the duty required of him. Arjuna is induced to give up his sour attitude towards political involvement. Śrī Krishna incited Arjuna to show renunciation in mood, rather than in action. This is karma yoga. It is natural to develop resentment after hearing that one does not have the waiver from the Supreme Being and that one must perform in the cultural field, even to kill relatives who offended the sense of justice of the Supreme Being.

While natural, such a sour attitude will not help in achieving our spiritual aspirations. In fact it will add to the problems before us. It will cause further disapproval from the Supervising Supreme Lord, as Śrī Krishna identified Himself in the *Gītā*.

Thus it is better to cast off the sour mood and face the unpalatable conditions, learning fast from Śrī Krishna how to perform karma yoga to His satisfaction. We should apply the renunciation mood consistently (nitya). Whether we are householders or preaching monks, we have to learn enough yoga whereby we can apply renunciation in our moods and be detached while performing. Then we would be easily freed from implication and unafraid of the potential for rash reactions from material nature.

The only problem facing us, then, is if the Supreme Lord harnesses us to His karma yoga work before we are trained sufficiently. Thereby faced with responsibilities for a family or congregation, we may not have sufficient yoga skill to display indifference to opposite features and to ignore natural prejudices and cravings. In such a situation we have to learn yoga in a short time and then apply it as directed by Śrī Krishna.

If He harnessed us to responsibilities before we have the yoga proficiency, we will not get it by wishful thinking or by another spiritual discipline like chanting His holy names, because He does not state anywhere in the *Gītā* that we can do that. We will have to learn yoga in a short time, by taking a course and keeping a firm steady practice as we derive from it, the required expertise.

The question remains as to why the Supreme Being would harness us to responsibilities, if He knows that we lack the yoga training. That question is there. However regardless of the answer, the fact remains that the responsibilities are upon us. Therefore we should promptly take up yoga practice.

सांख्ययोगौ पृथग्बालाः
प्रवदन्ति न पण्डिताः ।
एकमप्यास्थितः सम्यग्
उभयोर्विन्दते फलम् ॥५.४॥
sāṁkhyayogau pṛthagbālāḥ
pravadanti na paṇḍitāḥ
ekamapyāsthitaḥ samyag
ubhayorvindate phalam (5.4)

sāṁkhyayogau = sāṁkhya — Sāṁkhya ideas + yogau — and yoga practices; pṛthagbālāḥ — simple—minded people; pravadanti — they describe; na — not; paṇḍitāḥ — the perceptive speakers; ekam — one; apy = api — even; āsthitaḥ — practiced; samyag — correctly; ubhayor = ubhayoḥ — of either; vindate — one gets; phalam — result

It is the simple-minded people, not the perceptive speakers, who say that Sāṁkhya ideas and yoga practices are separate. Even if one method is practiced correctly, the practitioner gets the result of either. (5.4)

Commentary:

The Samkhya philosophical views and the haţha yoga practices are not really separate because ultimately a person who understands the Samkhya ideas intellectually, and who does not practice yoga, will have to take up yoga in order to realize what he understood intellectually. From the other perspective, one who mastered haţha yoga to the mystic extent, will, on his own, try to follow the philosophical outlay of the Samkhya ideas or he will be inspired to discover such ideas for himself. The two views are not separate. Simple—minded people who are childlike (pṛthagbālāh), regard the two systems as separate, because until one practices either one to a proficient stage, one cannot understand the complimentary nature of each process.

Those who think that spiritual life cannot be related to a physical system of exercise, have a negative bias towards haţha yoga. Those who feel that thinking and reasoning will ultimately lead nowhere, may focus on the physical postures in haţha yoga practice. Thus each of these persons might become antagonistic to the other. In actuality, these systems compliment one another. Śrī Krishna wanted Arjuna to know that the application of yoga to worldly life is related to renunciation of social activity. The two courses are not in opposition. If one completes the application of yoga to worldly life, he will be successful when he takes to renunciation. This was proven in the lives of the ancient yogi kings like Janaka.

The disciplined use of opportunities in a yogic mood is especially good at the stage when one lacks an exemption from cultural life. It facilitates one to move faster to the higher level where one gets the exemption and can totally renounce cultural life. Thus the two courses are complimentary.

यत्सांख्यैः प्राप्यते स्थानं
तद्योगैरपि गम्यते ।
एकं सांख्यं च योगं च
यः पश्यति स पश्यति ॥५.५॥
yatsāṁkhyaiḥ prāpyate sthānaṁ
tadyogairapi gamyate
ekaṁ sāṁkhyaṁ ca yogaṁ ca
yaḥ paśyati sa paśyati (5.5)

yat — whatever; sāṁkhyaiḥ — by the Sāṁkhya experts; prāpyate — is attained; sthānaṁ — the level; tad — that; yogair = yogaiḥ — by the yogis; api — also; gamyate — is reached; ekaṁ — one; sāṁkhyaṁ — samkhya; ca — and; yogaṁ — yoga; ca — and; yaḥ — who; paśyati — perceived; sa = saḥ — he; paśyati — sees

The level obtained by the Sāṁkhya experts is also reached by the yogis. Sāṁkhya and yoga are essentially one. He who perceives that really sees. (5.5)

Commentary:

Formerly, the Samkhyas were higher than the yogis because the Samkhyas became proficient in yoga and also charted the mystic terrain. They mastered both yoga practice and mystic insight. In modern times, however, many who pass as Samkhyas are not yogis at all. They pretend to be higher than the yogis, but in reality, they cannot be higher because they lack accurate mystic insight gained by yoga practice. They do have theoretical understanding, but abuse the ideas by propagating them without being proficient in yoga. Many of these pretender Samkhyas write commentaries on the *Bhagavad Gītā*, even some commentaries which are rated as standard text in a disciplic succession. Thus many people who read their literature become imprinted with wrong views about the *Gītā*.

The reason why the level obtained by the ancient Samkhya experts is also reached by the yogis is this: The Samkhyas already had yoga proficiency. The yogis, when they gain more proficiency, will find it necessary to acquire insights about the mystic and spiritual terrains. They will be students of the mystically-experienced Samkhyas who charted the subtle, causal and spiritual territories.

Then, Samkhya and yoga are essentially one, with yoga being the preliminary stage and insightful Samkhya being the advanced level occurring after the yogi becomes proficient. Thus as Śrī Krishna said, the person who perceives that really sees.

संन्यासस्तु महाबाहो
दुःखमाप्तुमयोगतः ।
योगयुक्तो मुनिर्ब्रह्म
नचिरेणाधिगच्छति ॥५.६॥
saṁnyāsastu mahābāho
duḥkhamāptumayogataḥ
yogayukto munirbrahma
nacireṇādhigacchati (5.6)

saṁnyāsaḥ — renunciation of opportunity; tu — indeed; mahābāho — O mighty man; duḥkham — difficulty; āptum — to obtain; ayogataḥ — without yoga—proficiency; yogayukto = yogayuktaḥ — yoga—proficient; munir = muniḥ — sage; brahma — spiritual level; nacireṇādhigacchati = nacirena — in no span of time + adhigacchati — reaches

Renunciation of opportunities is difficult to attain without yoga practice, O mighty man. In the nick of time, a yoga—proficient sage reaches the spiritual plane. (5.6)

Commentary:

Sannyasa nowadays means taking a special mantra and assuming preaching responsibilities. In the time of Śrī Krishna, sannyasa meant that, as a preliminary qualification, one had to be proficient in yoga practice. Nowadays yoga is shunned in some spiritual societies which award the sannyasa order to serious applicants. Times changed.

Arjuna wanted to renounce the opportunities presented to him by providence. Śrī Krishna very tactfully told Arjuna that the requirement for taking up sannyasa is a previous proficiency in yoga practice, not fear of a battle or cowardice in the face of having to discipline relatives on the warfield. In other words, we should not take sannyasa because we fear cultural involvements. Sannyasa is not for the man who is running away from responsibilities for women and children, nor is it for a man who hates women or who fears them because of the sexual energies which become impulsive in their association. Sannyasa is part of a maturity and advancement in yoga practice. In the nick of time, a yoga-proficient sage reaches the spiritual plane by his assumption of sannyasa because he and only he gets the waiver from cultural activity. As such his spiritual progress is sure and steady.

योगयुक्तो विशुद्धात्मा
विजितात्मा जितेन्द्रियः ।
सर्वभूतात्मभूतात्मा
कुर्वन्नपि न लिप्यते ॥५.७॥
yogayukto viśuddhātmā
vijitātmā jitendriyaḥ
sarvabhūtātmabhūtātmā
kurvannapi na lipyate (5.7)

yogayukto = yogayuktaḥ — one proficient in yoga; viśuddhātmā — one of purified self; vijitātmā — one who is self—controlled; jitendriyaḥ — one who has conquered his senses; sarvabhūtātmabhūtātmā = sarva – all + bhūta — being + ātma – self + bhūta – being + ātmā — self (sarvabhūtātmabhūtātmā — one who feels related to all beings); kurvan – acting; api — even; na — not; lipyate — is implicated

A person who is proficient in yoga, whose soul is purified, who is self—controlled, who conquered his senses, whose self feels related to all beings, is not implicated when acting. (5.7)

Commentary:

Even though these requirements are very hard to attain, many persons rate themselves to this verse. First, one must be proficient in yoga practice. This does not mean yoga practice in the past life. It means in the present, just as Arjuna and even Śrī Krishna were when this discourse occured. Second, one must have performed sufficient psychological austerities to have purified the subtle and causal forms and have controlled his psyche to the greatest degree. He should have already conquered his senses by the pratyāhār 5th step in yoga practice. His self should feel related to all beings. Then if such a person acts, he is not implicated culturally. Even though he remains tangled in worldly affairs, still, somehow he is not implicated in such a way as to tag him for follow—up existences in which he would have to accept haphazard transmigrations.

Śrī Krishna mentioned this to rid Arjuna of the fear of implication in the cultural field and to stress that an escape into the sannyasa order would carry even more hazards for a person who is unproficient in yoga practice, who has not mastered himself and has not served in the mission of the Supervising Universal Lord.

In these verses, Śrī Krishna systematically destroyed the idea that a man gets an exemption from cultural acts and becomes liberated just by taking the renounced order of life. Unless he possesses the yoga proficiency and especially unless he has the waiver from cultural acts, given to him by Śrī Krishna, he cannot become liberated. He would only acquire the disapproval of the Supervising Universal Lord.

नैव किंचित्करोमीति
युक्तो मन्येत तत्त्ववित् ।
पश्यञ्शृण्वन्स्पृशञ्जिघ्रन्न्
अश्नन्गाच्छन्स्वपञ्श्वसन् ॥५.८॥
naiva kiṁcitkaromīti
yukto manyeta tattvavit
paśyañśṛṇvanspṛśañjighrann
aśnangacchansvapañśvasan (5.8)

naiva = na — not + eva — indeed; kiṁcit— anything; karomīti = karomi — initiate + iti — thus; yukto = yuktaḥ — proficient in yoga; manyeta — he thinks; tattvavit — knower of reality; paśyañśṛṇvan = paśyan — seeing + śṛṇvan — hearing; spṛśañjighrann = spṛśan — touching + jighran — smelling; aśnan — eating; gacchan — walking; svapañśvasan = svapan — sleeping + śvasan — breathing

"I do not initiate anything." Being proficient in yoga, this is what the knower of reality thinks. While seeing, hearing, touching, smelling, eating, walking, sleeping and breathing, (5.8)

Commentary:

The knower of reality must be in such a state of mind, through yoga proficiency, not just by imagination or by belief or by hearing of it from another. He should see directly into reality to the extent of seeing that he does not initiate anything.

प्रलपन्विसृजन्गृह्णन्
उन्मिषन्निमिषन्नपि ।
इन्द्रियाणीन्द्रियार्थेषु
वर्तन्त इति धारयन् ॥५.९॥
pralapanvisṛjangṛhṇann
unmiṣannimiṣannapi
indriyāṇīndriyārtheṣu
vartanta iti dhārayan (5.9)

pralapan — talking; visṛjan — evacuating; gṛhṇan — holding; unmiṣan — opening the eyelids; nimiṣan — closing the eyelids; api — also; indriyāṇīndriyārtheṣu = indriyāṇi – senses + indriyārtheṣu — in the attractive objects; vartanta — interlock; iti — thus; dhārayan — considers

...while talking, evacuating, holding, opening and closing the eyelids, he considers, "The senses are interlocked with the attractive objects." (5.9)

Commentary:

This perception of the knower of reality, the tattvavit, is continuous for him. It is not a superimposition of what he reasoned or what his spiritual master told him in a convincing lecture. This is why Śrī Krishna used the term tattvavit. Tattva means the real state or true condition of something. In the Samkhya philosophy, these are itemized, beginning with the highest principles of the Supreme Spirit and ending with the lowest which are the solid materials.

To understand this intellectually and not to see it mystically does not constitute what it takes to be a tattvavit. When one reaches a stage where he has the mystic vision to perceive realities through his supercharged subtle body or directly by spiritual perception, while seeing, hearing, touching, smelling, eating, walking, sleeping, breathing, talking, evacuating, holding, opening and closing the eyelids, he will consider on the basis of direct perception, that his senses are interlocked with attractive objects.

ब्रह्मण्याधाय कर्माणि
सङ्गं त्यक्त्वा करोति यः ।
लिप्यते न स पापेन
पद्मपत्रमिवाम्भसा ॥५.१०॥
brahmaṇyādhāya karmāṇi
saṅgaṁ tyaktvā karoti yaḥ
lipyate na sa pāpena
padmapatramivāmbhasā (5.10)

brahmaṇy = brahmaṇi — on the spiritual level; ādhāya — putting on, focused on; karmāṇi — actions; saṅgaṁ — attachment; tyaktvā — having discarded; karoti — he acts; yaḥ — who; lipyate — affected; na — not; sa = saḥ — he; pāpena — by necessary violence; padmapatram = padma – lotus + patram — leaf; ivāmbhasā = iva — just as + ambhasā — by water

Being focused on the spiritual level, discarding attachments, his acts are not defiled by necessary violence, just as a lotus leaf is not affected by water. (5.10)

Commentary:

Such a person by his own vision, not by hearsay, will naturally discard attachments, because he sees the usual vision of the interlocking senses and objects. His actions would not be defiled, even by necessary violence as Arjuna is induced to commit on the warfield. He would then remain uncontaminated just as a lotus leaf does not soak up a liquid which is poured over it.

कायेन मनसा बुद्ध्या
केवलैरिन्द्रियैरपि ।
योगिनः कर्म कुर्वन्ति
सङ्गं त्यक्त्वात्मशुद्धये ॥५.११॥
kāyena manasā buddhyā
kevalairindriyairapi
yoginaḥ karma kurvanti
saṅgaṁ tyaktvātmaśuddhaye (5.11)

kāyena — with the body; manasā — with the mind; buddhyā — with the intellect; kevalair = kevalaiḥ — alone; indriyair = indriyaiḥ — by the senses; api — even; yoginaḥ — yogis; karma — cultural activity; kurvanti — they perform; saṅgaṁ — attachment; tyaktvā — having discarded; 'tmaśuddhaye = ātmaśuddhaye = ātma — self + śuddhaye — towards purification

With the body, mind and intellect, or even with the senses alone, the yogis, having discarded attachment, perform cultural acts for self—purification. (5.11)

Commentary:

This verse is of special interest to us as kriyā yogis. It is one of the few verses in which the term ātmaśuddhaye occurs. One other such verse is number 12 of Chapter Six. Kriyā yoga concerns this ātmaśuddhaye or purification of the ātma, except in this case, the word ātma means the psyche of the spirit.

As a general term, ātma means the spirit itself but in the purificatory actions the spirit is exempt. It has a psychic system which must be purified. Kriyā yoga specializes in such purity.

What we hear from Lord Krishna is very interesting. He said that the yogis, having discarded attachment, perform cultural acts for self purification. This means that so long as we do not have an exemption from Him, we must perform cultural activities or otherwise be baffled in some way or the other.

As capable mystics, the advanced yogis act with their body, mind, intellect or even with their senses alone or with all these combined. They do so for self purification. Thus a person cannot take sannyasa in the true sense unless he has purified himself sufficiently by the performance of detached cultural acts.

युक्तः कर्मफलं त्यक्त्वा
शान्तिमाप्नोति नैष्ठिकीम् ।
अयुक्तः कामकारेण
फले सक्तो निबध्यते ॥५.१२॥
yuktaḥ karmaphalaṁ tyaktvā
śāntimāpnoti naiṣṭhikīm
ayuktaḥ kāmakāreṇa
phale sakto nibadhyate (5.12)

yuktaḥ — proficient in yoga; karmaphalaṁ — reward of cultural activity; tyaktvā — having abandoned; śāntim — peace; āpnoti — obtains; naiṣṭhikīm — steady; ayuktaḥ — a person not proficient in yoga; kāmakāreṇa — by action which is motivated by desire; phale — in result; sakto = saktaḥ — attached; nibadhyate — is bound

The person who is proficient in yoga, and who abandons the rewards of cultural activity, obtains steady peace. The person who is not proficient in yoga, being attached to results, is bound by desire—motivated action. (5.12)

Commentary:

Those proficient in yoga respond differently to life's circumstances because they are situated in direct mystic perception. They are not acting merely on the basis of what is heard. Their psyche, especially the emotional part of it, is purified. They perform like robots just doing what is suggested by the Supervising Universal Lord. They are not bound by desire—motivated actions.

सर्वकर्माणि मनसा
संन्यस्यास्ते सुखं वशी ।
नवद्वारे पुरे देही
नैव कुर्वन्न कारयन् ॥५.१३॥
sarvakarmāṇi manasā
saṁnyasyāste sukhaṁ vaśī
navadvāre pure dehī
naiva kurvanna kārayan (5.13)

sarvakarmāṇi = sarva — all + karmāṇi — actions; manasā — with the mind; saṁnyasyāste = saṁnyasy (saṁnyasi) — renouncing + āste — he sits; sukhaṁ — happily; vaśī — director; navadvāre = nava – nine + dvāre — in the gate; pure — in the city; dehī — the embodied soul; naiva = na — not + eva — indeed; kurvan — acting; na — nor; kārayan — causing activity

Renouncing all action with the mind, the embodied soul resides happily within as the director in the nine—gated city, neither acting or causing activity. (5.13)

Commentary:

So long as we regard ourselves as performers, such a state of mind is inconceivable to us. We already feel that we are directors but we are possessed with the urge to direct what occurs externally. Śrī Krishna mentioned us as directors of the subtle organs of the psyche. Such organs are the intellect, mind, sensual energy and life force. However to be such a director, one must link with the Supervising Universal Lord and gain His approval for one's activities.

The nine-gated city is the combination of the physical and subtle forms. These comprise the living physical form with its nine openings of the two eyes, two ears, two nostrils, one mouth, one genital and one anus. Both in the liberated and conditioned states, the spirit does not act or cause activity. In the conditioned state, the spirit somehow or another becomes impressed with the idea that he is a performer; in the liberated state, by virtue of direct mystic perception, the spirit sees the actual motivators.

न कर्तृत्वं न कर्माणि
लोकस्य सृजति प्रभुः ।
न कर्मफलसंयोगं
स्वभावस्तु प्रवर्तते ॥५.१४॥
na kartṛtvaṁ na karmāṇi
lokasya sṛjati prabhuḥ
na karmaphalasaṁyogaṁ
svabhāvastu pravartate (5.14)

na — not; kartṛtvaṁ — means of action; na — nor; karmāṇi — actions; lokasya — of the creatures; sṛjati — he creates; prabhuḥ — the Lord; na — nor; karmaphalasaṁyogaṁ = karma – action + phala — consequence + saṁyogaṁ — cyclic connection; svabhāvaḥ — inherent nature; tu — but; pravartate — it causes

The Lord does not create the means of action, or the actions of the creatures, or the action—consequence cycle. The inherent nature causes this. (5.14)

Commentary:

This statement is useful only to kriyā yogis and not to ordinary religionists and believers who follow the general paths of religion which bear a belief in God as the ultimate creator of everything. Here Śrī Krishna plainly states that the Supreme Lord does not create the means for action, the various creature forms and the materials used in completing actions. Neither does He create the actions Himself, nor the action—consequence cycle which perpetually manifests through material nature and in it, on the gross and subtle planes of this existence. Śrī Krishna states that the inherent nature (svabhāva) does this.

What therefore is this inherent nature?

Some translators of the *Bhagavad Gītā* seem to think that the word prabhu in this verse pertains to the limited spirit who uses a particular body. In the next verse, such meaning proves faulty since the term vibhuh means the Almighty God and not any limited being. Prabhu cannot mean the limited spirit because realistically, he cannot be the producer of the world or of his own actions, since he is motivated by the subtle psychology which presses on him from all sides.

What is the inherent nature?

It is the nature of the energies involved in an activity. Everything has potency. Everything will exhibit expression and potential if given opportunity. In that sense everything is reactive. Everything is electric. All the various inherent natures are themselves the causes of the various activities. The Supreme Lord is for the most part, a by-stander in terms of gross, subtle and supersubtle mundane displays of creativity.

Kriyā yoga concerns itself with svabhāva of the soul itself by discovering the inherent nature (svabhāva) of the psyche. When through such mystic inquiry within the nature, one sorts his subtle energies, the subtle instruments and the spirit, then he reaches the stage of knowing that the inherent nature of everything is what causes activity. At that point one assumes the attitude of a sannyasi, one of complete detachment from the various gross and subtle materials. This all occurs on the mystic plane after one develops prāṇa vision and other types of mystic perception by the practice of haṭha yoga and prāṇāyāma.

नादत्ते कस्यचित्पापं
न चैव सुकृतं विभुः ।
अज्ञानेनावृतं ज्ञानं
तेन मुह्यन्ति जन्तवः ॥५.१५॥

nādatte = na — not + ādatte — perceives; kasyacit — of anyone; pāpaṁ — evil consequence; na — not; caiva = ca — and + eva — indeed; sukṛtaṁ — good reaction; vibhuḥ — the Almighty God; ajñānenāvṛtaṁ = ajñānena —

nādatte kasyacitpāpaṁ
na caiva sukṛtaṁ vibhuḥ
ajñānenāvṛtaṁ jñānaṁ
tena muhyanti jantavaḥ (5.15)

by ignorance + avṛtam — shrouded; jñānaṁ — knowledge; tena — through which; muhyanti — they are deluded; jantavaḥ — the people

The Almighty God does not receive from anyone, an evil consequence or a good reaction. The knowledge of this is shrouded by ignorance through which the people are deluded. (5.15)

Commentary:

This statement and the one in the previous verse verifies conclusively that one cannot develop a relationship with the Supreme Personality through the material energies. This is because the Supreme Being receives neither evil consequences nor a dividends. Thus the idea of being saved by God through His acceptance of our sins or through the acceptance of such sins by His agents, is an unreasonable proposition.

Now since the Supreme Person will not receive (nādatte) anything mundane, then how can we develop a relationship with Him to upgrade our status? Essentially, everything mundane remains with the mundane or stated differently, whatever portion of mundane energy we utilize can only be returned to the general pool of mundane force which is in existence. We cannot at any stage transport what is mundane into a purely spiritual situation. Thus it is factual, even from the scientific angle, that we cannot give to the Supreme Being something mundane.

The shrouding action (avṛtam) of material nature causes our intellect to perceive incorrectly. Thus we formulate many untrue views, especially about religion and about our relationship with God. These views are then publicized by our spiritual leaders and internalized by us. In this wayward manner, we become frustrated in the bid for heaven, life after life.

A yogi carefully and steadily frees himself from the systems of belief which are unsubstantiated by mystic vision. He sees through the purified intellect which is calibrated by the performance of haṭha yoga and prāṇāyāma, along with the advanced stages of yoga which are pratyāhār sense withdrawal, dhāraṇa concentration of subtle phenomenon and dhyāna contemplation on the supersubtle causal and spiritual realities and samādhi trance through which one is transported away from this mundane situation in all its aspects.

As by using only the human body, a human being sees clearly the material world before him, so the mystic yogi after having perfected prāṇāyāma and pratyāhār sense withdrawal sees through the subtle existence, and then through the causal and spiritual environments, which appear dark and void to others, even to believers in God.

No one can bargain with God for the redemption of pious credits generated in this world. Such credits have a value here on social and cultural levels, but God has no use for such financial or cultural assets. We may bargain with other limited beings or we may under God's supervision, utilise others and ourselves in the social, cultural and political fields. Still, when all is said and done, God has only superficial interest in this.

It means, therefore, that a kriyā yogi must become serious about turning away from the mundane world. Why should the yogi invest anymore in this world, if in fact God has no concerns here and if the concerns which God expresses here are cosmetic? With what is God concerned? In what world, does God pursue relationships? What is God's social status in that world?

ज्ञानेन तु तदज्ञानं
येषां नाशितमात्मनः ।
तेषामादित्यवज्ज्ञानं
प्रकाशयति तत्परम् ॥५.१६॥
jñānena tu tadajñānaṁ
yeṣāṁ nāśitamātmanaḥ
teṣāmādityavajjñānaṁ
prakāśayati tatparam (5.16)

jñānena — by experience; tu — however; tad — this; ajñānaṁ — ignorance; yeṣāṁ — of whom; nāśitam — removed; ātmanaḥ — of the self; teṣām — of them; ādityavaj = ādityavat — like the sun; jñānam — revelation; prakāśayati — causes to appear; tat – that; param — Supreme Truth (explained in two previous verses)

However, for those, in whose souls the ignorance is removed by experience, that revelation will cause the Supreme Truth to appear distinctly like the sun. (5.16)

Commentary:

With help from the Supreme Being, the individual living entity who is discontent with material existence, must evaluate his position, in an relationship with material nature, take hints from the Supreme being on how to erase that relationship, and then apply the divine advices for deliverance. He must work out his salvation. It will not occur by the Supreme Being's absorption of his sins or anything like that. The limited entity has to resolve his relationship with material nature by a careful application of austerities which counteract the hypnotic influence of material nature's hold on him. He must apply these himself as he is shown by the Supreme Being, His ultimate benefactor.

तद्बुद्धयस्तदात्मानस्
तन्निष्ठास्तत्परायणाः ।
गच्छन्त्यपुनरावृत्तिं
ज्ञाननिर्धूतकल्मषाः ॥५.१७॥
tadbuddhayastadātmānas
tanniṣṭhāstatparāyaṇāḥ
gacchantyapunarāvṛttiṁ
jñānanirdhūtakalmaṣāḥ (5.17)

tadbuddhayaḥ — those whose intellects are situated in that supreme truth; tadātmānaḥ — those whose spirits are focused on that Supreme Truth; tanniṣṭhāḥ — those whose reference is that supreme truth; tatparāyaṇāḥ — those who aspire to that supreme truth as the highest reality; gacchanty (gacchanti) — go + apunar – never again + āvṛttim — rebirth; jñana — experience + nirdhūta — removed + kalmaṣāḥ — faults

Those whose intellects are situated in that Supreme Truth, whose souls are focused on it, whose basic reference is that, whose faults are removed by the experience, who aspire to that as the highest reality, never go again to rebirth. (5.17)

Commentary:

This process of removing our faults by viewing the transcendence takes time. It is not part of a superstition nor part of a magical event occurring after meeting a guru or an adept of the kriyā path. Admittedly, we do have miraculous conversions in the kriyā system. And we do as neophyte yogis have elevating experiences from time to time, but the nature of the path is such that permanent gains come from consistent practice. Some practice for a long time before establishing that permanence. Others do so after only a short period. Regardless, it takes practice. We do not ascribe to radical experiences which change us for all time, since even when there are such experiences, we encounter relapses into old patterns.

In addition, our fallen condition is sufficient evidence that we can end up in a lower state at a future time. Thus we strive for the permanent aspects of elevation which come from individual practice. What we want from a yogi guru is the strength to maintain a consistent practice, for by that, all attainments will surely come, and they will come then in a permanent way.

For a yogi to directly see that the Supreme Being assume none of our sinful reactions or pious merits, his intellect must be capable of mystic insight. He must also see, visually, who does the handling. This means that he must have attained a very high mystic sensitivity by virtue of a firm and consistent yoga practice.

Śrī Krishna mentioned removal of the faults of the yogi. This means removing the fault of wrong perception whereby one sees, thinks or feels strongly that the Supreme Being creates the means of actions, the actions, and the action-consequence cycle. By such false thinking one rationalizes mentally or emotionally that the Supreme Lord would accept either our sins or credits. Such thinking is totally erroneous. Even though most religions flourish on such false thinking, it cannot lead to liberation from mundane conditioning.

The means of action are the various tools and materials used for manifestation of desires. These tools and materials are subtle and gross objects. In elementary religion,common belief is that God created these faculties. Actually these objects come about naturally by the proximity of both God and the limited spirits who eagerly contribute their attention for utilization of the objects.

Material nature is so responsive to the existential proximity of the spirits, that it is unnecessary for God to directly create the subtle and gross objects. The spirits have their own power. As soon as they are conscious in any surroundings or environment, they begin to act automatically, even without divine supervision.

The actions themselves do not come from the spirits but are motivated by the very superfine and subtle material energy called chitta in Sanskrit. This energy naturally links itself to the spirits and causes them to endorse whatever it motivates.

Some feel that God supervises the action—consequence cycle. Some statements of God, of Krishna, confirm this, but other statements of Krishna equally deny this. What, therefore, is the truth? Is it that material nature as a reactive, contained whole force, has within her potential, the ability to bear full consequential responsibility, for this creation, with or without God's supervision. Whatever is stirred up by the conjunction of the spirits and the super-subtle material nature, can and will be quelled or quieted by that same force sometime later.

As kriyā yogis, we need to reach a stage where we no longer see the Lord as the creator of actions. We should cease thinking and feeling that we can exchange our sins or credits for something from Him. It is simply not possible, except as a belief. God is just not concerned with it. Even though some lower divine beings may have expressed concern or may have said that God is, still He is not concerned. We must find another way to relate to Him. It cannot be a relationship on the basis of what we did in the subtle or gross mundane creations. The inherent nature (svabhāva) of the materials is the very same thing that causes the action-consequence cycle. A personal agent is unnecessary to distribute reactions for good or bad deeds. Admittedly there are personal agents involved, but more or less, these are not really necessary.

The Supreme Lord as He states here is not really involved. The belief in the necessity of an agent was denied by Śrī Krishna when He told His foster father, Nanda Gopa, that the Indra Devata, the supernatural person regulating rainfall, can only regulate it on the basis of the action and reaction equation and not independently. It all hinges on the inherent nature of the materials involved. Some of these materials are gross matter, some are subtle matter and some are supersubtle. In all cases, their inherent nature is the actual perimeter.

As kriyā yogis we want to escape of the action-consequence cycle, by removing ourselves or causing ourselves to be removed from it, not by appealing to God to take our pious credits or to remove from us the sinful reactions. We want to shift away from this faulty psychology which conditions us to think that God creates this mundane situation. Such a faulty vision naturally stops us from having the true relationship with God.

To avoid rebirth after using a physical body, one must be stationed in the Supreme Truth, before the time of death of that form. One cannot go to the Supreme Truth at the time of death, simply by being in a certain society and following its doctrines or worshiping its teacher or teachers and their favored Deity, even if such a Deity is Śrī Krishna. For not going again to rebirth, one should adjust the texture of one's consciousness such that one experiences the Supreme Truth while using a physical form. One's reference of consciousness must be the Supreme Truth by virtue of continuous mystic experience with that reality.

It is neither a matter of belief nor a system of theology or siddhanta. Such a siddhanta or an expounded theory of religion, does not situate one in the Supreme Truth even though it may facilitate the theoretical understanding of such truth, making one believe that such an understanding is the Supreme Truth itself. One must master the three higher states of yoga which are dhāraṇa mystic focus, dhyāna mystic contemplation and samādhi mystic trances, to decouple from all that pertains to this level of existence. Then, one can use psychic energies to develop the direct spiritual perception.

Those who do not do this will definitely go again for rebirth, regardless of whether they want to or not and regardless of whether they hoped to go to the spiritual places or not. They will again return to this world to be devotees of Krishna or to be whatever they were or whatever they desired to be in their past life. They will again leave a material body, lose their objective awareness and then again be drawn into a woman's body for formulating a baby form. They will gain focus in this world and use this world as the medium for theoretical understanding of the Supreme Truth, just as before. And they will more than likely, again forget their past birth. Thus they will be unable to realize what mistakes they made in the last birth and will, of necessity, assume the old dispositions.

विद्याविनयसंपन्ने
ब्राह्मणे गवि हस्तिनि ।
शुनि चैव श्वपाके च
पण्डिताः समदर्शिनः ॥५.१८॥
vidyāvinayasaṁpanne
brāhmaṇe gavi hastini
śuni caiva śvapāke ca
paṇḍitāḥ samadarśinaḥ (5.18)

vidyāvinayasaṁpanne = vidyā — learning + vinaya — trained + saṁpanne — accomplished; brāhmaṇe — in a brahmin; gavi — in a cow; hastini — in an elephant; śuni — in a dog; caiva = ca — and + eva — indeed; śvapāke — in a dog—flesh eater; ca — and; paṇḍitāḥ — scripturally—conversant mystic seers; samadarśinaḥ = sama – common factor + darśinaḥ — observing

In a learned, trained, accomplished brahmin, in a cow, an elephant, a dog, or a dog-flesh eater, the scripturally-conversant mystic seers observe a common factor. (5.18)

Commentary:

According to tradition in the time of Lord Krishna, a brahmin, had to be born in the family of an already recognized brahmin, whose family tree was traceable to a brahmin rishi, son of Lord Brahmā. Recently, some missionaries claimed that Śrī Krishna was unprejudiced in terms of caste and that a verse like this one, applies to a person who has brahmin qualities but who may not have been born in a brahmin family. Such opinions bear no weight even though some disciplic authorities relay them. Śrī Krishna spoke directly of the brahmin caste.

Śrī Krishna is certainly not prejudiced but in this verse He is using the traditional meaning. We must remember also that Śrī Krishna incited Arjuna to stick to his caste as a warrior and not to conveniently shift to the brahmin status. Yogic training is peculiar to the brahmin caste, because only they are permitted, by the Vedic tradition, to pursue the kind of lifestyle required for on-going successful yoga practice with exemption from the political, mercantile and servile realms. Arjuna had some of this yogic training in his youth and, later on, in his early manhood before the battle of Kurukṣetra, before the *Gītā* discourse. Still Śrī Krishna insisted that Arjuna use the emotional maturity acquired from yoga practice and complete his political duties as a warrior. Arjuna had to remain in his caste.

This verse applies to a person who is born in a brahmin family and who in addition, has the learning, training and accomplishment to substantiate his priestly and counseling authority. Here we talk of a person who got a brahmin body by birth, a body genetically formed from parents whose bodies came from a family line of caste brahmins. Here we discuss a spirit who picked up such a body by birth as contrasted to picking up a body with political, mercantile or servile tendencies. One who picked up a brahmin body, one who is learned, trained and accomplished, having been trained by his parents and by other brahmin-body people, and one who by that training performed activities that illustrate ideal brahmin qualities, is described in this verse.

This does not debar someone who picked up a lower body, one with political, mercantile or servile inclination. Such a person can change the body to make it have brahminical inclination but it would first require specific purificatory disciplines in the gross and subtle dimensions. He would require more than just learning, training and the resultant accomplishments which come from the ensuing practice. He would require reformation or change of his body's natural tendencies. Since reformation is not mentioned in this verse, it pertains specifically to a caste brahmin or a person who gets a body from parents who already have the brahminical qualities and whose physical genetic structure causes their babies to exhibit brahminical tendencies.

As kriyā yogis, we are not supportive of persons who believe in the brahmin caste to the extent that they feel that only persons who took birth from brahmin bodies can have brahminical qualities. All the same, we do not underrate such brahmin genetic bodies which have the brahmin tendency and which would make progression on the spiritual path easier for anyone who has or who gets such a body. Our view should be that regardless of the type of body a person takes, if he wants to make spiritual progress he can do so, provided he performs the austerities that apply to his case.

For instance, I took up a servile (shudra) body, which is practically, the lowest kind of human birth except for the body of an aborigine who has no education and is only trained in basic forest survival. This body came from a mother who had mercantile and secretarial skills and from a father who was a maritime navigator but who was an alcoholic for many years. Such a body is definitely not a brahmin form. However I took steps to reform the body. I had a greater degree of success in causing it to exhibit brahmin traits. Since this body did not get the education, training and resulting accomplishment in its youth, because it was not produced in that sort of environment, it lacked much. Some brahminical qualities filtered into this body from the subtle form which has those traits. This happened because of the reformatory steps taken and by some behavioral training given to this body by a grandparent.

Śrī Krishna stressed the learned, trained and accomplished caste brahmin as the higher species of life in the material setting, because such a body would exhibit the highest qualities consistently. A person like the writer for instance, who reformed his lower body such that it mostly behave like a brahmin, will by virtue of the power of material nature, revert to a lower behavior from time to time. In comparison with someone who has a caste brahmin form, which was educated, trained and accomplished, the writer's body would still be in a lower category, despite the additional reformatory disciplines (yoga kriyās) performed.

The point of this verse is that a scripturally-conversant mystic seer observes a common factor in the highest human body, in the cow, a very gentle creature, in the dog, a sometimes vicious animal, or in a dog-flesh eater, the lowest of human beings.

What is that common factor? How does the mystic seer perceive the similarity?

We can see that Śrī Krishna recognized the advantages and relative values of the various creature forms, as well as a special common factor which He did not define in this verse.

इहैव तैर्जितः सर्गो
येषां साम्ये स्थितं मनः ।
निर्दोषं हि समं ब्रह्म
तस्माद्ब्रह्मणि ते स्थिताः ॥५.१९॥
ihaiva tairjitaḥ sargo
yeṣāṁ sāmye sthitaṁ manaḥ
nirdoṣaṁ hi samaṁ brahma
tasmādbrahmaṇi te sthitāḥ (5.19)

ihaiva = iha — here in this world + iva (eva) — indeed; tair = taiḥ — by those; jitaḥ — conquered; sargo = sargaḥ — birth; yeṣāṁ — of whom; sāmye — in impartiality; sthitaṁ — established; manaḥ — mind; nirdoṣaṁ — faultless; hi — indeed; samaṁ — equally disposed; brahma — pure spirit; tasmāt — therefore; brahmaṇi — on the pure spiritual plane; te — they; sthitāḥ — established

Here in this world, birth is conquered by those whose minds are established in impartiality. Indeed, pure spirit is faultless and equally disposed. Therefore they are established on the pure spiritual plane. (5.19)

Commentary:

This impartiality deals with what is mentioned in the previous verse, the removal of one's psychology of the prejudices of various species of life. Each species has prejudices which give it certain advantages and disadvantages. As a spirit transmigrates among the species, he does so through the facility of a subtle body which houses or carries the various prejudices. In each subtle form, there are dispositions accumulated, embedded there for expression in the mundane existence.

In yoga by the grace of advanced teachers, we come to understand philosophically, and to actually perceive mystically that beyond the subtle body, there is the causal form which is filled with chitta, a very subtle energy. This subtle energy is the foundation of material existence. From this potency the subtle body is derived. Thus in the advanced stages one makes the endeavor to get away from the motivational force of emotions, which drives a spirit on and on in material existence.

The impartiality (samye) acquired by an advanced yogi allows him to see that each of the spirits inhabits one species or the other, assuming the advantages and disadvantages that accompany the particular subtle and gross forms. Seeing this on the mystic plane is not the same as reading about it in a book like this commentary. Seeing it is a mystic act that occurs after one performs the pertinent austerities in haţha yoga and prāṇāyāma, after mastering Kuṇḍalinī yoga and being far advanced in celibacy.

The vision of it causes one to desist from the struggle for existence and to work for the elimination of the subtle form and then the elimination of the chitta body, the causal form. Since the individual yogi must work for this all by himself, with the help of more advanced yogis, he cannot attain it merely by hearing. In fact the subtle and supersubtle mundane energies do not leave a living being who traverses the general paths of religion. They only desist if the individual applies himself effectively in the kriyā yoga.

This impartiality gives the yogi the advantage of not envying anyone in any lower or higher species of life. The yogi understands that the various disparities occur on the basis of preset conditions of material nature and preset positions in the spiritual existences. Thus he no longer resents anything. He abandons resentments and moves on to understand his relationship with material nature and with the divine beings. Once he sees his relationship, he realizes that his vision is somewhat clear, but not fully clarified, and so he applies himself to higher yoga. This is done under the directions of Lord Shiva who may instruct directly or may arrange for an advanced yogi to teach it.

The reason why Śrī Krishna, said that birth is conquered by those yogis who see the common factor in the highest, median or lowest species is this: Only such a yogi can become convinced to work hard in austerities for the stoppage of birth. Others will be unwilling to endeavor that much for freedom from these births. They will be prejudiced to various advantages and disadvantages which they have became familiar with in previous transmigrations.

These persons who are reluctant to perform the required austerities may or may not be devotees of Krishna, or may or may not be believers in a Supreme God. Those who hear of this and who become satisfied hearing of it to the extent that they do not feel the need to take up the austerities for clarity of mystic vision, will not attain freedom from birth but will become religious leaders, and will exploit others who seek this information.

It is interesting that Lord Śrī Krishna did not use the word ātma in this verse. He used the technical word, brahma, a word used repeatedly in the *Upanishads*. The technicality is this: The word ātma has negative connotations, indicating something that is transcendental but still has a contradictory bias towards material nature, while the word brahma has no such connotations.

Undoubtedly it is an enigma, a puzzle, as to how and why the ātma or individual spirit has a bias towards material nature and is therefore prejudiced against pure spirit or brahma. To show a distinction between the ātma and the brahma, the ātma is tagged as being a jiva or a limited spirit, which may be conditioned or influenced by its affiliation with the emotional material nature.

The *Upanishads* are famous for mantras which literally command the jiva, the individual spirit, to be the brahma or to be identical with the brahma and to give up all other association. The *Upanishads* command the spirit to be faultless and equally disposed just as Śrī Krishna stated in these verses. Thus the Upanishad gives out a mantra which states: You are that (pure spirit). Tat twam asi.

To become established in this way, the spirit must abandon or otherwise move its leaning in the direction of material nature. It must eliminate its need to absorb the advantages of those species of life to which it was introduced, over the millions and millions of years it was involved with material nature. Such an undertaking, of course, is a very fatiguing course for a living being. Thus, as it is laid out in the *Upanishads*, the goal of spiritual emancipation seems very impersonal and abstract.

This is because the spirit, as he is conditioned in material existence, is not accustomed to pure spirit or to the absolute detachment from the subtle material nature. Therefore he assumes that such a course is one of impersonalism. He feels that if he abandoned the emotional happiness present in material nature, he would strip himself of personality and all that it represents in the form of relationships with other conditioned and semi-conditioned beings.

To offset this fear of losing these relationships, the evolution of scriptures occurs naturally, as a movement from the *Upanishads* to the *Puranas* in which many stories about relationships with divine beings are described in great detail. While in the *Upanishads*, these relationships are not stressed and are hardly mentioned, in the *Puranas* they come on with full force and illustration. Thus people enjoy the Puranic episodes about easy liberation. They hope and believe that by the grace of God, they will be freed without any strenuous endeavor on their part.

Undoubtedly, a person who cannot yet mystically perceive that the spirits are harnessed to various psychic equipments which they use and which are powered both by their energy and by the cosmic emotions, cannot be free from these births. Mere belief in God will not free anyone from these births. Each spirit, if he requires such freedom, must work for it by super-psychological means.

Of course not every spirit works equally as hard for it. Some because of divine status and the releasing power which that gives them, will attain it without much endeavor. Hpwever, most ordinary spirits will have to endeavor by strenuous mystic means.

न प्रहृष्येत्प्रियं प्राप्य
नोद्विजेत्प्राप्य चाप्रियम् ।
स्थिरबुद्धिरसंमूढो
ब्रह्मविद्ब्रह्मणि स्थितः ॥५.२०॥
na prahṛṣyetpriyaṁ prāpya
nodvijetprāpya cāpriyam
sthirabuddhirasaṁmūḍho
brahmavidbrahmaṇi sthitaḥ (5.20)

na — not; prahṛṣyet — should become excited; priyaṁ — dear item or favorable circumstance; prāpya — having attained; na — no + udvijet — should detest; prāpya — having obtained; ca — and + apriyam — something unpleasant; sthira – stable; buddhiḥ — intelligent; asammūḍhaḥ — without confusion; brahmavid — a person who continually experiences the spiritual reality; brahmaṇi — on the spiritual plane; sthitaḥ — situated

Having attained a desired item or favorable circumstance, a person should not become excited. Having attained something unpleasant, he should not detest it. With stable intelligence, without confusion, a person who continually experiences the spiritual reality, remains situated on the spiritual plane. (5.20)

Commentary:

Śrī Krishna hinted at how we reach the level of attachment from the advantages and disadvantages of the various species of life. In other words, each of us has certain innate biases and prejudices acquired over millions upon millions of transmigrations. These have formed into dispositions that we carry in our subtle and causal forms, the elimination of which can be attained by steady practice of yoga as described by the Blessed Lord.

These are only hints. The actual method consists of more than just hearing and conceiving of what was heard. We just heard of it. From that, concepts of freedom will form but these will not free us. What are the actual methods for release?

So, when Arjuna presented his reasoning for not wanting to fight, those views were drummed up by his inner prejudices. Śrī Krishna destroyed Arjuna's confidence in that psychology by showing that what Arjuna said was not part of the reality, even though it was a concept in Arjuna's mind.

Śrī Krishna, briefly described the actual course of spirituality. Such a brief description is merely an overview. It does not have all details required for practice. Still some commentators and their followers have run with these sketches as if they acquired the whole course by hearing of it.

Some of the practice is given. For example, when one has a desired item or favorable circumstance, one should train to not become excited. But suppose in training oneself, one gets excited nonetheless, then what next? In kriyā yoga that happens initially. One hears of it as we hear in this verse, then one practices, and finds that he still becomes excited. Then one understands that he is not of the lucky few who apply the forceful dampening of the excitation once and for all. One realizes that one's inner nature must be transformed by some other method.

Śrī Krishna said that a person, seeing an end to the births should not become excited over desired or favorable items, but what happens if he does become excited repeatedly? What is the process for practice then? That person must realize that his nature is contrary to the higher development of eliminating the need of these births. How can one reach a state where his psychology desires an item dearly, and then he the spirit, remains unexcited nevertheless?

As it is unnatural not to become excited over something desired, so it is unusual not to detest that which is unpleasant. For the consistent practice of this, our psychology would have to be changed. It is insufficient to hear and to then pressure ourselves not to react or respond. We need a change of nature, a change of tendency for a permanent dispassion.

Stable intelligence or sthirabuddhir is a stable sensing organ in the subtle body, not just a state of stable understanding. The kriyā yogi mystically perceives the buddhi organ in the brain of the subtle form. Others merely think that it is their understanding, their analyzing faculty. When by practice of higher yoga, the yogi can stabilize his buddhi organ, then he continually experiences the supersubtle reality and becomes situated on the mystic plane. From there he attains higher perception of the causal and spiritual situations.

बाह्यस्पर्शेष्वसक्तात्मा
विन्दत्यात्मनि यत्सुखम् ।
स ब्रह्मयोगयुक्तात्मा
सुखमक्षयमश्नुते ॥५.२१॥
bāhyasparśeṣvasaktātmā
vindatyātmani yatsukham
sa brahmayogayuktātmā
sukhamakṣayamaśnute (5.21)

bāhya – external; sparśeṣv (sparśeṣu) — sensation; asakta – not attachéd; ātmā — soul; vindatyātmani = (vindati) — finds + ātmani — in the spirit; yat — who; sukham — happiness; sa = saḥ — he; brahmayogayuktātmā = brahma – spiritual plane + yoga — yoga process; yukta – linked + ātmā — spirit; sukham — happiness; akṣayam — non—fluctuating; aśnute — makes contact with

The person who is not attached to the external sensations, who finds happiness in the spirit, whose spirit is linked to the spiritual plane through yoga process, makes contact with the non-fluctuating happiness. (5.21)

Commentary:

Here again, the kriyā yogi must distinguish between the realization that comes from hearing or reading and mystic vision that comes from yoga practice. A kriyā yogi should not be satisfied with mere hearing or reading. He should not allow anyone to convince him that merely by hearing he will attain all vision in spiritual life.

After hearing that one will find happiness in the spirit by not being attached to the external sensation, a religious person may assume a discipline whereby he detaches himself immediately, whenever placed in a situation that generates attachments. This is the accomplishment from hearing. However in kriyā yoga, we want to practice beyond that stage, so that we perform psychological actions, which cause us not to be attached to external sensation. In other words, the austerities prompt a change in nature, so that we lose the urge for attachments.

In this verse Śrī Krishna mentioned brahma yoga. He refers to the yoga practice which takes a spirit to the brahman plane of existence. By this process the spirit genuinely turns away from the material situation and focuses itself on the spiritual plane through a mystic yoga process. If successful, the yogi forsakes the material happiness and the items and feelings which yield that. He takes to the plane of non-fluctuating happiness, a level of existence which is omnipresent but not always perceived by a limited spirit.

ये हि संस्पर्शजा भोगा
दुःखयोनय एव ते ।
आद्यन्तवन्तः कौन्तेय
न तेषु रमते बुधः ॥५.२२॥
ye hi saṁsparśajā bhogā
duḥkhayonaya eva te
ādyantavantaḥ kaunteya
na teṣu ramate budhaḥ (5.22)

ye — which; hi — indeed; saṁsparśajā — coming from sensual contact; bhogā — pleasures; duḥkhayonaya = duḥkha — pain + yonayaḥ — sources; eva — indeed; te — they; ādyantavantaḥ = ādy (ādi) — beginning + anta — ending + vantaḥ — possessed with; kaunteya — O son of Kuntī; na — never; teṣu — in them; ramate — delights; budhaḥ — a wise person

The pleasures that come from sensual contact are sources of pain. They have a beginning and ending, O son of Kuntī. A wise person never delights in them. (5.22)

Commentary:

At first one hears this type of instruction either from Śrī Krishna in the *Bhagavad Gītā*, or from a realized soul or his spokesman. A person can realize this and not even know it was expressed by Śrī Krishna long ago. One usually hears a truth like this and then tries to implement its meaning into one's life by philosophical analysis and by trying to stop the psyche from enjoying. This awkward discipline is not kriyā yoga. It is only a step towards the kriyā path. After one takes that step and repeatedly practices it, he comes to the conclusion that the mere hearing of these truths and the implementation of awkward haphazard disciplines on the self are ineffective because still the psyche does not rid itself of the tendency to enjoy what will be painful later. One then begins to look for the kriyā path.

Such a search for a teacher of kriyā yoga is usually futile. This is because there are so few kriyā masters using physical bodies. Instead of finding such a master, one finds many pretenders who, somehow or the other, acquire small or large followings and who are publicized as deliverers of fallen souls.

After sitting at the feet of such pretenders serving them getting any lasting results, finding that one's nature always reverts back to its pleasure-seeking ways, one at last begins to study one's own nature and then one locates a genuine teacher. As soon as a person begins to study his nature, and as soon as he realizes that problems originate from his own deficiencies, then a kriyā teacher is made available to him.

Conversely, sometimes without looking for a kriyā teacher one gets the association of one. This is due to a past life connection with the kriyā path or due to a twist of fate. Those with the past life connection, practice immediately after meeting the teacher; the others associate but do not practice. They hear about the path when others who are serious of it ask the teacher questions in their presence. They enjoy a social or even a casual relationship with the teacher but still they are not attracted to the kriyā path. They take the teacher for granted as a friend, lover, associate or relative according to the particular relationship providence affords.

It is interesting that, in this verse, Śrī Krishna made such an outlandish statement, telling us that the pleasures that come from sensual contact (samsparśajā) are sources of pain. What exactly does Krishna say here? Does He mean all the pleasure that comes from sensual contact? The Sanskrit word sparśa means touch or feeling. This would imply that all sensual contact leads to suffering. O what a statement!

Was Śrī Krishna also implying that since Arjuna allowed his psyche to range over the soldiers on the war field, suffering was the inevitable result of such sensual contact, a suffering which Arjuna felt when he broke down in tears and could no longer hold weapons. Śrī Krishna said that a budhah, a truly wise person, does not delight in such pain-yielding sensual contact.

शक्नोतीहैव यः सोढुं
प्राक्शरीरविमोक्षणात् ।
कामक्रोधोद्भवं वेगं
स युक्तः स सुखी नरः ॥५.२३॥
śaknotīhaiva yaḥ soḍhuṁ
prākśarīravimokṣaṇāt
kāmakrodhodbhavaṁ vegaṁ
sa yuktaḥ sa sukhī naraḥ (5.23)

śaknotīhaiva = śaknoti — can + iha – here on earth + iva (eva) — indeed; yaḥ — who; soḍhuṁ — to endure; prāk — before; śarīravimokṣaṇāt = śarīra — body + vimokṣaṇāt — from leaving; kāmakrodhodbhavaṁ = kāma — craving + krodha — anger + udbhavaṁ — basis; vegaṁ — impulsion; sa = saḥ — he; yuktaḥ — discipline; sa = saḥ — he; sukhī — happy; naraḥ — human being

The person who, before leaving the body, endures the craving—based, anger—based impulsions, is disciplined. He is a happy human being. (5.23)

Commentary:

Before practicing kriyā yoga and becoming successful at it, one practices this suggestion of Śrī Krishna, by remaining stationed at the same place in the psyche and just bearing on with the craving-based, anger-based impulsions. Yet, in doing this, one becomes not a happy human being but simply an austere one.

When in kriyā yoga practice, one learns how to shift from the lower plane where the craving-based, anger-based impulsions are formulated and when one shifts to a plane where one sees that the promised pleasure leads to responsibility which is psychological pain, then one takes more shelter in the higher plane and after prolonged practice, one exhibits the happiness described in this verse. Initially one becomes sober.

From soberness, one goes to the higher plane of spiritual security, where one is not threatened or ravished by material nature. All this must be accomplished before the death of the material body. This is not a promised state of salvation. It is the experience of the spiritual world and the supersubtle material landscapes. The person who accomplished this, has shifted from the mundane plane and experienced the subtle and supersubtle worlds and then the spiritual plane.

योऽन्तःसुखोऽन्तरारामस्
तथान्तर्ज्योतिरेव यः ।
स योगी ब्रह्मनिर्वाणं
ब्रह्मभूतोऽधिगच्छति ॥५.२४॥
yo'ntaḥsukho'ntarārāmas
tathāntarjyotireva yaḥ
sa yogī brahmanirvāṇaṁ
brahmabhūto
'dhigacchati (5.24)

yo = yaḥ — who; 'ntaḥsukho = antahsukhaḥ — he who is happy within; 'ntarārāmas = antarārāmas — he who is spiritually delighted; tathāntarjyotir (tathāntarjyotiḥ) = tathā — as a result + antarjyotiḥ — he who has brilliant consciousness within; eva — indeed; yaḥ — who; sa = saḥ — he; yogī — yogi; brahmanirvāṇaṁ — stoppage of disturbing sensuality and attainment of constant spirituality; brahmabhūto = brahmabhūtaḥ — absorption on the spiritual plane; 'dhigacchati = adhigacchati — he attains

The person who is happy within, who is spiritually delighted and as a result, experiences the brilliant consciousness, he, that yogi, experiences the stoppage of disturbing sensuality and attains constant spirituality in absorption on the spiritual plane. (5.24)

Commentary:

The brilliant consciousness, antar jyotih, is not a state of mind or pleasure. It is not just knowing that one is a devotee of Śrī Krishna, or that one can be happy because of divine association. This antar jyotih is a light seen within the psyche when the eyes are closed. It is a bright sheer luminescence. This comes about by deep meditation from much practice in the four higher states of yoga, which are pratyāhār sense withdrawal, dhāraṇa focus of the subtle power, dhyāna contemplation on the faculties of the subtle body and samādhi trance states which project a particular spirit out of this gross existence and lock him into higher levels.

The brilliant consciousness, antar jyotih, is experienced only after all disturbing aspects of sensuality and mentality are stopped, or as Śrī Patañjali said after the vrittis or mental movements cease.

When this happens, a luminescent light takes over the psyche, or so it seems. The spirit withdraws from the mundane level completely. All thoughts of religious chants and other religious symbols cease. It happens after his mentality and sensuality are quieted, away from all negative and positive impressions gained in this world, in the religious and irreligious way.

A kriyā yogi after striving for some time and often in the wrong way, becomes frustrated. Gradually with the help of advanced yogis whom he meets physically and in the astral dimensions, he gets on the right track and strives in the right way. This requires isolation. He must protect himself from those religious people who think that chanting holy names and viewing God's deity forms, is the total path of spirituality. These people discourage a deeper spiritual practice. These influences retard progression. In their association, one will never experience the antar jyotih (brilliant consciousness).

Some people think that by rattling off the name of God and by going to see the Deity dressed attractively and colorfully in the temple, they will have completed the spiritual course, and by that method, reach the place of Krishna, the kingdom of God. They are not interested in this antar jyotih (brilliant consciousness). Some of them regard it as impersonal. Others feel that it will be attained by them in the course of their services to the guru, temple and organizations to which they are affiliated.

For kriyā yoga, these belief systems are insufficient. We want to have that antar jyotih in real terms. Śrī Krishna, if He felt that we would get this brilliant consciousness by any other means, like chanting His holy names, or seeing His deity form, would have told us so in this verse. This antar jyotih (brilliant consciousness) comes from self purification, which is the aim of personal yoga practice. It may seem to be neophyte to those who feel that they have already attained the lotus feet of Śrī Krishna, but even so, it is the genuine first step in the process of attaining spiritual visions. The person described in this verse, the neophyte yogi who is just making some progress in higher yoga, does, as Śrī Krishna states, experience the stoppage of the disturbing sensuality and attains constant spirituality in absorption on the spiritual plane. There is no doubt about it. His focus shifts off the mundane plane of life, and all that pertains to religion on this plane now becomes irrelevant for him. Others, however, who are not as advanced try to engage him in religious services. They try to re-indoctrinate him and drag him to their religious services, which to them, are the ultimate spiritual discipline.

According to actions of providence, a neophyte yogi must sometimes cooperate with the enemies of yogis, and other times he is freed from them by providence. Then he runs away, takes isolation and secretly makes firm progress so that he can reach a place where the disturbing sensuality ceases as Patañjali indicated when he said that the vrittis must be totally curtailed for the summation of yoga. It is a great relief when such a neophyte yogi sits to meditate and then all thoughts stop for him, because he shifts off to a level where the thoughts cannot manifest, where they do not arise. He perceives only the sheer antar-jyotih, brilliant luminescent spiritual consciousness.

A neophyte yogi may seriously work with his psyche for hours on end, day after day, trying to figure out why the disturbing sensuality cannot be lifted or removed and why he cannot shift himself into the antar-jyotih luminescence; it is because of associating with religious and irreligious non-yogis.

लभन्ते ब्रह्मनिर्वाणम्
ऋषयः क्षीणकल्मषाः ।
छिन्नद्वैधा यतात्मानः
सर्वभूतहिते रताः ॥५.२५॥
labhante brahmanirvāṇam
ṛṣayaḥ kṣīṇakalmaṣāḥ
chinnadvaidhā yatātmānaḥ
sarvabhūtahite ratāḥ (5.25)

labhante — they attain; brahmanirvāṇaṁ — cessation of material existence and a simultaneous absorption in spirituality; ṛṣayaḥ — the seers; kṣīṇakalmaṣāḥ = kṣīṇa – terminates + kalmaṣāḥ — sins, faults; chinnadvaidhā = chinna — removed + dvaidhā — doubts; yatātmānaḥ = yata – restrained + ātmānaḥ — souls; sarvabhūtahite = sarva – all + bhūta — creatures + hite — in welfare; ratāḥ — joy

Those seers whose sins and faults are terminated, whose doubts are removed, whose souls are restrained, who find joy in the welfare of the creatures, attain a cessation of their material existence and a simultaneous absorption in spirituality. (5.25)

Commentary:

The seers, the rsayah, are not just devotees of Śrī Krishna, nor are they pure devotees of Krishna as the term pure devotee is usually defined in the modem era. These seers are yogi ascetics who attained the antar-jyotih brilliant consciousness, such that when they close their eyes, they can escape from the plane of thinking and enter into the luminescence and perceive supernaturally and spiritually.

Such yogis may or may not be devotees of Śrī Krishna. What qualifies them is their attainment of that mastership and not their devotee or non-devotee status. For such people, their sins and faults are terminated or are being drastically reduced, for it is only if one's sins and faults are terminated or are near terminated, that one can get the exemption from the disturbing sensuality (brahma nirvāṇam).

The removal of faults of the psychology (kṣiṇakalmaṣāh) is attained only by austerities in kriyā yoga. Other methods do a cosmetic service by removing the faults for the time being and then allowing them to be asserted again at a future time with greater force. It is a mystic technique that causes the removal of the faults since these faults come into the subtle body by virtue of pressure applied from the causal plane.

The removal of faults comes on by yoga practice, otherwise the faults leave and then return again and again. Consistent yoga practice, especially mastership of prāṇāyāma and application of a tight pratyāhār sensual energy withdrawal, is removes the faults in the psychology. That and nothing else works.

Śrī Krishna spoke of the removal of doubts. These are doubts about the effectiveness of the kriyā process and the fear of taking it up seriously. One is pressured by relatives and friends and even religious people and by devotees of the same Śrī Krishna, to look away from the eightfold process of yoga. In such association one develops doubts about yoga, especially about the slowness of its results and about the time and effort it will take to be successful. When such doubts are removed, the neophyte makes steady efforts and thus wards off the resistance that discouraged practice.

The result of all this is the cessation of one's material existence and a simultaneous absorption in spirituality, the very same thing that one's friends and relatives fear. They do not want any of their associates to be that serious about spiritual life. They do not like the idea of nirvāṇa, which means nir or not having anything to do with the material world or its superficial religions.

कामक्रोधवियुक्तानां
यतीनां यतचेतसाम् ।
अभितो ब्रह्मनिर्वाणं
वर्तते विदितात्मनाम् ॥५.२६॥
kāmakrodhaviyuktānāṁ
yatīnāṁ yatacetasām
abhito brahmanirvāṇaṁ
vartate viditātmanām (5.26)

kāmakrodhaviyuktānāṁ = kāma — desire + krodha — anger + viyuktānāṁ — of the separation from; yatīnāṁ — of the ascetics; yatacetasām — of those whose thinking is restrained; abhito = abhitaḥ — very close; brahmanirvāṇaṁ — cessation of material existence, assumption of enlightened spirituality; vartate — it is; viditātmanām — of those who understand the spiritual self

The cessation of material existence and assumption of enlightened spirituality is soon to be attained by those ascetics whose thinking is restrained, who understand the spiritual self and are seperated from desire and anger. (5.26)

Commentary:

This describes what is experienced at the beginning of the higher stages of kriyā yoga. At that point one's thinking is restrained. This means all thinking, including topics of devotional books, religious books and even philosophical topics, even thinking of the subject matters covered here in the *Gītā*. There is a time for learning from a teacher; then one has to practice. It is the practice that brings results. Invariably, what one learned is incorrect but one finds this only by practice. This is because one either learns from a teacher who was partially successful and who only knows the path to some extent, or one has a very experienced teacher but misunderstands him by virtue of having an imperfect mind. All this is cleared up only by practice whereby the faulty ideas are discovered.

After sufficient practice and sufficient reform and correction, one functions correctly. Then and only then, one's thinking becomes totally restrained. At this point, one sees the antar-jyotih (brilliant consciousness). Day after day according to the length of practice of seeing this, one develops an understanding of the spiritual self and becomes familiar with mystic geography so that one can shift to and locate that plane of spirituality, anytime one sits to meditate. As soon as the practicing yogi shifts back to this world to perform here socially or culturally or even religiously, he partially breaks his connection with the spiritual plane.

However, since he has a method of shifting back, if he does not get too involved in the social, cultural and religious physical world, he can shift over again when given the authority. Otherwise he has to work again to clean up his psychology before he can cross over again.

As soon as he shifts over to this side, the side we are accustomed to, he loses sight of the brilliant consciousness, but once he effectively shifts away from our side, he again returns to the brilliant consciousness. Thus until he can acquire a waiver from the Supreme Being, for non-participation in karma yoga, he will be shifting back and forth repeatedly. Anytime he returns to the social setting and becomes involved, he will lose touch for the time being, even though he may remember experiences in the antar-jyotih (brilliance consciousness).

The thinking is not restrained by mere stoppage of thinking, but rather by being in a certain position in reference to the buddhi organ which is the thinking compartment mechanism. From certain positions and only from those positions, mostly in the center of the head of the subtle body, the yogi can cause the buddhi organ not to carry out thinking or picturing operations. When this is done, the buddhi organ develops the ability to see, feel and be affected by the brilliant consciousness.

स्पर्शान्कृत्वा बहिर्बाह्यांश्
चक्षुश्चैवान्तरे भ्रुवोः ।
प्राणापानौ समौ कृत्वा
नासाभ्यन्तरचारिणौ ॥५.२७॥
sparśānkṛtvā bahirbāhyāṁś
cakṣuścaivāntare bhruvoḥ
prāṇāpānau samau kṛtvā
nāsābhyantaracāriṇau (5.27)

sparśān — sensual contact; kṛtvā — having done; bahir = bahiḥ — external; bāhyāṁś = bāhyān — excluded; cakṣuścaivāntare = cakṣuś — visual focus + ca — and = eva — indeed + antare — in between; bhruvoḥ — of the two eyebrows; prāṇāpānau — both inhalation and exhalation; samau — in balance; kṛtvā — having made; nāsābhyantaracāriṇau = nāsa – nose + abhyantara — within + cāriṇau — moving

Excluding the external sensual contacts, and fixing the visual focus between the eyebrows, putting the inhalation and exhalation in balance, moving through the nose, (5.27)

Commentary:

This is a primary goal in kriyā yoga practice. One must put himself, his pin-point identity, into such a position within the psyche that he can do this practice. This involves prāṇāyāma which is mentioned by Śrī Krishna as prāṇāpānau samau kṛtvā.

The relationship between the breath movement and the mind is that the movement of prāṇa in the subtle body causes the mind to lock and unlock its focus. This locking and unlocking action keeps the self fluctuating in reference to the mind. One objective in kriyā yoga is to keep the mind in conformity to the self. That is the exact opposite of the natural relationship of dependence of the self on the mind's mechanism. By mind, I mean the mind and its contents which are the buddhi organ and the related energies which affect its operation and calibration.

This Chapter Five is the curriculum of elementary kriyā yoga. Very few of readers of the *Bhagavad Gītā*, those in a disciplic succession from Śrī Krishna and those out of it, realize this. Generally, one cannot recognize kriyā yoga instructions, if one did not practice or has not practiced kriyā yoga recently in the present life. Usually a practice from a former life does not give one the updated recall required to recognize these directions for kriyā yoga.

Why did Śrī Krishna mention this locational technique to Arjuna at a time when Arjuna could not practice as the yogis do, and at a time when Śrī Krishna Himself discouraged Arjuna from going into isolation for yoga expertise? This is a good question. We must keep in mind however that both Śrī Krishna and Arjuna did perform these techniques successfully previously, before the battle encounter at Kurukṣetra. Thus in a sense, this is for Arjuna, a refresher course for Arjuna to recall what he recently mastered in kriyā practice.

The exclusion of the external sensual contacts (sparśān kṛtvā bahir bāhyāmś), when done to perfection, highlights for the yogi, the perfection of the 5th and 6th stages of yoga practice. These are pratyāhār sensual contact withdrawal and stoppage, and dhāraṇa inner attentive capture and focus. These are very advanced practices. One has to move beyond Deity worship which is considered by some as the ultimate advancement.

Even though Śrī Krishna, as well as divine people like Śrī Balarāma and Lord Shiva have manifested Themselves in Deity forms, still, in order to meet Them on the spiritual or transcendental side, one must forsake Their mundane manifestations. When this is done, then one can practice the final steps of yoga, in order to leave this zone and meet Them in Their spiritual locales. Deity worship which is the highlight of externally focused devotees, is itself preliminary in advanced yoga practice.

Those who feel that they will progress directly from Deity worship in this world to transcendental service in the spiritual world, do miscalculate. They will only come back into this world, because they failed to lift their focus from this side of existence. They failed the test indicated in this verse, about excluding the external sensual-contact including external sensual contacts with the Lord's manifestation on this side of existence.

One has to lift the mind from such contacts and focus through the supernatural openings which are found in the buddhi intellect organ in the head of the subtle body.

Śrī Krishna said that it is the visual focus, (cakṣus) which must be focused between the eyebrows. I give information from practical experience.

First of all the visual focus is a thing in itself. It is not the same as the soul's focus. Those two aspects are completely different. The soul's focus of his attentive power may be superimposed into the visual focus or into any other type of focus like touching, tasting and feeling. The soul's attentive focus is not an aspect of the buddhi organ but it is the singular sense of the ahankar (sense of initiative). When the soul's attentive force is unified with any other focus, the soul perceives through that sense, and the five sensual focuses are aspects of the buddhi intellect organ. It is the visual sense specifically that is cultivated in this practice of kriyā yoga which is given by Śrī Krishna is this verse.

Śrī Bābāji Mahasaya, a master kriyā yogi who uses a yoga siddha body, told me that in conjunction to this, a yogi who has difficulty curbing the visual sense, may use the naad continuous frequency sound which is usually heard in the vicinity of the right ear, as an anchor point from which to lock on to the visual sense when that is manifested by the buddhi organ.

The balancing of the inhalation and exhalation as these move through the airway, is a process that is given by many meditation teachers. They have their peculiar ways of explaining it. Essentially it is a subtle procedure, but it begins with physical practice. If the in-and-out breaths are not in balance, the mind does not settle down for meditation, and therefore higher meditation becomes impossible.

Some teachers say that one can easily transcend the restless mind and meditate but such an appraisal of the mind and its influence is an underestimation of our dependent relationship on the movements of the mind. Śrī Patañjali in his *Yoga Sūtras* alerted us that yoga success actually means a stoppage of the adjustments of the mind. That indicates that for yoga success, we must have an effective means of stopping the various types of natural operations of the mind. It cannot be otherwise as some teachers convincingly state.

The exclusion of sensual contacts does not mean that one excludes these only while meditating but also while acting in the world. One must be very detached and not allow the objects encountered to make too strong of an imprint or register on the mind, otherwise one will be unable to meditate effectively since the mind will, by its very nature, replay the strong impressions created in the form of imaginations, thinking, visual and sound effects like a television set.

The animation of the various impressions in the mind must be stopped entirely for successful yoga practice, exactly as Śrī Patañjali, the mahāyogī, suggested in his *Yoga Sūtras*.

यतेन्द्रियमनोबुद्धिर्
मुनिर्मोक्षपरायणः ।
विगतेच्छाभयक्रोधो
यः सदा मुक्त एव सः ॥५.२८॥
yatendriyamanobuddhir
munirmokṣaparāyaṇaḥ
vigatecchābhayakrodho
yaḥ sadā mukta eva saḥ (5.28)

yatendriyamanobuddhir = yata — controlled + indriya — sensual energy + mano (manah) — mind + buddhiḥ — intelligence; munir = muniḥ — wise person; mokṣaparāyaṇaḥ — one who is dedicated to achieving liberation; vigatecchābhayakrodho = vigata — gone away + icchā — desire + bhaya — fear + krodho (krodhaḥ) — anger; yaḥ — who; sadā — always; mukta — liberated; eva — indeed; saḥ — he

...the wise man, who is dedicated to achieving liberation, whose sensual energy, mind and intellect are controlled, whose desire, fear and anger are gone, is liberated always. (5.28)

Commentary:

Mokṣaparāyaṇah is the person who is dedicated (parāyaṇah) to liberation (mokṣa). This person sees that as the objective. Please notice that Śrī Krishna does not dislike this person. He does not deride this person or try to divert this person to bhakti yoga or devotion to Himself. Only such a person will want to go through the austerities of kriyā yoga and such a person may or may not be a devotee of Śrī Krishna.

The various living entities possess different aspirations. One has to know what he wants and one should strive to achieve that only.

Regardless of what this teacher says or that teacher says and regardless of the lineage which such persons advocate or represent, Śrī Krishna said that to be liberated always one must have the following qualifications:

- ✓ Being dedicated to achieving liberation as defined in this chapter by the methods given in this chapter (mokṣaparāyaṇah).
- ✓ Controlling the sensual energy, mind and intellect (yata).
- ✓ Eliminating desire, fear and anger (vigata).

भोक्तारं यज्ञतपसां
सर्वलोकमहेश्वरम् ।
सुहृदं सर्वभूतानां
ज्ञात्वा मां शान्तिमृच्छति ॥५.२९॥
bhoktāraṁ yajñatapasāṁ
sarvalokamaheśvaram
suhṛdaṁ sarvabhūtānāṁ
jñātvā māṁ śāntimṛcchati (5.29)

bhoktāraṁ — enjoyer; yajñatapasāṁ — of the religious ceremonies and austerities; sarvalokamaheśvaram = sarva – all entire + loka — world + maheśvaram — Supreme God; suhṛdaṁ — friend; sarvabhūtānāṁ — of all creatures; jñātvā — recognizing; māṁ — me; śāntim — spiritual peace; ṛcchati — attains

Recognizing Me, as the enjoyer of religious ceremonies and austerities, the Supreme God of the entire world, the friend of all creatures, he attains spiritual peace. (5.29)

Commentary:

This is a portrayal of the successful kriyā yogi who is a devotee of Lord Krishna. A kriyā yogi may attain everything that was listed in verses 17 through 28, provided he qualifies by the standards given in the respective verses. If, in addition to this, he recognizes Lord Krishna as the enjoyer of religious ceremonies and austerities, and as the Supreme God of the entire world, as well as the friend of the creatures, then he attains spiritual peace. As portrayed here, Śrī Krishna is the approving factor in this world.

CHAPTER 6

Yoga Practice*

श्रीभगवानुवाच
अनाश्रितः कर्मफलं
कार्यं कर्म करोति यः ।
स संन्यासी च योगी च
न निरग्निर्न चाक्रियः ॥६.१॥
śrībhagavānuvāca
anāśritaḥ karmaphalaṁ
kāryaṁ karma karoti yaḥ
sa saṁnyāsī ca yogī ca
na niragnirna cākriyaḥ (6.1)

śrī bhagavān — the Blessed Lord; uvāca — said; anāśritaḥ — not relying on; karmaphalaṁ — result of an action; kāryaṁ — obligation; karma — action; karoti — he fulfills; yaḥ — who; sa = saḥ — he; saṁnyāsī — renouncer; ca — and; yogī — yogi; ca — and; na — not; niragnir = niragniḥ — without a fire ceremony; na — nor; cākriyaḥ = ca — and + akriyaḥ — lacking physical activities

The Blessed Lord said: A person who fulfills obligatory action, without depending on the result of the action, is a renouncer and a yogi, not the one who is without a fire ceremony or who lacks physical activity. (6.1).

Commentary:

A person who avoids obligatory actions and uses yoga as an excuse to side-step social involvement, will not be successful in the practice. He will be bothered by vibrations which come from his neglect of duty. On the other hand, a person who takes up the obligations and who practices yoga in his spare time, will be successful on two fronts: both in yoga practice and in cultural duties. His yoga progress will be slow, but he will efficiently complete cultural duties. If he has a skillful teacher, who can advise him, he will perform the duties in a terminal way, so as to gradually, but surely, end his material existence. That will result in increased time for yoga practice, which will make his practice rapid and effective over a period of time.

Yoga practice cannot be an excuse to avoid mandatory social duties which come upon the yogi and which are endorsed by the Supreme Being, by Krishna. If a yogi avoids such duties, then we can know for sure that his yoga practice will not bear fruitful results. The case of Arjuna is clear: He wanted to move away from socio-political duties but Śrī Krishna would have none of it. Śrī Krishna insisted that Arjuna use his emotionally-hardened nature, gained from yoga practice, and apply himself in the performance of duties in the Kuru civil war.

As Śrī Krishna did not excuse his dear friend Arjuna, so it is hardly likely that he will excuse any of us. We have to complete the duties to His satisfaction so that ultimately He may grant the exemption from such duties. Then, we may get into a full time practice. In the meantime, we can use any spare time to master techniques given to us by advanced teachers of the craft.

**The Mahābhārata contains no chapter headings. This title was assigned by the translator on the basis of verse 12 of this chapter.*

Śrī Krishna, in this verse, banished any fool-hardy ideas we might have about renunciation. A person is not renounced merely because he has no physical activity or because he does not participate in religious rituals. Renunciation is more of a psychological attitude. It is best demonstrated when we see a person who consistently fulfills obligatory action without depending upon or being motivated by the desired results of such activity.

It is the psychological stance of renunciation that denotes a true renunciate, not just what he does or does not do physically.

यं संन्यासमिति प्राहुर्
योगं तं विद्धि पाण्डव ।
न ह्यसंन्यस्तसंकल्पो
योगी भवति कश्चन ॥६.२॥
yaṁ saṁnyāsamiti prāhur
yogaṁ taṁ viddhi pāṇḍava
na hyasaṁnyastasaṁkalpo
yogī bhavati kaścana (6.2)

yaṁ — that which; saṁnyāsam — renunciation; iti — thus; prāhur = prāhuḥ — the authorities define; yogaṁ — applied yoga; taṁ — it; viddhi — know; pāṇḍava — Arjuna Pandava; na — not; hy = hi — indeed; asaṁnyastasaṁkalpo = (asaṁnyastasaṁkalpaḥ) = asaṁnyasta — without renunciation + saṁkalpaḥ — intention; yogī — yogi; bhavati — becomes; kaścana — anyone

That which the authorities define as renunciation, know it as applied yoga, O Arjuna Pandava. Indeed, no one becomes a yogi without an intention for renunciation. (6.2)

Commentary:

The authorities mentioned here are the Upanishad sages. These persons became famous either as theistic yogis, ritualistic yogis or as philosophical yogis.

Renunciation, Śrī Krishna said, is actually applied yoga. In other words, renunciation is a psychological stance gained after perfecting yoga to a greater degree whereby one is freed from having to respond to the pleasures and pains of material existence, as well as to gains and losses.

Indeed, Śrī Krishna said, no one becomes a yogi without intention for renunciation. In other words, no one can persist in yoga practice unless he or she is motivated for renunciation. The desire or intention (sankalpa) for renunciation is itself the motivation which makes a person take up and persist with the rigors and regiments of yoga. All the same, there are many persons who gain recognition as sannyasis, but who do not perform yoga and who have absolutely no intention of doing so. Some of these abhor yoga and think that it is unnecessary, but they do feel that one should have a detached psychology. In the time of Śrī Krishna, however, being a yogi implied having a drive for renunciation, and being known as a renunciant indicated that one was proficient in yoga.

आरुरुक्षोर्मुनेर्योगं
कर्म कारणमुच्यते ।
योगारूढस्य तस्यैव
शमः कारणमुच्यते ॥६.३॥
ārurukṣormuneryogaṁ
karma kāraṇamucyate
yogārūḍhasya tasyaiva
śamaḥ kāraṇamucyate (6.3)

ārurukṣor = ārurukṣoḥ — of one who strives; muner = muneḥ — of a philosophical man; yogaṁ — yoga expertise; karma — cultural activity; kāraṇam — the means; ucyate — it is remembered; yogārūḍhasya — of one who mastered yoga; tasyaiva = tasya — of him + iva (eva) — indeed; śamaḥ — tranquil method; kāraṇam — the means; ucyate — it is remembered

For a philosophical man who strives for yoga expertise, cultural activity is recommended. For one who has mastered yoga already, the tranquil reserved method is the means. (6.3)

Commentary:

This is a contrasting description of a beginner yogi and an advanced one. Basically, the advanced one has a waiver from the Supreme Being, from Śrī Krishna Himself, such that the advanced yogi does not have to fulfill cultural obligations. He is exempt from such involvement.

The beginner has no such waiver. He should, in fact he must, take up cultural duties in earnest but in such a mood as to complete them in a terminal way. Other people who are not kriyā yogis also take up cultural activity but they perform in such a way as to expand their involvements and to create bases for more sociology.

There is another technicality. The advanced yogi who is presently fitted into a beginner's role, must also complete cultural duties, because for one reason or the other, he is now stuck down on the material plane, and must, by providence, work for a new waiver. Even though this yogi was perfected in a past life or in many past lives, for one reason or the other, he again came down into gross manifestation and became involved. Somehow whatever waiver he earned before, was retracted by the Supreme Being.

Again, that yogi must work to get out of the material world. However, this beginner who is actually an advanced yogi in his subtle body, will get out of the material world quickly, because in his subtle and causal forms, he carries a blueprint for the grand escape. By instinct he knows how to satisfy the Supreme Being by doing the assigned duties. His sudden and abrupt release from this existence is guaranteed.

It is interesting that in this verse Lord Krishna left aside those who are not philosophical. Actually this is consistent with the Upanishadic attitude, for the sages of that era stressed philosophy, particularly the Samkhya philosophy which was mentioned by Śrī Krishna in Chapter Three:

śrībhagavānuvāca
loke'smindvividhā niṣṭhā purā proktā mayānagha
jñānayogena sāṁkhyānāṁ karmayogena yoginām (3.3)

The Blessed Lord said: In the physical world, a two-fold standard was previously taught by Me. O Arjuna, my good man. This was mind regulation by the yoga practice of the Sāṁkhya philosophical yogis and the action regulation by the yoga practice of the non-philosophical yogis. (3.3)

Basically what Śrī Krishna stated is that persons who are not philosophically inclined, who are not munis, will not take to renunciation and thus, even if they take up yoga practice, they will not have a strong motive for perfecting it. As such, they will, more than likely not progress to the advanced stage.

If however, a person has a philosophical outlook, and if in addition, he strives for yoga expertise, he is advised to perform cultural activities. When however one masters yoga, one naturally gets the waiver from the Supreme Being and thus the tranquil reserved method, which consists of the three last stages of yoga, is the means.

Śrī Krishna informed that Arjuna, despite his philosophical nature was a beginner at the cultural application of yoga . Arjuna should take up cultural activity. And perhaps later on, when Arjuna mastered the higher stage of yoga, he would acquire the divine waiver and take up the higher states of yoga without having to be culturally involved. This does not mean that a neophyte may not practice the advanced stages, but if he practices in earnest and advances rapidly, he will still have to participate culturally. He should not take to the tranquil reserved method just to avoid assigned duties. He may practice higher yoga in his spare time only. There should be no attempt to use it to side-step or avoid assigned duties.

यदा हि नेन्द्रियार्थेषु
न कर्मस्वनुषज्जते ।
सर्वसंकल्पसंन्यासी
योगारूढस्तदोच्यते ॥ ६.४ ॥
yadā hi nendriyārtheṣu
na karmasvanuṣajjate
sarvasaṁkalpasaṁnyāsī
yogārūḍhastadocyate (6.4)

yadā — when; hi — indeed; nendriyārtheṣu = na — not + indriyārtheṣu — in attractive objects; na — not; karmasv = karmasu — in performance; anuṣajjate — feels attached; sarvasaṁkalpasaṁnyāsī = sarvasaṁkalpa — all motivations + saṁnyāsī — discarding; yogārūḍhas — proficient in yoga practice; tadocyate = tada — then + ucyate — it is said

Indeed, when having discarded all motivations, a person feels no attachment to attractive objects or to performance, he is said to be proficient in yoga practice. (6.4)

Commentary:

Sarva sankalpa means all motivations or all intentions for exploiting material existence. When having discarded all such intentions by the required purity, and when in actuality a person feels no attachment to attractive objects in this world or to the performance, then he is said to be proficient in yoga (yogārūḍhas).

There are many, many motivations in the nature of a living being. These come from the chitta (subtle emotional energy) in the causal form. That causal form is actually the root source of the material existence. This chitta, super-subtle pranic energy, trickles into the subtle body and, from there, activates our gross and subtle forms for fulfillments. It utilizes the life force, intellect and sense of initiative (ahankāra) in the struggle against other living beings and against any opposing forces launched by material nature at large.

These motivations are subdued to an extent by the desire for renunciation, a desire which Śrī Krishna said, forms the basis for persistent practice. Even though the desire for renunciation does help a yogi to persist in the practice, it does not eradicate or remove all his mundane desires which are forced on by the causal body. It is yoga practice and the purity derived from it that causes the yogi to distance his spirit from the causal form and its motivational powers.

What Śrī Krishna described in this verse is the advanced stage, when the yogi becomes detached not only from his gross and subtle bodies but from his causal form and its contents. Such a yogi definitely has a waiver from all social, cultural and political involvements in this world. Unlike Arjuna at that stage of his life when this discourse was given, such a yogi does not participate in battles and entangling social matters.

On one hand, the material world is absolutely necessary and on the other it is absolutely unnecessary. The advanced yogi described in this verse reached the stage of seeing how unnecessary this world is. Since his view is genuine, he is exempt from the social world. He does not have to perform karma yoga as King Janaka and others did, and as was mandatory for Arjuna. He does not have to help God, help Krishna, in His self-appointed world-reforming task.

उद्धरेदात्मनात्मानं
नात्मानमवसादयेत् ।
आत्मैव ह्यात्मनो बन्धुर्
आत्मैव रिपुरात्मनः ॥६.५॥
uddharedātmanātmānaṁ
nātmānamavasādayet
ātmaiva hyātmano bandhur
ātmaiva ripurātmanaḥ (6.5)

uddhared = uddharet — should elevate; ātmanā — by the self; 'tmānaṁ = ātmānam — the self; nātmānam = na — not + ātmānam — the self; avasādayet — should degrade; ātmaiva = ātmā — self + eva — only; hyātmano = hyātmanaḥ = hy (hi) — indeed + ātmanaḥ — of the self; bandhur = bandhuh — friend; ātmaiva = ātmā — self + eva — as well; ripur = ripuḥ — enemy; ātmanaḥ — of the self

One should elevate his being by himself. One should not degrade the self. Indeed, the person should be the friend of himself. Or he could be the enemy as well. (6.5)

Commentary:

This is the whole idea behind kriyā yoga, that of striving with the self to help the self to get up and out of material existence. It is the self that must give the most help to the self. By self we mean the spirit as well as its psychological equipments which are apart from it within the nature but still in close proximity to it.

According to how we relate to our psychology, according to how we control it, we either befriend ourselves or operate as self-enemies, but it is not a matter of external actions. Kriyā yoga concerns the mystic side of existence. Physical actions, insofar as they reflect what we do on the mystic side, have great value but physical actions which look good physically, but depart from what we do on the mystic side, are misleading and deter spiritual advancement. In kriyā yoga, we stress the mystic side. Thus we take austerities which directly increase mystic perception and give effective control of the psyche.

बन्धुरात्मात्मनस्तस्य
येनात्मैवात्मना जितः ।
अनात्मनस्तु शत्रुत्वे
वर्तेतात्मैव शत्रुवत् ॥६.६॥
bandhurātmātmanastasya
yenātmaivātmanā jitaḥ
anātmanastu śatrutve
vartetātmaiva śatruvat (6.6)

bandhur = bandhuḥ — friend; ātmā — personal energies; 'tmanas = ātmanas — of the self; tasya — of him; yenātmaivātmanā = yena — by whom + ātmā — self + eva — indeed + ātmanā — by the self; jitaḥ — subdued; anātmanas — of one who is not self—possessed; tu — but; śatrutve — in hostility; vartetātmaiva = varteta — it operates + ātmā — self + eva — indeed; śatruvat — like an enemy

The personal energies are the friend of the person by whom those energies are subdued. But for one whose personality is not self-possessed, the personal energies operate in hostility like an enemy. (6.6)

Commentary:

Jitah means to conquer or subdue, to bring under control. Here as opposed to modern slogans, Śrī Krishna states flatly that by force only, do the personal energies of the self become friendly to the self. They do not do so by charm. One must study the various parts of the psyche, know their operations and plan how to mystically bring them under the spirit's control. Then they become friendly to the spiritual aspirations of the self; otherwise they will continue to operate in a spiritually destructive way.

What are the personal energies? These are distinct parts of the subtle and causal bodies, consisting of the life force, the mind chamber, the buddhi organ, the sense of initiative and the chitta subtle energy. These five, with their offshoots, are the psyche of a spirit. These must be controlled on their own planes. They cannot be controlled by physical endeavor, even though they may be temporarily charmed or stunned. These continue with their traits unless they are dealt with on the mystic level. Hence the necessity for austerities which increase mystic perception.

जितात्मनः प्रशान्तस्य
परमात्मा समाहितः ।
शीतोष्णसुखदुःखेषु
तथा मानावमानयोः ॥६.७॥
jitātmanaḥ praśāntasya
paramātmā samāhitaḥ
śītoṣṇasukhaduḥkheṣu
tathā mānāvamānayoḥ (6.7)

jitātmanaḥ — of the self—controlled person; praśāntasya — of the person who is peaceful; paramātmā — the directive part of the self; samāhitaḥ — composed; śītoṣṇasukhaduḥkheṣu = śīta — cold + uṣṇa — heat + sukha — pleasure + duḥkheṣu — in pain; tathā — also; mānāvamānayoḥ = māna — honor + avamānayoḥ — in dishonor

The directive part of a self—controlled, peaceful person remains composed in the cold, heat, pleasure, pain, and also in honor and dishonor. (6.7)

Commentary:

This is all kriyā yoga terminology. It pertains to those who practice, not others. Even if others are devotees of Śrī Krishna, they cannot have the required expertise. We must bear in mind that Arjuna was an accomplished yogi. It is appropriate for Śrī Krishna or for any teacher of the craft to speak of it to him. Arjuna is quite familiar with the kriyā path, even though he was baffled in its application to political life.

Before being schooled in the art of karma yoga, Arjuna thought that kriyā yoga was an art unto itself without application to the social field. This meant that those who taught him the craft did not spell out details of its application to worldly life. His teachers were brahmins with exemptions, who were not politically involved.

By nature, a brahmin thinks it preposterous to use kriyā yoga in the political field but it appears that Śrī Krishna approved that usage for those who came into this manifestation with bodies from non-brahmin parents. Śrī Krishna advertised the path of karma yoga as His own yoga.

In this verse, Śrī Krishna further incited Arjuna to fight, bringing to Arjuna's attention, that if he was truly advanced, he would, as the directive part of himself, remain composed in cold, heat, pleasure, pain, honor and dishonor. Arjuna would have emotional maturity because of yogic application. His emotions would be hardened. He would not break down in tears as he did. If he had a duty to fight on the battlefield, as stipulated by supernatural directors like Śrī Krishna, then he would do so without wincing, with full detachment.

As a notation for kriyā yoga, we must take the meaning of the Sanskrit term paramātmā, seriously. This term generally means Supersoul or Supreme Soul. Ātma means soul or spirit. Param means supreme, super or higher. Here Śrī Krishna used the term in reference to the other parts of the psyche. In this verse, I translated paramātmā as the directive part of the self. This directive part is the spirit itself in conjunction with its sense of initiative, which is termed ahankāra in Sanskrit. Translators usually take the term ahankāra to mean false ego. I translated that as sense of initiative. Ahankāra is not a term used in this particular verse, but the directive part of the self who uses a causal or subtle body is indeed the self in conjunction with the sense of initiative. That directive part of a self-controlled and peaceful person, of an accomplished kriyā yogi, remains composed in the various psychological, environmental and social situations.

ज्ञानविज्ञानतृप्तात्मा
कूटस्थो विजितेन्द्रियः ।
युक्त इत्युच्यते योगी
समलोष्टाश्मकाञ्चनः ॥६.८॥
jñānavijñānatṛptātmā
kūṭastho vijitendriyaḥ
yukta ityucyate yogī
samaloṣṭāśmakāñcanaḥ (6.8)

jñānavijñānatṛptātmā = jñāna — knowledge + vijñāna — realized experience + tṛpta — content + ātmā — self; kūṭastho = kūṭasthaḥ — stable; vijitendriyaḥ = vijita — subdued + indriyaḥ — sensual energy; yukta — disciplined in yoga; ityucyate = ity (iti) — thus + ucyate — is called; yogī — yogi; samaloṣṭrāśmakāñcanaḥ = sama — same + loṣṭra — lump of clay + aśma — stone + kāñcanaḥ — gold

The yogi who is satisfied with knowledge and realized experience, who is stable and who has conquered his sensual energy, who regards a lump of clay, a stone or gold in the same way, is said to be disciplined in yoga. (6.8)

Commentary:

This is the standard for judging whether a yogi completed the course of yoga successfully. For him to be an advanced yogi, he must be satisfied with knowing spiritual and material knowledge as well as with spiritual and material experience which he realized in terms of what was described by the Samkhya philosophy. One who is not knowledgeable and who has no mystic experience to substantiate what he speaks of, is not a successful yogi.

We will go over this list of qualifications in detail. At first in material existence, one realizes that he has a material body. Once this occurs, one finds that the material body is useful for obtaining information from others. This information is called knowledge. The question is: Why is it that the soul forgets his past life and his stay in the world hereafter? Why is it that his memory of those experiences does not remain within conscious purview? Why does a baby not remember its past life in an old body or in some type of body somewhere else, and even just existing without a gross form?

The answer to the puzzle is contained in the question itself, since the memory of the activities and identity held in a past life, is different to the spirit itself. The memory is not stored in the spirit but rather in the buddhi organ of the spirit. It is also stored in the causal body but only as a compressed impression. Unless the compressed impression is converted, it cannot be realized as it was experienced in history.

Just as the memory of a person's birth is stored in the form of birth records in a government office and can be retrieved by a clerk familiar with the filing system, so the memory of past life events is retrievable but one must have the proper subtle tools to access it.

Generally, a baby cannot remember past lives because the spirit in a baby form is not in a position to read the files. Those records are kept in the buddhi organ in the subtle body and in the causal form as well, except that in the causal compartment, the memory is compressed into pranic energy. One cannot read that unless one is a mahāyogī. We understand that Gautama Buddha penetrated the causal level and was able to translate it, and see his past lives in this sector of existence, but that is quite unusual. Even though it is possible, it is hardly likely that any of us will do that. I have seen Śrīla Yogeshwarananda reviewing information that was compressed on the causal plane but while observing him, I could not translate the compressed information.

Generally as soon as one develops self awareness, one feels different from the family one was born into and different from the society and alternately, one feels very unified with it but from a different objective view. This happens when one's body reaches about nine to twelve years of age. At that time however, due to social and cultural pressures, one is pushed or shoved to get an education. Under such pressure one gathers knowledge from relatives, teachers and friends. One does this in the race for survival. At first one feels that this is a race for the survival of one's body, because one may feel so identical with the body, that one thinks that one is the body. Thus the information that one usually accumulates has to do with social and cultural achievement. Generally adults ask a twelve-year-old boy or girl this question: What do you want to be when you grow up?

As far as they are concerned the person is his body. Thus they try to motivate the person to strive to be someone great. They know from recent experience, that if one does not strive, one will, more than likely, turn out to be an ordinary human being with insufficient livelihood.

Later on because of spasms in the subtle body, because of irregularities, one begins to question the bodily concept of life. This happened to Lord Buddha. It happens to many others as well. However the relatives and friends are usually expert in hushing anyone who inquires about anything beyond the bodily concept. A few of us, a handful, persist in such inquiry.

Because of spasms in the memory of the subtle body, we begin to feel uneasy in the materialistic societies which our parents so carefully created and maintained. Thus we begin to wonder about the supernatural. We look for books, mystic yogis, advanced religious teachers, anyone or anything that gives us some idea of the transcendence which is behind the material world.

Even though our relatives and friends may have us locked into the materialistic scene which they love so much, still we regularly escape from it, because the subtle body can by its own ability, leave the physical form while it sleeps. Thus dreaming is the most basic form of transcending the physical world. Even if the government imprisons a man, still they cannot keep his subtle body from separating from the gross form which they restricted in a prison. The subtle body escapes on its own power. It also returns to the physical body on its own power, so much so that usually, the spirit has no control over this.

The acquirement of a basic education from parents and teachers serves the social and cultural purpose but it does little for spiritual realization. When, however, one begins to apply the information practically and one sees how to translate knowledge into action on the material plane, one begins to see that it is responsibility which controls the material level of existence. In Sanskrit this responsibility is called dharma.

Responsibility is also called bhārah in Sanskrit but bhārah also means load or weight. As soon as a sober person understands that responsibility is a psychological weight to be carried, he seeks to give it up. Some who are not sober, the materialistic entities, are either eager to manage responsibility or to carry it with a resentful attitude and use intoxicants to relieve the resulting stress.

From this same sense of responsibility, comes an inquiry into the purpose of cultural life. When a person inquires into this, he encounters a paradox because he sees that many of those before him, his elders and ancestors, carried similar loads until the death of their bodies. What then is the purpose of carrying such a load? What will one get if he loses his body while enduring the responsibilities? Since all material bodies must perish sooner or later and since the psychological loads are on-going, the question of how one will be awarded for managing and carrying those psychic weights remains unanswered. Is it merely a function of nature? Will there be a payoff in the world hereafter or in this world after taking another body? Where and when will a man be rewarded for carrying the load of social, cultural or political duties?

Some living entities, who are too comfortably adapted, do not pry into such inquiries. They willingly serve in the course of responsibilities until their bodies perish. They just hope for the best. They are satisfied to exist under these conditions. They leave the mystery of existence to itself.

However in this *Bhagavad Gītā*, we see that Lord Krishna pushed Arjuna to carry the load of responsibility which Arjuna inherited by taking birth in the Kuru family. Śrī Krishna explained to Arjuna that there would be a payoff either in this world or in the next. We may recall that the psychological weight of it overcame the determination of Arjuna, when he broke down in tears. His heart nearly burst apart as his emotions swelled and rushed out of it, when he tottered on the chariot and almost fell over in a swoon. Śrī Krishna then retrieved Arjuna from that state. He showed Arjuna how and when one would get the rewards of carrying responsibility or bearing dharma. Śrī Krishna said:

hato vā prāpsyasi svargaṁ jitvā vā bhokṣyase mahīm
tasmāduttiṣṭha kaunteya yuddhāya kṛtaniścayaḥ (2.37)

Either be killed and achieve the angelic world, or having conquered, enjoy the nation. Therefore stand up and be decisive, O son of Kunti. (2.37)

As soon as one understands that he will be rewarded for carrying out the social, cultural or political obligations which are laid before him by family members, teachers and government officials, one must determine if it is worth the effort. To Arjuna, before he was lectured to by Śrī Krishna, it was not worth the while. Arjuna said:

na ca śreyo'nupaśyāmi hatvā svajanamāhave
na kāṅkṣe vijayaṁ kṛṣṇa na ca rājyaṁ sukhāni ca (1.31)
kiṁ no rājyena govinda kiṁ bhogairjīvitena vā
yeṣāmarthe kāṅkṣitaṁ no rājyaṁ bhogāḥ sukhāni ca (1.32)
ta ime'vasthitā yuddhe prāṇāṁstyaktvā dhanāni ca
ācāryāḥ pitaraḥ putrās tathaiva ca pitāmahāḥ (1.33)
mātulāḥ śvaśurāḥ pautrāḥ syālāḥ saṁbandhinastathā
etānna hantumicchāmi ghnato'pi madhusūdana (1.34)
api trailokyarājyasya hetoḥ kiṁ nu mahīkṛte
nihatya dhārtarāṣṭrānnaḥ kā prītiḥ syājjanārdana (1.35)

And I can imagine no benefit in killing off my kinfolk in battle. I do not desire victory, O Krishna, or political power, or good feelings. (1.31)

What value to us would there be with political control of a nation, O Chief of the cowherds? What use would there be with the enjoyable aspects or with life? Those in whose interest, the political control, the enjoyments and pleasures, were desired by us, (1.32)

...(they) are armed in battle formation, having left aside their lives and financial assets. These are revered teachers, fathers, sons and also grandfathers, (1.33)

...brothers of our mothers, fathers of our wives, grandsons, brothers-in-law, and also their relatives. O slayer of Madhu, I do not desire to slay them even though they are intent on killing, (1.34)

...even for political control of the three sectors of the universe, how then for the earth? What joy should be had by killing the sons of Dhṛtarāṣṭra? (1.35)

This opinion and feeling of Arjuna is fine, if there was no God in charge of the world and if there were no supernatural beings more powerful than us and able to hinder us. According to Śrī Krishna, Arjuna had no viable alternative. This is what Śrī Krishna said:

svadharmamapi cāvekṣya na vikampitumarhasi
dharmyāddhi yuddhācchreyo'nyat kṣatriyasya na vidyate (2.31)

And considering your assigned duty, you should not look for alternatives. In fact, for the son of a king, there is no other duty which is better than a righteous battle. (2.31)

This means that there is a specific duty which we must perform in order to stay in the grace of the Supreme Being. Thus there is really no alternative but to do it, and we should do it as a service to the Supreme Person and for no other reason. It does not have to make sense, other than being what is approved by the Supreme Being. At the same time, such a service of responsibility is not really fulfilling to the soul, because even though it is endorsed by the Supreme Being, even by Śrī Krishna, still it deals with the maintenance of bodies in this world. It is not exclusively meant for the spirit.

Karma yoga for all it is, and even for all that Śrī Krishna advocated it as being, even as He called it, mat yoga or His system of discipline, is not the be-all and end-all. It is just something that must be done, because so long as this world is in vogue, it is required. So long as material bodies are required by us for spiritual realization, karma yoga or yogicly-managed cultural participation has value.

Still, the question remains as to what else is to be gained in this world. Is there anything eternal here? Are we supposed to keep taking bodies while forgetting our past lives, on and on and on? What else is there?

Śrī Krishna made it clear in Chapter Two, that Arjuna would be rewarded for cultural acts which were approved by the Supreme Being. Arjuna would be rewarded in this world or in the subtle material world. Such a subtle world is not the spiritual world and from such a world one must again descend to this gross level, to again inhabit another material body, to again generate the required piety and get the same approval for one's cultural acts. Is this all?

Since cultural skill leads to the subtle material heavens and since from that location, one will again have to come back to this world, we are left to ask if there are any other locales. Where else can we go? What must be done to get to other places?

The factor that triggers our interest in going to some other place is vijñānam or experience. Vijñānam has various phases according to how we are focused when experiencing in the material world. In the lower phases, we rationalize all experience in terms of gross material existence. We interpret everything in terms of this one life. By that we distort the existence. This distortion occurs within the mind. Since we cannot consciously recall previous lives, we rationalize everything that occurs around us in terms of current interpretations. Thus we live by mental miscalculations.

If there were no dreams, no subtle world experienced when our subtle body separates from the gross one, we would be satisfied with rationalizing everything within the present context. That is the situation of the animals. Their mentality is primitive and thus for them, life is very simple indeed. Animals, too, have dreams but animals do not have an up-to-date memory system even in terms of this life. They do not compare, contrast and try to make sense of dream experiences. We do, hence our experience of the subtle world triggers an inquiry into the subtle part of existence. It causes us to be more objective, to stand apart even from dreams. This gives us a glimpse of the transcendence.

Since others before us, and since we ourselves in past lives, explored the dream world and reached certain conclusions, that information comes down to us now as speculations, philosophy and as descriptions of the mystic world. These descriptions stimulate us to make further inquiry and to further experience the subtle existence. The experience culled from this process is the higher stage of vijñānam, known as transcendental experience. Anything that transcends the gross life is regarded as being supernatural but that which transcends even the subtle is known as the spiritual.

After experiencing some subtle realities and knowing for sure by the experiences and by the testimony of more advanced yogis, one either remains stagnant in spiritual progress or advances by performing yoga austerities which clarify and allow greater mystic vision. One who stagnates usually takes a religious process that gets him nowhere but provides a false sense of security. Some others who become stagnant shun the established religions and either establish a new one or join an old spiritual society. Some others who are stagnant merely hang around in material existence without affiliation to anything whatsoever. These usually feel that the whole world is a zoo not to be taken seriously.

The stability of a kriyā yogi is based on his anchorage in the spiritual plane. This experience varies according to the yogi's level of advancement and is connected to conquering the sensual energy as mentioned in this verse. Conquering the sensual energy is the 5th step of yoga practice. Becoming stable, kuţastho, is the 6th step. These are pratyāhār and dhāraṇa focus. When the yogi can withdraw his sensual energies and contain his buddhi organ so that it avoids the gross physical world or the near-to-gross but subtle dimension, then he has mastered the 5th step.

From that he advances to the 6th step which is dhāraṇa, focus of his will into the focusing power of the buddhi organ. When the two parts align and the buddhi's focus remains still, then the yogi gains a steady perception into the world beyond the physical.

Only by the discipline of advanced kriyā yoga can one reach the stage where he puts aside clay, stone and gold as being all the same materials produced in material existence by atomic juxtaposition; otherwise one must use these substances in various prejudiced ways according to their relative values in time and place, according to the social, cultural or political demands in the various species of life.

In the religious field also, one must maintain prejudices to the various substances as one tries to create beautiful images of the Lord, architecturally fascinating temples and the various other trappings that surround formal worship. In advanced yoga, all this is put aside for internal purification and the internal vision which follows it. Thus when we see a person who is satisfied with general knowledge, but who has mystic experiences, who is stable in his focus on realities beyond the gross and subtle energies, who has conquered his sensual energy, and who regards the various materials, as being essentially the same, being void of real value, then we have found a person, who is disciplined in response to this world by the mastership of yoga.

सुहृन्मित्रार्युदासीन
मध्यस्थद्वेष्यबन्धुषु ।
साधुष्वपि च पापेषु
समबुद्धिर्विशिष्यते ॥६.९॥

suhṛnmitrāryudāsīna = suhṛn (suhṛd) — friend + mitra — acquaintance + ary (ari) — enemy + udāsīna — indifferent; madhyasthadveṣyabandhuṣu = madhyastha — evenly disposed + dveṣya — enemy + bandhuṣu — to kinsmen; sādhuṣv = sādhuṣu — in

suhṛnmitrāryudāsīna
madhyasthadveṣya bandhuṣu
sādhuṣvapi ca pāpeṣu
samabuddhirviśiṣyate (6.9)

saintly people; api — also; ca — and; pāpeṣu — in sinful people; samabuddhir = samabuddhiḥ — one who exhibits balanced judgement; viśiṣyate — be regarded with distinction

A person who is indifferent to friend, acquaintance, and enemy, who is evenly-disposed to enemies and kinsmen, who exhibits balanced judgment towards saintly people or sinful ones, is to be regarded with distinction. (6.9)

Commentary:

This distinction indicates a divine person who is descended into the human world or a human being who has attained a divine status by yoga practice. In either case, the distinction is due. Such a person deserves admiration. He does not have to be a devotee of Krishna but he must exhibit the behavior described in this verse.

योगी युञ्जीत सततम्
आत्मानं रहसि स्थितः ।
एकाकी यतचित्तात्मा
निराशीरपरिग्रहः ॥६.१०॥
yogī yuñjīta satatam
ātmānaṁ rahasi sthitaḥ
ekākī yatacittātmā
nirāśīraparigrahaḥ (6.10)

yogī — yogi; yuñjīta — should concentrate; satatam — constantly; ātmānam — on the self; rahasi — in isolation; sthitaḥ — situated; ekākī — alone; yatacittātmā = yata — controlling + citta — thinking + ātmā — self; nirāśīr — without desire; aparigrahaḥ — without possessions

In isolation, the yogi should constantly concentrate on the self. Being alone, he should be of controlled thinking and subdued self without desire and without possessions. (6.10)

Commentary:

Some commentators contend that the word kuţastho in verse 6 means the Supreme Absolute Truth, the Supreme Personality of Godhead. However, one should note the context, where in this verse 10, the focus is given as the self (ātmānam). This keeps in line with the Upanishadic procedures, of focusing on the self for self-discovery by mystic experience, and then focusing that self on the brahman spiritual energy.

As the kriyā yogis have always established, the word kūṭastho refers to steady focus on the ātma. This is done in isolation, both physical and psychological confinement, whereby one is not distracted by physical or subtle objects. This is the stage of samādhi trance to lock on to other worlds. In this verse, controlled thinking does not mean control of all thought other than on Lord Krishna or a divine person. It actually means a complete cessation of thinking as indicated in the Śrī Patañjali Yoga Sutras. Only by such a stoppage can the buddhi organ revert to mystic visual perception.

Some say that thinking cannot be stopped. This is true on the normal level of consciousness. If one masters prāṇāyāma, he may switch his buddhi organ to a higher frequency whereby the thinking ceases. As such, this practice can only be achieved by a person who mastered prāṇāyāma. Others, whether devotees of Krishna or non-devotees, cannot accomplish a total stoppage of thought because when one tries to control it with the present level of consciousness, one finds that he cannot.

Even for us as kriyā yogis, we find that when we do prāṇāyāma and then do meditations immediately after, we experience stoppage of thinking. If we meditate at other times, we usually can decrease but not totally stop the thinking patterns.

A yogi must be without desire and without possessions. Only then, will his mind be free of its tendency to care for and protect whatever he owns. The yogi sheds desires and possessions because he finds them to be obstructive to meditation. When he tries to meditate, he finds that the mind cannot release itself from such things nor can he release the mind unless in fact, he sincerely gave up the items. As a matter of necessity, and for the sake of progressing further, he gives them away.

Desires, too, are a psychological possession. These are even harder to give up than physical assets. The yogi in his meditative research, finds out that desires have weight. They are a commodity on the psychological plane.

After trying and trying and trying again to meditate and failing at it, being nudged by desires which arise as picturizations and ideas, the yogi decides to shed them. Thus he takes the instruction of the great yogi teachers more seriously.

Eka means one. Ekaki means being alone. Other paths require a congregation. Here in kriyā practice, being alone is important. This is a singular way of discipline. One cannot progress in kriyā yoga unless one works with oneself alone.

शुचौ देशे प्रतिष्ठाप्य
स्थिरमासनमात्मनः ।
नात्युच्छ्रितं नातिनीचं
चैलाजिनकुशोत्तरम् ॥ ६.११ ॥
śucau deśe pratiṣṭhāpya
sthiramāsanamātmanaḥ
nātyucchritaṁ nātinīcaṁ
cailājinakuśottaram (6.11)

śucau — in clean; deśe — in place; pratiṣṭhāpya — fixing; sthiram — firm; āsanam — seat; ātmanaḥ — of his self; nātyucchritaṁ = na — not + atyucchritaṁ — too high; nātinīcam = na — not + atinīcam — too low; cailājinakuśottaram = caila — cloth + ajina — antelope skin + kuśa — kusha grass + uttaram — underneath

In a clean place, fixing for himself a firm seat which is not too high, not too low, with a covering layer of cloth, antelope skin and kusha grass underneath, (6.11)

Commentary:

Modern yogis come from every class of human society, from the priestly and philosophically-inclined folk, to the administrative and martial kind, to the mercantile types and the laboring class. Nowadays no one is barred from yoga lessons. If you want to do yoga you merely have to find a teacher and learn from him or her. Formerly, however, in the time of Śrī Krishna, it was not easy for a person to learn yoga if he was not in the higher three castes. Those in the highest caste learned much more than the others.

Formerly, if a person was not born in the brahmin caste, the technicalities of higher yoga practice, the three last stages of yoga, were not taught to him. It was very difficult to discover these techniques. Śrī Krishna's stipulation about a clean place (śucau deśe), pertains to the brahmin caste. Traditionally, they are meticulous about cleanliness and have elaborate rituals for it, which border on superstitions. However, a modern yogi would do well to honor this regulation for cleanliness of his living place.

If he lives simply, he will find it easy to keep a clean place and servants or a maid will be unnecessary. In an unelaborate setting, cleanliness becomes very easy. The place for sitting should be firm. It should not be too comfortable to the material body. This means that one should avoid cushions. In the early days, yogis sat on a layer or two of natural material. Later on in history, some yogis who became famous after entering samādhi and who then took many disciples, were induced by wealthy followers to sit on very soft cushions, but this is not part of yoga practice. It is part of the influence which flows back from materialistic disciples.

The seat should be neither too high nor too low. In other words, it should not be below ground level or much above. It should have a covering layer of cloth that is not thick. Śrī Krishna recommends antelope skin, even though Lord Shiva, the master of yogis, is known for his tiger skin seat. Śrī Krishna advised that kusha grass, be placed underneath the antelope skin. We should now study text 11 of Chapter Five again:

kāyena manasā buddhyā kevalairindriyairapi
yoginaḥ karma kurvanti saṅgaṁ tyaktvātmaśuddhaye (5.11)

With the body, mind and intelligence, or even with the senses alone, the yogis, having discarded attachment, perform cultural acts for self-purification. (5.11)

This means essentially that once we realize that we lack a waiver from cultural activities, we commit to doing whatever is assigned by the Supreme Being, but we must do it with detachment, otherwise the results of the actions will find us and will again drag us back to material existence. By acting as destined with detachment, we commit terminal actions, which lead to the end of a person's material existence.

It is important to discard attachment while doing one's duty as stipulated by Śrī Krishna or by His agent or by providence which is His representative. Previously, under the strain of mental ideas and emotional pressures, we acted with attachment. Now we must change that. After acting with attachment and after getting adverse and uncomfortable returns, we got disgusted (nirveda). That disgust produced in our nature, a sense of renunciation, whereby we no longer wanted to participate. By that reluctance, we turned away from the cultural scene, but since we did not get a waiver, that rejection of duty produced complications.

Śrī Krishna brought it to our attention that we must follow in the footsteps of the great yogis who successfully departed material existence. They did yoga and they also performed cultural actions with detachment. Both aspects are necessary. The whole *Bhagavad Gītā*, when studied carefully, provides serious instruction on how to get out of material existence, if one lacks a waiver from cultural acts. It is for the neophyte yogis. Other people do not understand these instructions because they are not committed to abandoning material existence.

What we understand from these two essential verses (5.11 and 6.12), is this: We must perform assigned or destined cultural activities with detachment. We must take up the yoga process for psychological purification. These two things are absolutely necessary in order to get the cultural exemption and reach the stage of having a full time yoga practice that culminates in nirvāṇa, as described previously by Śrī Krishna:

eṣā brāhmī sthitiḥ pārtha naināṁ prāpya vimuhyati
sthitvāsyāmantakāle'pi brahmanirvāṇamṛcchati (2.72)

This divine state is required, O son of Pṛthā. If a man does not have this, he is stupefied. At the time of death, the full stoppage of mundane sensuality and the attainment of divinity is attained by one who is fixed in this divine state. (2.72)

labhante brahmanirvāṇam ṛṣayaḥ kṣīṇakalmaṣāḥ
chinnadvaidhā yatātmānaḥ sarvabhūtahite ratāḥ (5.25)

Those seers whose sins and faults are terminated, whose doubts are removed, whose souls are restrained, who find joy in regarding the welfare of the creatures, attain a cessation of their material existence and a simultaneous absorption in spirituality. (5.25)

तत्रैकाग्रं मनः कृत्वा
यतचित्तेन्द्रियक्रियः ।
उपविश्यासने युञ्ज्याद्
योगमात्मविशुद्धये ॥६.१२॥
tatraikāgraṁ manaḥ kṛtvā
yatacittendriyakriyaḥ
upaviśyāsane yuñjyād
yogamātmaviśuddhaye (6.12)

tatraikāgraṁ = tatra — there + ekāgram — single—focused; manaḥ — mind; kṛtvā — having made; yatacittendriyakriyaḥ = yata — controlled + citta — thought + indriyakriyaḥ — sense energy; upaviśyāsane = upaviśya — seating himself + āsane — in a posture; yuñjyād = yuñjyāt — should practice; yogamātmaviśuddhaye = yogam — to yoga discipline + ātma — self + viśuddhaye — to purification

...being there, seated in a posture, having the mind focused, the person who controls his thinking and sensual energy, should practice the yoga discipline for self-purification. (6.12)

Commentary:

Ātmaviśuddhaye, the purification of the psyche or the purification of the spirit (ātma) while it is in conjunction with the psyche, is discussed in two verses of the *Gītā*, this one and verse 11 of the previous chapter:

kāyena manasā buddhyā kevalairindriyairapi
yoginaḥ karma kurvanti saṅgaṁ tyaktvātmaśuddhaye (5.11)

With the body, mind and intelligence, or even with the senses alone, the yogis, having discarded attachment, perform cultural acts for self-purification. (5.11)

The ātma or spirit is causeless and eternal, as Śrī Krishna defined and as the Upanishadic sages upheld throughout the Upanishad literature. Śrī Krishna described the ātma to Arjuna in this way in Chapter Two:

na jāyate mriyate vā kadā cin nāyaṁ bhūtvā bhavitā vā na bhūyaḥ
ajo nityaḥ śāśvato'yaṁ purāṇo na hanyate hanyamāne śarīre (2.20)

This embodied soul is not born, nor does it die at any time, nor having existed will it not be. Being birthless, eternal, perpetual and primeval, it is not slain in the act of killing the body. (2.20)

As neophyte kriyā yogis, the self-purity verses in consideration, namely verse 12 of this Chapter along with verse 11 of Chapter Five, are to us, the most important statements in the *Bhagavad Gītā*. Our primary concern is self-purification. When we achieve that we can seek devotion to Krishna. Without that ātmaviśuddhaye, purification of the psyche, our devotion to Krishna, love for Krishna, and relationship with Krishna has little or no value since it is an impure offering, something that Krishna will not accept. It would be our pious credits or impious demerits coming to us as returns from material nature and Śrī Krishna strongly denies accepting there in a previous verse:

nādatte kasyacitpāpaṁ na caiva sukṛtaṁ vibhuḥ
ajñānenāvṛtaṁ jñānaṁ tena muhyanti jantavaḥ (5.15)

The Almighty God does not receive from anyone, an evil consequence or a good reaction. The knowledge of this is shrouded by ignorance through which the people are deluded. (5.15)

Many people feel that their offerings to Śrī Krishna are being accepted and that this denial verse applies only to non-devotees, people without a confirmed sentiment to Him, people who have not joined, surrendered to or patronized a disciplic succession which came down from Him. However, until a person can relinquish his pious and impious returns from material nature, he will be unable to attract Śrī Krishna's attention.

For us, the neophyte kriyā yogis who know for sure that our priority is self purification, we must study this verse 12 along with verse 11 of Chapter Five very carefully, to see what we must do for self purification. These two verses are the crux of the matter for us at this stage. We should not be diverted by anything else. Devotion to Śrī Krishna, for all it is extolled to be, can very well wait. There is no point in running after it if we are not purified, especially since our impurity will not go away merely by impure devotional services. Those who feel that from the impure stage a human being can cultivate devotion and become pure just by doing that, will gain very little from this commentary.

Let us review this verse 12 again:

tatraikāgraṁ manaḥ kṛtvā yatacittendriyakriyaḥ
upaviśyāsane yuñjyād yogamātmaviśuddhaye (6.12)

...being there, seated in a posture, having the mind focused, the person who controls his thinking and sensual energy, should practice the yoga discipline for self-purification. (6.12)

This does not mean that a person sits in a lotus posture or in an easy pose and just tries to focus his mind on an object. It does not mean that he controls his thinking and sensual energy (yatacittendriyakriyah) by sheer will power. It really means that after mastery of the āsana postures in haţha yoga and prāṇāyāma methods, the person can now focus his buddhi organ which is housed in his mind. Simultaneously, due to his increase in pranic energy by prāṇāyāma, he can control his thinking faculty and subtle sense organs, which are all parts of the buddhi organ in the head of the subtle body.

One cannot do this practice effectively unless one masters āsana postures and prāṇāyāma. It is simply impossible. This is why great souls took to yoga practice in the time of the *Upanishads*, in the time of the production of the Puranic literature and afterwards, even today. Without yoga, when we sit to meditate, we get nowhere or we only get a glimpse now and again. However, when we change the normal energy in the mind and substitute higher energy, we can focus the buddhi organ in such a way as to see beyond this world. This is not imagination but it is the use of the tool which constructs imagination. That tool is part of the buddhi organ which is in the head of the subtle body.

Purification of the psyche (ātmaviśuddhaye) is precisely what is described in this verse. T his is the purpose of elementary kriyā yoga, to control the thinking faculty and sensual energies. Before one can control the mind's functions and stop these from impulsive operations, one must purify the life force by haţha yoga. This includes the perfection of celibacy yoga.

समं कायशिरोग्रीवं
धारयन्नचलं स्थिरः ।
संप्रेक्ष्य नासिकाग्रं स्वं
दिशश्चानवलोकयन् ॥ ६.१३ ॥
samaṁ kāyaśirogrīvaṁ
dhārayannacalaṁ sthiraḥ
saṁprekṣya nāsikāgraṁ svaṁ
diśaścānavalokayan (6.13)

samam — balanced; kāyaśirogrīvaṁ = kāya — body + śiro (śiraḥ) — head + grīvam — neck; dhārayan — holding; acalam — without movement; sthiraḥ — steady; saṁprekṣya — gazing at; nāsikāgraṁ = nāsikā — nostril + agram — tip; svam — own; diśaścānavalokayan = diśaḥ — the directions + ca — and + anavalokayan — not looking

Holding the body, head and neck in balance, steady without movement, gaze at the tip of the nose, not looking in any other direction. (6.13)

Commentary:

Note that Śrī Krishna does not designate Himself as the focus here. He gave a description for purity of the personal energies of the psyche and not for anything else. For this, one must do yoga as described.

Nāsikāgram means gazing at the tip of the nose. Still, some commentators, even as accomplished yogis, say that it is the bridge or highest point on the nose. However the highest point on the nose is given as a point of focus in another verse in the *Gītā* as follows:

sparśānkṛtvā bahirbāhyāṁś cakṣuścaivāntare bhruvoḥ
prāṇāpānau samau kṛtvā nāsābhyantaracāriṇau (5.27)

Excluding the external sensual contacts, and fixing the visual focus between the eyebrows, putting the inhalation and exhalation in balance, moving through the nose... (5.27)

In Chapter Five, Śrī Krishna spoke of fixing the visual focus between the eyebrows; now, he speaks of focusing at the tip of the nose because a yogi must, as a preliminary procedure, purified his life force and get it to express itself primarily into his head.

The methods for this are taught in Kuṇḍalinī yoga which raises the electricized life force. The tip of the nose is electrically connected to the base of the spinal column where the life force resides. In tantric yoga and in Kuṇḍalinī yoga which are related, one learns how to awaken this life force.

It is not sufficient to master buddhi yoga which includes the focus of the visual power into the eyebrows. One should master Kuṇḍalinī yoga beforehand; otherwise one will fail to master buddhi yoga. Therefore, those who state that nāsikāgrama practice in this verse 13 of Chapter Six means focus between the eyebrows as described in verse 27 of Chapter Five, can only be correct if it is implied that persons doing this successfully have already raised their Kuṇḍalinī energy.

The kuṇḍalinī chakra occasionally rises of her own accord, but as a habit she returns to the base of the spine to focus on digestion, sexuality, excretion and mobility. Thus we are speaking of a permanent reorientation or a permanent flow of her energy up the spine into the brain and the buddhi organ.

A great yogi who assisted me in yoga practice, Śrīla Yogeshwarananda, told me from his position on the divide between the astral and causal levels, that holding the body, head and neck in balance is only possible for a person who has mastered celibacy yoga. He said that others can practice sitting in lotus posture with their body, head and neck in an apparent straight line, but they are not really in that position unless they have mastered celibacy. This mastership of celibacy comes about simultaneously with the mastery of Kuṇḍalinī chakra.

Gazing at the tip of the nose as described, will not produce the intended result unless the practitioner completes celibacy and Kuṇḍalinī yoga. That is what my readers should know. These practices of celibacy and Kuṇḍalinī yoga are preliminary. By gazing as described, an accomplished celibate produces a bindu or pin-point representation of the life force into the buddhi organ. This stabilizes the sensual energies so that they do not go hunting for sexual adventures, which usually are their most treasured pursuit.

प्रशान्तात्मा विगतभीर्
ब्रह्मचारिव्रते स्थितः ।
मनः संयम्य मच्चित्तो
युक्त आसीत मत्परः ॥६.१४॥
praśāntātmā vigatabhīr
brahmacārivrate sthitaḥ
manaḥ saṁyamya maccitto
yukta āsīta matparaḥ (6.14)

praśāntātmā = praśānta — pacified + ātmā — self; vigatabhīr (vigatabhīḥ) = vigata — gone away + bhīḥ — fear; brahmacārivrate — in the vow of sexual restraint; sthitaḥ — established; manaḥ — mind; saṁyamya — controlling; maccitto = maccittaḥ — though fixed on Me; yukta — disciplined; āsīta — should sit; matparaḥ — devoted to Me

With a pacified self, free from fears, with a vow of sexual restraint firmly practiced, with mind controlled and having Me in his thought with his mind concentrated, he should sit, being devoted to Me as the Supreme Objective. (6.14)

Commentary:

The stipulation about being alone (ekākī) and being isolated, not only applies to materialistic associations but also to association with disciples and fellow seekers. Thus in kriyā yoga, the whole layout of disciplines is completely different from other paths which encourage fellowship. This fellowship of other seekers who are pursuing the same beliefs and who aspire for the same objectives is sometimes called sadhusaṅga or satsaṅga, which means the fellowship or saṅga of sadhus, the good men, the pious people and of the sat, the reality-seekers or true-blue religionists.

It is believed that one should pursue the course of ekākī isolation only when one is in the neophyte stage of practicing under the direction of a yoga guru at his ashram. The belief extends further to suggest that once one has mastered the disciplines, he should gradually end the isolation and take disciples to train them as he was taught. However, these beliefs are more or less ideas of non-kriyā yogis.

Sir Paul Castagna, an associate of the writer, noted that the arrowhead of the *Gītā*, its piercing point, is that one must tread on the path of no return and, with that attitude, forget oneself through life's circumstances. This is kriyā yoga, where the yogi is so isolated that he feels as if he will not return to this life and to the affiliations that accompany it. Indeed he feels that he is alone. That is in tune with the *Gītā*, because we see that even with Śrī Krishna on the chariot, Arjuna had to decide for himself alone, what he would do. Even though prompted by Śrī Krishna, He had to do it alone.

Arjuna, alone, had to battle the various relationship energies within his nature that concerned many people present at the Kurukṣetra confrontation. From within his psyche he had to say to these people, "I am sorry I cannot relate to you. I cannot render sympathy. I have to destroy your body. Who are you? I do not know you. You are not my uncle, teacher or friend. You are the enemy of dharma, the enemy of righteousness. It is regrettable, seeing you in that way. I am duty bound to discipline you."

The idea of having disciples and the plan for taking these is not really part of kriyā yoga, though it is a necessity in some cases. In fact, it is a part of karma yoga, the same yoga which Śrī Krishna insisted Arjuna take up at Kurukṣetra. While those with political obligations, people like Arjuna, must take up karma yoga in the fashion of the legendary King Janaka, so we must take up karma yoga by taking disciples, which means taking responsibility for the kindergarten stage of kriyā practice of others. Is this then a distraction? It certainly is. Only those who are enamored of responsibility and who have an appetite for fame and being honored, will not view the acceptance of disciples as an impediment on the kriyā path.

Being ekākī, being alone, is disrupted when one takes disciples. Therefore a guru should not lose sight of that fact. Arjuna sensed that being at Kurukṣetra was a diversion from his yoga objectives. As such, he asked Śrī Krishna about the contradiction between renunciation of the material world and assumption of responsibilities in its social realm. Śrī Krishna responded and stressed that there was a relationship between the two and that a person like Arjuna must, like King Janaka, utilize yoga expertise in the worldly scene because he had no exemption to do otherwise.

We also have no exemption and sometimes take disciples. Hence, we should keep that to a minimum and not sacrifice our isolation altogether. We must know for certain that in the kriyā path, this isolation is a psychological one, more so than physical. In the advanced stages it is an isolation from sensual stimuli for the conservation of energy to gain complete mastery of the 5th stage of yoga, pratyāhār (sense withdrawal).

Does this writer have disciples? Sure he does. As the writer of two commentaries on *Bhagavad Gītā,* disciples are there. In this situation, I do not institute myself as being important or more important than the disciplines I showed them. This is how I maintain the ekāki isolation. Otherwise my practice would be demolished by my need for fame, adoration and prominence.

Do I initiate disciples? No, I do not do so because the kriyā path does not require it as do other systems. Is anyone my official disciple? No,because in the kriyā path the student's official teacher is his practice and his connection with Lord Shiva or some other mahāyogī, even Lord Krishna. I am just an agent, a medium to convey information. If Lord Shiva asks me to instruct someone I do so but not because I directly care about the person. It is Lord Shiva's concern, not mine. My problem is how to complete the disciplines introduced to me.

If I see Lord Shiva initiate someone in the astral world, if that person is not conscious of participating, and if instructed, I might describe the experience to that person but otherwise I do not have any connection with initiations. We should note that Arjuna was promptly and unofficially, without ceremony, initiated in the transcendental science of the *Bhagavad Gītā* by Śrī Krishna, suddenly and without rehearsal or preparation. It was not in a temple. There were no groups of smiling people walking around chanting the holy names of Krishna or anything like that. It was an on-the-spot discourse.

How many other disciples did Śrī Krishna make on the occasion? Ask yourself that question.

If having disciples means that I instruct someone in the path of kriyā and then I leave him alone to follow the disciplines, and periodically check with him and that is all, then yes: I do have disciples.

युञ्जन्नेवं सदात्मानं
योगी नियतमानसः ।
शान्तिं निर्वाणपरमां
मत्संस्थामधिगच्छति ॥६.१५॥
yuñjannevaṁ sadātmānaṁ
yogī niyatamānasaḥ
śāntiṁ nirvāṇaparamāṁ
matsaṁsthāmadhigacchati (6.15)

yuñjan — disciplining; evaṁ — as described; sadā — continuously; 'tmānaṁ = ātmānam — himself; yogī — yogi; niyatamānasaḥ — one who has a subdued mind; śāntiṁ — spiritual security; nirvāṇaparamāṁ = nirvāṇa — extinction of mundane affinity + paramām — highest living state; matsaṁsthām — existentially positioned with Me; adhigacchati — achieves

Disciplining himself continuously as described, the yogi who has a subdued mind, experiences spiritual security. He achieves the extinction of mundane affinity as he simultaneously attains the highest living state. He achieves an existential position with Me. (6.15)

Commentary:

It would be impossible for the yogi to discipline himself continually (sadā) as described, unless he maintains the ekākī (isolation) stipulation. We have seen this repeatedly, where a yogi after advancing a little or after mastering the 8th and final stage of yoga, samādhi (trance consciousness), changes, takes disciples and then spends so much time teaching, explaining, building boarding houses and so on that he stops the kriyā practice entirely. Some of these teachers begin teaching meditation and deprive their students of the elementary stages of yoga which are so necessary for a thorough and complete success.

If I am to discipline myself continuously, I would have to maintain the practice even while taking disciples and that would not be possible unless my association with disciples was minimal and if the disciples could live on their practice, and not require constant association with me. This is the jist of it. In this case, the practice of yoga itself must take precedence and must be the adorable spiritual teacher and not the teacher himself. The teacher himself must be a student and must conduct a personal practice on a full time basis. He must not make himself available for adoration, worship and such honors, because the time this would take is the same time required for practice. His studentship must be maintained. He must continue his higher stage of practice to advance it and cannot spend much time reviewing lower stages with disciples. They must have the enthusiasm and stamina to individuallycomplete their lessons of yoga, with him checking their practice infrequently in a way that does not jeopardize his disciplines.

The subdued mind with spiritual security is the completion of the 5th stage of yoga practice with a foothold on the 6th stage. This is the completion of the pratyāhār sensual energy withdrawal practice and the stabilization of the mind on other dimensions. The mind in this case means the whole mind compartment with its contents and the buddhi sensing subtle mechanism. The main challenge is the buddhi organ which utilizes the general sensing power of the mind to tune into excitements. At first the yogi must train the intellect and the mind not to range over things in the gross dimension, especially things of a sexually-attractive nature.

The bit about the spiritual security (śāntim) concerns the yogi's newly-found freedom from the gross sensations which were pulling his body here and there before he perfected the pratyāhār sense withdrawal practice. He finds peace in the focus of his buddhi organ into a subtle dimension which visually unfolds into an open sky which is out of this world. Some say that this is a glimpse into the spiritual sky but other advanced yogis like Śrīla

Yogeshwarananda do not agree. They say it is just a supersubtle dimension and that the yogi has higher levels to attain.

The view into the other world does not carry with it the pulling and yanking nudges which we are subjected to when we meet attractive objects here. The buddhi organ which is always jumpy in its sensual response in this world, settles down peacefully when the view to the other world is opened widely. Thus some yogis remain gazing inwards like this for minutes, hours or even days according to their particular abilities. During that time, the usual thoughts, ideas and mental picturizations which concern this world, do not occur. Thus some yogis say that the imaginations of the mind stop once and for all. This is psychological peace (śāntim).

Such yogis have achieved the extinction of mundane affinity, at least for the time being, for we see that some still return to conditional life even after attaining such states. This return is mostly due to taking on disciples. Some are helpless when disciples find them, become fond of them, rely on them, and praise them, telling them what a savior they will be. Unfortunately many such potential disciples exist for the careless yogi. One who sticks to the kriyā path in all earnest, cannot be victimized by disciples because he will maintain the association of greater yogis, who will keep him tied to his practice and to further advancement. This does not mean that he will not take disciples, but he will not allow them to indulge him in the savior or messiah image.

Śrī Krishna said that a successful yogi, one who mastered all that we described so far, does become existentially positioned with Krishna. In other words, he does reach the spiritual world and does display a spiritual body as himself.

Note that Śrī Krishna never says that such a great soul should pose as His representative or anything like that. Kriyā yoga is not for such purposes. It is exactly as it stated for self purification, psyche purity (ātmaviśuddhaye) and then for attaining an existential stance that is similar to Śrī Krishna's (matsamsthām).

नात्यश्नतस्तु योगोऽस्ति
न चैकान्तमनश्नतः ।
न चातिस्वप्नशीलस्य
जाग्रतो नैव चार्जुन ॥ ६.१६ ॥

nātyaśnatastu yogo'sti
na caikāntamanaśnataḥ
na cātisvapnaśīlasya
jāgrato naiva cārjuna (6.16)

nātyaśnatas = na — not + atyaśnatas — of too much eating; tu — but; yogo = yogaḥ — yoga; 'sti = asti — it is; na — not; caikāntam = ca — and + ekāntam — solely; anaśnataḥ — of not eating at all; na — not; cātisvapnaśīlasya = ca — and + atisvapna — too much sleeping + śīlasya — of habit; jāgrato = jāgrataḥ — of staying awake; naiva = na — nor + eva — indeed; cārjuna = ca — and + arjuna — Arjuna

But Arjuna, yoga practice does not consist of eating too much. And it is not the practice of not eating at all, or the habit of sleeping too much or staying awake either. (6.16)

Commentary:

Yoga practice is not haphazard fasting or irregular sleeping. The yogi works with nature, studies nature and then adjusts his schedule accordingly. It is not that he stops eating suddenly, stops sleeping and avoids the routine. Fasting in yoga practice is done in conjunction with āsana postures for efficient blood circulation in the body, prāṇāyāma breath methods for more intake of fresh air into the gross body, pratyāhār sensual withdrawal for relief from the fatiguing excitements ever present in the world, dhāraṇa intellect concentration for training the buddhi organ to stop procuring fulfillments in this world, and samādhi fixation practice to transfer one's interest into the spiritual sky.

A yogi's diet is regulated by yoga practice. As he advances his diet changes on the basis of his āsana postures, breath increase methods and life force reliability in terms of the life force being freed from extra chores like over-eating, sensual excitements, and varied focus on worldly life. A yogi's diet is controlled daily by his continuous disciplines as stressed in the previous verse.

A yogi's sleeping consists of subtle activities in the astral world and on other levels beyond it where he meets more advanced yoga teachers for instructions. His sleeping also consists of meditations. It consists of allowing the life force to do its rejuvenation work on the gross body. Sometimes in the subtle world, a yogi meets with disciples who take advice from him while his body rests and is cared for by the attentive recharging life force.

Sleep has a good use for a yogi. There is no reason for him to avoid it altogether. He has use for it, for transferring his attention to the subtle side of existence.

युक्ताहारविहारस्य
युक्तचेष्टस्य कर्मसु ।
युक्तस्वप्नावबोधस्य
योगो भवति दुःखहा ॥६.१७॥
yuktāhāravihārasya
yuktaceṣṭasya karmasu
yuktasvapnāvabodhasya
yogo bhavati duḥkhahā (6.17)

yuktāhāravihārasya = yukta — regulated + āhāra — eating + vihārasya — of leisure; yuktaceṣṭasya = yukta — disciplined + ceṣṭasya — of endeavor; karmasu — in duties; yuktasvapnāvabodhasya = yukta — disciplined + svapna — sleep + avabodhasya — of waking; yogo = yogah — yoga practice; bhavati — is; duḥkhahā — distress—removing

For a person who is regulated in eating and in leisure, who is disciplined in the endeavor of duties, who is moderate in sleeping and waking, for him, the yoga practice is a distress-remover. (6.17)

Commentary:

Yoga practice serves also as a distress-remover (duhkhahā). Many modern people take to yoga practice for that very reason, for the removal of psychological and physical stress. However one cannot be successful in higher yoga if one is merely motivated to do it for the removal of hassles. Even though this is a byproduct of yoga practice, still it should not be the motive for performing yoga. Śrī Krishna explained the proper motive when he discussed renunciation in verse 2 of this chapter:

yaṁ saṁnyāsamiti prāhur yogaṁ taṁ viddhi pāṇḍava
na hyasaṁnyastasaṁkalpo yogī bhavati kaścana (6.2)

That which the authorities define as renunciation, know it as applied yoga, O Arjuna Pandava. Indeed, no one becomes a yogi without an intention for renunciation. (6.2)

Thus the intention before doing advanced yoga must be to renounce the material situation and to relieve one's dependence on it.

The distress-removing power of yoga is clearly demonstrated to us in the life of the great yogis. It shows us that by regulating eating, leisure, endeavor, sleeping and waking, yoga practice produces health and freedom from hassles. When yoga takes grip of one's life, eating, leisure, endeavor, sleeping and waking change in a way that makes it easy for the life force to protect the body. This life force expresses itself through involuntary but necessary actions in the body, actions like eating, sleeping, breathing and so on. The life force is curbed and assisted by a successful Kuṇḍalinī yoga practice.

Śrī Krishna included duties (karmasu) just to remind Arjuna that renunciation of destined actions is not part of true yoga practice. Performance of duties is included in the yoga effort. It facilitates yoga either immediately or in the long run.

यदा विनियतं चित्तम्
आत्मन्येवावतिष्ठते ।
निःस्पृहः सर्वकामेभ्यो
युक्त इत्युच्यते तदा ॥६.१८॥
yadā viniyataṁ cittam
ātmanyevāvatiṣṭhate
niḥspṛhaḥ sarvakāmebhyo
yukta ityucyate tadā (6.18)

yadā — when; viniyataṁ — tightly controlled; cittam — thought; ātmany = ātmani — in the spiritual core self; evāvatiṣṭhate = eva — alone + avatiṣṭhate — is attentive; niḥspṛhaḥ — free from desire; sarvakāmebhyo (sarvakāmebhyaḥ) = sarva — all + kāmebhyaḥ — from cravings; yukta — proficient in yoga; ity = iti — thus; ucyate — is said; tadā — then

When with tightly controlled thought, he is attentive to his spiritual core self alone, being freed from desires and from all cravings, he is said to be proficient in yoga. (6.18)

Commentary:

A person cannot, inside his psychology, be attentive to his spiritual self or to the spiritual self of anyone else, even of the Supreme Soul, if his thoughts are not tightly squeezed out. Sometimes it happens, that all of a sudden, a yogi or non-yogi, has a vision of the Supreme Soul or a higher entity or his own self, spontaneously and causelessly, without doing yoga practice. That happens, but it only happens momentarily and very infrequently. It does not persist except as a memory.

I have had such experiences but these are not sufficient for a consistent spiritual life. On the other hand, advanced yoga gives one that consistent spiritual life with steady on-going supernatural and spiritual perceptions. Kriyā yoga holds no attraction for those satisfied with infrequent glimpses of spiritual life. They are unwilling to do the austerities.

When one has a sudden divine revelation as sometimes happens even to the most ordinary people, at that time, the haphazard or organized thoughts pertaining to this world are squeezed out. This occurs not by personal endeavor, but by a divine grace. However, a person who has the desire for kriyā yoga is the type of person who cannot depend on that kind of once-in-a-while grace. Such a person depends mainly on the type of divine grace which spurs him on to complete the kriyā disciplines day after day, resulting in a more consistent communication with divinity.

By effective practice he gains the power to control thoughts, the power to squeeze them out of his mind, the power to situate himself in a place within his psyche where the thoughts do not arise and from where he can operate the mystic vision.

These verses which describe the psychological means to develop self focus for purification and for knowing the self, do not support the contention that self discovery is not a priority. The idea, that self discovery is in the package of Krishna-consciousness, and therefore does not have to be worked on or achieved separately, is a completely new opinion. It is not derived from the *Bhagavad Gītā*, a text in which Śrī Krishna in some chapters, verse after verse, drives home the importance of working for it by mystic practice.

Citing verses from Śrīmad Bhāgavatam and from elsewhere, particularly from Bengali scriptures which describe the life of Lord Caitanya Mahāprabhu, some preachers explain that the gopi cowherd damsels of Vṛndāvana did no meditations in self focus to attain direct service to Śrī Krishna. Some even cite Arjuna who they contend got his perfection merely by being a friend of the Lord.

Nonetheless, a person who is attracted to kriyā yoga and who by nature, feels the need for it, should not be diverted by these arguments. If a person is satisfied hearing of the gopis, or Arjuna and of others in that way, then he should stick to that process for the results promised and for the fulfillments he would receive there. Otherwise, one should pay close attention to these verses in the *Gītā*, take up their practice and follow the methods given by Śrī Krishna.

In Patañjali *Yoga Sūtras*, the description of the culmination of yoga practice is sketched. That exposition tallies completely with these verses of the *Bhagavad Gītā*: That proficiency in yoga is key-noted by the control of the mento-emotional energies and the resulting self-focus, along with freedom from desires and cravings. In other words, the proficiency is known to a yogi who departed the normal consciousness which is saturated with desires, cravings, and random thoughts.

यथा दीपो निवातस्थो
नेङ्गते सोपमा स्मृता ।
योगिनो यतचित्तस्य
युञ्जतो योगमात्मनः ॥६.१९॥

yathā dīpo nivātastho
neṅgate sopamā smṛtā
yogino yatacittasya
yuñjato yogamātmanaḥ (6.19)

yathā — as; dīpo = dīpaḥ — lamp; nivātastho (nivātasthaḥ) = nivāta – windless + sthaḥ — situated; neṅgate = na — not + iṅgate — flickers; sopamā = so (sāḥ) — this + upamā — in comparison; smṛtā — recalled; yogino = yoginaḥ — of the yogi; yatacittasya — of a person whose thinking is restrained; yuñjato = yuñjataḥ — of practicing; yogam — yoga; ātmanaḥ — of the self

This comparison is recalled: A lamp in a windless place which does not flicker, and a yogi of controlled thought who performs disciplines in relation to the spiritual self. (6.19)

Commentary:

The comparison between a lamp in a windless place and the successful yogi, pertains to full success of the four higher stages of yoga, namely pratyāhār sense withdrawal, dhāraṇa mental focus of the attention through the stilled buddhi organ, dhyāna contemplation of what is experienced in the other worlds, and samādhi trance stages where the yogi locks into the other world for extended periods of time. In the pratyāhār sense withdrawal stage, the yogi retracks his interest from the turbulent environment of this world. He does so gradually over a period of time of mystic practice where he trains his psyche to ignore what it finds as delightful. This includes some painful delights, which though painful, bring a perverted pleasure to the psyche.

A yogi with a waiver from cultural activity progresses much faster than one who has to act in the world. Thus, those who act in the world should continue the kriyā disciplines day after day and still tend to the cultural duties assigned. Such a person should be content with his lot of slow progression. His main objective is to get the waiver but he knows that if he does not efficiently carry out his cultural obligations, he will never get the exemption. Thus he tends to cultural duties with great care, listening for hints on how to perform in a terminal way.

It is doubtful that any of us can perfect yoga fully while we perform karma yoga. We must get the waiver so that we can be free for full time practice. All the same, if we do not get the waiver we would be unsuccessful if we neglect cultural duties and substitute yoga practice in its place. This is actually the lesson of the *Gītā* and the objection that Śrī Krishna made to Arjuna's plan, which was to avoid unpalatable cultural obligations. Admittedly the cultural environment is a living threat to a yogi and it is a grim reminder of the sure course of this world of rounds of births and deaths without relief. Nevertheless, we must comply with the demands of the Supreme Being for our participation in His world-saving mission which Śrī Krishna described in Chapter Four:

yadā yadā hi dharmasya glānirbhavati bhārata
abhyutthānamadharmasya tadātmānaṁ sṛjāmyaham (4.7
paritrāṇāya sādhūnāṁ vināśāya ca duṣkṛtām
dharmasaṁsthāpanārthāya saṁbhavāmi yuge yuge (4.8)

Whenever there is a decrease of righteousness, O son of the Bharata family, and when there is an increase of wickedness, then I show Myself. (4.7)

For protecting the saintly people, to destroy the wicked ones, and to establish righteousness, I come into the visible existence from era to era. (4.8)

We should understand that the Supreme Being does not intend to lift a finger to protect the world, even though He defines such sovereignty as His self-appointed duty. In fact He wants everyone else to share in the responsibility. Thus He claims to have organized four castes. We heard of this in Chapter Four:

cāturvarṇyaṁ mayā sṛṣṭaṁ guṇakarmavibhāgaśaḥ
tasya kartāramapi māṁ viddhyakartāramavyayam (4.13)

According to the distribution of habits and work tendencies, the four career categories were instituted by Me. Know that I am never required to participate. (4.13)

Since He says that He is never required to participate, it implies that we should do the work. It is a matter of discovering our allotment, executing it promptly and then getting a waiver from Him. Without the waiver, the full success of yoga practice will elude us. Destiny has a way about it, where it does not allow a yogi to be successful in practice, if he does not have the waiver from cultural activities.

As I stated before, in the pratyāhār sense withdrawal state, the yogi retracts his interest from the sensually-turbulent environment of this world, so that gradually through mystic practice, his psyche becomes trained not to feed on the sense objects. However, for those of us who are duty-bound to cultural life, we cannot really perfect this practice, and therefore our attempt at the three higher stages of yoga will be incomplete. We will not reach the culmination until we gain the waiver. I want to be clear on this, because I do not want to mislead anyone. I myself, at the time of writing these commentaries, am in the status of not being able to reach full culmination.

The fact that I took up the task of writing these commentaries, despite my condition of incomplete yoga practice, is not my fault. I was inspired to write this by Śrī Śrī Krishna - Balarāma Deities, by Lord Shiva and also by Śrī Bābāji Mahasaya of kriyā yoga lineage.

Whatever I need to know for this purpose that I have not perfected in myself, will be told to me or will be shown to me. In addition I can draw on previous completions of yoga in previous lives, information which is stored in my higher subtle body. Thus readers need not harbor any doubts nor be despaired. Śrī Krishna, Śrī Balarāma, Lord Shiva and Śrī Bābāji Mahasaya wanted me to write these purports for the sake of clarification for those who are struggling in the elementary kriyā practice and who are discouraged because of the objections raised by people who feel that yoga should not be practiced.

In the pratyāhār process one tries to quiet down the turbulent sensual environment but one finds that such a task is impossible. When one understands this, one tries to calm oneself in order to make one's psyche become non-responsive. This takes time to complete. In that practice one has to do battle in his mind, with thoughts, picturizations, expanding ideas, as well as with seed desires which come from the subconscious, from the causal body and which continually seep into the subtle form, in the buddhi organ, expanding there and forcing the psyche to act in the material world for fulfillments. This is a big struggle within the psyche. Some kriyā yogis considered this struggle to be so vital, that they took the *Bhagavad Gītā* and said that it is only symbolic of this struggle, that Śrī Krishna represents the self in charge of the psyche and that Arjuna represents this or that within the self. Thus the self must be victorious within and not on a battlefield like Kurukṣetra.

It is certainly a struggle within the psyche but it is a struggle outside of it as well. A conquest within the psyche is a sure indication of a conquest outside in terms of effective renunciation of cultural opportunities.

Once the pratyāhār stage is mastered, the yogi proceeds to the next level, in which he focuses his attention deliberately through the visual energy of the buddhi organ. This is a very technical procedure that cannot be forced by will power. That is the problem with its practice.

In the kriyā path many teachers stress the meditation or focus on the brow chakra, the third eye, the eye that opens up between the eyebrows of the practicing yogi, but such a focus will bear no result for most practitioners because it does not open by will power or merely wanting to see through it.

The 6th stage of yoga, that of dhāraṇa concentration of the will through the buddhi organ, is not perfected by sheer will power or a desire to succeed or by long long hours of practice without the proper technique. Those of us who lack a waiver from cultural activities will only be allowed so many seconds or minutes for this practice daily. The Supreme Being has set the psychological environment in such a way, as to prevent us from stilling the buddhi organ completely, and without stilling it, we cannot engage or focus our will into the visual energy.

Concentration at the third eye with or without eyes tilted upwards is certainly a good practice but the yogi will not have the result if he does not practice in a particular way. He must master Kuṇḍalinī yoga, celibacy yoga and, to a great extent, purity-of-character yoga, otherwise he will not succeed because his buddhi organ will not be quieted. It will be full of mundane impressions and will be goaded and harassed by the impure life force. Seed desires which seep in from the subconscious and the external reality will press upon it and command it to act in the physical and subtle material worlds even against the yogi's will.

This writer heard and followed some of the advice given by some kriyā teachers about focusing on the third eye. I now state that most do not know what they are lecturing on. First, before one can focus effectively, one has to isolate and arrest the visual energy of the buddhi organ. I was trained in this by Śrīla Yogeshwarananda in the subtle world. He used to enter the top of my subtle body and instruct me in this. One must first get hold of the visual energy of the buddhi organ. This indicates that one must know that organ and be able to grasp subtle objects just as if they were gross things. To ultimately be successful in brow chakra meditation, one has to be very advanced.

Once the yogi can locate the visual energy of the buddhi organ, he can focus his will power or attention through it. That is a practice of dhāraṇa concentration. Depending on the yogi's stage of practice and his psychology, he focuses on what is required for success at that stage. It is not stereotyped. Some yogis focus on supernatural persons, some on divine persons, some on mahāyogī teachers, some on the supersubtle world at random, some on the causal world, some on the spiritual world, and some even on objects of this gross dimension.

Śrī Bābāji Mahasaya instructed me to write down that when at first one finds the visual energy, then gradually by daily practice, one is able to hold it and to focus one's attention through it. One sees, as Śrī Paramhansa Yogananda states, a bluish sky. Śrī Bābāji said that some yogis see a very bright blinding light which is hard to stare at. He said that some yogis are captured by that light and remain looking inward at it for a long time, while their physical form remains motionless and their breath becomes suspended. Some, he said, see a bright five-pointed star which keeps their attention anchored to it. Some others must focus on the star for it to remain in their view. He said that persons who have no exemption from cultural acts will be unable to hold the visual energy for long, since the buddhi organ, being prompted by compelling disturbances, will shift back. Such yogis should endeavor for the practice and should take care with cultural duties so that later when waived, they would have cultivated the habit of meditation.

Dhyāna contemplation, the 7th stage of yoga, is a closing stage, just before reaching the samādhi stage. This 7th stage closes out for the yogi, the beginning mystic practice which he struggled to master. A struggle for mastery over sensual energy withdrawal and sensual energy containment occurs because the material world binds one hand-and-foot to the disturbing sensual mechanism. In the material world, one remains bound, so much so, that even those regarded as being religious expect that a saintly person will continue with formal worship ceremonies. If anyone turns away from this and strives for success in kriyā yoga, he must ward off both the religious people and the irreligious people. Thus in the stage of dhyāna contemplation of what is seen and perceived in other ways in the supersubtle world, the yogi gets relief from the psychologically strenuous practices of the pratyāhār sense withdrawal and dhāraṇa focus of his attention through the curbed buddhi organ.

Because Lord Vishnu took it upon Himself to come into gross manifestation to attract and to inspire us to meet Him in the spiritual world, some devotees worship His icon, believing they will go to the transcendental places merely by that Deity worship, as described in the *Puranas* and subsidiary literatures. So when a devotee of Krishna becomes attracted to yoga practice, and his interest in Deity worship decreases as he dedicates more time to yoga, fanatic devotees who do not understand the intention of the Deity appearance, object and issue discouraging and hostile energies to deter the yogi-devotee and to bring him back to the Deity ceremonies. They feel that they are doing him a favor, saving him from the risk of impersonalism.

Unfortunately, these non-yogi devotees miss the entire point of Lord Vishnu's descent, which is to inspire the devotees to rise above this material world so they can meet Lord Vishnu on another side of existence. Lord Vishnu came to get us to take up the kriyā practices through which we can meet Him the highest plane, the spiritual side. The non-yogi devotees do not understand this. They feel they know everything about

Lord Vishnu. Hence a yogi-devotee quietly goes away from them, to abide by the stipulation of isolation (ekākī), so that he can really please Lord Vishnu by leaving the Lord's physical manifestation on this side in order to reach the Lord as He is, on another side. Those who feel that suddenly at the time of death, their physical profile which the subtle body carries, will disappear, will have a rude awakening, when they discover that their outlook remains the same and they must come back into this world to become devotees of the Deities again.

The dhyāna contemplation stage is the stage at which a yogi-devotee steadies himself on whatever becomes perceptible to him on the other side. Over a long period of such practice he gets to see Lord Vishnu there. He steadies the focus and then he is able to enter into samādhi trance to anchor his psyche in that place. Such a person will, at the time of death, follow the same course of escape and leave this material world. How the others, the non-yogi devotees, will do it, only they and their teachers know, because what they are doing is not at all scientific. It is based on hopes and beliefs. Still, hopes and beliefs do have power and therefore we do not deny their claims, but hopes and beliefs are not a definite process.

Whatever was contemplated during the dhyāna stage will be encountered in the samādhi trance stage. While in the dhyāna stage, there was a deliberate focus on these other worlds and the objects perceived there, in the samādhi stage the focus is nondeliberate without any effort whatsoever. Thus in that stage, the yogi is relieved from having to apply himself in a focusing way. He can just cast all his energy, his entire spiritual psyche, into the causal or spiritual environment as the case may be.

The comparison is made to the yogi, who has attained samādhi trance and whose attentive energies are no longer disturbed and distracted by the sensuality in this world. This sensuality includes the Deity form of Lord Vishnu. The Puranic histories attest to this. Lord Kapila flatly stated that Deity worship is part of the neophyte bhakta stage. It is a fact that persons like Dhruva and Nārada, persons who are extolled and followed by all yogi and non-yogi devotees of Lord Vishnu, did leave aside their Mūrtis and steady themselves on samādhi and then focus on the spiritual body of Lord Vishnu. Somehow, most modern devotees of Lord Vishnu ignore these facts and bombast or discourage yogi devotees who strive for attainment.

यत्रोपरमते चित्तं
निरुद्धं योगसेवया ।
यत्र चैवात्मनात्मानं
पश्यन्नात्मनि तुष्यति ॥६.२०॥
yatroparamate cittaṁ
niruddhaṁ yogasevayā
yatra caivātmanātmānaṁ
paśyannātmani tuṣyati (6.20)

yatroparamate = yatra — where + uparamate — it stops; cittaṁ — thinking; niruddhaṁ — restraint; yogasevayā = yoga – yoga discipline + sevayā — by practice; yatra — where; caivātmanā = ca — and + eva — indeed + ātmanā — by the self; 'tmānaṁ = ātmānam — the self; paśyan — seeing; ātmani — in the self; tuṣyati — is satisfied

At the place where being restrained by yoga practice, thinking stops, and at the place where the yogi perceives the self by the self, he is satisfied in the self. (6.20)

__Commentary:__

Cittam niruddham is restraint (niruddham) of the supersubtle emotional energy which filters in from the causal body into the subtle one and which triggers the disturbing sensuality which keeps all conditioned beings both theist and atheist alike, ever busy with desires in the material world. This was also discussed by Śrī Patañjali in the *Yoga Sūtras* where he stated that the culmination of yoga is the restraint of the chitta energy.

Śrī Krishna speaks of the place (yatra) where the disturbing sensuality stops and where the yogi gets free of the psychology of the subtle and causal bodies, so that he can find out who exactly he is. What place is this? Where is it located? The answer is found in kriyā yoga practice, when in the 6th stage of the practice, that of dhāraṇa focus, one finds the dimensional and psychological location from which one can focus attention through the blank visual sense of the buddhi organ. This is not a physical place at all. It cannot be discovered while peering out of the material body on the material world, or even while peering on Deity forms of the Supreme Lord. This place is only found by internalization.

Those who are hung up on the Deity form and think that Deity worship is the culmination of their spiritual life, cannot understand this verse. They feel that yoga is inferior and is simply hard labor for nothing. On the contrary, Śrī Krishna stressed yoga over and over again in so many verses of Chapters Five and Six and elsewhere.

सुखमात्यन्तिकं यत्तद्
बुद्धिग्राह्यमतीन्द्रियम् ।
वेत्ति यत्र न चैवायं
स्थितश्चलति तत्त्वतः ॥६.२१॥
sukhamātyantikaṁ yattad
buddhigrāhyamatīndriyam
vetti yatra na caivāyaṁ
sthitaścalati tattvataḥ (6.21)

sukham — happiness; ātyantikaṁ — continuous; yat = yad — which; tad — this; buddhigrāhyam — grasp by the intellect; atīndriyam — beyond the mundane senses; vetti — he knows; yatra — whereabout; na — not; caivāyam = ca — and + eva — indeed + ayam — this; sthitaścalati = sthitaḥ — established + calati — he shifted; tattvataḥ — the reality

He knows the whereabouts of that continuous happiness, which is grasped by the intellect and which is beyond the mundane senses. And being established, he does not shift from that reality. (6.21)

Commentary:

This is all a technical description of the high end of kriyā yoga practice. At this point, the attention of the spirit, passing through the pinpoint of his initiative, is focused through one of the senses of the buddhi organ. Being established there, one does not shift from that reality (tattvatah).

What is focused on there is superior to everything we perceive here; one does not shift back here unless one is compelled. Thus some yogis who attain this do come back into this world, because they are forced by the way of providence. Some do not return at all, as they are permitted to permanently depart.

यं लब्ध्वा चापरं लाभं
मन्यते नाधिकं ततः ।
यस्मिन्स्थितो न दुःखेन
गुरुणापि विचाल्यते ॥६.२२॥
yaṁ labdhvā cāparaṁ lābhaṁ
manyate nādhikaṁ tataḥ
yasminsthito na duḥkhena
guruṇāpi vicālyate (6.22)

yaṁ — which; labdhvā — having attained; cāparaṁ = ca — and + aparaṁ — other; lābhaṁ — attainment; manyate — he thinks; nādhikam = na — not + adhikam — greater; tataḥ — than that; yasmin — which; sthito = sthitaḥ — established; na — not; duḥkhena — by distress; guruṇāpi = guruṇā – by deep + api — also; vicālyate — is drawn away

And having attained that, he thinks there is no greater attainment. Being established in that, he is not drawn away, even by deep distress. (6.22)

Commentary:

This applies to those who do come back here. Since they had that experience and since they practiced sufficiently to attain steadiness in touch with those high realities, they no longer have the same attraction to this place as before. Thus they are not drawn away from that higher level, even if subjected to deep distress. They keep in touch with that even when obligated or induced to participate in social and cultural affairs.

Indirectly, Śrī Krishna said that if Arjuna was that advanced of a yogi, he would do his duty as a warrior even when faced with the prospect of mundane distress, a prospect Arjuna faced at Kurukṣetra. From so many angles, Śrī Krishna proved that Arjuna was not in the spiritual view.

तं विद्याद्दुःखसंयोग —
वियोगं योगसंज्ञितम् ।
स निश्चयेन योक्तव्यो
योगोऽनिर्विण्णचेतसा ॥६.२३॥
taṁ vidyādduḥkhasaṁyoga —
viyogaṁ yogasaṁjñitam
sa niścayena yoktavyo
yogo'nirviṇṇacetasā (6.23)

tam — this; vidyād = vidyāt — let it be understood; duḥkhasaṁyoga = duḥkha – emotional distress + saṁyoga — emotional identity with; viyogaṁ — separation; yogasaṁjñitam = yoga – mastery of yoga + saṁjñitam — recognized as; sa = saḥ — this; niścayena — with determination; yoktavyo = yoktavyaḥ — to be practiced; yogo = yogah — yoga; 'nirviṇṇacetasā (anirviṇṇacetasā) = anirviṇṇa – not depressed + cetasā — with thought

Let it be understood that this separation from emotional distress is the mastery of yoga. This yoga is to be practiced with determination and without depressing thought. (6.23)

Commentary:

A key note of successful yoga practice is renunciation. This was described in verse 2 of Chapter Six:

yaṁ saṁnyāsamiti prāhur yogaṁ taṁ viddhi pāṇḍava
na hyasaṁnyastasaṁkalpo yogī bhavati kaścana (6.2)

That which the authorities define as renunciation, know it as applied yoga, O Arjuna Pandava. Indeed, no one becomes a yogi without an intention for renunciation. (6.2)

Another key note is the separation from emotional distress. Arjuna, though he mastered yoga to a greater degree, did not master it enough to realize the distinction between his spirit and his emotional nature. One's emotional nature is part of a cosmic system of sympathetic feelings. Even though it is in the psyche, one should keep a distance from it. This distance is kept by the emotional-hardening developed in advanced yoga practice.

Here Śrī Krishna tactfully revealed that the yogic accomplishments of Arjuna did not include a thorough detachment within. Śrī Krishna hinted that Arjuna needed to complete the yoga course but without any depressing thoughts whatsoever. Arjuna had to continue the practice and keep away from the energies which produced depressing thoughts.

Many neophyte yogis fail to pass over this hurdle and remain affected by the depressing thoughts. Many thereby turn away from yoga. Many more will do the same in the future. That depression, which comes from the required psychological isolation, is so powerful and penetrating that it stops a neophyte from going any further on the kriyā path. It causes him to turn about and submit to social and cultural demands. This Chapter Six is an overview of the kriyā yoga practice.

संकल्पप्रभवान्कामांस्
त्यक्त्वा सर्वानशेषतः ।
मनसैवेन्द्रियग्रामं
विनियम्य समन्ततः ॥६.२४॥
saṁkalpaprabhavānkāmāṁs
tyaktvā sarvānaśeṣataḥ
manasaivendriyagrāmaṁ
viniyamya samantataḥ (6.24)

saṁkalpaprabhavān = saṁkalpa — motive + prabhavān — produced; kāmāṁs — cravings; tyaktvā — having abandoned; sarvān — all; aśeṣataḥ — without exception; manasaivendriyagrāmaṁ = manasā — by mind + eva — indeed + indriyagrāmaṁ — the total sensual energy; viniyamya — controlling; samantataḥ — completely

Abandoning without exception, all desires which are produced from motivation, and completely restraining the total sensual energy by the mind, (6.24)

Commentary:

This is another advanced stage in kriyā practice when the yogi locates himself in such a place (yatra, B.G. 6.20) that the motivation energy in the causal body no longer seeps into the subtle form to motivate it for social and cultural acts. When he is located in the right place within the psychology, then the mind does not accommodate external sensual energy and does not allow the intellect to send rays into the outer world. The nature of the mind changes completely. It keeps the sensual energy depolarized from this world with a distinctive lack of attraction to the excitements.

शनैः शनैरुपरमेद्
बुद्ध्या धृतिगृहीतया ।
आत्मसंस्थं मनः कृत्वा
न किंचिदपि चिन्तयेत् ॥६.२५॥

śanaiḥ śanairuparamed
buddhyā dhṛtigṛhītayā
ātmasaṁsthaṁ manaḥ kṛtvā
na kiṁcidapi cintayet (6.25)

śanaiḥ śanair (śanaiḥ) — little by little; uparamed = uparamet — should withdraw from sensual activity; buddhyā — by intelligence; dhṛtigṛhītayā = dhṛti – firmness + gṛhītayā — grasped; ātmasaṁsthaṁ = ātma – spiritual self + saṁsthaṁ — fixed; manah — mind; kṛtvā — having made; na — not; kiṁcit — anything; api — even; cintayet — should think

...little by little, with a firm grasp by the intelligence, he should withdraw from sensual activity. Having made his mind to be fixed on the spiritual self, he should not think of anything. (6.25)

Commentary:

Śrī Krishna regressed to give Arjuna some lessons. It appears that Arjuna was integrated in the stage of kriyā practice where the yogi masters pratyāhār sense withdrawal and then begins to practice the dhāraṇa focus. Arjuna was then accelerated to a higher state by the boost of his brother Yudhiṣṭhira and his grandfather Vyāsadeva. However when their assistance was withdrawn, Arjuna was left to himself at the 5th stage, the pratyāhār practice.

This is worthy of notation. If we take a boost from a kriyā master, that boost does not reflect our actual status. The only thing that indicates true progression is individual practice. Boosts or shaktipat or whatever we may call it, grace and mercy and all these influences, are not the true progression. One has to make one's own endeavor. Only that would be permanently ingrained.

To continue the yoga practice, Śrī Krishna instructed that little by little, with a firm grasp over the operation of intellect, Arjuna should withdraw from sensual activity. This is the pratyāhār or 5th stage. When this is mastered, one gains fixity on the psychology which leads to a controlling relationship with it.

यतो यतो निश्चरति
मनश्चञ्चलमस्थिरम् ।
ततस्ततो नियम्यैतद्
आत्मन्येव वशं नयेत् ॥६.२६॥
yato yato niścarati
manaścañcalamasthiram
tatastato niyamyaitad
ātmanyeva vaśaṁ nayet (6.26)

yato yato = yataḥ yataḥ — wherever; niścarati — wanders away; manaścañcalam = manas — mind + cañcalam — drifting; asthiram — unsteady; tatastato = tatastataḥ — from there; niyamyaitad = niyamya — restrain + etad — it; ātmany (ātmani) — in the self; eva — indeed; vaśam — control; nayet — should direct

To wherever the unsteady, drifty mind wanders, from there he should restrain it. He should direct the mind to control it in the self. (6.26)

Commentary:

This is the 5th. stage of yoga practice. It is surprising in a way that Arjuna, a person who attained samādhis in the Himalayas and who visited the Swārga paradise of Indra, was by himself, in his personal endeavors only on the 5th stage. But that was the case. Thus without the boost of Yudhiṣṭhira and Śrīla Vyāsadeva, Arjuna acted cowardly when he faced relatives at Kurukṣetra. These are valuable lessons about personal practice.

In this verse, the word mind means the mind chamber and its contents, which are the buddhi organ and the initiative. These must be steadied from their drifty wanderings. The yogi tries to do this and then he discovers that he has to be located in a certain place in the psyche for achievement. He also discovers that a counterproductive life style contributes to psychosis. With this understanding he makes certain adjustments.

प्रशान्तमनसं ह्येनं
योगिनं सुखमुत्तमम् ।
उपैति शान्तरजसं
ब्रह्मभूतमकल्मषम् ॥६.२७॥
praśāntamanasaṁ hyenaṁ
yoginaṁ sukhamuttamam
upaiti śāntarajasaṁ
brahmabhūtamakalmaṣam (6.27)

praśāntamanasaṁ = praśānta — psychologically pacified + manasaṁ — mind; hyenaṁ = hy (hi) — indeed + enam — him; yoginaṁ — yogi; sukham — happiness; uttamam — superior; upaiti — experiences; śāntarajasaṁ = śānta — calmed + rajasam — emotion; brahmabhūtam — spiritual level; akalmaṣam — free from bad tendencies

Indeed, being psychologically pacified, the yogi, whose emotions are calmed, who is on the spiritual plane, who is free from bad tendencies, experiences superior happiness. (6.27)

Commentary:

This psychological pacification is not a trick of settling down the mind, or reducing its stress by quietness, exposure to nature scenes, calming music or chanting many rounds of holy names. This pacification comes from escaping the sensual environment which we are presently engaged. When the yogi shifts off, pierces through and focuses his attention and his buddhi organ mechanism into the other sky, then he gets this pacification. After mastering pratyāhār sensual energy withdrawal and then practicing dhāraṇa concentration of the initiative into the focusing power of the buddhi organ, the yogi reaches this stage.

In this case, the yogi's emotions are calmed, because he was transferred to another plane of existence, a place free from the troublesome nature which occurs on the human level of social existence. His transfer to that plane, however, is temporary, because inevitably he returns to this level to deal with others, for purposes of teaching and for ending entanglements for which he has no exemption or waiver.

In his own psyche, because he has left aside or slipped beyond the troublesome emotional zone, it has subsided like a raging angry sea which spent all its violent energy and returned to calmness. However, if again the yogi is put into a turbulent condition by arrangement of destiny, his emotional being will again become agitated. He will again be subjected to the violent moods which are symptomatic of being agitated in the material world. The potential for such behavior is always there on that level.

The freedom from bad tendencies (akalmasam) comes from effective kriyā practice which the yogi performed before he reached the advanced stages. These cause changes in his character, such that he does not cheat, steal, connive or manipulate others. Most of all he does not neglect self-critique. This self-critiquing technique is a hallmark of kriyā practice, in which the yogi gets an energy from higher yogis, to turn his critical energy onto himself. When he applies this consistently it causes changes in his character, which regulate his behavior in such a way to make him into a veritable saint. Thus as Śrī Krishna says, such a yogi attains the superior happiness (sukham uttamam).

युञ्जन्नेवं सदात्मानं
योगी विगतकल्मषः ।
सुखेन ब्रह्मसंस्पर्शम्
अत्यन्तं सुखमश्नुते ॥६.२८॥
yuñjannevaṁ sadātmānaṁ
yogī vigatakalmaṣaḥ
sukhena brahmasaṁsparśam
atyantaṁ sukhamaśnute (6.28)

yuñjan — applying yoga disciplines; evaṁ — thus; sadā — constantly; 'tmānaṁ = ātmānam — the self; yogī — yogi; vigatakalmaṣaḥ — free from faults; sukhena — easily; brahmasaṁsparśam — contacting the spiritual plane; atyantaṁ — endless; sukham — happiness; aśnute — attains

Applying the yoga disciplines constantly to the self, the yogi being freed from faults, easily contacting the spiritual plane, attains endless happiness. (6.28)

Commentary:

This again is stressed by Śrī Krishna, about the constant application of the yoga disciplines. This is the method whereby one does not stop the practice but continues on and on, day after day, accumulating the skill of yoga. Unless one is motivated strongly, one cannot do this. Without the constant application one cannot be successful. Yoga practice, though it is primed by help from senior yogis and from the Supreme Being, will flounder if one does not habitually do it and make it the top priority in one's life.

Even though Śrī Krishna described some very high stages of practice, still in so many verses, He stressed the required constancy of effort. Sadā means always or on-going.

We should note that Śrī Krishna, unlike many of those teachers who came down in His succession recently, does stress the application of the yoga disciplines to the self (yunjan evam sadātmānam). Śrī Krishna for His own glorification could have put Himself here as the object of the disciplines but we see that He puts the self of the yogi ('tmānam/ātmānam). Elsewhere in the *Gītā*, Lord Krishna will stress Himself but here for the purpose of defining what yoga is, He stresses the self of the practitioner. It is not that the practitioner is unable to properly focus on Śrī Krishna initially. Nor is it true that by initially focusing on Krishna, the self will be purified. That is totally wrong. Unfortunately, it is a working belief of many leading and following devotees of Śrī Krishna who push the idea with convincing arguments.

Exactly how such preachers dismiss so many verses, which stress the focus of the self and the application of yoga disciplines, is a mystery to this commentator. These people dodge and weave their way out of these verses with a skill that even a yogi admires. However we have to stick to this verse and to what was originally said to Arjuna. By applying the yoga disciplines constantly to the self, the yogi, being freed from faults, easily contacting the spiritual plane, attains endless happiness.

सर्वभूतस्थमात्मानं
सर्वभूतानि चात्मनि ।
ईक्षते योगयुक्तात्मा
सर्वत्र समदर्शनः ॥६.२९॥

sarvabhūtasthamātmānaṁ
sarvabhūtāni cātmani
īkṣate yogayuktātmā
sarvatra samadarśanaḥ (6.29)

sarvabhūtastham — existing in all mundane creature forms; ātmānaṁ — spirit; sarvabhūtāni — all creatures; cātmani = ca — see + ātmani — in the self; īkṣate — he sees; yogayuktātmā — one who is proficient in yoga; sarvatra — in all cases; samadarśanaḥ — seeing the same

With a spirit existing in every creature, and with every creature based on a spirit, a person who is proficient in yoga, perceives the same existential arrangement in all cases. (6.29)

Commentary:

Interestingly, even though Śrī Krishna gave so many technical details about yoga, still He had no intention of allowing Arjuna to pursue the completion of its practice at the time of the Battle of Kurukṣetra. Śrī Krishna, as the Supreme Being, would not give Arjuna a waiver or exemption from cultural life at that stage of Arjuna's life. It means therefore that Arjuna had to keep this information in mind, like a student who is given a textbook for a class which he will take later. However, those of us who have a full or partial exemption from the cultural world, can use any or all of this information, depending on the amount of time we are allowed for practice.

This vision of similarity is mentioned frequently in the *Bhagavad Gītā*. We have to remember this and apply this idea whenever Śrī Krishna speaks of the similarity. Other types of similarities exist, but Śrī Krishna mentions this particular one which is also stressed in the *Upanishads*. Sometimes, commentators and readers of the *Bhagavad Gītā* substitute the other similarities and pass that off either on audiences or on themselves as being the ones

Śrī Krishna mentioned. As kriyā yogis we should not make such mistakes. We gain nothing from Śrī Krishna by hijacking His words and attaching our preferred meanings.

This vision is obtained by someone who is proficient in yoga and by no other person. Others might get the vision now and again, but not consistently. It is only by yoga practice, that one usually gets vision in that way. By the use of drugs as many modern youths do, by the use of prayers and chants, by injury to the brain and nerves, a person might, in some cases, get this vision but it will not be consistent or lasting.

Proficiency in yoga (yogayukta) is required for the consistency. In this vision one sees the same existential arrangement of a spirit attached psychologically to a mind and life force, with or without a gross body. We can understand this intellectually but that is not the same as seeing it visually on the mystic plane, where one sees subtle objects like the life force and the buddhi organ, and where through the sense of initiative, one sees the spirit reflected as a bright spherical light. This existential arrangement is the same in the case of each spirit, even though spirits do vary in their efficient usage of the psyche and in their existential power levels.

यो मां पश्यति सर्वत्र
सर्वं च मयि पश्यति ।
तस्याहं न प्रणश्यामि
स च मे न प्रणश्यति ॥६.३०॥

yo māṁ paśyati sarvatra
sarvaṁ ca mayi paśyati
tasyāhaṁ na praṇaśyāmi
sa ca me na praṇaśyati (6.30)

yo = yaḥ — who; mām — me; paśyati — sees; sarvatra — in all forms; sarvam — all creatures; ca — and; mayi — in Me; paśyati — sees; tasyāham = tasya — his + aham — I; na — never; praṇaśyāmi — I am out of range; sa = saḥ — he; ca — and; me — my; na — never; praṇaśyati — he is out of view

To him who sees Me in all forms and who sees all creatures in reference to Me, I am never out of range, and he is never out of My view. (6.30)

Commentary:

Śrī Krishna switched to a higher vision which is seen by more advanced yogis. There are others who have learnt about this and who were taught to believe this. They become convinced that Śrī Krishna is in every form but are not consistent in the application of such learning. They do not actually see this when they look through their gross eyeballs. Their subtle vision does not function on the mystic plane.

According to the Vedic version, this is the vision of the Paramātmā Supersoul or the Antaryami inner monitor of each being. This Person, it is said, exists in the causal body of every living being and is about the size of a thumb if He is perceived directly. He is said to have four arms and has a very pleasing appearance and is adorned with clothing, garlands, and jewels. This Person appears on the causal plane, existing there in the causal section of the psyche of every living being. Each living being who has a subtle body, has this Person abiding in the causal form which is the support and origin of that subtle body.

There is no question of perceiving this Supersoul if one has not perceived the causal body. In fact most religious people cannot perceive their own subtle form. Yes, many people have a belief in it, but most of them do not have the perception. Therefore there is no question of knowing their causal form and hence many of us cannot see this Supersoul directly.

Generally Śrī Krishna remains beyond range of the human beings because they are too grossly aware and hardbound in their focus on this gross world. Since Śrī Krishna is not manifested in a living physical form as He was in the time of Arjuna, many of us cannot perceive Him, except through His contact from the *Bhagavad Gītā* and the other scriptures which illustrate His life and teachings.

A small group of human beings make contact with Śrī Krishna's Deity form, which is a non-living physical form. Physically such a form is non-living, but on the mystic plane, He is very active. Because that physical form of the Deity of Śrī Krishna appears as a non-living physical form, many people have difficulty believing that the Deity is indeed Śrī Krishna.

सर्वभूतस्थितं यो मां
भजत्येकत्वमास्थितः ।
सर्वथा वर्तमानोऽपि
स योगी मयि वर्तते ॥६.३१॥
sarvabhūtasthitaṁ yo māṁ
bhajatyekatvamāsthitaḥ
sarvathā vartamāno'pi
sa yogī mayi vartate (6.31)

sarvabhūtasthitam — existentially situated in all creatures; yo = yaḥ — who; māṁ — Me; bhajaty = bhajati — he honors; ekatvam — in harmony; āsthitaḥ — established; sarvathā — in various circumstances; vartamāno = vartamānaḥ — existentially situated; 'pi = api — although; sa = saḥ — he; yogī — yogi; mayi — in Me; vartate — he remains in touch

Although moving in various circumstances, the yogi who is established in that harmony, who honors Me as being existentially situated in all creatures, remains in touch with Me. (6.31)

Commentary:

The stages of this realization begin with seeing the existence of a spirit harnessed with a set of psychological equipments. When this becomes firmly rooted by constant practice, in mystic yoga, then the person moves to a higher vision of seeing the Supreme Self, Śrī Krishna, alongside the spirit in each form. This Supreme Self is seen as the same Pervading Personality, even though the spirits are all different individual souls.

When at first one sees the spirits who are harnessed with the psychological equipments, one faces the components of personality and then one goes into a state of shock. These components of personality expose the myth of the cultural person, the so-called human being. Here it is rather a combination of a spirit and various psychic equipments with a socio-cultural overcoating. This makes the yogi want to laugh at the presumption of the social designations. He specifically smiles when he sees so many entities who pose as eternal spiritual masters and who have disciples toting such a doctrine and harassing the public about something that is totally untrue. A person may rise to power as a spiritual master and not even be qualified as such. Another person may qualify as a spiritual master and not have a single disciple.

The social designations, including that of "spiritual master", are for the most part, a farce. Most of them are not perpetual. Seeing this on the mystic plane, when seeing the components of the so-called personality of each human being, the yogi desires to laugh. However since he has a practice to maintain, he does not become preoccupied with these perceptions.

In between the stage of seeing the spirits harnessed to the psychological equipments and that of seeing the Supreme Being who resides in each of the psyches, there is an interim stage not mentioned in this overview by Śrī Krishna. The interim stage is the realization that all spirits and their psychological hook-ups (equipments) are efficiently conducted by material nature. This vision gives the yogi an added boost of detachment, especially when he sees the awesome all-encompassing power of material nature.

Even though the vision of the All-pervading, All-penetrating Supreme Being is a higher vision that comes at a later stage, still the vision of material nature's control is important in causing the yogi to develop the highest degree of dispassion. When this material nature is seen, the yogi realizes that he does not have the power to match it. Thus he desists from trying to save the world all by himself. This dispassion does not give him an exemption from cultural work but it does free him from a bloated sense of compassion.

This is important because a person who is not freed from his own hang-ups cannot advance far in yoga. He will go a little way and then become stagnant, or he will go a little way and then keep practicing day after day without making progress, even for years. So long as the neophyte yogi does not get rid of his own sense of compassion or does not become detached from it, he cannot reach the advanced stage. In the back of his mind, he will feel that the Supreme Being sponsors violence.

The violence in the world and the disparities that we see are certainly being sponsored, but not by the Supreme Being, only by material nature, or by what Śrī Krishna called the inherent nature (svabhāva):

na kartṛtvaṁ na karmāṇi lokasya sṛjati prabhuḥ
na karmaphalasaṁyogaṁ svabhāvastu pravartate (5.14)

The Lord does not create the means of action, or the actions of the creature, or the action consequence cycle. But the inherent nature causes this. (5.14)

Until the yogi can see this directly, he cannot really accept it. This is because he has not seen that the so-called personalities are a hodge-podge or quilted combination of spirits, and their subtle psychologies. This subtle psychology is a combination of various mystic equipments, like life force, buddhi organ, mind compartment, causal body and a sense of initiative.

An engine in whole consists of various parts. It is not partless and can be dismantled. Similarly, the human personality as we call it in normal usage, is nothing but a spirit and some psychic parts. A yogi is first shocked into these considerations when by the grace of a steady practice of his own and by guidance from great yogis, he is shown his own buddhi organ as merely a mystic mechanism. When he begins to see subtle objects just as clearly as he can distinguish physical things, then he understands this.

In this verse, Śrī Krishna spoke of the yogi who moves about in various circumstances. It appears from this that the yogi surpassed the stage of having to stay at one place for disciplines and meditation. In other words, this yogi mastered even the samādhis and is free to travel about any and everywhere. He is so advanced that being in the various social environments cannot cause him to digress. His spiritual vision is so constant, so permanently a part of his normal stage of mind, that the world is no threat to him. This is an advanced yogi.

Even though like other commentators I give remarks on these advanced stages, which are beyond the stage where I practice now, still what I say has value because I can remember my former practice of these stages. At present I am commissioned by Śrī Bābāji Mahasaya to give this commentary. In addition whatever I would need to write down will come into my consciousness automatically by the grace of either Śrī Krishna, Śrī Baladeva, Lord Shiva, Śrīla Yogeshwarananda, Śrī Bābāji Mahasaya, Śrī Agastya Muni, Lord Hanumānji and others who are conversant with the practices. Recently, on October 15th of 2001, I asked Sriman Bharat Patel to procure for me, the *Bhagavad Gītā* commentary of Śrī Paramhansa Yogananda. I am supposed to receive that in a few days. The reason is this: Śrī Bābāji Mahasaya told me that my commentary is a continuation of the commentary which was written by Śrī Paramhansaji. According to Śrī Bābāji Mahasaya, Paramhansaji was commissioned by him to write that *Gītā* but for one reason or the other, it did not fulfill the whole task. Hence this became necessary. There was also a published work along the same line, by Śrīla Satyeshwarananda. In any case, as another agent of Śrī Bābāji Mahasaya, I present the Mahasaya's ideas and intentions as they relate to Śrī Krishna's teachings.

When the yogi becomes very very advanced, and when the samadhis which he experienced, are embedded in his consciousness, then he begins to see the Supreme Being everywhere. It is said that Śrī Aurobindo, a yogi in India, did in fact reach this stage. From what I recall in my past lives when I perfected this, one gets from this a special happiness to be able to see that Supreme Being everywhere. One hardly sees the limited spirits in that stage, not even one's own self. One not only sees God then, but one sees exactly how God does not relate to what is going on in the social world. This vision is different to the vision of the Universal Form which Śrī Krishna showed Arjuna. This vision is similar to working in a modern factory. In such a factory there might be hundreds of workers on the ground floor, doing various tasks, busily meeting assigned quotas and putting various things together. As a worker, one is occupied with the tasks assigned. One hardly thinks of the owner of the factory. Then one day one looks up and sees someone on a higher floor, who merely watches everything. He sees some workers who are lazily doing their tasks, some who sabotage the factory, some who are very efficient and others who are idle or arguing with a foreman. The owner just looks and does not interfere. Of course, if a worker sees the owner in such a detached mood that employee is bound to wonder. After all, why does the owner not interfere to chastise some workers and to reward others? Why is he so detached? One smiles when one realizes too that the owner is aware of the fact that one has seen him, while the vast majority of other workers do not even know of the owner's existence on that higher floor. Who is that owner of the enterprise? Where is he from? What category is he in? What is his relationship with each and every worker and the foremen who are so concerned about the enterprise, even more so than the owner himself?

आत्मौपम्येन सर्वत्र
समं पश्यति योऽर्जुन ।
सुखं वा यदि वा दुःखं
स योगी परमो मतः ॥६.३२॥
ātmaupamyena sarvatra
samaṁ paśyati yo'rjuna
sukhaṁ vā yadi vā duḥkhaṁ
sa yogī paramo mataḥ (6.32)

ātmaupamyena = ātma — self + aupamyena — by reference; sarvatra — in all cases; samaṁ — similarity; paśyati — he sees; yo = yaḥ — who; 'rjuna = arjuna — Arjuna; sukhaṁ — pleasurable sensations; vā — or; yadi — regardless; vā — or; duḥkhaṁ — painful sensations; sa = saḥ — he; yogī — yogi; paramo = paramaḥ — highest; mataḥ — considered as

He who, in reference to himself, sees the same facilities in all cases, regardless of pleasure or painful sensations, he, O Arjuna, is considered as the highest yogi. (6.32)

Commentary:

Even though he mentioned the higher realization in the previous verse, still Śrī Krishna returned to the foundational vision of seeing that a spirit is harnessed to psychic equipments in each of the creature forms. Many spiritual masters profess that this realization is very basic and that a person need not strive for it in particular. In their view, the vision of Śrī Krishna with two hands in a transcendental body, as the archa vigraha sanctified duly-installed Mūrti icon in the temple, is better and will include these baseline views. However such opinions are their ideas only and not Śrī Krishna's. Repeatedly through the *Gītā*, this vision of the similarity in each of the creature forms, comprising of a spirit and a psychology which amounts to spirit and psychic equipments, is stressed by Śrī Krishna.

This refers neither to the intellectual idea of this nor the understanding and mere acceptance of it. It is a direct mystic perception, seeing a spirit and viewing his psychic equipments in broad psychic daylight. The person who sees like this consistently, who has developed his yoga practice that far, and whose buddhi organ became so introverted as to convert its imagination-faculty into psychic vision, is considered to be the highest yogi (yogī paramah matah). He completed the eightfold yoga course through its system of disciplines.

This verse 32 is Lord Krishna's completion of the curriculum for yoga, but we will hear more as Arjuna requests details.

अर्जुन उवाच
योऽयं योगस्त्वया प्रोक्तः
साम्येन मधुसूदन ।
एतस्याहं न पश्यामि
चञ्चलत्वात्स्थितिं स्थिराम् ॥६.३३॥
arjuna uvāca
yo'yaṁ yogastvayā proktaḥ
sāmyena madhusūdana
etasyāhaṁ na paśyāmi
cañcalatvātsthitiṁ sthirām (6.33)

arjuna – Arjuna; uvāca — said; yo = yah – who; 'yaṁ = ayaṁ — this; yogas — yoga practice; tvayā — by you; proktaḥ — explained; sāmyena — by comparative similarity; madhusūdana — O slayer of Madhu; etasyāhaṁ = etasyā — of this + aham — I; na — not; paśyāmi — see; cañcalatvāt — due to shiftiness; sthitiṁ — position; sthirām — standard

Arjuna said: O slayer of Madhu, due to a shifty vision, I do not see this standard position of a comparatively similar view which is yielded by this yoga practice, declared by You. (6.33)

Commentary:

It is due to shifty vision (cañcalatvāt), but that shiftiness is the normal course in creature existence. Arjuna was correct. We discover this truth when we attempt to meditate before mastering prāṇāyāma. Those who meditate without first mastering prāṇāyāma are simply joking about the process, for their shifty mind will not allow the liberty of directly and correctly perceiving the psychic phenomena. So long as the intellect is taking energy from lower levels, it cannot stop this shiftiness.

A person can look at whatever Deity he likes even the properly-installed, properly-sanctified Deity of Śrī Krishna. He can chant whatever name of God that suits his fancy. He can be a loyal member to his religious group, but unless he can make his mind take in a higher level of energy, it will not be stable. It will be shifty. Despite the proposal of shifting from one idea of Krishna to another, on and on, in the declared system of Krishna Consciousness, he will still not develop the luminous consciousness described. His mystic perception will still not be clear.

Even though Śrī Krishna, the Supreme Being, was standing next to Arjuna, still Arjuna could not see the spirits being harnessed to various similar psychic equipments in each of the bodies of the soldiers before him. He could not see Śrī Krishna as the detached over-

Lord of all these creature forms. Still today, many devotees of Krishna allow themselves to be convinced that they will see this merely by seeing the Deity of Śrī Krishna, by calling the name of Krishna and by fulfilling the missionary ambitions of spiritual masters. The beliefs become rooted through the hypnotic influence of these gurus.

Arjuna, the dear friend of Śrī Krishna, the eternal friend of the Lord, who travels with the Lord here and there continually, admitted that he did not see the comparatively similar view of the creatures which Śrī Krishna described as being a product of successful yoga practice. Still, others have stated that if we become their disciples and convince others to do likewise, we will automatically see all this. It is a wonder indeed!

चञ्चलं हि मनः कृष्ण
प्रमाथि बलवद्दृढम् ।
तस्याहं निग्रहं मन्ये
वायोरिव सुदुष्करम् ॥६.३४॥

cañcalaṁ hi manaḥ kṛṣṇa
pramāthi balavaddṛḍham
tasyāhaṁ nigrahaṁ manye
vāyoriva suduṣkaram (6.34)

cañcalam — unsteady; hi — indeed; manaḥ — the mind; kṛṣṇa — Krishna; pramāthi — troubling; balavat — impulsive; dṛḍham — resistant; tasyāham = tasya — of it + aham — I; nigraham — controlling; manye — I think; vāyor = vāyoḥ — of the wind; iva — compared to; suduṣkaram — very difficult to accomplish

Unsteady indeed is my mind, O Krishna. It is troublesome, impulsive and resistant. I think that controlling it is comparable to controlling the wind. It is very difficult to accomplish. (6.34)

Commentary:

This accurately describes a mind with no recourse but to take in energy from lower levels. This is why prāṇāyāma is necessary for it enables the mind to take in energy from higher levels. From the lower levels one cannot really improve on the nature of the mind. The nature of its energy intake determines how it functions. If a higher energy, a higher form of prāṇa, is absorbed, then the mind's shiftiness stops. The key here is not the mind, or the spirit who tries to regulate it, but the subtle energy, prāṇa, which the mind ingests. Prāṇāyāma, the 4th step of yoga is necessary if we want consistent success in yoga practice. Other methods of yoga or religion or whatever, cannot do much to make the mind take in higher types of energy.

Arjuna had controlled his mind like that before when he performed yoga and entered into samādhi but sitting there on the chariot at Kurukṣetra, he lost touch with that ability. Since his previous success in yoga, he had dropped to a much lower level of mental energy intake. He was back to our usual level of consciousness. Was Arjuna *Krishna Conscious* as it is defined today by some authorities? He certainly was. And still, he could not get his mind to that plane where he could see the comparatively similar psychological situation of the creatures. It is a mystery, how we who do not have Śrī Krishna before us physically, will be able to bypass yoga and reach the higher stage.

श्रीभगवानुवाच
असंशयं महाबाहो
मनो दुर्निग्रहं चलम्।
अभ्यासेन तु कौन्तेय
वैराग्येण च गृह्यते ॥६.३५॥
śrībhagavānuvāca
asaṁśayaṁ mahābāho
mano durnigrahaṁ calam
abhyāsena tu kaunteya
vairāgyeṇa ca gṛhyate (6.35)

śrībhagavān – the Blessed Lord; uvāca — said; asaṁśayam — undoubtedly; mahābāho — O powerful man; mano = manah — the mind; durnigraham — difficult to control; calam — unsteady; abhyāsena — by practice; tu — however; kaunteya — O son of Kuntī; vairāgyena — by the indifference to response; ca — and; gṛhyate — it is restrained

The Blessed Lord said: Undoubtedly, O powerful man, the mind is difficult to control. It is unsteady. By practice, however, O son of Kuntī, by indifference to its responses, also, it is restrained. (6.35)

Commentary:

Abhyāsena means, *by practice,* to control the mind as stipulated in yoga. It does not mean using other methods to control the mind which were not designed or discovered by the Upanishadic yogi sages. One must use yogic methods to control the mind, otherwise one will not be successful. In addition, one must become indifferent to the mind's responses to the various stimuli the mind encounters in the material world. This all takes time to implement. The mind does not give up easily. Anyone who hopes for success must practice for some time to get sustaining results. Otherwise one will get limited success and then regress terribly and be baffled again and again.

Unless a person is serious, he will not attain mind control. He must also be granted at least a partial waiver by the Supreme Being, so that he can find the time to practice. One must use whatever quality time one has to cultivate yoga. If one does this, mind control methods that are effective will be automatically earned or inspired into one's mind.

These mind control techniques directly involve controlling or holding the mind in order to stop it from random thoughts, imaginations and ideas without having to substitute in the mind, mantras and various sounds. In other words, by these techniques one can actually stop the mind from its vrittis or adjustments without having to use crutches or preferred diversions. When the mind is stopped from its thoughts, imaginations and ideas, then one's brow chakra operates and finally in the higher stages, one's spiritual vision opens up. The brow chakra is an eye in the subtle body, but when the spiritual vision opens, that is an entirely different type of vision. Both of these are attained when one is able to control the mind without using sounds and various other diversions or preferred indulgences.

Vairāgyena, indifference to responses, comes gradually after the yogi realizes that so long as he exposes the mind or allows the mind to expose itself to the sensual objects, he must endure its regurgitation of the residual impressions. Not wanting to repeatedly clean the mind and vent the absorbed impressions, he begins to tighten the intake of the senses, so that many impressions do not enter. Then, eventually, he realizes that he is working against himself by leaving the mind to its own devices and he seeks psychological isolation, ekākī (B.G. 6.10).

Since the yogi lacks a full waiver from the Supreme Being, from Śrī Krishna, and must be culturally involved to a degree, he monitors his mind closely when in sensually-charged or excitement-charged environments. In this way he absorbs a minimal amount of sensual impressions and has less clearing and venting of the mind to do when he sits for his pratyāhār and other meditation practices. It all takes time and individual effort.

असंयतात्मना योगो
दुष्प्राप इति मे मतिः ।
वश्यात्मना तु यतता
शक्योऽवाप्तुमुपायतः ॥६.३६॥
asaṁyatātmanā yogo
duṣprāpa iti me matiḥ
vaśyātmanā tu yatatā
śakyo'vāptumupāyataḥ (6.36)

asaṁyatātmanā = asaṁyata —undisciplined + ātmanā — by the self; yogo = yogaḥ — yoga; duṣprāpa — difficult to master; iti — thus; me — my; matiḥ — opinion; vaśyātmanā = vaśya — disciplined + ātmanā — by the self; tu — however; yatatā — by endeavor; śakyo = śakyaḥ — possible; 'vāptum = avāptum — to acquire; upāyataḥ — by effective means

For the undisciplined person, yoga is difficult to master. This is My opinion. For the disciplined one, however, by endeavor, it is possible to acquire the skill by an effective means. (6.36)

Commentary:

To be a yogi, one must be able to endeavor and one must have an effective means. Those who cannot earn their spiritual progress may take to other paths. It all depends on the nature of the individual. The psychology of a spirit is to a degree conditioned by material nature. Yoga, therefore, is not for everyone.

अर्जुन उवाच
अयतिः श्रद्धयोपेतो
योगाच्चलितमानसः ।
अप्राप्य योगसंसिद्धिं
कां गतिं कृष्ण गच्छति ॥६.३७॥
arjuna uvāca
ayatiḥ śraddhayopeto
yogāccalitamānasaḥ
aprāpya yogasaṁsiddhiṁ
kāṁ gatiṁ kṛṣṇa gacchati (6.37)

arjuna — Arjuna; uvāca — said; ayatiḥ — undisciplined person; śraddhayopeto = śraddhayopetaḥ = śraddhayā — by faith + upetaḥ — possesses; yogāccalitamānasaḥ = yogāc (yogāt) — from yoga practice + calita — deviated + mānasaḥ — mind; aprāpya — not attain; yogasaṁsiddhiṁ — yoga proficiency; kāṁ — what; gatiṁ — course; kṛṣṇa — Krishna; gacchati — he goes

Arjuna said: What about the undisciplined person who has faith? Having deviated from yoga practice, having not attained yoga proficiency, what course does he take, O Krishna? (6.37)

Commentary:

The yati is the disciplined person, referring to those who have a consistent tendency for discipline. Some of us have the patience required to proceed with and wait for the results of yoga practice. Others are more hasty and seek paths which promise quicker results and do not require as much isolation and endeavor. Some human beings cannot tolerate the long isolation required for success in yoga. Such persons must always be in a group effort. They are reliant on belief and faith in what they cannot experience. Arjuna asked about the undisciplined yogi, the ayati. He credited that yogi's faith in yoga but lack of proficiency. What course would such a person take? This question highlights the fact that besides those yogis with disciplined nature and those non-yogis who are faith and belief reliant, there is also those with some tendency for the discipline of yoga but who are also faith reliant. These people are uncomfortable in the faith-belief religious systems and they are not fully compatible to yoga disciplines. As a result they left faith-belief systems to take up yoga practice but they lacked the disciplinary persistence required to succeed. Hence they left aside the practice and took another course. What are the alternatives for such people?

The indication is that Arjuna asked about himself here. Few commentators on this verse realize this. Most seem to think that Arjuna asked this question out of sympathy for fallen yogis. Actually, Arjuna is talking about himself and about no one else. It is Arjuna who learned yoga, succeeded at it and then let the practice go lax. He lost touch with it and could not apply it at Kurukṣetra when he faced the emotional crisis which buckled his knees.

कच्चिन्नोभयविभ्रष्टश्
छिन्नाभ्रमिव नश्यति ।
अप्रतिष्ठो महाबाहो
विमूढो ब्रह्मणः पथि ॥६.३८॥
kaccinnobhayavibhraṣṭaś
chinnābhramiva naśyati
apratiṣṭho mahābāho
vimūḍho brahmaṇaḥ pathi (6.38)

kaccin = kaccid — is he; nobhayavibhraṣṭaś = na — not + ubhaya — both + vibhraṣṭaḥ — lost out; chinnābhram = chinna — faded + abhram — cloud; iva — like; naśyati — lost; apratiṣṭho = apratiṣṭhaḥ — without foundation; mahābāho — O Almighty Kṛṣṇa; vimūḍho = vimūḍhaḥ — baffled; brahmaṇaḥ — of the spirituality; pathi — on the path

Is he not like a faded cloud, lost from both situations, like being without a foundation? O Almighty Krishna: He is baffled on the path of spirituality. (6.38)

Commentary:

It is not that a person doing yoga will of necessity have to return to social, cultural or political work, as Arjuna had to. Some yogis will not have to do that. Some can continue with the practice with a waiver from the Supreme Being. Such persons, with the waiver, would not do karma yoga, as is being demanded of Arjuna.

These questions of Arjuna bring to relevance the importance of continuing the practice, even after intense sessions and even after being in association of a great yoga teacher. Regardless of whether one has the exemption or not, it is important to continue the practice; otherwise, a yogi will resume cultural life with full force and forget the yoga perspective.

In this verse, Arjuna described his own condition. He may as well have used the first person and stated: "What about me? I practiced yoga and have faith in religion. Having deviated from yoga by getting involved in cultural life, and thus having not attained the yoga proficiency, what course would I take if my body dies, O Krishna? Am I not like a faded cloud, lost from what is spiritual and lost from the cultural field as well? I am without a foundation in either process, O almighty Krishna. I am baffled in both respects."

This brings to mind Arjuna's original request of Śrī Krishna:

kārpaṇyadoṣopahatasvabhāvaḥ
pṛcchāmi tvāṁ dharmasaṁmūḍhacetāḥ

yacchreyaḥ syānniścitaṁ brūhi tanme
śiṣyaste'haṁ śādhi māṁ tvāṁ prapannam (2.7)

As a mercy prone man, overcome by these feelings of pity, with my sense of duty clouded by mental confusion, I ask You to tell me with certainty, what is preferable. I am a student of Yours. Instruct me, who is submitted to You. (2.7)

Arjuna also wanted this clarification:

arjuna uvāca
saṁnyāsaṁ karmaṇāṁ kṛṣṇa punaryogaṁ ca śaṁsasi
yacchreya etayorekaṁ tanme brūhi suniścitam (5.1)

Arjuna said: You approved renunciation of social activity and also mentioned the application of yoga to worldly life. Which one of these is better? Tell me this with certainty. (5.1)

एतन्मे संशयं कृष्ण
छेत्तुमर्हस्यशेषतः।
त्वदन्यः संशयस्यास्य
छेत्ता न ह्युपपद्यते ॥६.३९॥
etanme saṁśayaṁ kṛṣṇa
chettumarhasyaśeṣataḥ
tvadanyaḥ saṁśayasyāsya
chettā na hyupapadyate (6.39)

etan = etad — this; me — of mine; saṁśayam — doubt; kṛṣṇa — Krishna; chettum — remove; arhasy = arhasi — you can; aśeṣataḥ — without reminder, fully; tvadanyaḥ = besides you; saṁśayasyāsya = saṁśayasya — of doubt + asya — of this; chettā — remover of doubt; na — not; hy (hi) — indeed; upapadyate — he exists

You can, O Krishna, remove this doubt of mine fully. Besides You, no other remover of doubt, exists here. (6.39)

Commentary:

At this point, Arjuna was still confused. He remained uncertain of his course, despite receiving so much information from Śrī Krishna about the path of yoga and its application to cultural life. Arjuna was still uncertain about what he should do.

Arjuna already asked these questions using other words and speaking from other perspectives. Thus we see that it is not easy to get back on the spiritual track.

Arjuna accepted Śrī Krishna as the only person who could remove doubts, but Śrī Krishna was unable to this point, to remove such uncertainties completely. Now, Arjuna appealed for a more convincing demonstration by Śrī Krishna.

श्रीभगवानुवाच
पार्थ नैवेह नामुत्र
विनाशस्तस्य विद्यते ।
न हि कल्याणकृत्कश्चिद्
दुर्गतिं तात गच्छति ॥६.४०॥
śrībhagavānuvāca
pārtha naiveha nāmutra
vināśastasya vidyate
na hi kalyāṇakṛtkaścid
durgatiṁ tāta gacchati (6.40)

śrībhagavān – the Blessed Lord; uvāca — said; pārtha — O son of Pṛthā; naiveha = na – neither + eva — indeed + iha — here on earth; namutra = na — nor + amutra — above in the celestial regions; vināśaḥ — loss; tasya — his; vidyate — it is realized; na — not; (hi) — indeed; kalyāṇakṛt — performer of pious acts; kaścid — anyone; durgatiṁ — into misfortune; tāta — O ideal one; gacchati — goes down permanently

The Blessed Lord said: O son of Pṛthā, it is realized that neither here on earth nor above in the celestial regions, does the unaccomplished yogi lose his skill. Indeed, O dear Arjuna, no performer of virtuous acts, goes down permanently into misfortune. (6.40)

Commentary:

Both the skill of yoga practice, as well as the skill of the application of yoga to cultural or political life (karma yoga), remains in the subtle body of the ascetic. It is never lost. It is activated according to the kind of environment he is providentially situated in. When the ascetic is in the heavenly world, he applies himself according to what providence requires of him there. Instincts and tendencies surface in his mind automatically. He then acts or reacts accordingly. The ascetic does not have to consciously remember any skill which is stored in his subtle form. The skills are activated by pressures of providence which are beyond his control. Thus there is no chance that yogic or cultural skill will be lost at any time.

This does not mean that the yogi will always have a conscious grip of his memory. He may lose it. However its storage in the subtle body as an instinct or tendency, assures that it can be retrieved. It is the same for all other living entities who use subtle forms.

Those who habitually, life after life, seek to enact pious activities, the kalyāṇakṛts, cannot sink down permanently into degradation. By their very nature, they will strive to come out of such situations. Thus there is no chance of them being degraded forever. The force of pious activities is always sufficient to buoy them upwards in material existence and to push them further into spiritual inquiry.

प्राप्य पुण्यकृताँल्लोकान्
उषित्वा शाश्वतीः समाः ।
शुचीनां श्रीमतां गेहे
योगभ्रष्टोऽभिजायते ॥ ६.४१ ॥
prāpya puṇyakṛtāṁllokān
uṣitvā śāśvatīḥ samāḥ
śucīnāṁ śrīmatāṁ gehe
yogabhraṣṭo'bhijāyate (6.41)

prāpya — obtaining; puṇyakṛtām — of the performer of virtuous acts; lokān — celestial places; uṣitvā — having lived; śāśvatīḥ — many, many; samāḥ — years; śucīnām — of the purified person; śrīmatām — of the prosperous person; gehe — in the social circumstance; yogabhraṣṭo = yogabhraṣṭaḥ — fallen from yoga; 'bhijāyate = abhijāyate — is born

After obtaining the celestial places where the virtuous souls go, having lived there for many, many years, the fallen yogi is born into the social circumstances of the purified and prosperous people. (6.41)

Commentary:

Though temporarily elevated to the celestial places, still this yogi is considered fallen. He did not obtain the far-fetched objective of yoga which is to exit material existence altogether. Instead, after passing from his body, he entered a zone in which he could not continue the disciplines. He assumed a body which could only enjoy the subtle paradises. This is a fallen state for the yogi.

His assumption of that heavenly body is an indication that his yoga practice was not complete, since on the basis of his psychology for enjoyment, he took such a body. This yogi will have to take another human form and again work to purify himself of the need for such bodies which deprive him of discrimination and support a mentality of enjoyment. Fortunately due to austerities in previous human births on earth-like planets, this yogi gets the opportunity to take birth in families of prosperous or purified people. Some yogis, according to tendency, may take birth in a wealthy family that only has a tiny bit of purity.

Others take birth in families which have great purity but very little wealth. It all depends on the nature of the particular yogi and the social opportunities available when he is compelled to take another physical body.

The main idea is that his yoga practice which was repeatedly disrupted has a cumulative effect over a period of lives. As such, nothing is more important than his yoga practice. His sojourn in heaven and even his endurance of hellish places or hard times, are merely disruptions to yoga. By the grace of providence, by the facility set on in the creation by the Supreme Being, Śrī Krishna, the yogi benefits from his incomplete attempts at yoga. Thus his instinct for the practice surfaces repeatedly in each earthly life.

अथ वा योगिनामेव
कुले भवति धीमताम् ।
एतद्धि दुर्लभतरं
लोके जन्म यदीदृशम् ॥ ६.४२ ॥
atha vā yogināmeva
kule bhavati dhīmatām
etaddhi durlabhataraṁ
loke janma yadīdṛśam (6.42)

atha vā — alternately; yoginām — of the yogi; eva — indeed; kule — in the family situation; bhavati — is born; dhīmatām — of the enlightened people; etad — this; dhi = hi — indeed; durlabhataram — difficult to attain; loke — in this world; janma — birth; yad — which; īdṛśam — such

Alternately, he is born into a family of enlightened people. But such a birth is very difficult to attain in this world. (6.42)

Commentary:

The enlightened people, dhīmatām, are super yogis, who maintain either a householder lifestyle or who are monks with appreciative affiliation for advanced householders. The yogi who gets his birth in such a situation is fortunate indeed. He receives the most valuable sort of human birth. From such a birth, this yogi can hardly fail to complete the austerities.

That birth gives the yogi the advantage of a body inclined to yoga practice and the required disciplines. That alone is a winning grace for him. The psychological environment of such parents is the ideal situation for him.

We read in the Śrīmad Bhāgavatam, that Lord Vishnu regularly took a body from such yogi parents, who do the austerities to perfection. In fact, it appears that Lord Vishnu will only take a body from such parents and from no one else. When his parents are not yogis, it means that they were perfected yogis in past births. Both his mother and father are usually mahāyogīs. Thus for an ordinary entity to get such a birth, is indeed a very special occurrence.

तत्र तं बुद्धिसंयोगं
लभते पौर्वदेहिकम् ।
यतते च ततो भूयः
संसिद्धौ कुरुनन्दन ॥ ६.४३ ॥
tatra taṁ buddhisaṁyogaṁ
labhate paurvadehikam
yatate ca tato bhūyaḥ
saṁsiddhau kurunandana (6.43)

tatra — there; tam — it; buddhisaṁyogam — cumulative intellectual interest; labhate — inspired with; paurvadehikam — from a previous birth; yatate — he strives; ca — and; tato = tataḥ — from that time; bhūyaḥ — again; saṁsiddhau — to perfection; kuru—nandana — O dear son of the Kurus

In that environment, he is inspired with the cumulative intellectual interest from a previous birth. And from that time, he strives again for yoga perfection, O dear son of the Kurus. (6.43)

Commentary:

Such a high-charged environment where one's parents are mahāyogīs, has great value. One is immediately inspired not only by their example but by one's own cumulative interest in yoga, from the last birth when one performed austerities. This reinforces the need to be serious about yoga practice. This sort of environment was awarded to Shuka, the son of Śrīla Vyāsadeva. Otherwise if one takes birth in some other type of family, he will unavoidably suffer a regression, in proportion to how little or how much yoga the parents perform. The fortunate yogi who gets the preferred birth, does not have a counterproductive childhood environment. He does not have to spend time cleaning his psychology of unwanted aspects to which he was exposed in infancy and in schools

Of course, this description does not apply to most of us. We know all too well that the vast majority of us did not get such births. It is hardly likely that we may get one in the near future. It is, however, interesting to know what sort of birth we might acquire if we advance far in the practice in one lifetime.

पूर्वाभ्यासेन तेनैव
ह्रियते ह्यवशोऽपि सः ।
जिज्ञासुरपि योगस्य
शब्दब्रह्मातिवर्तते ॥ ६.४४ ॥
pūrvābhyāsena tenaiva
hriyate hyavaśo'pi saḥ
jijñāsurapi yogasya
śabdabrahmātivartate (6.44)

pūrvābhyāsena = pūrva — previous + abhyāsena — by practice; tenaiva = tena — by it + eva — indeed; hriyate — he is motivated; hy (hi) — indeed; avaśo = avaśaḥ — without conscious desire; 'pi = api — even; saḥ — he; jijñāsuḥ — persistently inquiring; api — even; yogasya — of yoga; śabdabrahmātivartate = śabda – spoken description + brahma — spiritual reality + ativartate — instinctively sees beyond (śabdabrahma – Vedas)

Indeed, by previous practice, he is motivated, even without conscious desire. He who persistently inquires of yoga, instinctively sees beyond the Veda, the spoken description of the spiritual reality. (6.44)

Commentary:

This describes persons like Shuka, the son of Vyāsadeva. It gives us the idea of the condition of the mind of a yogi, who takes a body as an infant of mahāyogī parents. Others who fit into this category are Śrī Ganesha and Śrī Kartikeya, the sons of Lord Shiva, as well as Śrī Pradyumna and Śrī Aniruddha, the son and grandson of Śrī Krishna. Only a few people get such births, so we need not fantasize over it. It is sufficient to understand the kind of birth environments achieved by such great souls. We should not be resentful but should instead work as we are and do our best to complete the practice with utmost determination and power.

We are also motivated without conscious desire but not as much as the great souls. Our motivation is disrupted by distractions from our birth environment as well as by our impure minds. Our progress is slower. Our awakening occurs in a much more delayed and sporadic manner.

We also persistently inquire of yoga. We do ponder the incentive posture of the *Vedas* and other scriptures. We too want to go beyond mere conceptions of the spoken description of the spiritual reality, but we cannot make such rapid progress as the advanced yogis. We can however admire those yogis from a distance, since they have all facilities working for them. Śrīla Yogeshwarananda Yogiraja suggested that for those of us who do not get such a birth, we may follow in his footsteps in leaving our birth environment and sincerely, with determination, striving for completion of the yoga austerities. He said:

> ***"Providence will not always facilitate a yogi. But a yogi should not resent destiny. Instead the yogi should invest energy in the practice, and so forge his way to success. He should not leave aside yoga at any stage. He should take help from more advanced yogis and get their ideas for techniques which he should practice for further advancement. Even though Śrī Krishna glamorized the ideal birth for a yogi in these verses, still that does not mean that most yogis will get this ideal parentage. Thus one should not be dismayed because of taking a disagreeable birth."***

प्रयत्नाद्यतमानस्तु
योगी संशुद्धकिल्बिषः ।
अनेकजन्मसंसिद्धस्
ततोयाति परां गतिम् ॥ ६.४५॥
prayatnādyatamānastu
yogī saṁśuddhakilbiṣaḥ
anekajanmasaṁsiddhas
tatoyāti parāṁ gatim (6.45)

prayatnāt — from steady effort; yatamānaḥ — consistently controlled; tu — but; yogī — yogi; saṁśuddha — thoroughly cleansed; kilbiṣaḥ — bad tendencies; anekajanmasaṁsiddhas = aneka — not one + janma — birth + saṁsiddhaḥ — perfected; tato = tataḥ — from then onwards; yāti — reaches; parāṁ — supreme; gatim — goal

From a steady effort and a consistently controlled mind, the yogi who is thoroughly cleansed of bad tendencies, who is perfected in many births, reaches the supreme goal. (6.45)

Commentary:

This verse supports what Śrīla Yogeshwarananda said. It takes many births for a person to complete yoga practice. This is because of the shortness of a human lifetime. Some ancient yogis held off death of their bodies for sometime, in order to complete the practice using the same body. For most of us that will not occur. Sometimes one hears reports of yogis who live in ancient bodies which are two hundred, five hundred or a thousand years old. In fact it is believed that Śrī Bābāji Mahasaya uses such a physical body. However I can tell you here that Śrī Bābāji does not use such a body at all. He uses a yoga siddha subtle body. He does appear to yogis whose third eye (brow chakra) or whose buddhi organ visual power is stabilized. It is a superstition to think that he uses a physical form that is so many hundreds of years old but which appears to be like that of a sixteen year old boy. His body is subtle, being made of sunlight.

Unless one is Lord Vishnu or Lord Shiva, one will more than likely take many many births to accomplish the yoga austerities. When Lord Vishnu or Lord Shiva takes on a human form, their example of a sudden and sure perfection is not an example that any of us can follow. Thus it is a sheer fantasy when devotees of Lord Vishnu or Lord Shiva think that they can get out in one life, without having a cumulative previous practice. One cannot get out of this material existence without performing individual penances and without taking up the relevant mystic kriyās. It is simply impossible. The divine beings like Lord Vishnu, Lord Shiva, Lord Krishna, Lord Balarāma and others can get out instantly without the pre-qualifications but not others. Others will return repeatedly in human or animal forms just as they have done in the present birth.

Śrī Bābāji Mahasaya said this:

"These six chapters of the Bhagavad Gītā are an introduction to the course of kriyā yoga. In five chapters, namely Chapters Two through Six, Śrī Krishna sketched out the course of kriyā yoga, from the neophyte to the terminal or advanced stages. By a careful study of this information one can get some idea of what it would take to be a kriyā yogi."

तपस्विभ्योऽधिको योगी
ज्ञानिभ्योऽपि मतोऽधिकः ।
कर्मिभ्यश्चाधिको योगी
तस्माद्योगी भवार्जुन ॥६.४६॥
tapasvibhyo'dhiko yogī
jñānibhyo'pi mato'dhikaḥ
karmibhyaścādhiko yogī
tasmādyogī bhavārjuna (6.46)

tapasvibhyo = tapasvibhyaḥ — to the other types of ascetics; 'dhiko = adhikaḥ — is superior; yogī — yogi; jñānibhyo = jñānibhyaḥ — to the masters of the philosophical theory; 'pi = api — also; mato = mataḥ — is considered to be; 'dhikaḥ = adhikaḥ — is superior; karmibhyaḥ — to the ritual performers; cādhiko (cādhikaḥ) = ca — and + adhikaḥ — is better than; yogī — yogi; tasmād = tasmāt — hence; yogī — yogi; bhavārjuna = bhava — be + arjuna — Arjuna

The yogi is superior to other types of ascetics; he is also considered to be superior to the masters of philosophical theory, and the yogi is better than the ritual performers. Hence, be a yogi, Arjuna. (6.46)

Commentary:

The previous verse describes the perfected yogi as one who completed the course and reached the supreme goal (parām gatim). Śrī Krishna gave His opinion that such a yogi is superior to the other types of ascetics, better than the masters of philosophical theory who have not practiced or perfected yoga and better than the ritual performers. Then Śrī Krishna advised Arjuna to be a yogi. Before this verse, it seems that Śrī Krishna veered Arjuna away from the ascetic life, but now Śrī Krishna tells Arjuna to be a yogi.

At that time and place, at the battlefield of Kurukṣetra, Arjuna was to apply his already acquired skill of yoga to the performance of cultural activities in the matter of participating in a civil war, to solve a quarrel between the princes, Yudhiṣṭhira and Duryodhana. It is clear that the perfected yogi is the best of the ascetics.

योगिनामपि सर्वेषां
मद्गतेनान्तरात्मना ।
श्रद्धावान्भजते यो मां
स मे युक्ततमो मतः ॥६.४७॥
yogināmapi sarveṣāṁ
madgatenāntarātmanā
śraddhāvānbhajate yo māṁ
sa me yuktatamo mataḥ (6.47)

yoginām — of the yogis; api — also; sarveṣāṁ — of all these; madgatenāntarātmanā = madgatena — attracted to me + antarātmanā — with his soul; śraddhāvān — full of faith; bhajate — worships; yo = yaḥ — who; mām — me; sa = saḥ — he; me — to me; yuktatamo = yuktatamaḥ — most devoted; mataḥ — is regarded

Of all yogis, the one who is attracted to Me with his soul, who worships Me with full faith, is regarded as being most devoted to Me. (6.47)

Commentary:

Śrī Krishna introduced the value of devotion to Him by worship of Him and attraction to Him with the yogi's soul. Some yogis are not attracted to Śrī Krishna, but they still gain some transcendental goal according to their individual natures, as realized at the time of liberation. Those yogis who are attracted to Śrī Krishna with their souls, and who worship Him with full faith, are regarded by Him as being His best devotees.

There are four aspects mentioned in verse 45 for the yogi's complete success. These are steady effort (prayatnāt), a consistently controlled mind (yatamānas), thorough cleansing of bad tendencies (samśuddha kilbisah) and perfection as a result of cumulative austerities in many births. There is not one word here about a flash salvation, just after one birth with grace only or only because of being a devotee of Śrī Krishna.

If one is not inclined to steady effort (prayatnāt), then he cannot be a yogi, and in fact, he will not be attracted to the path at all. Yoga concerns itself with the cleansing of bad tendencies, and Śrī Krishna indicated in Chapter Five text 11 and Chapter Six text 12 that one must perform cultural acts for associative purification while also performing yoga for personal purity. Through these efforts, the bad tendencies do go away after many lives.

CHAPTER 7

Krishna: The Ultimate Reality*

श्रीभगवानुवाच
मय्यासक्तमनाः पार्थ
योगं युञ्जन्मदाश्रयः ।
असंशयं समग्रं मां
यथा ज्ञास्यसि तच्छृणु ।७.१॥
śrībhagavānuvāca
mayyāsaktamanāḥ pārtha
yogaṁ yuñjanmadāśrayaḥ
asaṁśayaṁ samagraṁ māṁ
yathā jñāsyasi tacchṛṇu (7.1)

śrībhagavān — the Blessed Lord; uvāca — said; mayy = mayi — in Me; āsaktamanāḥ — attention absorbed in; pārtha — O son of Pṛthā; yogam — yoga; yuñjan — practicing; madāśrayaḥ= mad — on me + āśrayaḥ — being dependent; asaṁśayaṁ — without doubt; samagraṁ — fully; māṁ — Me; yathā — as; jñāsyasi — you will know; tac = tad — this; chṛṇu = śṛṇu — hear

The Blessed Lord said: With attention absorbed in Me, O son of Pṛthā, practicing yoga, being dependent on Me, you will know of Me fully without a doubt. Hear of this. (7.1)

Commentary:

This deals with understanding who Śrī Krishna is, how He affects the living beings, what part He plays in the destiny of the yogi and His demands upon the living entities. Sometimes there is a mix-up between the purpose of yoga and this understanding of who Krishna is, but in the *Gītā*, Śrī Krishna did not confuse these issues. Yoga and its initial purpose which is purification of the psyche (B.G. 6.12) is not mixed up with this knowing of Śrī Krishna.

At the advanced stages and at those stages only, a yogi really understands who Krishna is and understands what demands are being made by Krishna. The process of knowing Śrī Krishna is part of advanced kriyā practice, after one has already mastered some stages of higher yoga and decides to apply the expertise to learning something about Him.

To have the attention as absorbed in Śrī Krishna, a yogi should have already mastered the 5th and 6th stages of practice. These are the stages of pratyāhār sensual energy withdrawal and dhāraṇa focus of the attention into the visual energy of the buddhi organ.

One must practice yoga consistently (yogam yuñjan). That means that yoga is the main process of spiritual discipline, not chanting or temple functions and other procedures, which are highly advertised nowadays. One must be dependent on Śrī Krishna. This dependence on Him was not explained in great detail yet in the *Gītā*, but it means that one must be in tune with Krishna and with great yogins who are very close to Him. Then the yogi will know Krishna fully without a doubt. In this chapter, Śrī Krishna gave details on how to do this.

**The Mahābhārata contains no chapter headings. This title was assigned by the translator on the basis of verse 7 of this chapter.*

Those who say that yoga is not necessary for knowing Krishna, have bypassed these statements and substituted information given elsewhere by Śrī Krishna and by others. However these instructions are for the yogis, especially for us on the kriyā path. There is no contention. If someone can follow in the footsteps of the gopis of Vṛndāvan, who were absorbed in Śrī Krishna without yoga practice, then all good fortune will find that person. For that person, yoga is unnecessary but for those of us who cannot follow the gopis, this *Bhagavad Gītā* discourse is there as it was delivered to Arjuna, with methods that we can implement, methods described by Śrī Krishna Himself.

ज्ञानं तेऽहं सविज्ञानम्
इदं वक्ष्याम्यशेषतः ।
यज्ज्ञात्वा नेह भूयोऽन्यज्
ज्ञातव्यमवशिष्यते ॥७.२.
jñānaṁ te'haṁ savijñānam
idaṁ vakṣyāmyaśeṣataḥ
yajjñātvā neha bhūyo'nyaj
jñātavyamavaśiṣyate (7.2)

jñānam— information; te — to you; 'ham = aham — I; savijñānam — with experience; idam — this; vakṣyāmy (vakṣyāmi)— I will explain; aśeṣataḥ — without deleting anything; yaj = yad — which; jñātvā — having known; neha = na — not + iha — in this world; bhūyo = bhūyaḥ — further; 'nyaj = anyat — other; jñātavyam — to be discovered; avaśiṣyate — is left

I will explain the information and give the experience to you without deleting anything. Having known that, no other experience would be left to be discovered in this world. (7.2)

Commentary:

Śrī Bābāji Mahasaya instructed me to write that the first five chapters of Śrī Krishna's speech to Arjuna, Chapter Two through Chapter Six, are a detailed sketch of kriyā yoga. The purpose of the *Gītā* speech was to prompt Arjuna to apply what he already mastered in yoga to worldly affairs, to the political conflict of the Kuru people. Now in Chapter Seven, the tone changes. Śrī Krishna shifted away from yoga and spoke about the yogi's familiarity with Him. Śrī Krishna attributes this as the highest information and the highest experience to be gained by a yogi. Arjuna got the information and the experience behind it. Śrī Krishna said that with such experience no other evidence would be required in this world.

मनुष्याणां सहस्त्रेषु
कश्चिद्यतति सिद्धये ।
यततामपि सिद्धानां
कश्चिन्मां वेत्ति तत्त्वतः ॥७.३॥
manuṣyāṇāṁ sahasreṣu
kaścidyatati siddhaye
yatatāmapi siddhānāṁ
kaścinmāṁ vetti tattvataḥ (7.3)

manuṣyāṇām — of human beings; sahasreṣu — in thousands; kaścid — someone; yatati — strives; siddhaye — to psychological perfection; yatatām — of those who endeavor; api — even; siddhānām — of those who are perfected; kaścin = kaścid — someone; mām — me; vetti — comprehends; tattvataḥ — in truth

Someone, in thousands of human beings, strives for psychological perfection. Of those who endeavor, even of those who are perfected, someone knows Me in truth. (7.3)

Commentary:

Many people strive for psychological perfection, motivated by one reason or another. Śrī Krishna said that only one or two get to know Him. So what is so special about knowing

Śrī Krishna? Furthermore, Śrī Krishna said that of those who are perfected (siddhānām), only one or two know Him in truth. In other words, a person can attain psychological perfection and still not know much about Śrī Krishna.

भूमिरापोऽनलो वायुः
खं मनो बुद्धिरेव च ।
अहंकार इतीयं मे
भिन्ना प्रकृतिरष्टधा ॥७.४॥
bhūmirāpo'nalo vāyuḥ
khaṁ mano buddhireva ca
ahaṁkāra itīyaṁ me
bhinnā prakṛtiraṣṭadhā (7.4)

bhūmir = bhūmiḥ — solid substance; āpo = āpaḥ — liquid substance; 'nalo = analaḥ — flames; vāyuḥ — gas; kham — space; mano = manaḥ — mindal energy; buddhir = buddhiḥ — intelligence; eva — indeed; ca — and; ahaṁkāra — initiative; itīyam = iti — thus + iyam — this; me — My; bhinnā — apportioned; prakṛtir = prakṛtiḥ — mundane energy; aṣṭadhā — eight—sectioned

Solid substance, liquid substance, flame, gas, space, mindal energy, intelligence, and initiative are My apportioned, eight—sectioned mundane energy. (7.4)

Commentary:

This is data from the Samkhya philosophy. Somehow the prakṛti, subtle mundane energy, has become diversified into eight constituents, which we experience as solids, liquids, fiery emanations, gases, skies, or rarefied spaces, mindal energy, very subtle intellectual organs in the subtle body and a sense of initiative which causes the display of individuality.

Śrī Krishna claimed that these eight factors are His mundane energy. He made a claim of possession. Getting to know Śrī Krishna includes understanding that He is the Supreme Proprietor. This is something that Śrīla Bhaktivedanta Swami stressed over and over again, on the basis of statements like these made by Śrī Krishna and others.

Since this is the first statement made by Śrī Krishna about the yogi getting to know Him, it means that the first thing a yogi discovers is that the subtle and gross mundane energies have a supreme proprietor. That information, that experience, greatly restricts what the yogi can do. If a yogi gets the psychological perfection for himself, and if he does not get this information and experience about Śrī Krishna, he might assume that the gross and subtle materials have no absolute owner. As soon as one sees that all these materials have an owner, then and there, one's exploitive perspective changes. An owner implies the need for permission to use the resources. Thus a yogi who is a realized devotee of Krishna will not be an exploiter unless instructed by the Lord to utilize materials.

Of course if one has attained psychological perfection, then he should have no need to exploit. At least this is how the logic goes. In reality, psychological perfection may not wipe out this need. The need to exploit is so engrained, that even after getting the psychological perfection, a legitimate need to exploit will remain. Thus the question is how to fulfill that need without becoming implicated in natural and supernatural crimes.

अपरेयमितस्त्वन्यां
प्रकृतिं विद्धि मे पराम् ।
जीवभूतां महाबाहो
ययेदं धार्यते जगत् ॥७.५॥

apareyam = apara — inferior + iyam — this; itas = itaḥ — besides; tv = tu — but; anyām – another; prakṛtiṁ — energy; viddhi — know; me — of Me; parām — higher; jīvabhūtām — the hosts of individual spirits; mahābāho — O

apareyamitastvanyāṁ
prakṛtiṁ viddhi me parām
jīvabhūtāṁ mahābāho
yayedaṁ dhāryate jagat (7.5)

strong man; yayedam = yaya — through which + idam — this; dhāryate — is sustained; jagat — universe

That is inferior. But, O strong man, know of My other higher energy which consists of the hosts of individual spirits, through which this universe is sustained. (7.5)

<u>*Commentary:*</u>

A shocking proposal is announced for the first time in the *Gītā* — that of Śrī Krishna's claim of the individual spirits as his superior grade of property. Ownership by Śrī Krishna extends to the spirits as well as to their psychologies. The psychologies were indicated in the previous verse, by His announcement of the ownership of all mental, intellectual and decisive energies. Śrī Krishna now goes a step further to announce royalty over the spirits as well. What does this mean to an aspiring yogi? One meaning is clear: One might get psychological perfection to a greater degree and not realize Krishna's sovereignty. That was explained in verse 3 of this chapter. The other clarification is that even if one attains psychological perfection, it may not resolve any misunderstandings about one's relationship with Śrī Krishna. If, as He says, He is the Supreme Proprietor, then what are our obligations to Him? What do you do if Someone owns you?

To add complexity to the matter, Śrī Krishna gave information in the last sentence of the Sanskrit, stating that we sustain the universe. What does that mean? Usually someone injects a piece of separate information for a particular purpose. Śrī Krishna, without ambiguity, said, "yayedaṁ dhāryate jagat," that we are the ones through which this universe is sustained.

It means that he pointed Arjuna back to His stipulation that Arjuna must act in the cultural field for completing karma yoga or yogicly-detached action in the world under His direction. He wants us to sustain the world as directed by Him, just as He directed Arjuna. Of course, we naturally find ourselves in a sustaining position on a micro level in this world, but still Śrī Krishna is speaking about such sustaining energy, being responsive to His mandate.

एतद्योनीनि भूतानि
सर्वाणीत्युपधारय ।
अहं कृत्स्नस्य जगतः
प्रभवः प्रलयस्तथा ॥७.६॥
etadyonīni bhūtāni
sarvāṇītyupadhāraya
ahaṁ kṛtsnasya jagataḥ
prabhavaḥ pralayastathā (7.6)

etadyonīni = etad — this + yonīni — multiple origins; bhūtāni — the creatures; sarvāṇīty = sarvāṇi — all + ity (iti) — thus; upadhāraya — understand; aham — I; kṛtsnasya — of the entire; jagataḥ — of the universe; prabhavaḥ — cause of production; pralayaḥ — cause of the destruction; tathā — as well

This higher energy functions as the multiple origins of all creatures. Understand this. I am the cause of production as well as destruction of the entire universe. (7.6)

<u>*Commentary:*</u>

A yogi whose attention is absorbed in Śrī Krishna, who continues practicing yoga, and who is dependent on Krishna, begins to know Krishna in the way described in this verse. His knowledge however is not bookish, as in hearing the *Bhagavad Gītā* but rather it is by mystic experience of these truths. There is a huge difference between those who hear this, believe and form conceptions of it, and those who see this with direct vision on mystic and spiritual planes, as developed through yoga practice.

While generally, we regard the spirits as their bodies and when we hear of the difference between the spirit and the body, we try to understand what we hear and try to act accordingly, the mystic yogi directly perceives the spirits as energizers of the various bodies. This yogi may go further to see Śrī Krishna as the remote cause of the production and destruction of the material world. In the interim periods of creation, when various creature forms are manifested in the gross and subtle levels, the individual spirits serve as immediate origin points for the various creature forms. But ultimately Śrī Krishna is the remote cause. He gave more details elsewhere in the *Gītā*.

मत्तः परतरं नान्यत्
किंचिदस्ति धनंजय ।
मयि सर्वमिदं प्रोतं
सूत्रे मणिगणा इव ॥७.७॥
mattaḥ parataraṁ nānyat
kiṁcidasti dhanaṁjaya
mayi sarvamidaṁ protaṁ
sūtre maṇigaṇā iva (7.7)

mattaḥ — than myself; parataram — higher; nānyat = na — not + anyat — other; kiṁcid — anything; asti — is; dhanaṁjaya — O conqueror of rich countries; mayi — on Me; sarvam — all; idam — this; protam — strung; sūtre — on a thread; maṇigaṇā — pearls; iva — like

O conqueror of rich countries, no other reality is higher than Myself. All this existence relies on Me, like pearls strung on a string. (7.7)

Commentary:

Here Śrī Krishna made a claim as the highest reality and as the central factor in everything, indicating that He is the Support of everything, just as pearls rely on the continuity and supporting force of a thread.

How does this apply to kriyā yoga? It applies in the advanced stages for those kriyā yogis who feel a connection with Śrī Krishna or who have heard of the *Bhagavad Gītā* and who want to validate if the declarations made in that text. After one perfects the disciplines sufficiently to purify one's psychology, one will naturally perceive higher beings like Śrī Krishna. Then one will inquire into the function of such beings and try to understand one's relationship with them.

रसोऽहमप्सु कौन्तेय
प्रभास्मि शशिसूर्ययोः ।
प्रणवः सर्ववेदेषु
शब्दः खे पौरुषं नृषु. ॥७.८॥
raso'hamapsu kaunteya
prabhāsmi śaśisūryayoḥ
praṇavaḥ sarvavedeṣu
śabdaḥ khe pauruṣaṁ nṛṣu(7.8)

raso = rasaḥ — taste; 'ham = aham — I; apsu — in water; kaunteya — O son of Kuntī; prabhāsmi = prabhā — light + asmi — I am; śaśisūryayoḥ — of the sun and moon; praṇavaḥ — of the sacred syllable Om; sarvavedeṣu — in all the Vedas; śabdaḥ — sound; khe — in the atmosphere; pauruṣam — manliness; nṛṣu — in men

I am represented as taste in water, O son of Kuntī. I am signified as light in the moon and sun, as the sacred syllable Om in all the Vedas, as the sound in the atmosphere, as the manliness in men. (7.8)

Commentary:

Śrī Krishna describes in how the yogi, who is dependent on Him, begins to see His influence in the material creation. The first factor is nourishment represented by the taste of water. This nourishment is for the creature forms. Water also has a subtle counterpart and thus pertains to the subtle creatures. This is not nourishment of the spirit but rather nourishment of the psyche and its production, the gross body.

The second factor is energy, which is represented as the light of the sun and moon. By energy, the nourished bodies move hither and thither.

Sound follows after energy. Once a body is nourished and energized in an environment, it makes sounds. In the *Vedas*, in the Upanishad, the sound *Om* is considered to be supreme. In the time of Arjuna, yogis used *Om* as the primary repetitive sound. Śrī Krishna said that He was identified by that sacred utterance.

After a body makes a sound, it seeks status. Thus Śrī Krishna identified Himself with manliness. That power is the chauvinistic attribute of the creature forms.

The lesson for us as kriyā yogis is this: First we become purified. That means psychological purification. We have to work with the eight-staged yoga process. Once we achieve purity of the psyche, then we may, if we feel a dependence on Śrī Krishna or if our yoga teachers, feel so, lock into the existence of Śrī Krishna to see what sort of relationship we have with Him and what relationship He has with the material world.

The mahāyogīn Markandeya Rishi is an example of a yogin who successfully traversed this course. He conducted research into Śrī Krishna's relationship with the material world. In this seventh chapter, we will get the curriculum for those yogins who become purified in their psyche and progress to the next stage which is to see, mystically, how Śrī Krishna is behind all mundane manifestation. Some yogins like Śrīla Yogeshwarananda of Gangotri, not feeling that dependence on Krishna, do this research in terms of the brahman spiritual energy. These see that energy as the background behind all such phenomena. Such yogis, despite their success, may not agree that Śrī Krishna is the Supreme Being, the parambrahman.

Each yogin will approach this stage according to his nature and according to what realizations and mystic insights he experienced. It is not stereotyped. The common way is this: First the yogi purifies his psychology by haṭha yoga and by mystic means. Then he turns and looks to see how the material energy is electrified by either the Supreme Personality or by the Supreme Primal Cause.

पुण्यो गन्धः पृथिव्यां च
तेजश्चास्मि विभावसौ ।
जीवनं सर्वभूतेषु
तपश्चास्मि तपस्विषु ॥७.९॥
puṇyo gandhaḥ pṛthivyāṁ ca
tejaścāsmi vibhāvasau
jīvanaṁ sarvabhūteṣu
tapaścāsmi tapasviṣu (7.9)

puṇyo (puṇyaḥ) — wholesome; gandhaḥ — odor; pṛthivyām — in the earth; ca — and; tejaḥ – brilliance; cāsmi = ca — and + asmi — I am; vibhavasau — in the sun; jīvanam — life; sarvabhūteṣu — in all creatures; tapaścāsmi = tapaḥ — austerity + ca — and + asmi — I am; tapasviṣu — in the ascetics

I am represented as wholesome odor in the earth. I am sensed by the brilliance in the sun, by the life in all creatures. I am indicated by the austerity of the ascetics. (7.9)

Commentary:

The wholesome odor of the earth is discovered in meditation to be the source of agricultural soil. This dirt is the substance in which vegetation flourishes. A yogi in researching origins of subtle prāna, checks on these things, in his bid to realize the influences which prevail over his psyche. Two investigations arise, one regarding the supernatural beings who regulate the subtle and gross resources, and one regarding who originally infused the supersubtle mundane energy with so many varieties of simple and complex materials.

In these mystic investigations a yogi accesses a subconscious store of information and finds times when he used lower bodies. Sometimes when doing this, a yogi slips into the subconscious of other persons and goes through experiences they had in lower bodies. There are three subconscious areas. Two are in the subtle body and one is in the causal form. To go back millions and millions of years, a yogi has to extract imprints from the causal body and bring these near the subtle form for translations and sensible experiences.

A good way to investigate what Śrī Krishna said about the wholesome odor of the earth (puṇyo gandhah pṛthivyām ca) is to recall to the time when one might have used a boar or pig form. These forms smell various types of earth, more sensitively than a human.

When going back into pig forms a yogi sometimes finds that there is an interest in the use of tusks. This may also be investigated, as to how tusks form in the skulls of certain mammals, how horns and antlers form, and how the energies, needs and intentions in the causal body which bring these factors into existence. In this way, in his meditations, a yogi sees the root cause of these material existences. Or as Śrī Krishna so tacitly stated, once having known this, no other experience would be left to be known.

A yogi researches like this to see who is ultimately responsible for the formation of these creature forms. Is it the actual living entity harnessed to the psychic equipment? Is there some ultimate personality who is the Supreme Cause? Is it an energy which operates to utilize the spirit's continuously-produced energy? What is the cause?

According to what Śrī Krishna told Arjuna, Śrī Krishna is Himself the cause. A yogi may investigate this. Śrī Krishna is not the only one to make such a claim. Throughout the world, there were different revelations of this to various sages and prophets. Others made similar claims about such proprietorship and about being the Foundation of the world. Is it Śrī Krishna as He claims? Or is it Someone Else? Does it really matter if it is Śrī Krishna or Someone Else?

The brilliance of the sun and the life of earthly creatures are related since the sun is the source of our planet. Whatever materials exist here, initially came from the sun. The life energy in our bodies is created from sun energy, both from the sunlight we experience now and from the explosions which cause pieces of the sun to be blasted away from it and then to form planets like this earthly one.

Is there a personality behind all this? The scientific community finds no evidence of a personal cause who triggers the explosion which causes the sun to accrete various planets. In yoga practice, a yogi sometimes gets an experience where his subtle body becomes so energized that it changes into a sunlight form. This means that his limbs and facial features are made out of sunlight. When one is translated into such a body, one sees myriads of other beings in such sunlight forms.

Sometimes if the sun's environment permits, a yogi shoots up to the sun planet and experiences the life that transpires there. There are buildings, streets and civilizations on the sun planet but it is all being done with the sunlight energy only. There are varying hues of color of that energy. In such experiences one does not necessarily see Śrī Krishna but one does see other powerful supernatural beings who supervise those worlds.

When one does Kuṇḍalinī yoga, he develops prāṇa vision. This happens when the Kuṇḍalinī energy is purified to a degree. By prāṇa vision one sees the chakras or energy-gyrating centers on the subtle spinal column and in various other parts of the body. Sometimes, all of a sudden, one sees miniature supernatural people moving about. This may be astonishing when they are first seen. These forms are tiny, one or two inches in height.

Sometimes these persons, desiring to be unseen, move out of a yogi's vision. Sometimes they act as if they are unaware that the yogi perceived them. Sometimes one of these persons leaves a yogi's body and another higher one comes into it and sits on a lotus seat on a particular chakra. Sometimes a yogi becomes terribly frightened when he sees these persons. He begins to wish that he never started yoga practice. Other yogis become joyful to see such persons and feel that the vision of them is a sign of sure success. These are not hallucinations. Such miniature bodies actually do exist in other dimensions.

After doing Kuṇḍalinī yoga for some time, and then mastering it, the yogi begins to track that Kuṇḍalinī or life force to see how it is formulated and to eliminate it, because it is the energy which sponsors creature survival, something the yogi wants to be exempt from eventually. However, eliminating the Kuṇḍalinī force requires approval of higher personalities like Lord Shiva and Lord Krishna. At a certain point, the yogi realizes that there is only so much he can do for his own liberation. He seeks out the other persons who have the final say in his bid for freedom.

Another mystery of this creation is the animation of creature forms (jīvanam sarvabhūteṣu). Even though the yogis see the comparative similarity in all creatures, still there is another mystery to be solved, which is the distribution of a higher sustaining energy. The advanced yogis track this energy to see where it is sourced.

In advanced yoga, in rare sessions of samādhi, a yogi sometimes, all of a sudden, sees this energy coming in from a great distance. He rates it as cosmic power which emanates from a super brilliant source of white light with a slight bluish tint. This light is blinding to the yogi when he first sees it. It has a cooling influence which is like moonlight. In this verse Śrī Krishna makes a claim as the source of that sustaining energy, which in conjunction with the individual spirits, animates all creature forms.

Sages like Markandeya Rishi had samādhis in which they saw Śrī Krishna providing that sustaining force. Śrīla Vyāsadeva, the writer of the *Bhagavad Gītā*, was one such mahāyogī. Sometimes however it appears that Lord Shiva sends out the energy from his body. Some yogins like Parāśar Muni attributed Lord Vishnu as the person who does this.

Another important research is the austerity of the ascetics. In kriyā, we sometimes trace our will to practice to certain mahāyogīs. For instance, this writer traced many of his motivations and initiative for yoga to persons like Lord Krishna, Lord Balarāma, Lord Shiva, Lord Ganesh, Lord Hanumān, Lord Padmanabha, Śrīla Yogeshwarananda, Śrī Bābāji Mahasaya, Swami Shivananda and Śrī Śrī Lakṣmī-Nārāyaṇa. In some cases like that of Śrī Bābāji Mahasaya, I traced Lord Shiva's influence in him. I know for sure that Lord Krishna inspired my affiliation with Lord Balarāma who in turn sent me over to study from Lord Shiva, who sometimes puts me under the care of his students who are mahāyogīs. By this, I made some considerable progress. Exactly how Lord Krishna is the direct motivator of all asceticism of the ascetics, is a mystery to me but I have no reason to disbelieve it. As it is with divine beings, one cannot expect to trace every aspect of the influence. Unless a yogi can enter certain special samadhis, which pertain to specific researches, he cannot trace out all the details. It is left to him to inquire from mahāyogīs who have personally seen the truths.

बीजं मां सर्वभूतानां
विद्धि पार्थ सनातनम् ।
बुद्धिर्बुद्धिमतामस्मि
तेजस्तेजस्विनामहम् ॥७.१०॥
bījaṁ māṁ sarvabhūtānāṁ
viddhi pārtha sanātanam
buddhirbuddhimatāmasmi
tejastejasvināmaham (7.10)

bījam — primary cause; mām — Me; sarvabhūtānām — of all creatures; viddhi — know; pārtha — O son of Pṛtha; sanātanam — primeval; buddhir = buddhiḥ — intelligence; buddhimatām — of the geniuses; asmi — I am; tejaḥ — splendor; tejasvinām — of the splendrous things; aham — I

Know me as the primeval, primary cause of all creatures, O son of Pṛthā. I can be inferred as the intelligence of the geniuses and glimpsed by the splendor of the splendrous things. (7.10)

Commentary:

The special facilities of the subtle and gross mundane creature forms (bhūtānām) is a subject of research for the yogi who reaches the stage of causal existence. From there a yogi looks back into the subtle and gross world and begins to understand how the creature forms arise from a conjunction of causal mundane energy and the spirits.

What, however, is the force that causes the spirits to conjoin with the causal energy? A yogi needs to research this so that he can decode his own affiliation with material nature and understand those living entities who are still time-bound here. Those yogis who do not understand this by direct mystic perception, fall back into the material world, where they function as gurus or saviors. Some of them intensify their austerities and adopt causal forms which do not produce any subtle or gross bodies. They remain on the causal level for billions of years.

In this verse 10, Śrī Krishna declared Himself as the primeval primary cause of the creature forms. This means that He is the cause of the conjunction between the limited spirits and the causal energy. It is left to the particular mystic to verify this. The main point of kriyā yoga is to move away from the system of believing only and to develop mystic perception, to view the Reality behind the subtle and gross mundane existence.

There is a supreme genius that can be inferred by anyone who witnesses the various levels of scholarship exhibited by various entities in mundane existence. Sometimes we see that a particular individual outclasses all others in a particular field. Likewise it is possible that there is a person could excel above all others in all skills. Śrī Krishna indicated Himself as that person. A yogi can investigate this by studying the nature of Śrī Krishna. One would have to know Śrī Krishna personally to verify this. That would be the way of kriyā yoga. In this we are open-minded to scriptural statements but we also seek direct perception of these admittances. Simply put, by direct experience all of one's misgivings are removed. Some feel that the uncertainties are removed by believing alone but that is not the case. By self-conviction, doubts are superficially removed.

The yogi must research those splendrous things which attracted his sense strongly before he became resistant to and disinterested in the forms of mundane energy. He must do this in order to fully release himself, for unless one understands how these things are formulated and displayed, and how one's nature becomes responsive to them, one will more than likely remain spellbound.

बलं बलवतां चाहं
कामरागविवर्जितम् ।
धर्माविरुद्धो भूतेषु
कामोऽस्मि भरतर्षभ ॥७.११॥
balaṁ balavatāṁ cāhaṁ
kāmarāgavivarjitam
dharmāviruddho bhūteṣu
kāmo'smi bharatarṣabha (7.11)

balam — strength; balavatām — of the strong; cāham = ca — and + aham — I; kāmarāgavivarjitam = kāma — selfish desires + rāgavivarjitam — free from passionate urges; dharmāviruddho = dhārmaviruddhaḥ = dharma — Vedic rules of morality + aviruddhaḥ — not opposed to; bhūteṣu — in creatures; kāmo = kāmaḥ — romance; 'smi = asmi — I am; bharatarṣabha — powerful son of the Bharatas

I am indicated as the strength of the strong, which is free from selfish desire and passionate urges. I am supportive of romance which is not opposed to the Vedic rules of morality, O powerful son of the Bharata family. (7.11)

Commentary:

The root cause of God's interest in this world is explained in this verse in a roundabout way. This is connected to how Śrī Krishna described His self-appointed task in verses 7 and 8 of Chapter Four:

yadā yadā hi dharmasya glānirbhavati bhārata
abhyutthānamadharmasya tadātmānaṁ sṛjāmyaham (4.7)
paritrāṇāya sādhūnāṁ vināśāya ca duṣkṛtām
dharmasaṁsthāpanārthāya saṁbhavāmi yuge yuge (4.8)

Whenever there is a decrease in righteousness, O son of the Bharata family, and where there is an increase in wickedness, then I show Myself. (4.7)

For protecting the saintly people, to destroy the wicked ones, and to establish righteousness, I come into the visible existence from era to era. (4.8)

A kriyā yogi researches this, to know the extent of his obligation in terms of responsible living and its enforcement in subtle and gross mundane conditions. In seeking to get a waiver from cultural activities, a yogi encounters many hindrances both from limited entities and the supernatural people. Therefore it becomes necessary to see how responsibility is formulated in this world.

A kriyā yogi, once he reaches the 5th stage of yoga, that of pratyāhār sense withdrawal, learns how to buffer the influence of the limited entities who repeatedly take material bodies and who usually assume predominance in human society. Such buffering power of the yogi is then discovered to be insufficient for warding off cultural duties. The yogi experiences another greater influence which motivates him directly and which reaches him through others when the selfish interest of materialistic people is reinforced by it. This influence is bifurcated or split into two parts. One sees this in deep meditation. One part comes from material nature. The other part comes from supernatural and divine personalities.

It is not simply coming from one Supreme Being like Śrī Krishna. In fact it is traceable to many supernatural and divine persons, who are much more powerful than the yogi and who can limit his advancement. Seeing this on the mystic plane, the kriyā yogi tries to settle with the various powerful persons so that he can achieve his objective in the long term.

The yogi understands that God is not completely free from the responsibility for events in this world. Thus the yogi himself is not free either and can only get a waiver from the

Supreme Being if somehow that Supreme Personality finds some other usefulness for him. Otherwise, regardless of whether one is a yogi or not, one will have to keep coming back into these worlds and assuming some type of assigned or circumstantial responsibility according to the time and the place.

Seeing that the Supreme Being and various divine and supernatural personalities are molding this world, using mundane potencies to enforce their will, the yogi retreats and silently observes how they influence the situation. Seeing that they try to rule limited beings, the yogi decides once and for all, to work harder for his own purification and to leave all other matters alone. This causes an intensification in kriyā yoga practice.

Sometimes this plan of the yogi is thwarted by the will of a supernatural or divine personality and the yogi acquiesces because he knows that resistance may result in a greater setback for his practice. In a sense, Arjuna faced such a situation, where he could not bring himself to participate in what was presented to him by destiny. He did not want to cooperate. At the same time, Arjuna could not see that his desires would be thwarted. Luckily for him, the Supreme Being, Śrī Krishna, showed that the most efficient way to attain his objectives was to cooperate with Providence which was personified as Śrī Krishna.

Kāmo is a power which generally opposes kriyā yoga. Kāmo or kāmah means lusty power or romantic energy. Since this power to generate creature forms, it has a positive aspect. Śrī Krishna claims that He is not opposed to the moral use of such power. A yogi advoctes celibacy but he realizes that sexual intercourse is a necessity for some. In fact, even the yogi cannot get a body in these realms except through intercourse. Thus it is both a negative aspect and a sacred activity. Some very advanced entities and the supernatural people do assume bodies in some of these realms without sexual intercourse but that is the exception. Generally one gets a body through sexual interplay, the mixing of energies between male and female. A yogi tracks the sexual power to understand its beneficial and degrading use. He knows well, that it is the power through which he may take another physical body. He also sees that the Supreme Being is behind responsible sexual activity and that the Supreme Being discharges grace energies into irresponsible sexual activity in order to offset the neglectful parents and to invest positive energies in the children produced.

ये चैव सात्त्विका भावा
राजसास्तामसाश्च ये ।
मत्त एवेति तान्विद्धि
न त्वहं तेषु ते मयि ॥७.१२॥
ye caiva sāttvikā bhāvā
rājasāstāmasāśca ye
matta eveti tānviddhi
na tvahaṁ teṣu te mayi (7.12)

ye — which; caiva — and indeed; sāttvikā — perceptive clarity; bhāvā — states of being; rājasāḥ — enthusiasm; tāmasāśca = tāmasāḥ — depression + ca — and; ye — which; matta — from Me; eveti = eva — indeed + iti — thus; tān — them; viddhi — know; na — not; tv = tu — but; aham — I; teṣu — in them; te — they; mayi — on Me

Regarding the states of being, which are perceptive clarity, enthusiasm, and depression, know that they are produced by Me. But I am not based in them. They are dependent on Me. (7.12)

<u>*Commentary:*</u>

The active influence or state of the most subtle form of material energy is another subject of research for kriyā yogis. This is necessary to understand how one is influenced by these forces. Where do these energies derive their penetrating power? Why is the spirit sexually disposed towards the subtle mundane potency?

The three influences which inhabit a limited spirit are other spirits, the Supreme Being and the mundane potencies. It is not hard to accept the influence of fellow spirits; nor is it hard to trace that. An in—depth study of the Gītā gives one the ability to recognize the influence of the Supreme Lord. What about the subtle mundane potencies? It is necessary for the yogi to trace out how he accepts its influence. He must first sort out the Supreme Lord's part, as well as his natural affinity. Whatever is traceable to God cannot be adjusted by the yogi, unless the Lord awards an exemption. On the other hand, whatever is caused by his own natural affinity may be adjusted totally or partially, all depending on the category of the yogi's spirit.

Śrī Krishna stated that the manifested states of being, which are perceptive clarity, enthusiasm and depression, are produced by Him, yet He remains independent from them. They are dependent on Him in so far as their manifestations are being maintained. Elsewhere Śrī Krishna points out that the primal mundane energy is an eternal reality, brahman. He also mentions the affinity of the spirits for the mundane energy.

His production of the objective world with its sexualized forms which lead us to submit to its suggestions, does not solve or explain our affinity for it. Someone may produce an item, a commodity for instance, but that does not mean people will be automatically attracted to it. Manufacturers, for instance, invent many products which are not sold because the public has no desire for the items. Meanwhile, other products are eagerly consumed by human beings.

Śrī Krishna remains apart from His production of manifested mundane energy, so what about our repeated attempts to integrate ourselves with the same. We cannot successfully tag Śrī Krishna with the responsibility for subtle matter's influence over us, except to say that He is the producer. In this case, in kriyā yoga, we investigate the cause of our affinity with matter. Can we eradicate part or all of it? This is researched in deeper states of meditation, when the yogi penetrates into the causal level where the first display of the prakṛti energy occurs, and where our intimacy with that energy emerges first. It would not be possible to get out of the material world, unless such a puzzle is solved; our affinity for the subtle mundane energy will remain and will keep us in its proximity for absorption of its ideas. As a creeper leans on a tree and cannot develop a tendency to stand on its own, so the mundane energy leans on the spirit and is incapable of relinquishing its tendency to cling for support. And in turn, as trees may desire that creepers should use their standing power, so the spirit desires that the mundane potency draw its power for usage. These aspects must be researched by the yogi.

Devotees of Śrī Krishna who have no interest in yoga and who find that yoga is unnecessary or a distraction to their cultivation of a loving relationship with Him, glorify the aspect of Śrī Krishna's independence from material nature. They proudly declare His resistance. For a kriyā yogi, this resistance, though admirable, is not the issue. The issue is our condition of affinity with these energies. We as kriyā yogis, at least the writer, is also a devotee of Śrī Krishna but that fact does not solve the problem of my attraction to the mundane energy, for that attraction exists side by side and apart from my attraction to Śrī

Krishna. Understanding this, I work to eliminate the affinity to prakṛti if that is possible. If it is not, then the question of its minimization remains.

त्रिभिर्गुणमयैर्भावैर्
एभिः सर्वमिदं जगत् ।
मोहितं नाभिजानाति
मामेभ्यः परमव्ययम् ॥७.१३॥
tribhirguṇamayairbhāvair
ebhiḥ sarvamidaṁ jagat
mohitaṁ nābhijānāti
māmebhyaḥ paramavyayam (7.13)

tribhir = tribhiḥ — by three; guṇamayair = guṇamayaiḥ — by mundane influence produced; bhāvair = bhāvaiḥ — by states of being; ebhiḥ — by these; sarvam — all; idam — this; jagat — world; mohitam — stupified; nābhijānāti = na – not + abhijānāti — recognizes; mām — Me; ebhyaḥ — than these; param — higher; avyayam — unaffected

All this world is stupefied by the three states of being, which are produced by the mundane influence. The world does not recognize Me, Who is higher than these energies and Who is unaffected. (7.13)

Commentary:

This is exactly the point. It is difficult to bypass the mundane potency. The purpose of kriyā yoga is for each of the practitioners to find a way to abandon material nature. Each yogi must find a particular way based on his affinity, because each of us is attracted by a particular flavor of material nature. We are stupefied by the three states of being which are produced by it.

One discovers the stupefying nature of the mundane potencies when one tries to perfect the 5th stage of yoga and then move to the 6th stage. One can remain there for a very long time if one does not master prāṇāyāma and be awarded of a simple lifestyle by virtue of a waiver from cultural activity. One struggles in meditation to remove oneself from the constantly—arising thoughts and picturizations, which are produced effortlessly and continually by the imagination. This prohibits one from entering samādhi.

Sometimes suddenly, one sees mystically through the perceptive eye of the buddhi organ, but that is not by virtue of control. It happens by climatic influences, rather than by control. That is unsatisfactory.

Some devotees of Śrī Krishna, the non-yogis, feel that since they accept and recognize Śrī Krishna as being higher than the mundane potencies and since they know by His declarations that He is unaffected, they will not be stupefied. They have a system of using mundane potencies in Krishna's devotional service as they define it.

A kriyā yogi has no business in such a system. We look at the situation squarely. We realize that we must directly do something to lessen and ultimately end the stupefaction. If that is not possible, then at least we want to decrease our relationship with material nature.

The question as kriyā yogi devotees of Śrī Krishna is this: What does Śrī Krishna's permanent elevation above the mundane potency have to do with us? How does that relate to us?

दैवी ह्येषा गुणमयी
मम माया दुरत्यया ।
मामेव ये प्रपद्यन्ते
मायामेतां तरन्ति ते ॥७.१४॥
daivī hyeṣā guṇamayī
mama māyā duratyayā
māmeva ye prapadyante
māyāmetāṁ taranti te (7.14)

daivī — supernatural; hy = hi — indeed; eṣā — this; guṇamayī — quality—controlled; mama — of Me; māyā — magical display; duratyayā — difficult to transcend; mām — Me; eva — indeed; ye — who; prapadyante — they rely on; māyām — bewitching energy; etām — this; taranti — they can see beyond; te — they

Indeed this quality-controlled illusion of Mine is supernatural and difficult to transcend. Only those who rely on Me, can see beyond this bewitching energy. (7.14)

Commentary:

The quality controlled mundane energy is on-going. It does not cease merely because one entity becomes liberated from it. Those who are not yet liberated and who are advanced enough may penetrate beyond it to see its controller, Śrī Krishna, the Supreme Person as He described Himself. Likewise a successful transcendentalist may see beyond it to see an all-pervading spiritual energy. The vision beyond the material world should not be a philosophy or a belief but an actual perception similar to physical vision is so.

Śrī Krishna, as the Supreme Person, flatly states that the bewitching quality-controlled illusion is difficult to transcend. It presses upon the limited entities from all sides, not only grossly but subtly. It blinds whatever little mystic perception we might have. In meditation, in attempts at meditation, it presses itself upon the yogi and thwarts him, keeping him ever occupied with its sounds, ideas and picturizations, such that he cannot activate the reality-piercing vision.

Due to the difficulties encountered when trying to transcend the quality-controlled illusion, some devotees ignore yoga practice and try to convert the illusion into something divine. They hope that Śrī Krishna will have mercy and miraculously allow them to transcend this illusion. Using verses like this to support that belief, such devotees say that because they are now relying on Śrī Krishna, He will arrange for them to see beyond this world which is His lower creation. They feel that He will lift the veil of illusion, so that they can see His transcendental body.

The problem with this view is that it hinges on the reliance on Śrī Krishna. Can a person who is bound up in this world, be fully reliant on Śrī Krishna while he is bound and while he uses mundane energy for all offerings to Śrī Krishna?

This reliance on Śrī Krishna also means reliance for instructions on how to perform purificatory austerities, but some feel it is an emotional reliance only, which excludes yoga practice and only extracts devotional service from the devotee. This devotional service manifests by preaching to others and doing devotional services for temples and their related upkeep, while being supporting and honoring popular preachers who initiate preaching programs to evangelize Śrī Krishna's name. This meaning for the reliance on Śrī Krishna ignores many verses in the *Gītā*, where Śrī Krishna tells Arjuna to take up certain austerities. For us as kriyā yogis, the reliance on Śrī Krishna is one through which we derive strength to take up the purificatory actions and attitudes which cause our psyches to be purified and make our natures increasingly compatible with Śrī Krishna and other supernatural and divine beings, who assist us in the quest for salvation.

न मां दुष्कृतिनो मूढाः
प्रपद्यन्ते नराधमाः ।
माययापहृतज्ञाना
आसुरं भावमाश्रिताः ॥७.१५॥
na māṁ duṣkṛtino mūḍhāḥ
prapadyante narādhamāḥ
māyayāpahṛtajñānā
āsuraṁ bhāvamāśritāḥ (7.15)

na — not; mām — Me; duṣkṛtino = duṣkṛtinaḥ — evildoers; mūḍhāḥ — confused; prapadyante — they take shelter; narādhamāḥ — lowest of human beings; māyayāpahṛtajñānā = māyayā — by misconception + apahṛta — erased + jñānā — discrimination; āsuram — corrupted; bhāvam — existence; āśritāḥ — attached

The confused evildoers, the lowest of human beings, those whose discrimination is erased by misconceptions, do not take shelter of Me. They are attached to a corrupted existence. (7.15)

Commentary:

Some use this statement to verify their status as devotees, drawing a demarcation, as this verse indicates, between two camps, those of devotees and nondevotees. The nondevotees are regarded as being evil rascals who do not take shelter of Krishna, as this verse states, and who subsequently become attached to a corrupted existence.

This verse applies to kriyā yogis, who can fall into one of two categories as either devotees or non-devotees of Śrī Krishna. If the kriyā yogi chooses to practice without worshipping Krishna, then he is still, as verse 7.17 will state, informed and constantly disciplined. The missing key ingredient is his devotion to Krishna or his willingness to take shelter in Krishna. Unless he becomes devoted to Krishna, his practice will be corrupted or degraded in the advanced stages, even if he not a confused evildoer. Similarly, a disciplined and successful kriya yogi who normally takes shelter in Krishna while living at a Krishna temple, engaged in temple service, can at anytime allow his mind to become inattentive to spirituality. At that point, he falls under the mundane energy and once again becomes a low human being.

चतुर्विधा भजन्ते मां
जनाः सुकृतिनोऽर्जुन ।
आर्तो जिज्ञासुरर्थार्थी
ज्ञानी च भरतर्षभ ॥७.१६॥
caturvidhā bhajante māṁ
janāḥ sukṛtino'rjuna
ārto jijñāsurarthārthī
jñānī ca bharatarṣabha (7.16)

caturvidhā — four kinds; bhajante — worship; mām — Me; janāḥ — people; sukṛtino = sukṛtinaḥ — good people; 'rjuna = arjuna — Arjuna; ārto = ārtaḥ — distressed person; jijñāsur = jijñāsuḥ — inquisitive person; arthārthī — needy person; jñānī — informed person; ca — and; bharatarṣabha — O bullish man of the Bharata family

Four kinds of good people worship Me, O Arjuna: the distressed one, the inquisitive one, the needy one, and the informed one, O bullish man of the Bharata family. (7.16)

Commentary:

Sukṛtino (sukṛtinah) means good (su) acting (kṛtino). These persons instinctively commit the majority of their activities from a pious motivation. It does not mean that all these people are perfect but rather that they are predominantly pious, kind, concerned and affectionate. Śrī Krishna sorted these personalities into four large groups, stating that they are the four kinds of good people who worship Him.

There is no clarification in this verse as to whether some of the good people do not worship Krishna. There is no clarification as to whether some of them worship other supernatural and divine beings other than Krishna. It is clear that Śrī Krishna sorts his devotees into four groups as described:

- ✓ *Those who are in distress for one reason or the other and who approach Śrī Krishna for assistance to get relief from the misery which assails them. This can be physical or psychological affliction.*
- ✓ *Those who are inquisitive, being curious to know about Śrī Krishna, about the material world, about the spiritual world and about the relationship that they have with any of this. Such a devotee may or may not get serious about spiritual life but he has a liking for Śrī Krishna which keeps him close to the Lord in one way or other.*
- ✓ *Those who are needy, wanting one thing or another, either physical things or psychological aspects like peace of mind and emotional security.*
- ✓ *Those who are informed about the position of Śrī Krishna and who had some transcendental experiences through which they know this material existence is superficial and that the real life is based on spiritual reality.*

These four kinds of people are among the devotees of Śrī Krishna. Sometimes they conflict with each other. Sometimes a great one among each of the four types emerges as a popular figure. He polarizes his group and may harass the devotees of the other categories.

Most of the kriyā yogis come from the last group mentioned, the informed persons who have mystic insight. Some, a handful of kriyā yogis, have come from the other groups. Usually a person cannot practice kriyā consistently unless he is, by nature, inclined to mysticism. Kriyā yoga depends on personal practice. It does not act prejudicially upon anyone. It is not a guru—honoring type of institution. It is a practicing craft.

Ocassionally, throughout the history of the kriyā yoga lineages, some as gurus have attracted followers who are not mystically-inclined. This occurs because a certain kriyā teacher may have a tendency for fame. Somehow that fame-lover may master kriyā to a greater degree and then relapse into his basic nature which contains the need for popularity. To legitimize such greed for fame, he poses as a savior of mankind or a person who does the most wonderful thing for humanity. All of that is, of course, not part of kriyā. It represents the failure of that yogi to alter his psychology altered by the method of kriyā which he practiced.

तेषां ज्ञानी नित्ययुक्त
एकभक्तिर्विशिष्यते ।
प्रियो हि ज्ञानिनोऽत्यर्थम्
अहं स च मम प्रियः ॥७.१७॥
teṣāṁ jñānī nityayukta
ekabhaktirviśiṣyate
priyo hi jñānino'tyartham
ahaṁ sa ca mama priyaḥ (7.17)

teṣām — of these; jñānī — the informed man; nityayukta — constantly disciplined in yoga; ekabhaktir = ekabhaktiḥ — one who is singularly devoted; viśiṣyate — is distinguished; priyo = priyaḥ — fond; hi — indeed; jñānino = jñāninaḥ — of the informed person; 'tyartham = atyartham — very; aham — I; sa = sah — he; ca — and; mama — of Me; priyaḥ — fond

Of these, the informed man who is constantly disciplined in yoga, being singularly devoted, is distinguished indeed. I am fond of this person and he is fond of Me. (7.17)

Commentary:

In the previous verse, Śrī Krishna listed the informed devotee among the four types who worship Him. Most kriyā yogis come from this informed group but not all informed persons are not attracted to yoga. Some feel that it is a waste of time. They are philosophically-minded just as the kriyā devotees, but they feel that a philosophical interest in Śrī Krishna and the mysteries of existence does not have to be supplemented by yoga practice. They hope to attain perfection just by reading about Krishna's pastimes and by intellectually grasping their preferred translations and commentaries of the *Bhagavad Gītā*, by preaching to others about it and by serving a spiritual master whom they regard as a pure devotee.

Many of these philosophically-inclined devotees take the route charted out by Lord Śrī Caitanya Mahāprabhu but there are others who follow different religious leaders and incarnations of Godhead and who exhibit the same preference for avoiding yoga. Lord Śrī Caitanya Mahāprabhu did not extol the kriyā path. He was silent on it. Therefore for those of us who are to follow His process, there are hardly any instructions coming from His mouth about it.

The distinguished devotee, as listed in this verse, is the one who is philosophically-inclined, constantly disciplined in yoga and singularly devoted to Śrī Krishna. This means that kriyā yogis who are not solely devoted to Krishna are not in the category described in this verse, nor are devotees of Krishna who are not constantly disciplined in yoga as defined in Chapter Six. This verse does not apply to neophyte kriyā yogis who are devotees of Krishna, because such devotees would not be constantly disciplined in yoga yet, nor would they have Śrī Krishna as their single object of focus. It is only in the very advanced stages of kriyā yoga practice, that anyone would be capable of such concentration. Śrī Krishna said that He was fond of such a person and such a person adores Him.

Of note, is the acclaim given to the gopis of Vṛndāvana, who are rated by Lord Śrī Caitanya Mahāprabhu as being the highest, dearest devotees of Śrī Krishna. They did not perform yoga austerities in that lifetime. In the *Gītā*, the love of the gopis is not given much acclaim at all but their affection for Śrī Krishna is rated in the Śrīmad Bhāgavatam even by Śrī Shuka, the son of Śrīla Vyāsadeva, who was himself a mahāyogī. Some commentators interpreted the gopis into many of these *Gītā* verses, which have to do with affection for Śrī Krishna, but they did that after muting the yoga requirements.

It was later on with the emergence of other Vaishnava scriptures like the Gītā Govinda and the Śrī Caitanya Caritāmṛta, that the love of the gopis was explained in detail and was rated as the highest, most elevated, most endearing love for Śrī Krishna.

However, as kriyā yogis, we adhere to the *Gītā*. We have no objection to the acclaim for the gopis. We admire their devotion, but we follow the path of kriyā yoga.

Even Śrī Uddhava personally observed the affection and steadfast concentration of the gopis, but still he did not follow their path. In fact he was instructed by Śrī Krishna to follow the kriyā path which Śrī Krishna described to him when Śrī Maitreya Rishi was listening earnestly for hints on how to complete the practice as a devotee of the Lord. In several breaks in the lectures that Śrī Krishna gave Uddhava, Uddhava pleaded for another path to the lotus feet of Śrī Krishna but just as Krishna insisted that Arjuna follow the karma yoga course, so He insisted that Uddhava follow the kriyā path. Thus it is a fact that some devotees will attain perfection through the kriyā facility.

उदाराः सर्व एवैते
ज्ञानी त्वात्मैव मे मतम् ।
आस्थितः स हि युक्तात्मा
मामेवानुत्तमां गतिम् ॥७.१८॥

udārāḥ — exalted; sarva — all; evaite = eva — indeed + ete — these; jñānī — informed person; tv = tu — but; ātmaiva = ātmā – personal self + eva — indeed; me — of Me; matam — is considered; āsthitaḥ — situated with; sa = saḥ — he; hi — truly;

udārāḥ sarva evaite
jñānī tvātmaiva me matam
āsthitaḥ sa hi yuktātmā
māmevānuttamāṁ gatim (7.18)

yuktātmā — one who is disciplined in yoga practice; mām — Me; evānuttamām = eva — indeed + anuttamām — supreme; gatim — objective

All these are exalted people, but the informed one is considered to be my personal representative. Indeed, he who is disciplined in yoga practice, situated with Me as the Supreme Objective. (7.18)

Commentary:

This verse gives us the definition of a pure devotee of Krishna. This may not fit into the definitions given in other Vaishnava scriptures like the Śrī Caitanya Caritāmṛta, but no one can deny that this was given by Śrī Krishna to Arjuna. It is very clear that this person, the informed devotee who is constantly disciplined in yoga, being singularly devoted to Krishna, is distinguished amongst the devotees and is considered as Śrī Krishna's personal representative.

If anyone qualified as the spiritual master who represented Śrī Krishna, this would be the person. Where can we find such a person whose kriyā practice is that advanced and who is singularly devoted to Śrī Krishna? Many have come and many still come, touting themselves as Krishna's pure representative. Most of these are not great yogis. Some of them have not practiced kriyā yoga in their present birth. They claim that because they are attracted to Krishna purely and fully, they performed all the yogas completely in previous transmigrations.

Without contesting all this, those of us who follow the kriyā route must stick to what is here for kriyā yogis. These guidelines are clear. This is our object, to be disciplined in yoga practice and to be situated spiritually with Krishna as the Supreme Objective. We must realize that ours is not an impersonal course because we are persons. There are advanced persons ahead of us. Besides that, there are supernatural and divine persons existing who are worthy of veneration and praise. Thus we should stick to the personal way and, under the direction of great yogins, move closer and closer to our objective by the very method of a consistent and steady practice, which causes psychological purification and opens spiritual vision.

As instructed by Śrī Bābāji Mahasaya, I checked each of the verses and commentaries on the *Gītā* which was presented by Śrī Paramhansa Yogananda. However, I find little there that I can draw for this commentary. This is due to the fact that Śrī Paramhansaji's edition focuses on establishing his institution of Self Realization Fellowship. In addition, he tried to put himself in place as a world savior. In any case, he somehow came to me in a subtle form and discussed some of the verses with me. He wanted me to definitely state that the *Bhagavad Gītā* contains the description of kriyā yoga.

Much of the information which I give about kriyā practice in these commentaries and in other books, was not rendered plainly by Śrī Paramhansaji because he hailed from a kriyā lineage that operated differently. By their tradition, one had to serve a spiritual master personally before one received such information. However I received commission from Śrī Bābāji Mahasaya, the leader of the same lineage. He gave me commission to describe the practices in detail and to make it available to anyone who desired to know of it, even if such a person does not accept me as an authority and even if such a person is disinclined to doing anything to assist me in the publications of these literatures.

Another mahāyogī, Śrīla Yogeshwarananda, inspired that I write down everything by keeping close track of every detail of my progress and then compose books based on the notes. Śrīla Yogeshwarananda adopted me as his disciple. Sometimes he used my brahmarandra subtle head as a living space. In that way I have gained his association. Just as important, Śrī Paramhansa Yogananda did wonders to create an interest in kriyā yoga on a worldwide basis and for this we are appreciative.

बहूनां जन्मनामन्ते
ज्ञानवान्मां प्रपद्यते ।
वासुदेवः सर्वमिति
स महात्मा सुदुर्लभः ॥७.१९॥
bahūnāṁ janmanāmante
jñānavānmāṁ prapadyate
vāsudevaḥ sarvamiti
sa mahātmā sudurlabhaḥ (7.19)

bahūnām — of many; janmanām — of births; ante — at the end; jñānavān — the informed devotee; mām — Me; prapadyate — surrenders to; vāsudevaḥ — son of Vasudeva; sarvam — everything; iti — thus; sa = saḥ — he; mahātmā — great soul; sudurlabhaḥ — hard to locate

At the end of many births, the informed devotee surrenders to Me, thinking that the son of Vasudeva is essential to everything. Such a great soul is hard to locate. (7.19)

Commentary:

Many teachers of Krishna Consciousness said or indicated that one does not need to delay surrender for many births. Their idea is that if one surrenders now to a bonafide spiritual master, one could bypass this clause about a surrender after many births. However I feel that their proposition is a farce. Here is why:

By nature, a living entity has to work through a certain amount of his attraction to material nature. His attraction to Śrī Krishna does not deny or remove his attraction to material nature or any other supernatural or divine personages. The attraction to material nature is a reality. The attraction to other divine persons is a fact as well. The attraction to material nature will not go away merely because the attraction to the divine personages is highlighted. In fact, it will just remain dormant. It will arise again to divert one from the loving sentiment for divine personalities. Thus one has to work out that attraction until it ceases.

The formula for this is given in Chapter Five text 11 and Chapter Six text 12 as follows:

kāyena manasā buddhyā kevalairindriyairapi
yoginaḥ karma kurvanti saṅgaṁ tyaktvātmaśuddhaye (5.11)

With the body, mind and intelligence, or even with the senses alone, the yogis, having discarded attachment, perform cultural acts for self-purification. (5.11)

tatraikāgraṁ manaḥ kṛtvā yatacittendriyakriyaḥ
upaviśyāsane yuñjyād yogamātmaviśuddhaye (6.12)

...being there, seated in a posture, having the mind focused, the person who controls his thinking and sensual energy, should practice the yoga discipline for self purification. (6.12)

These are the formulas. If love of Krishna was the formula, Śrī Krishna would have told both Arjuna and Uddhava about it. In fact Uddhava had the love of Krishna and suggested it as the means but Krishna pushed off the proposal and directed Uddhava to take up kriyā yoga. Similarly, Arjuna was not allowed any devotionalism at all.

From this, we can honestly deduce that whatever is stated in the *Gītā*, cannot be deleted by anyone. It must be adhered to, and even if someone waivers it, still as kriyā yogis, we must stick to it.

Clearly it is stated that after many births, the advanced kriyā yogi surrenders to Krishna, seeing that Śrī Krishna is the essential factor in all the existences. One cannot do this before reaching the advanced stage. Those who claim otherwise are mistaken because we cannot fully surrender until we are fully purified. It is impossible. So long as we have not cleansed our nature's attachment to the mundane reality, we cannot surrender fully to Krishna, because a part of our nature will necessarily and inherently remain in reserve. That part cannot be wished away merely by loving Krishna from an impure level. It has to be worked out because it is only operative in the mundane environment. Millions or billions of years may unfold without expressing that lowly part but it will remain in tact, in dormancy until there is opportunity to express it and work out its desires. This is why it takes many, many births.

Hearing that Krishna is the essential factor in all these existences, does not mean that we can surrender to Krishna fully either. After hearing we surrender in part. It will remain so until we acquire the full purity, which is acquired by working out our mundane affinity in the practical day-to-day physical world, as well as in the subtle mundane world. Kriyā yoga is not fools' gold. It is not for attracting followers or promising salvation. It is exactly for the purity of psychology by the methods declared in verse 11 of Chapter Five and verse 12 of Chapter Six as quoted.

A great soul like the one described in this verse, is indeed hard to locate, for the very reason that only a few such persons would be physically present on the planet at a time. And such a person because of his singular devotion and intense focus on Śrī Krishna would not be interested in becoming the spiritual master of anybody, or posing in this world as a great revivalist or any such thing.

कामैस्तैस्तैर्हृतज्ञानाः
प्रपद्यन्तेऽन्यदेवताः ।
तं तं नियममास्थाय
प्रकृत्या नियताः स्वया ॥७.२०॥
kāmaistaistairhṛtajñānāḥ
prapadyante'nyadevatāḥ
taṁ taṁ niyamamāsthāya
prakṛtyā niyatāḥ svayā (7.20)

kāmaiḥ — by desires; taistair = taihtaiḥ — by whose, by these, contrary; hṛtajñānāḥ — persons whose experience is overshadowed; prapadyante — they plead with; 'nyadevatāḥ = anyadevatāḥ = anya — other + devatāḥ — supernatural rulers; taṁtam — this or that; niyamam — religious procedures; āsthāya — following; prakṛtyā — by material nature; niyatāḥ — restricted; svayā — by their own

Persons whose experience was overshadowed by contrary desires, plead with other supernatural rulers, following this or that religious procedure, being restricted by their own material nature. (7.20)

<u>Commentary:</u>

This is a key verse for understanding our relationship with material nature. Here Śrī Krishna denounces those who by contrary desires and by their own relationship with material nature worship various supernatural beings, devatas. This also applies to devotees of Krishna who do not practice yoga, as well as the neophyte kriyā yogis who are devotees. Anytime that we are pulled under by the influence of material nature, as Arjuna was before

Śrī Krishna adjusted him, we fall under the influence of contrary desires and succumb to material nature, to the degree that we have a leaning towards those mundane energies.

Prakṛtyā svayā means our own material nature or our intimate relationship with material nature. Directly or indirectly, consciously or unconsciously, we do shift our reliance away from the Supreme Being to lesser authorities like the various supernatural beings who are called devatas in Sanskrit. This is because the Supreme Being does not give facility for contrary desires. To fulfill these, we must take shelter of lesser authorities. The existence consists of both personal and impersonal energies. At all times, both factors interplay in the fulfillment of desires. Hence we cannot avoid taking shelter of others who more advanced than us or of energies which supplement our deficiencies. A personalist stance does not eliminate the necessity of relying on impersonal energies. Similarly, an impersonalist attitude does not eliminate the reliance on personalities. Both factors are permanently intertwined.

The restriction through which one clings to material nature and must remain under its mandate, for usefulness to it, comes on by a natural affection of a spirit to material nature. The purpose of kriyā yoga is to break such an attraction, if possible, or at least minimize it. It all depends on one's category as a spirit. Some spirits cannot fully break the connection, while others can. Those who cannot release fully from it, can perform kriyā yoga to decrease it.

The overshadowing potency (hṛta) of material nature upon a spirit, is based on the spirit's absorption of material nature's conceptions and subsequent digesting in his mind the various possibilities for further expression of mundane ideas. Thus kriyā yoga, at least a main portion of it, entails curbing the imagination, which is a faculty of the buddhi organ. When the imaginations cease, then the kriyā yogi develops the eye of knowledge which is not understanding but an actual mystic eye through which one perceives subtle, causal and spiritual objects with clarity, just as one would clearly perceive a gross object through the physical eyes.

यो यो यां यां तनुं भक्तः
श्रद्धयार्चितुमिच्छति ।
तस्य तस्याचलां श्रद्धां
तामेव विदधाम्यहम् ॥ ६.२१ ॥
yo yo yāṁ yāṁ tanuṁ bhaktaḥ
śraddhayārcitumicchati
tasya tasyācalāṁ śraddhāṁ
tāmeva vidadhāmyaham (7.21)

yo yo = yaḥ yaḥ — whoever; yāṁ yām— whatever; tanum — deity form; bhaktaḥ — devotedly worship; śraddhayārcitum = śraddhayā — with belief + arcitum — to worship; icchati — desires; tasya – of him; tasyācalām = tasya — of him + acalām — unwavering; śraddhām — confidence; tām — it; eva — indeed; vidadhāmy = vidadhāmi — allow; aham — I

I grant unwavering faith to anyone, who with belief, wants to devotedly worship any worshipable deity form. (7.21)

Commentary:

That Śrī Krishna will do such a thing is dangerous for a kriyā yogi, for it means that if a yogi is impure, he may develop an attachment to a supernatural being who might not discipline him in his interest. Of course in the long run, the yogi would learn from mistakes. Instead of correcting and chastising a neophyte kriyā yogi, Śrī Krishna would allow him (vidadhāmi) to take advice from a lesser personality who will not instruct him in his interest, so that the neophyte might, in the end, learn by mistakes.

A key term is unwavering faith (acalām śraddhām). If one has such faith in a deity or teacher, and if that person does not lead one in the right direction, then actually Śrī Krishna will not obstruct it. He would allow it. He waits until one has learnt a lesson. Sometimes when someone is shown the correct action under the kriyā yoga course, he rejects it forthright as not in his interest At the same time, for varying reasons, others come forward and show him what appears to be a much better course. This course leads to more perplexity, and this can go for many many births.

स तया श्रद्धया युक्तस्
तस्या राधनमीहते ।
लभते च ततः कामान्
मयैव विहितान्हि तान् ॥७.२२॥
sa tayā śraddhayā yuktas
tasyā rādhanamīhate
labhate ca tataḥ kāmān
mayaiva vihitānhi tān (7.22)

sa = saḥ — he; tayā — with this; śraddhayā — by faith; yuktaḥ — endowed; tasyārādhanam = tasya — of this + ārādhanam — worshipfully petitioning a deity; īhate — thinks of; labhate — gets; ca — and; tataḥ — from that; kāmān — desires; mayaiva = maya — by Me + eva — indeed; vihitān — permitted; hi — truly; tān — them

Being endowed with this confidence, he thinks of worshipfully petitioning the deity and gets from that source, his desires, as those fulfillments are permitted by Me. (7.22)

Commentary:

Even though it appears that Śrī Krishna discussed the situation of other persons, from the kriyā perspective, he mentions only us, the neophyte kriyā yogis. He says that when we are endowed with confidence in others who may not be particularly interested in our purification, but who appear so, we petition those persons or forces and get fulfillments, in so far as these are permitted by Him. When this happens, the liabilities stay with us and not with Śrī Krishna. The pains, aches, hassles, distresses and even the resulting enjoyments remain with us. Śrī Krishna is apart from it.

अन्तवत्तु फलं तेषां
तद्भवत्यल्पमेधसाम् ।
देवान्देवयजो यान्ति
मद्भक्ता यान्ति मामपि ॥७.२३॥
antavattu phalaṁ teṣāṁ
tadbhavatyalpamedhasām
devāndevayajo yānti
madbhaktā yānti māmapi (7.23)

antavat — something with an end, short—lived; tu — but; phalam — results; teṣām — of them; tad — this; bhavaty = bhavati — it is; alpamedhasām — of those with little intelligence; devān — supernatural rulers; devayajo = devayajaḥ — those who worship the supernatural rulers; yānti — go; madbhaktā — those who worship Me; yānti — go; mām — to Me; api — surely

But for those with little intelligence, the result is short—lived. The worshippers of the supernatural rulers go to those gods. Those who worship Me, surely go to Me. (7.23)

Commentary:

For those with little intelligence? Who did Śrī Krishna speak about? It is you and me as well as those who exhibit very little intelligence most of the time. We sometimes act as if we possess the same ignorance which we are quick to recognize in others who are not as evolved and who are not in as high of an existential category as ourselves.

For us, when we reject the kriyā course and take energies from those not interested in serious adherence to that path, the results are short lived and we are off-track. At those times, we do go to those supernatural rulers, and when and if we get back on track, then we go to Śrī Krishna. In this way we take a zig-zag course. This will go on until we reach the advanced stages and are no longer pulled away from the disciplines described in the *Gītā*.

अव्यक्तं व्यक्तिमापन्नं
मन्यन्ते मामबुद्धयः ।
परं भावमजानन्तो
ममाव्ययमनुत्तमम् ॥७.२४॥
avyaktaṁ vyaktimāpannaṁ
manyante māmabuddhayaḥ
paraṁ bhāvamajānanto
mamāvyayamanuttamam (7.24)

avyaktam — that which is beyond the sensual range; vyaktim — that which is grossly perceived; āpannam — within range, limited; manyante — they think; mām — Me; abuddhayaḥ — unintelligent ones; param — higher; bhāvam — being; ajānanto = ajānantaḥ — not realizing; mamāvyayam = mama — of Me + avyayam — imperishable; anuttamam — supermost

Though I am beyond their sensual range, the unintelligent think of Me as being limited to their gross perception. They do not realize My higher existence which is imperishable and supermost. (7.24)

Commentary:

This pertains to those in the time of Krishna and to those human beings right now who find it hard to believe that Śrī Krishna is what He claims to be. In the time of Śrī Krishna, Duryodhana for instance, attested repeatedly that Śrī Krishna was a cheap magician and nothing else. Duryodhana did not accept these declarations.

On the other hand, some devotees of Śrī Krishna deny His assumption of a material body, claiming that there was no such form and that Śrī Krishna's earthly body is spiritual.

Śrī Krishna, by the statement issued in this verse, does verify a material body for Himself, stating that unintelligent persons in His own time think of Him as being limited to what they perceived grossly. In other words they felt that Śrī Krishna was no more than the material body He manifested. They did not realize His imperishable and supermost higher existence .

The question is however: Who among us actually saw the imperishable and supermost form of Śrī Krishna? How can we verify it? We may believe in Śrī Krishna, accepting His self-acclaim, but that still does not give us the spiritual perception through which we can verify what He said.

This again calls for the kriyā yoga practice to be consistently performed by us, so that we can develop the spiritual perception. At first, by kriyā yoga, we aim for psychological purification but it does not end there. It advances further into what Śrī Krishna introduced in this Chapter Seven. Here he explained applied kriyā yoga, or mystic techniques which decipher the mysteries of existence.

नाहं प्रकाशः सर्वस्य
योगमायासमावृतः ।
मूढोऽयं नाभिजानाति
लोको मामजमव्ययम् ॥७.२५॥

nāham = na — not + aham — I; prakāśaḥ — visible; sarvasya — of everyone; yoga – yogically self—controlled + māyā — mystic power + samāvṛtaḥ — shielded; mūḍho = mūḍhaḥ — stupified; 'yam = ayam — this; nābhijānāti = na — not + abhijānāti —

nāhaṁ prakāśaḥ sarvasya
yogamāyāsamāvṛtaḥ
mūḍho'yaṁ nābhijānāti
loko māmajamavyayam (7.25)

recognizes; loko = lokaḥ — population; mām — Me; ajam — not subjected to birth shocks; avyayam — not liable to existential pressures of change

I am not visible to everyone, because I am shielded by My yogicly, self—controlled mystic powers. This stupefied population does not recognize Me as not being subjected to shocks of birth and not being liable to existential pressures of change. (7.25)

Commentary:

The fact that Śrī Krishna used a material body in the time of Arjuna is again confirmed in this verse, where people saw Śrī Krishna physically. Duryodhana and others who were hostile to Krishna and who rejected His divinity, saw His material form. What was invisible to them was His imperishable and supermost form described in the previous verse as mamāvyayam anuttamam.

Realistically, until we can understand our own spiritual existence, we cannot in fact understand Śrī Krishna. We can believe in Śrī Krishna at any stage but real perception of His spiritual form cannot occur if we do not have objective experience of our spirituality apart from the gross and subtle material forms.

Śrī Krishna's imperishable and supermost form is not visible to everyone, because He is shielded by His yogicly, self-controlled mystic power. In fact, a limited spirit cannot even understand or perceive his own spiritual form, because he is restricted by the portion of material nature which is attuned to his spirit and which uses up his attention continuously.

A clear distinction is made between the limited spirits and the Supreme Being, Śrī Krishna, when He says that the stupefied population does not recognize Him as not being subjected to shock of birth and not being liable to existential pressures of change. In other words, what affects us, the limited spirit, does not affect Śrī Krishna. That is His claim.

Again, mere belief in Śrī Krishna's ability to transcend the limitations we face, is not the same as actually perceiving this by mystic vision. Those who become satisfied merely by hearing of this, usually remain stagnant with that acceptance.

The kriyā yogis, though they are sometimes condemned as being too inquisitive, push beyond mere belief and get direct mystic perception but only in the advanced stages of practice, long after they have mastered seven of the eight steps of kriyā yoga. It is in the last stage, that of samādhi practice, that the kriyā yogis are able to perceive this.

वेदाहं समतीतानि
वर्तमानानि चार्जुन ।
भविष्याणि च भूतानि
मां तु वेद न कश्चन ॥७.२६॥
vedāhaṁ samatītāni
vartamānāni cārjuna
bhaviṣyāṇi ca bhūtāni
māṁ tu veda na kaścana (7.26)

vedāham = veda — know + aham — I; samatītāni — the departed souls; vartamānāni — the living creatures; cārjuna = ca — and + arjuna — Arjuna; bhaviṣyāni — those who are to be born; ca — and; bhūtāni — creatures; mām — Me; tu — but; veda — recognizes; na — not; kaścana — anyone

I know the departed souls and the living creatures, O Arjuna, as well as those beings who are to be born. But no one recognizes Me. (7.26)

Commentary:

A yogi with some mystic perception, who at least completed the 5th stage of pratyāhār sense withdrawal, can understand Śrī Krishna's perspective by his own experience of knowing the past, present and future to a limited degree. A person who completed the 5th stage holds some objective perception of his past life as well as that of others.

As the Supreme Being, Krishna must know of the entities who departed, those who use gross bodies and those who will take birth in the future. That would be an easy perception for Him.

A kriyā yogi knows a little of this in so far as he is advanced. Sometimes a kriyā yogi is shown his own past life or that of another personality but it is shown only for the sake of advancement. Most of the past lives were whimsical histories, that do not necessarily add to our spiritual quest. The meaningful past lives hold significance but the impressions of those existences are carried only in our subtle and causal forms. By special mystic techniques, a kriyā yogi access his past austerities and invoke in his psyche, liberating energies which free him from current perplexities and impediments. This is all done by the direction given to any of us by the mahāyogīs, like Lord Shiva, as well as by our consistent practice.

इच्छाद्वेषसमुत्थेन
द्वंद्वमोहेन भारत ।
सर्वभूतानि संमोहं
सर्गे यान्ति परंतप ॥७.२७॥
icchādveṣasamutthena
dvaṁdvamohena bhārata
sarvabhūtāni saṁmohaṁ
sarge yānti paraṁtapa (7.27)

icchādveṣasamutthena = icchā — liking + dveṣa — disliking + samutthena — through the urge; dvandvamohena = dvandva — two—fold sensuality + mohena — by the delusive influence; bhārata — O man of the Bharata family; sarvabhūtāni — all beings; saṁmoham — delusion; sarge — at the beginning of the creation; yānti — they are influenced by; paraṁtapa — O scorcher of the enemy

O man of the Bharata family, at the beginning of any creation, all beings are influenced by delusion through the urge of liking or disliking and by the delusive influence of the two—fold sensuality. So it is, O scorcher of the enemy. (7.27)

Commentary:

And in echo, I say, "So it is, fellow yogis." We must accept this. This is the very reason why we are here again, taking more material bodies, willingly or unwillingly, in the effort to complete the practice. Whatever progress we made before, was erased to some extent by the corrosive action of the two-fold sensuality, which caused us to again be degraded and again recover lost ground.

So it is indeed, O scorcher of the unimportant external enemies! When we leave aside those unimportant enemies and see to the enemy of our own degraded psychology, we will obtain success. By introspection and careful study of what we require for success, and by proper application, we will succeed.

The urge of liking and disliking is expressed forcefully by the buddhi organ in the brain of the subtle body but the life force in the trunk of that form is the real driving force that gives it the extra boost required for impulsive actions. Until we can get away from this influence, our spiritual life will be nil. It is plain and simple. No amount of belief in anything can dismiss the influence of the delusive energy. It is eradicated by purification of our psychology, through ridding our natures of lower energies.

येषां त्वन्तगतं पापं
जनानां पुण्यकर्मणाम् ।
ते द्वंद्वमोहनिर्मुक्ता
भजन्ते मां दृढव्रताः ॥७.२८॥
yeṣāṁ tvantagataṁ pāpaṁ
janānāṁ puṇyakarmaṇām
te dvaṁdvamohanirmuktā
bhajante māṁ dṛḍhavratāḥ (7.28)

yeṣām — of whom; tv = tu — but; antagatam = anta — terminated + gatam — gone; pāpam — sinful propensity; janānām — of people; puṇyakarmaṇām — of persons of righteous actions; te — they; dvandvamohanirmuktā = dvandva — two—fold + moha — delusion + nirmuktā — free from; bhajante — worship; mām — Me; dṛḍhavratāḥ — those who maintain firm vows of austerity

But those people whose sinful propensities are terminated, whose actions are righteous, who are free from the two—fold delusion, who are maintaining firm vows of austerity, do worship Me. (7.28)

Commentary:

Who are these people? They are certainly not us, because all of our sinful propensities are not terminated. Certainly some of our bad propensities are terminated, but some others lie dormant for manifestation under certain favorable conditions. This verse describes those who have completed the path of kriyā yoga to perfection. Their psychologies are completely cleansed and their sinful propensities are completely terminated. So for us to go about trying to clean up society and help others with their sinful nature is ludicrous indeed. We have our natures to clean. Only some of our actions are righteous, not all. Every so often we fall into a really vicious behavior or into a so—called pious activity that is, in truth, the most vicious of acts, just as Arjuna under the banner of kindness to relatives, fell under the cruelty of neglecting their spiritual and moral progression.

We are not maintaining firm vows all the time, only some of the time. We do worship Śrī Krishna faithfully but only some of the time. It is the delusive influence of the dual sensuality that effectively distracts us. Any yogi can perform a simple test to check his focus by closing his eyes in a quiet place and by trying to concentrate the intellect. He will find that it does not remain stable. Every so often, more often than not, he is diverted to something which the mind effortlessly conceives. When the kriyā yogi discovers that he was diverted he may try to refocus again. Why is it that he cannot realize that he is diverted when the diversion starts? Why is it that he realizes a little later on that he was shifted from focus, like a man who planned to travel across the sea in a northerly direction and who did not realize that his boat turned to a southerly course.

जरामरणमोक्षाय
मामाश्रित्य यतन्ति ये ।
ते ब्रह्म तद्विदुः कृत्स्नम्
अध्यात्मं कर्म चाखिलम् ॥७.२९॥
jarāmaraṇamokṣāya
māmāśritya yatanti ye
te brahma tadviduḥ kṛtsnam
adhyātmaṁ karma cākhilam (7.29)

jarāmaraṇamokṣāya = jarā — bodily deterioration + maraṇa — bodily death + mokṣāya — to permanent release; mām — Me; āśritya — being dependent; yatanti — strive; ye — who; te — they; brahma — spiritual existence; tad — this; viduḥ — they know; kṛtsnam — complete; adhyātmam — Supreme Self; karma — cultural activity; cākhilam = ca — and + akhilam — entirely

Those who, being dependent on Me, strive for permanent release from bodily deterioration and death, know this spiritual existence completely, as well as the Supreme Spirit and the value of cultural activity. (7.29)

Commentary:

Dependence on Śrī Krishna? Sure! But for how much of the time? How many hours of my life was I dependent? Here we do not discuss a belief or demonstration of that dependence by holding membership in a certain institution affiliated with Śrī Krishna but rather, our actual personal dependence, our direct absorption in Śrī Krishna.

We do strive for permanent release from bodily deterioration, but we strive as allowed which depends on the amount of diversion imposed by the disturbing sensuality.

At present we cannot know the spiritual existence completely. We are beginning to understand the Supreme Spirit and Śrī Krishna is emphasizing the value of cultural activity as He sees it and as He demands our cooperation with His view of it. He is not ready to grant us a full waiver from it, no more than He was willing to give the exemption which Arjuna craved but could not procure.

साधिभूताधिदैवं मां
साधियज्ञं च ये विदुः ।
प्रयाणकालेऽपि च मां
ते विदुर्युक्तचेतसः ॥७.३०॥

sādhibhūtādhidaivaṁ māṁ
sādhiyajñaṁ ca ye viduḥ
prayāṇakāle'pi ca māṁ
te viduryuktacetasaḥ (7.30)

sādhibhūtādhidaivam = sa — with + adhibhūta — Lord of mundane beings + adhidaivam — Lord of the supernatural rulers and powers; mām — Me; sādhiyajñam = sa — with + adhiyajñam — Supreme Master of religious discipline; ca — and; ye — who; viduḥ — they know; prayāṇakāle — at the time of final departure from the body; 'pi = api — even; ca — and; mām — Me; te — they; vidur = viduḥ — know; yuktacetasaḥ — those with concentrated mental focus

Those who know Me as the Lord of mundane beings, Lord of the supernatural rulers and powers, and Supreme Master of religious disciplines, and who know Me even at the time of the final departure from the body, are the ones who know Me with concentrated mental focus. (7.30)

Commentary:

Certainly the above is true and we will get a glimpse of it in the coming verses. Śrī Krishna, it appears, set the guidelines for our deliverance from material nature. No one else can tell us something contrary to this. We need not fool ourselves or be fooled by others who present something else, even if such proposals appears palatable to us.

In conclusion, I feel that this chapter is a bit discouraging even to the serious neophytes. However, the truth is the truth. In so far as Śrī Krishna is the Supreme Personality, we should consider what He said. If we want to be successful, it would be in our interest to take Him seriously and apply ourselves fittingly to His demands. I found many surprise statements in this chapter. I am, to an extent, amazed by Śrī Krishna's insistence on so many details regarding how we should relate to Him and consider Him. This chapter is quite stunning!

CHAPTER 8

Another Invisible Existence*

अर्जुन उवाच
किं तद्ब्रह्म किमध्यात्मं
किं कर्म पुरुषोत्तम ।
अधिभूतं च किं प्रोक्तम्
अधिदैवं किमुच्यते ॥८.१॥
arjuna uvāca
kiṁ tadbrahma kimadhyātmaṁ
kiṁ karma puruṣottama
adhibhūtaṁ ca kiṁ proktam
adhidaivaṁ kimucyate (8.1)

arjuna – Arjuna; uvāca — said; kim — what; tad — this; brahma — spiritual reality; kim — what; adhyātmam — Supreme Soul; kim — what; karma — cultural activity; puruṣottama — Supermost Personality; adhibhūtam — sum total gross reality; ca — and; kim — what; proktam — authoritatively described as; adhidaivam — Supreme Supernatural Person and Power; kim — what; ucyate — is described

Arjuna said: What is this spiritual reality? What is the Supreme Soul? What is cultural activity, O Supermost Personality? Concerning the sum total gross reality, how is that described authoritatively? And speaking of the Supreme Supernatural Person and Power, what is that described to be? (8.1)

Commentary:

In a remark before his translation and commentary on Chapter Eight, Śrī Paramhansa Yogananda wrote that Arjuna was bewildered by some terms used by Śrī Krishna in Chapter Seven. Arjuna graciously asked for clarification.

Arjuna inquires about brahma (spiritual reality). This is an old question, asked by disciples of ancient sages and answered at great length in the Upanishads. In fact most of the explanations in the Upanishads are an exposition on the brahma.

Arjuna asks about the Supreme Soul, the adhyātman, and about the Supermost Personality, Puruṣottama. He asked about the sum total gross reality (adhibhūtam) and about the Supreme Supernatural Person and Power (adhidaivam).

Why such questions? How does this relate to Arjuna's duty as a warrior?

**The Mahābhārata contains no chapter headings. This title was assigned by the translator on the basis of the verse above*

अधियज्ञः कथं कोऽत्र
देहेऽस्मिन्मधुसूदन ।
प्रयाणकाले च कथं
ज्ञेयोऽसि नियतात्मभिः ॥८.२॥
adhiyajñaḥ kathaṁ ko'tra
dehe'sminmadhusūdana
prayāṇakāle ca kathaṁ
jñeyo'si niyatātmabhiḥ (8.2)

adhiyajñaḥ — Supreme Regulator of religious ceremonies and disciplines; katham — how; ko = kaḥ — who; 'tra = atra — here; dehe — in the body; 'smin = asmin — in this; madhusūdana — O slayer of Madhu; prayāṇakāle — at the time of departure from the body; ca — and; katham — how; jñeyo = jñeyaḥ — to be known; 'si = asi — you are; niyatātmabhiḥ = niyata – subdued + ātmabhiḥ — by persons

Who is the Supreme Regulator of religious ceremonies and disciplines? How is He located here in this body, O killer of Madhu? And how, at the time of departure from the body, are You to be known by those persons who are subdued? (8.2)

Commentary:

Śrī Krishna already told Arjuna that He was that Person, the Supreme Soul, the Supermost Personality, the Supreme Supernatural Person, the Supreme Regulator of religious ceremonies and discipline. Thus Arjuna became baffled in the last chapter which described a stage of very advanced practice, in its application to knowing, by direct experience, the mysteries of the Godhead.

Arjuna was baffled and so are we. Initially we came to yoga for self purification and mystic perceptive clarity. Now the Supreme Teacher says that we have to do more. After self purification, we have to apply ourselves to understanding the Supreme Person in respect to His functioning ways in this world.

Are we supposed to know Śrī Krishna at the time of departure from our bodies? Arjuna inquired of this because Śrī Krishna indicated that they should know Him with concentrated mental focus (yuktacetasah).

श्रीभगवानुवाच
अक्षरं ब्रह्म परमं
स्वभावोऽध्यात्ममुच्यते ।
भूतभावोद्भवकरो
विसर्गः कर्मसंज्ञितः ॥८.३॥
śrībhagavānuvāca
akṣaraṁ brahma paramaṁ
svabhāvo'dhyātmamucyate
bhūtabhāvodbhavakaro
visargaḥ karmasaṁjñitaḥ (8.3)

śrībhagavān – the Blessed Lord; uvāca — said; akṣaram — unaffected; brahma — spiritual reality; paramam — supreme; svabhāvo = svabhāvaḥ — personal nature; 'dhyātmam = adhyātmam — supreme soul; ucyate — it is said; bhūtabhāvodbhavakaro = bhūtabhāva – existence of mundane forms + udbhava – production + karo (karaḥ) — causing; visargah — creative power; karmasaṁjñitaḥ = karma — cultural activity + saṁjñitaḥ — is known

The Blessed Lord said: The spiritual reality is unaffected and supreme. The Supreme Soul is described as a personal existence Who causes the production of the mundane world. Cultural action is known as creative power. (8.3)

Commentary:

Since before the Upanishadic period, aksharam brahma became famous as the Supreme (paramam). Many yogis see this spiritual reality as the Ultimate and do not take seriously the claims of Śrī Krishna as being identical with and governing over that power. Some who are not kriyā yogis also regard that reality as the Supreme and take lightly, or totally disregard Śrī Krishna's claims.

The connection between the akṣaram brahma (spiritual reality) and the Supreme Personality is not clarified from a position in the material world, because there is a causal zone through which one must see before one can understand the spiritual reality.

As such Śrī Krishna established that the Supreme Soul (adhyātma) was described as a personal existence Who causes the production of the mundane world. There is no other way to really know the Supreme Soul from this side of existence.

Initially, the knowledge of a spiritual world is irrelevant because we must deal with the subtle and gross mundane reality. We cannot escape it by wishful thinking or by our beliefs. No matter what a human being believes, he or she must deal with the material body, with the displacement from it at its death, and with the assumption of another mundane form automatically regardless of whether one wants one or not. The puzzle of material existence is the first thing to solve out. We have to deal with personal and impersonal forces. Thus, those who only see it from a personal perspective miss out on the impersonal causes. Both personal and impersonal factors are involved in our material bondage.

We can understand this from the material body. Sometimes a doctor is needed to effect healing in the body. Another time, the same doctor may state that he can do nothing and that the body must heal itself. As such, there are times for a personal involvement and times for an impersonal one, all depending on how the energies were combined in the first place.

For human beings, the material world was created for cultural actions and for the resulting realizations which we get from the involvements. These realizations lead to the need for liberation from the cultural scene. Śrī Krishna claims that He created this world with such intentions.

अधिभूतं क्षरो भावः
पुरुषश्चाधिदैवतम् ।
अधियज्ञोऽहमेवात्र
देहे देहभृतां वर ॥८.४॥

adhibhūtaṁ kṣaro bhāvaḥ
puruṣaścādhidaivatam
adhiyajño'hamevātra
dehe dehabhṛtāṁ vara (8.4)

adhibhūtam — sum total gross reality; kṣaro = kṣaraḥ — ever—changing; bhāvaḥ — nature; puruṣaścādhidaivatam = puruṣa — master of the world + ca — and + adhidaivatam — Lord of the Supernatural rulers and powers; adhiyajño = adhiyajñaḥ — the Supreme Regulator of religious ceremonies and disciplines; 'ham = aham — I; evātra = eva — indeed + atra — here; dehe — in the body; dehabhṛtām vara — O best of the embodied souls

The sum total gross reality is ever—changing nature. The master of the world is the Lord of the supernatural rulers and powers. O best of the embodied souls, I, Who exist here in the body, am the Supreme Regulator of religious ceremonies and disciplines. (8.4)

Commentary:

We must contend with adhibhūtanam or the sum total gross reality. Because we are limited spirits, it is too large of a reality for us to subdue. What we can do, however, is to control our response to it. A big part of kriyā yoga concerns the cultivation of detachment, but such detachment only lasts if the kriyā yogi changes his diet of energies. If he remains on a diet of lower energies, he will perpetually seek detachment without ever retaining it. It is not a matter of willpower. One must replace the lower energies and take in a higher quality of energy from the gross and subtle environment.

Once a kriyā yogi understands that he cannot change the functions of particular types of energy, he accelerates his course by saving his controlling energy to fight the psychological need for lower involvements. At first he has no recourse but to imbibe higher material energies. This occurs on the gross and subtle levels. For instance on the gross level he stops eating certain types of food. He does not eat flesh; he does not eat hot spicy foods. He adopts these restrictions to facilitate the practice. Initially he is given a guideline for vegetarian and fruit-based meals, along with dairy products. Later when his practice matures, the practice itself dictates what he should eat.

In the subtle world, he also follows suit to regulate and change the subtle intake of energy according to the stages of practice. He does whatever is necessary for success. Different yogis at different stages eat different things according to the dictates of their practice. There is a similarity in the meals and the times of eating but there may be specific differences.

The sum total gross reality cannot be baffled by a yogi. In fact that energy is also regarded as being a reality and even the Supreme Being can only adjust it so much. Thus a yogi leaves aside that energy and tends only his response to it. His response and that alone is something he may adjust.

A limited being contends with natural and supernatural forces. Both of these are personified and un—personified. According to Śrī Krishna, there is a Lord of the world, who supervises the forces and powers. A kriyā yogi must understand and recognize that influence and get waivers from those supernatural people who control the exit from these lower worlds.

Śrī Krishna identified Himself as one who exists in the body of every creature and who regulates the religious ceremonies and disciplines. Arjuna wanted to know how one could see such a person who resides in every creature form. Where does that person reside? In which dimension? How is He to be related to? How is he perceived?

अन्तकाले च मामेव
स्मरन्मुक्त्वा कलेवरम् ।
यः प्रयाति स मद्भावं
याति नास्त्यत्र संशयः ॥८.५॥
antakāle ca māmeva
smaranmuktvā kalevaram
yaḥ prayāti sa madbhāvaṁ
yāti nāstyatra saṁśayaḥ (8.5)

antakāle — at the end of life; ca — and; mām — Me; eva — in particular; smaran — remembering; muktvā — giving up; kalevaram — body; yaḥ — who; prayāti — departs the body; sa = saḥ — he; madbhāvam — My condition of existence; yāti — is elevated; nāsty (nasti) = na — not + asti — is; atra — here; saṁśayaḥ — doubt

If at the end of one's life, one recalls Me in particular, as one gives up the body, one is elevated to My condition of existence. There is no doubt about this. (8.5)

Commentary:

This does not apply to any and everybody or even every devotee of Krishna. It applies particularly to the practicing yogi, who performs the disciplines of yoga described thus far in the *Gītā*. We must remember that Arjuna questioned about the yogi who is subdued:

adhiyajñaḥ kathaṁ ko'tra dehe'sminmadhusūdana
prayāṇakāle ca kathaṁ jñeyo'si niyatātmabhiḥ (8.2)

Who is the Supreme Regulator of religious ceremonies and disciplines? How is He located here in this body, O killer of Madhu? And how, at the time of departure from the body, are You to be known by those persons who are subdued? (8.2)

Someone else may attain Śrī Krishna at the time of death but in context of the previous chapters, this verse applies specifically to those who are disciplined and persistent in practice.

यं यं वापि स्मरन्भावं
त्यजत्यन्ते कलेवरम् ।
तं तमेवैति कौन्तेय
सदा तद्भावभावितः ॥८.६॥
yaṁ yaṁ vāpi smaranbhāvaṁ
tyajatyante kalevaram
taṁ tamevaiti kaunteya
sadā tadbhāvabhāvitaḥ (8.6)

yaṁ yam — whatever; vāpi = va – or + api – also; moreover; smaran — recalling; bhāvam — texture of existence; tyajaty = tyajati — abandons; ante — in the end; kalevaram — the body; taṁtam — that that; evaiti = eva — indeed + eti — is projected; kaunteya — O son of Kuntī; sadā — always; tad — that + bhāva — status of life + bhāvitaḥ — being transformed

Moreover, whatever texture of existence is recalled when a person abandons his body in the end, to that same type of life, he is projected, O son of Kuntī, always being transformed into that status of life. (8.6)

Commentary:

The texture of existence recalled at death is the same general consciousness which the person exhibits and identifies with during the life of his body. It is not a sudden call for help from a divine being or a convenient state of mind adopted just before dying. Even if the spirit in the dying body takes recourse to a religious life at that time, still his usual consciousness will form the basis for his next existence.

A yogi should seek to always adopt the proper life style. He should not think that he may, when near to death, suddenly adopt a religious, holy or austere life. He must understand that the overall texture of his consciousness determines his status. He needs to cultivate subtle perception while using the gross body. He will not suddenly adopt those perceptions at the time of death.

Many incentive scriptures convey the idea that a person can, all of a sudden, take a divine form at the time of death, if only that person calls on the name of the Supreme Lord or seeks refuge in a divine person or representative of the Lord. A kriyā yogi should leave all such statements aside. He should work to ensure that the texture of his consciousness during the life of his body is harmonious with what he aims for in the hereafter.

तस्मात्सर्वेषु कालेषु
मामनुस्मर युध्य च ।
मय्यर्पितमनोबुद्धिर्
मामेवैष्यस्यसंशयः ॥८.७॥
tasmātsarveṣu kāleṣu
māmanusmara yudhya ca
mayyarpitamanobuddhir
māmevaiṣyasyasaṁśayaḥ (8.7)

tasmāt — therefore; sarveṣu — at all; kāleṣu — at times; mām — Me; anusmara — remember; yudhya — fight; ca — and; mayy = mayi — on Me; arpitamanobuddhir (arpitamanobuddhiḥ) = arpita — anchor + manobuddhiḥ — mind and intelligence; mām — to Me; evaiṣyasy (evaiṣyasi) = eva — indeed + eṣyasi — will be with; asaṁśayaḥ — without doubt

Therefore, at all times, remember Me and fight. Anchor your mind and intelligence on Me. You will be with Me without doubt. (8.7)

Commentary:

This verse is designed to boost Arjuna's spirit and assure him of continued divine association with Krishna even if his body died. He would have it by virtue of the friendship and relationship he had with Śrī Krishna. Furthermore, Arjuna was counseled to remember Krishna while fighting in the battle of Kurukṣetra and to anchor his mind and intelligence on Śrī Krishna. Some feel that this means to anchor the general mental sphere and the calculative analyzing faculty but it really means that Arjuna was to focus his buddhi organ and sensual energy upon Krishna, in the way done by yogis.

In this verse, Śrī Krishna again urged Arjuna to fight. He gave a personal guarantee that Arjuna need not fear losing divine association. Arjuna would have it, after leaving his body, just as he had it before, as part of his life style and as part of the texture of his consciousness.

अभ्यासयोगयुक्तेन
चेतसा नान्यगामिना ।
परमं पुरुषं दिव्यं
याति पार्थानुचिन्तयन् ॥८.८॥
abhyāsayogayuktena
cetasā nānyagāminā
paramaṁ puruṣaṁ divyaṁ
yāti pārthānucintayan (8.8)

abhyāsa – practice;. yoga — yoga; yuktena — by discipline; cetasā — by the mind; nānyagāminā = na – not + anya –other + gāminā — by venturing outward; paramam — supreme; puruṣam — person; divyam — divine; yāti — one goes; pārthānucintayan = pārtha — son of Pṛthā + anucintayan — deeply meditating

With a mind that does not venture outwards, which is disciplined by yoga practice, a person goes to the divine Supreme Person, while deeply meditating, O son of Pṛthā. (8.8)

Commentary:

Now after giving that instruction to Arjuna alone, Śrī Krishna described how such an instruction is practiced by the advanced yogis. This is not how it is done by devotees of Śrī Krishna who are not practicing kriyā yoga. Others take assurance from this verse, but as it was spoken, it applies only to very advanced yogis.

Abhyāsayoga yuktena means by the discipline of yoga practice. How possibly can a commentator say that this is not yoga but that it is devotional service? This is an advanced kriyā yoga practice of anucintayan, deep meditation. This means the 7th and 8th stages of practice, that of dhāraṇa focus of the soul's will through the buddhi organ and the samādhi trance states.

Nanyagāminā means with a mind that does not venture outwards through the gross body. This cannot be Deity Worship. Rather, it is a shutting down of the sensual orifices in so far as they venture outwards for anything physical, including sacred physical objects. This means that the yogi mastered the 5th stage of yoga namely the pratyāhār sense withdrawal, where his buddhi organ retracted its sensual orifices from the gross reality and from the subtle objects which induce it to dwell on the gross levels. These are clearly yoga techniques.

In this verse, Śrī Krishna described a state attained by the advanced yogi. This is not for Arjuna on the battlefield but it is described to enlighten him on what the yogis do. This is one way in which they go to the divine Supreme Person, Who is Śrī Krishna Himself.

Do they go to the physical Śrī Krishna Who stood near to Arjuna on the chariot? The answer is yes, they do go to that Person, not to His physical body. They go to His spiritual form. Such yogis have no reason to avoid Śrī Krishna merely because He used a miracle—working physical form. The physical form used by Śrī Krishna is no bar to His divinity. It did not detract from His sovereignty as the divine Supreme Person.

कविं पुराणमनुशासितारम्
अणोरणीयांसमनुस्मरेद्यः ।
सर्वस्य धातारमचिन्त्यरूपम्
आदित्यवर्णं तमसः परस्तात् ॥८.९॥
kaviṁ purāṇamanuśāsitāram
aṇoraṇīyāṁsamanusmaredyaḥ
sarvasya dhātāram acintyarūpam
ādityavarṇaṁ tamasaḥ parastāt (8.9)

kavim — the person who knows everything; purāṇam — the most ancient; anuśāsitāram — the supreme supervisor; aṇor (aṇoḥ)— than the atom; aṇīyāṁsam — more minute; anusmared (anusmaret)— should meditate on; yaḥ — who; sarvasya — of all; dhātāram — supporter; acintya — unimaginable + rūpam — form; ādityavarṇam = āditya –radiance + varṇam — category; tamasaḥ — grossness; parastāt — distinct form

He who meditates on the Person Who knows everything, the most ancient of people, the Supreme Supervisor, the most minute factor, the one with unimaginable form, with a radiant body, free of grossness, (8.9)

Commentary:

This again is a description of kriyā yoga. Śrīla Vyāsadeva, his son Shuka, and his spiritual teacher Nārada were examples of such yogis. Another person, even if he is a devotee of Śrī Krishna, even if he is an established popular, disciple—making spiritual master in the disciplic succession from Śrī Krishna, cannot meditate in this exacting way. For him it would not be possible.

Śrī Caitanya Mahaprabhu used to be absorbed in the Krishna pastimes with the gopis, activities occuring in a spiritual dimension somewhere else, but Śrī Caitanya Mahāprabhu did not perform any yoga practice at that time, nor is there a record of him doing so during that advent. However, this does not mean that others who are devotees of Lord Caitanya are entering such pastimes in the same way. Most are not even if they imagine so. Śrī Krishna Caitanya, even without a record of yoga practice, definitely entered the spiritual world but that does not mean that this verse and all that was described in Chapter Seven, pertains to entering the spiritual dimensions without having mastered yoga. These verses definitely express what happens when one masters yoga. Lord Caitanya's pastimes do not negate these verses, or erase them, or take out the yoga practice as stressed.

The meditations described in this verse are done in deep samādhi trances and in piercing mystic perceptions. These are not done merely by understanding and accepting Bhagavad Gītā with confidence. The yogi focuses on the Person Who knows everything, the Supreme Being, The Supreme Personality of Godhead. The ascetic can do so insofar as he is permitted by that Supreme Person. The yogi may or may not know that this person is Śrī Krishna but regardless, if he is that advanced, He may in focused trance, understand the whereabouts and the spreading influence of that divinity.

The yogi tracks back in time to find the most ancient of people, the first person to manifest in the material energy after that energy became quiescent in the last time cycle. That first person is the Supreme Person because He has the most objectivity. He survives with the most objective awareness. For a yogi to do this, he has to be very very advanced. His consciousness has to be stilled sufficiently to detect very subtle phenomena on the causal plane of life.

The yogi then checks on the Person Who is the Supreme Supervisor, the most minute person in terms of His penetrating influences, the one with an unimaginable form, Who has a radiant divine body with spiritual limbs and senses and Who, indeed, is free from the need for grossness.

प्रयाणकाले मनसाचलेन
भक्त्या युक्तो योगबलेन चैव ।
भ्रुवोर्मध्ये प्राणमावेश्य सम्यक्
स तं परं पुरुषमुपैति दिव्यम् ॥८.१०॥
prayāṇakāle manasācalena
bhaktyā yukto yogabalena caiva
bhruvormadhye prāṇam āveśya samyak
sa taṁ paraṁ puruṣamupaiti divyam (8.10)

prayāṇakāle — at the time of death; manasācalena = manasā — by the mind + acalena— by unwavering; bhaktyā — with devotion; yukto = yuktaḥ — connected; yogabalena — with psychological power developed through yoga practice; caiva = ca — and + eva — indeed; bhruvor = bhruvoḥ — of the two eyebrows; madhye — in the middle; prāṇam — energizing breath; āveśya— having caused to enter; samyak — precisely; sa = saḥ — he; tam — this; param — supreme; puruṣam— person; upaiti — he goes; divyam — divine

...and that meditator who even at the time of death, with an unwavering mind, being connected devotedly, with psychological power developed through yoga practice, and having caused the energizing breath to enter between the eyebrows with precision, goes to the divine Supreme Person. (8.10)

Commentary:

Some experts at samādhi meditation do not mention the divine Supreme Person as part of their experience. Such meditators, though successful at the yoga process, do not encounter that Supreme Personality. Thus they accredit a transcendental energy which is infallible and supreme. To them, this energy is the Supreme Cause. Here Śrī Krishna described the meditation of his devotee who is expert at the yoga process. Such a person must have devotion to Śrī Krishna (bhaktyā), along with an unwavering mind and psychological power developed through yoga practice (yogabalena). He must be an expert at centering his attention into the buddhi organ seeing facility. That is a purely mystic procedure developed through expertise in prāṇāyāma and concentration.

By stating that the yogi devotee must cause the energizing breath enter between the eyebrows with precision, Śrī Krishna directly implied that such a yogi devotee must have perfected the Kuṇḍalinī and celibacy yoga techniques; only a person who has perfected these can execute that with precision at the time of death.

यदक्षरं वेदविदो वदन्ति
विशन्ति यद्यतयो वीतरागाः ।
यदिच्छन्तो ब्रह्मचर्यं चरन्ति
तत्ते पदं संग्रहेण प्रवक्ष्ये ॥८.११॥
yadakṣaraṁ vedavido vadanti
viśanti yadyatayo vītarāgāḥ
yadicchanto brahmacaryaṁ caranti
tatte padaṁ saṁgraheṇa pravakṣye (8.11)

yad — which; akṣaram — imperishable; vedavido = vedavidaḥ — knowers of the Veda; vadanti — they described; viśanti — they enter; yad — which; yatayo = yatayaḥ — ascetics; vītarāgāḥ — free from cravings; yad — which; icchanto = icchantaḥ — desiring; brahmacaryam — life of celibacy; caranti — they follow; tat = tad — this; te — to you; padam — process; saṁgraheṇa — in brief; pravakṣye — I will explain

I will briefly explain the process to you, which the knowers of the Veda describe as imperishable, which the ascetics who are free from cravings enter and who desiring to be transferred there, they follow a life of celibacy. (8.11)

<u>*Commentary:*</u>

Śrī Krishna, knowing that Arjuna was interested in the perfection of yoga, explained in brief what the devotional yogis and non-devotional ones attain.

There are various destinations which are described as imperishable locales for the spirits to attain. It is not just one place. To go to such places by self endeavor one must be free from cravings and must follow a life of celibacy which is highlighted by a continual striving for spiritual experience, for engaging with the brahma level of life in any of its phases. Devotion to Śrī Krishna should be there but it is not necessary in all cases, for it depends on the nature of the yogi. Some have the devotional nature. Others do not, all depending on their spirit category. Even though Śrī Krishna repeatedly mentions devotion to Himself, He does not ridicule or ignore the accomplishments of those who are not His devotees but who are successful yogis nonetheless.

सर्वद्वाराणि संयम्य
मनो हृदि निरुध्य च ।
मूर्ध्न्याधायात्मनः प्राणम्
आस्थितो योगधारणाम् ॥८.१२॥
sarvadvārāṇi saṁyamya
mano hṛdi nirudhya ca
mūrdhnyādhāyātmanaḥ prāṇam
āsthito yogadhāraṇām (8.12)

sarvadvārāṇi = sarva – all + dvārāṇi — entrances; saṁyamya — controlling; mano = manaḥ — mind; hṛdi — in the core of consciousness; nirudhya — confining; ca — and; mūrdhny = mūrdhni — in the brain; ādhāyātmanaḥ = ādhāya — situating + ātmanaḥ — of the soul; prāṇam — energizing breath; āsthito = āsthitaḥ — remain fixed; yogadhāraṇām — yoga concentration

Controlling all openings of the body, and restricting the mind in the core of consciousness, situating the energizing energy of the soul in the brain, remaining fixed in yoga concentration, (8.12)

<u>*Commentary:*</u>

Yogadhāraṇām pertains to the 6th stage of yoga, which is concentration in mystic yoga practice. This stage cannot be perfected merely by concentration. It is only perfected when one masters prāṇāyāma and the pratyāhār sensual energy withdrawal, which are the 4th and 5th stages. Some feel that they can concentrate themselves and their lives on Śrī Krishna without completing the yoga process, which they regard as a waste of time. Their teachers explain that instead of spending years trying to perfect yoga, they should instead directly apply themselves to Krishna's devotional service.

However for those who have the inclination to kriyā yoga, such advice is insufficient, for we find that the full purity does not develop merely by missionary activities, Deity Worship, and chanting of Śrī Krishna's name. The essential energy in the psyche remains the same in our case. Recognizing this, we strive for soul purification as described in Chapter Five verse 11 and Chapter Six verse 12:

kāyena manasā buddhyā kevalairindriyairapi
yoginaḥ karma kurvanti saṅgaṁ tyaktvātmaśuddhaye (5.11)

With the body, mind and intelligence, or even with the senses alone, the yogis, having discarded attachment, perform cultural acts for self—purification. (5.11)

tatraikāgraṁ manaḥ kṛtvā yatacittendriyakriyaḥ
upaviśyāsane yuñjyād yogamātmaviśuddhaye (6.12)

...being there, seated in a posture, having the mind focused, the person who controls his thinking and sensual energy, should practice the yoga discipline for self purification. (6.12)

Despite claims to the contrary, one cannot control all the openings of the body without doing yoga practice. In fact, the system of control mentioned in this verse as mūrdhnyādhāyātmanaḥ prāṇam, is the placement of the energizing energy of the soul into the brain. This is kuṇḍalinī yoga whereby the life force rises into the brain, up and away from the base chakra, the mulādhara region.

The restriction of the mind in the core of consciousness is initiated by a mystic process in the dhāraṇa 6th stage of yoga. It is completed in the 7th stage which is dhyāna. This is a purely mystic procedure. It cannot be done by just imagining it or sitting to meditate without first mastering the lower stages. It takes deliberate practice. It is not achieved merely using one's material body to worship Krishna, preach about Him, chant His names and follow an authority in the disciplic succession.

ओमित्येकाक्षरं ब्रह्म
व्याहरन्मामनुस्मरन् ।
यः प्रयाति त्यजन्देहं
स याति परमां गतिम् ॥८.१३॥
omityekākṣaraṁ brahma
vyāharanmāmanusmaran
yaḥ prayāti tyajandehaṁ
sa yāti paramāṁ gatim (8.13)

om — the uttered sound om; ity = iti — thus saying; ekākṣaram — one syllable; brahma — spiritual reality; vyāharan — chanting; mām — Me; anusmaran — meditating on; yaḥ — who; prayāti — passes on; tyajan — renouncing; deham — body; sa = saḥ — he; yāti — attains; paramām — supreme; gatim — objective

...uttering *Om,* the one—syllable sound which represents the spiritual reality, meditating on Me, the yogi who passes on, renouncing the body, attains the highest objective. (8.13)

Commentary:

Nowadays many non—yogi devotees of Śrī Krishna, leaders of the disciplic succession which stem from Him, deride *Om* and discourage followers from using it for the purposes stated in this verse. Some of them say that *Om* gives one an impersonalist objective and does not lead to the Supreme Person. However, this verse is clear in its acclaim for the chanting of the one- syllable sound, *Om*.

A person who is advanced and who utters *Om* while meditating on Śrī Krishna, passes on from this world while renouncing the body and he or she attains the highest objective. The life energy, mind and buddhi organ are fully concentrated and the sense of initiative is focused on reaching and keeping association with Śrī Krishna in the spiritual dimension.

अनन्यचेताः सततं
यो मां स्मरति नित्यशः ।
तस्याहं सुलभः पार्थ
नित्ययुक्तस्य योगिनः ॥८.१४॥
ananyacetāḥ satataṁ
yo māṁ smarati nityaśaḥ
tasyāhaṁ sulabhaḥ pārtha
nityayuktasya yoginaḥ (8.14)

ananyacetāḥ — one whose mind does not go to another focus; satatam — perpetually; yo = yaḥ — who; mām — Me; smarati — he remembers; nityaśaḥ — constantly; tasyāham = tasya — to him + aham — I; sulabhaḥ — easy to reach; pārtha — O son of Pṛthā; nityayuktasya — of one who is constantly disciplined in yoga; yoginaḥ — of the devotee

He whose mind does not go to another focus at any time, who thinks of Me constantly, for that yogi who is constantly disciplined in yoga, I am easy to reach, O son of Pṛthā. (8.14)

Commentary:

This is a description of the ideal yogi devotee of Śrī Krishna. For such a person, Śrī Krishna is easy to reach because he transcended the mundane energies and perceives the spiritual realities. Such a yogi has a definite way of reaching the Supreme Lord. He does not depend on an uncertain path to salvation. By virtue of advanced practice he experiences the salvation even when using a gross body.

मामुपेत्य पुनर्जन्म
दुःखालयमशाश्वतम् ।
नाप्नुवन्ति महात्मानः
संसिद्धिं परमां गताः ॥८.१५॥
māmupetya punarjanma
duḥkhālayamaśāśvatam
nāpnuvanti mahātmānaḥ
saṁsiddhiṁ paramāṁ gatāḥ (8.15)

mām — Me; upetya — approaching; punarjanma — rebirth; duḥkhālayam = duḥkha — misery + ālayam — location; aśāśvatam — shifty; nāpnuvanti = na — not + apnuvanti — subjected to; mahātmānaḥ — great souls; saṁsiddhim — perfect; paramām — supreme; gatāḥ — gone

Approaching me in this way, those great souls who went to supreme perfection are not subjected to rebirth in this shifty, miserable location. (8.15)

Commentary:

This mentions the yogi devotees of Śrī Krishna who became perfected before the time of Śrī Krishna and Arjuna. Such persons passed through the stage of self purification and progressed successfully through the advanced stage of applying their yogic insight to the Supreme Person.

आ ब्रह्मभुवनाल्लोकाः
पुनरावर्तिनोऽर्जुन ।
मामुपेत्य तु कौन्तेय
पुनर्जन्म न विद्यते ॥८.१६॥
ā brahmabhuvanāllokāḥ
punarāvartino'rjuna
māmupetya tu kaunteya
punarjanma na vidyate (8.16)

ā — up to; brahmabhuvanāl = brahmabhuvanāt — to Brahmā's world; lokāḥ — populations; punarāvartino = punarāvartinaḥ — subjected to repeated birth and death; 'rjuna = arjuna — Arjuna; mām — Me; upetya — approaching; tu — but; kaunteya — O son of Kuntī; punarjanma — impulsion of rebirth; na — not; vidyate — is experienced

Up to Brahmā's world, the populations are subjected to repeated births and deaths, O Arjuna. But in approaching Me, rebirth is not experienced, O son of Kuntī. (8.16)

Commentary:

Birth and death means repeated manifestation and relinquishment of forms in various dimensions. In some dimensions of this mundane existence, one's body does not die as a material one would on this planet; nor is one's body born in the same way. For instance in some subtle worlds, one does not take an infant form from an embryo. One's body appears there suddenly and begins to function as an adult form from the beginning. Then when the time for leaving that level is manifested, one suddenly disappears from there. Thus there is no death of the body in the earthly sense.

The Brahmā mentioned in this verse is the agent for creating these worlds in which we presently reside. He creates the environmental conditions by his conceptual energy which manipulates the subtle and gross materials, just as a great industrialist creates conditions of living for workers of a large industrial enterprise. Brahmā's situation is varied and widespread. In comparison to us, Brahmā is a god. If, though, we learn how to transcend Brahma's situation, we may approach Lord Krishna, the Supreme Lord.

One who transcends Brahmā's world, both his subtle and gross territories, does not have to take rebirth or reappearance in Brahmā's environments. That person attains something higher and is purged of the need for these lower manifestations.

Some devotees of Krishna, especially those who are not practicing yogis, get the idea that Brahmā is irrelevant and cannot keep them time bound, provided they take shelter of Lord Krishna, by taking directions from a pure devotee spiritual master who descended from Lord Caitanya. However the matter is not so simple.

Brahmā certainly has the power to keep them bewildered. Whatever they do, that is not an advanced kriyā yoga practice, is itself happening within the territory of Brahmā and under Brahmā's watchful gaze. Worshipping Śrī Krishna, without mastering advanced yoga, still leaves the worshippers under Brahmā's jurisdiction. It is a mistake to think that merely by worshipping Śrī Krishna's Deity form and chanting His name and by accepting a non—yogi spiritual master who hails from Lord Caitanya, one has transcended Brahmā. To transcend Lord Brahmā, one has to do more than that.

सहस्रयुगपर्यन्तम्
अहर्यद्ब्रह्मणो विदुः ।
रात्रिं युगसहस्रान्तां
तेऽहोरात्रविदो जनाः ॥८.१७॥

sahasra — one thousand + yuga — time cycle + paryantam — limit; ahar — day; yad — which; brahmaṇo = brahmaṇaḥ — of Brahmā; viduḥ — they know; rātrim — night; yugasahasrāntāṁ = yuga — time cycle + sahasra — one thousand + antam — end; te

sahasrayugaparyantam
aharyadbrahmaṇo viduḥ
rātriṁ yugasahasrāntāṁ
te'horātravido janāḥ (8.17)

— they; 'horātravido (ahoratravidaḥ) = ahoratra — day and night + vidaḥ — knowers; janāḥ — people

Those who know the day of Brahmā, which has a limit of one thousand time cycles, and the night of Brahmā, which ends in a thousand time cycles, are the people who know day and night. (8.17)

Commentary:

Knowing of the day and night of Brahmā is knowing the cosmic time cycles and their operational influence on the limited beings like you and me. One does not experience this merely by reading scripture or by hearing from a spiritual master who has intellectually grasped the concepts from the Śrīmad Bhāgavatam and related scriptures. This knowing is gained by samādhi trance states in which one perceives the time gaps and sees how Brahmā's mystic power operates. This has nothing to do with intellectual understanding of the data given by Śrī Krishna and by others.

It is described that during the day of Brahmā, this host of subtle and gross creatures lives and during his night they perish for a time, until he rises again and reenacts the creation.

In yoga we research the relevance of Brahmā. He is not a person we can easily dismiss. In that research one realizes that one's objectivity is dependent on the conscious mind of Brahmā. If his energy collapses, ours would lose conscious form too. Seeing this, a yogi if he is able and if he is existentially qualified, learns how to eliminate reliance on Brahmā and be transferred to a more stable divine being.

That stable being is one's pre-existence source which may or may not be Lord Krishna or one of the Vishnu people or the Shivas. The point is that one will know who it is when one reaches that stage. One must accept that person, even if before, one believed in another person as one's pre-existence source. There are many devotees who declare Lord Krishna as their pre-existence source. They do this by saying statements like, "Everyone is a servant of Krishna." This is said because Lord Śrī Caitanya Mahāprabhu stressed it.

However, such persons may find that their pre—existence source is not Lord Krishna, even though He is the Ultimate Person. Non—yogi devotees usually deride practices like Kuṇḍalinī yoga but it is in Kuṇḍalinī yoga that one learns the preliminary discipline for moving from one type of reliance to another. It begins by shifting the life force from the lower chakras to the higher ones. Then later when that is mastered, one shuts down the entire Kuṇḍalinī chakra and retreats into the buddhi organ. One goes further to retract that organ until one can do what Śrī Krishna suggests here about shifting the reliance from the Creator God Brahmā to Śrī Krishna Himself.

अव्यक्ताद्व्यक्तयः सर्वाः
प्रभवन्त्यहरागमे ।
रात्र्यागमे प्रलीयन्ते
तत्रैवाव्यक्तसंज्ञके ॥८.१८॥
avyaktādvyaktayaḥ sarvāḥ
prabhavantyaharāgame
rātryāgame pralīyante
tatraivāvyaktasaṁjñake (8.18)

avyaktād = avyaktāt — from the invisible world; vyaktayaḥ — the visible world; sarvāḥ — all; prabhavanty = prabhavanti — they are produced; aharāgame — at the beginning of Brahma's day; rātryāgame — at the beginning of Brahma's night; pralīyante — they are reverted back; tatraivāvyaktasaṁjñake = tatra — at the time + eva — indeed + avyakta — invisible world + saṁjñake — is understood as

When the day of Creator Brahmā begins, all this visible world is produced from the invisible world. When his night comes, the manifested energies are reverted back into the invisible world. (8.18)

Commentary:

The mental power of Brahmā, his psychological grip on our situation, and the fact that presently we are dependent on his consciousness, is clearly described in this verse. It is not easy to elude the grasp of Brahmā. For one thing, if Śrī Krishna was personally conducting everything, why is it that Brahmā is so instrumental in this case? Why is Brahmā in charge of the environments? The answer is, of course, that Śrī Krishna is not personally doing everything here. And furthermore Śrī Krishna's interest is not predominantly involved here. He is concerned about other places which are beyond Brahmā's locale.

It is only a naïve or simple-minded devotee who thinks that just by a belief in Krishna or by a belief in one of Krishna's devotees, one will, all of a sudden, transcend Brahmā's influence. This is mostly wishful thinking. If we stop to consider it, we will see that, to us, Brahmā is God for all practical purposes. It is like comparing our local sun to another luminary which is millions of times brighter. The comparison has little value because in our present circumstance, the local sun is sufficient. We do not need a much brighter sun because we can only absorb so much energy from this one. If you can only consume two grains of salt each day, seeing a mountain of salt has little value over seeing one hundred pounds.

At present those who are quite satisfied with the Krishna Deity Form, and who stress that such material forms are spiritual, are not interested in taking up the austerities of kriyā yoga to go higher. Thus their complaint about the yogi devotees is useless. If one is happy with the Deity Form and is satisfied to wait till the time of death to see Krishna's spiritual body, then it means that one is satisfied with Brahmā's arrangements of which the Śrī Krishna Deity form is a part. Such forms are created out of the materials Brahmā produced.

As Śrī Krishna stated, when the day of Creator Brahmā begins, all this visible world is produced from the invisible existence. When his night comes, the manifested energies are reverted back into the invisible world. That is it.

One cannot avoid this, merely by acclaiming oneself as a devotee of Śrī Krishna. Theway out is by a purely mystic process that transcends Brahmā's super-mystic process. Śrī Krishna could really care less if we get out of Brahmā's jurisdiction or not. Devotees of Śrī Krishna, particularly, the non-yogi devotees, put themselves on a pedestal as being so special to Śrī Krishna that He will personally take them out of Brahmā's world. They are in for a rude awakening because unless they are serious enough to take up kriyā practice, they will not get out. They will remain under Brahmā's jurisdiction. Even people like Nārada, accomplished yogis, are still under Brahmā's control. What about others who are much less and who have no yogic accomplishments, averse to even the yoga that is described in the *Bhagavad Gītā*?

The invisible world, known by the term avyakta in Sanskrit, is ignored by many non—yogi devotees. They feel that if one focuses on the Deity Form of Śrī Krishna and on the recommended devotional services, then one would not have to deal with the invisible existence at all. In their view this avyakta (invisible energy) is impersonal. Their idea is for an abrupt transference from this visible material and subtle existence to the visible perceptible spiritual existence of the Vaikuntha spiritual world.

Hearing of the transference, these non-yogic devotees hope that by not wasting time on yoga disciplines and its related strenuous austerities, they will, all of a sudden at the time of death, be transferred from the Vaikuntha temple environment created by their spiritual master in this world, to the real Vaikuntha in the spiritual world. However this is, for the most part, a fantasy. To cross from here to the spiritual world, one must first cross over the same avyakta (invisible energy) from which this material world emerged.

The avyakta invisible energies, even if they are rated as being of impersonal potency, are the very same energies from which Brahmā produced this subtle and gross universe. For his liberation a living entity will have to perceive that energy, and discern his connection to it, and figure out the why and how of his attachment to it. Unless such attachment is removed, he will never become liberated, no matter how he rants and raves about being a devotee of Śrī Krishna or any other Vishnu or Shiva personality.

The connection between a limited spirit and that avyakta invisible energy is very strong. It existed before the beginning of time, before this universe formed. Freedom from it is not an easy accomplishment for any limited being. One should not fantasize about Śrī Krishna's deliverance of oneself, because it is factual that Śrī Krishna is not that eager about our deliverance from the control of Brahmā, otherwise we would have been delivered long, long ago. It is not yesterday that we began this course in material existence. It was millions upon millions, trillions upon trillions of years before. Up to now Śrī Krishna has not delivered us. A yogi considers this and takes the needful action in all seriousness for the practice of the disciplines which are described in brief thus far in the *Bhagavad Gītā*.

भूतग्रामः स एवायं
भूत्वा भूत्वा प्रलीयते ।
रात्र्यागमेऽवशः पार्थ
प्रभवत्यहरागमे ॥८.१९॥
bhūtagrāmaḥ sa evāyaṁ
bhūtvā bhūtvā pralīyate
rātryāgame'vaśaḥ pārtha
prabhavatyaharāgame (8.19)

bhūtagrāmaḥ — multitude of beings; sa = saḥ — this; evāyam = eva — indeed + ayam — this; bhūtvā bhūtvā — repeatedly manifesting; pralīyate — is shifted out of visibility; rātryāgame — at the arrival of Brahma's night; 'vaśaḥ = avaśaḥ — happening naturally; pārtha — O son of Pṛthā; prabhavaty = prabhavati — it comes into existence; aharāgame — on the onset of Brahma's day

O son of Pṛthā, this multitude of beings which is repeatedly manifested, is naturally shifted out of visibility at the arrival of each of Brahmā's nights. It again comes into existence at the onset of Brahmā's day. (8.19)

Commentary:

Bhūtvā means coming into being again and again, repeatedly, ongoing for many trillions of times, just like germs which are repeatedly being killed and re—manifested by varying temperature changes in a pond due to intolerable coldness and livable warmth. That is our present situation. This is nothing new. The Supreme Being, if He were to take an action at all, would have done so long ago. It is not that some new incarnation can actually change our condition merely by appearing here. We have to work for deliverance through permanent change of our nature and by erasure of our relationship with material nature. Such a relationship is very private, very confidential. Mentally forgetting or minimizing it will not eliminate it. In fact, that will cause it to be impressed upon us with greater force at the nearest opportunity.

It is very difficult to get out of Brahmā's jurisdiction and to be free from the reliance on his mind. Being a devotee of Krishna does not necessarily cause a person to be freed from

Brahmā's mental mystic manifesting powers. When Brahmā's night comes, we phase out for the time being because we do not have the power to keep ourselves in objective consciousness without the support of his self—consciousness.

The fact remains that Śrī Krishna is interested in making us conform to cultural duties so that He does not have to take care of it Himself. We see this because He tried to get Arjuna to take up duties which if not completed, Śrī Krishna would have to complete Himself or assign to someone else. In the end, the Pandavas, Arjuna included, had to resort to yoga practice to elevate themselves above this world. They had to work for it individually. It was not given to them by Śrī Krishna, except that He arranged that they were pre—trained in the techniques by Vyāsa and other mahāyogīns.

A kriyā yogi cannot afford to ignore Brahmā, the Creator God, or the avyakta invisible energy from which Brahmā produces these manifested energies. To transcend all this, one has to understand how Brahmā operates and how the avyakta invisible energy functions to produce these worlds. Most of all, one needs to understand the very confidential relationship one has with the primal mundane energy.

परस्तस्मात्तु भावोऽन्यो
ऽव्यक्तोऽव्यक्तात्सनातनः ।
यः स सर्वेषु भूतेषु
नश्यत्सु न विनश्यति ॥८.२०॥
parastasmāttu bhāvo'nyo
'vyakto'vyaktātsanātanaḥ
yaḥ sa sarveṣu bhūteṣu
naśyatsu na vinaśyati (8.20)

paraḥ — high; tasmāt — than this; tu — but; bhāvo = bhāvaḥ — existence; 'nyo = anyaḥ — another; 'vyakto = avyaktaḥ — invisible; 'vyaktāt = avyaktāt — than the unmanifest state of the dissolvable creation; sanātanaḥ — primeval; yaḥ = which; sa = saḥ — it; sarveṣu — in all; bhūteṣu — in creation; naśyatsu — in the disintegration; na — not; vinaśyati — is disintegrated

But higher than this, there is another invisible existence, which is higher than the primeval unmanifested states of this dissolvable creation. When all these creatures are disintegrated, that is not affected. (8.20)

Commentary:

Some Vaishnava Acharyas or gurus, in disciplic succession, preach that we should ignore the avyakta invisible existence, but they do not provide sufficient justification. Why should we ignore the energy from which Brahmā produced these worlds or the higher potency (paras avyakta) which remains as it is and which is not used by Brahmā? The Acharyas feel that anything invisible is not worth the research and will lead to endless speculation and guessing. Śrī Krishna described the world from which He came, the world in which His special locale is permanently manifested. Some accomplished yogins like Śrīla Yogeshwarananda stated that they could not find such a world beyond the causal level, but other yogins attested to it. There are two unmanifested energies, one from which Brahmā produces this world and the other from a border territory between the primal mundane energy and the manifested spiritual territories which Śrī Krishna describes as being His locales.

These unmanifested energies must be crossed before one can reach Krishna's place. One can compare this to penetrating the earth's atmosphere. Objects entering the earth's atmosphere from outer space must have an effective heat shield or they will burn up during the flight through the outer edges of the atmosphere. A variety of heat shields were designed to date for use in manmade reentry vehicles. Without them, return from outer space would be impossible. In the same way, a yogi who has no mystic perception to understand how unmanifest energies and manifest existences are layered, bordered and zoned, cannot consciously go to Krishna's place.

If our current objective awareness is dependent on Brahmā's waking state, then we need him in order to objectively perceive anything. We will not suddenly be free to transcend Brahmā's influence at the time of death and go to Śrī Krishna. The basic process of Kundalini yoga helps in developing a resistance to Brahmā and in developing a way to shift reliance to Śrī Krishna, Lord Shiva, or someone else. However, until we perfect the relevant mystic techniques, we will necessarily remain under Brahmā's jurisdiction.

Through the change in consciousness, the invisible material energy is affected slightly when Brahmā produces this world, but the invisible spiritual energy is not affected. Within that invisible spiritual energy lie the spiritual places of Śrī Krishna, other Vishnu personalities, and Lord Shiva. At present it is invisible because we lack the sense perception to view it, just as one cannot see in the dark without the aid special night vision equipment. In a sense, it is already before us, but we do not see it. We regard it as void just as scientists regard the invisible dark matter as one massive void.

This spiritual world of Krishna which non-yogi devotees strongly desire and acclaim, is itself invisible to their sense perception. Still they fantasize and enjoy imaginations of what it might be, based on descriptions in scripture. No one, not even a devotee of Śrī Krishna can go there unless he develops the subtle body, the causal form and then the spatial spiritual form, which exhibits no limbs and senses, and finally the spiritual body with limbs and senses. This will not happen overnight or at the time of death or by a miracle. It occurs by undertaking the yoga disciplines described thus far in the Gītā.

अव्यक्तोऽक्षर इत्युक्तस्
तमाहुः परमां गतिम् ।
यं प्राप्य न निवर्तन्ते
तद्धाम परमं मम ॥८.२१॥
avyakto'kṣara ityuktas
tamāhuḥ paramāṁ gatim
yaṁ prāpya na nivartante
taddhāma paramaṁ mama (8.21)

avyakto = avyaktaḥ — invisible world; 'kṣara = akṣara — unalterable; ity = iti — thus; uktaḥ — is declared; tam — it; āhuḥ — authorities say; paramām — supreme; gatim — objective; yam — which; prāpya — attaining; na — not; nivartante — return here; tad — that; dhāma — residence; paramam — supreme; mama — My

That invisible world is unalterable, so it is declared. The authorities say that it is the supreme objective. Attaining that, they do not return here. That place is My supreme residence. (8.21)

Commentary:

The contrast between the primal mundane energy and the spiritual energy is denoted by two Sanskrit terms, namely kṣara and akṣara. This means that one is alterable and the other is not. Both energies are eternally existent but the spiritual one is described by great sages and by the Supreme Being, Śrī Krishna, as being unaffected. How then can we explain that the limited spirit is part of the akṣara manifestation? If the limited spirit is affected by the material energy, then its unalterableness is put to question. Elsewhere in the *Gītā (15.16)*, Śrī Krishna explained the limited spirits who become conditioned perpetually, are positioned between the absolute and the relative.

More or less, while trapped in a conditioned state, the limited spirits are superficially affected by their close proximity to the primal mundane energy. Unfortunately, some spiritus remain eternally in such proximity. Thus for them the superficial affectation is eternal. Heat radiated from one object may be absorbed by another cooler item. Similarly the spiritual energy which continually radiates from the limited conditioned entities, you and me, is perpetually being absorbed by the primal mundane energy, both when we are conscious and unconscious. The proximity to material nature is something we contend with perpetually.

पुरुषः स परः पार्थ
भक्त्या लभ्यस्त्वनन्यया ।
यस्यान्तःस्थानि भूतानि
येन सर्वमिदं ततम् ॥८.२२॥
puruṣaḥ sa paraḥ pārtha
bhaktyā labhyastvananyayā
yasyāntaḥsthāni bhūtāni
yena sarvamidaṁ tatam (8.22)

puruṣaḥ — person; sa = saḥ — this; paraḥ — supreme; pārtha — O son of Pṛthā; bhaktyā — by a devotional relationship; labhyaḥ — attainable; tv = tu — but; ananyayā — not by any other; yasyāntaḥsthāni = yasya — of which + antaḥsthāni — existing within; bhūtāni — beings; yena — by which; sarvam — all; idam — this; tatam — energized

That Supreme Person, O son of Pṛthā, is attainable through a devotional relationship and not by any other means. Within His influence, all beings exist. By Him, all the universe is energized. (8.22)

Commentary:

In very clear terms, Śrī Krishna explained how to attain a personal relationship with the Supreme Person (puruṣah parah) in His locale. To do so, one needs a devotional relationship (bhaktyā) that is formed not through a mundane type of devotion but a devotion which comes from a spirit purified by yoga practice as Śrī Krishna described.

On one hand, advanced yoga practice must be there, and on the other, devotion must be there, coming from the purified spirit and going to the Supreme Person, Śrī Krishna. Both factors must be present. The implication are huge. Yoga practice is required for purification of the psyche, but alone it is *not* enough for obtaining that Supreme Person. Therefore, so many yogis attain greater or lesser degrees of purification but lack a devotional relationship with Śrī Krishna, because they do not have bhaktyā (devotion) to the Supreme Person as described in this verse.

Śrī Krishna, like many spiritual masters who existed in His disciplic succession, stated that by no other means but devotion is He attained. This does not qualify impure affection from an unpurified psyche as true devotion. Thus as kriyā yogis, we agree with that requirement and, at the same time, recognize the folly of those who cut yoga practice from the Gītā and substitute devotion in its place. We also recognize that the gopis of Vṛndāvana or Lord Caitanya, persons who actually attained the Supreme Person without yoga practice, are in a different category. Their example is testimony to the fact that some do attain the Supreme Person with bhaktyā because they have purified psyches from the very beginning. For us, the contaminated beings, we must adopt the yoga practice.

Here in the *Bhagavad Gītā*, the purification of the psyche was stressed for six chapters thus far, from Chapter Three through this chapter; only then was devotion mentioned in no uncertain terms. We follow this system as Śrī Krishna presented it to Arjuna, because our tendency is to practice kriyā yoga for self purification and then to apply that purified psyche in devotion.

After preaching tirelessly to Arjuna about the elementary and then the very advanced stages, Śrī Krishna reveals the final requirement, that for kriyā yogis, none of them will attain the Supreme Person without having a devotional relationship; there is no other means. In other words, the kriyā yogi may attain this or that, he may be satisfied with this transcendental accomplishment or with that, but he will not attain the Supreme Person unless he has devotion for that God. This is final. We cannot argue the point.

To clarify what He meant, Śrī Krishna defined that Supreme Person as the one in whose influence, all beings exist, the one Who energizes the universe. So even if one does not believe this person is Śrī Krishna, still one can understand the position of that person based on the definition.

The suggestion here is that the advanced yogi will have to go further in mystic perception to trace and identify that person whose influence penetrates all beings and locales.

यत्र काले त्वनावृत्तिम्
आवृत्तिं चैव योगिनः ।
प्रयाता यान्ति तं कालं
वक्ष्यामि भरतर्षभ ॥८.२३॥
yatra kāle tvanāvṛttim
āvṛttiṁ caiva yoginaḥ
prayātā yānti taṁ kālaṁ
vakṣyāmi bharatarṣabha (8.23)

yatra — where; kāle — in time; tv = tu — but; anāvṛttim — not return; āvṛttim — return; caiva = ca — and + eva — indeed; yoginaḥ — yogis; prayātā — departing; yānti — go; tam — this; kālam — time; vakṣyāmi — I will tell; bharatarṣabha — O bullish man of the Bharata family

O bullish man of the Bharata family, I will tell you of the departure for the yogis who do or do not return. (8.23)

Commentary:

After telling how an advanced yogi would develop a relationship with Him and thereby migrate to His kingdom, in His association, Śrī Krishna returned to the main topic under discussion, which is the route of the kriyā yoga disciplines. Again we see that most of the discourse addresses the practice of yoga, at least so far up to this eighth chapter. Devotion to Krishna is high on the list of accomplishments of the yogis and its function is to facilitate a yogi's desire to attain Krishna's supreme residence.

Śrī Krishna spoke of the bodily departure for those yogis who return to take another material form and those who do not come back into the cycle of births and deaths.

Śrī Paramhansa Yogananda, the famous kriyā yogi, wrote in his commentary to the next three verses, 8.24—26, that this is mostly symbolic. He does not attest to these as actual restrictions on a yogi in regards to the time of the year when a yogi should or should not depart from his body. However we cannot follow the tone of Śrī Paramhansaji because the *Upanishads* testify also to these restrictions for the yogis. This writer also had mystic experiences which verify the limitations.

Another group of commentators, and for totally different reasons, disavow those verses (B.G. 8.24—26) in so far as they would restrict devotees of Krishna who are in their disciplic successions. According to this group, restriction pertaining to the sun or moon would not deter sincere devotees of Krishna who follow Krishna's pure devotee or who follow Lord Caitanya Mahāprabhu. However, again we cannot accept this denial of what Śrī Krishna said.

By distorting the next verse (8.27), these commentators substitute the word devotee for the word yogi and state that a devotee does not have to regard these seasonal planetary restrictions. However even though this is accepted by many readers of such commentaries, it makes no sense at all. Let us consider the verses:

अग्निर्ज्योतिरहः शुक्लः
षण्मासा उत्तरायणम् ।
तत्र प्रयाता गच्छन्ति
ब्रह्म ब्रह्मविदो जनाः ॥८.२४॥
agnirjyotirahaḥ śuklaḥ
ṣaṇmāsā uttarāyaṇam
tatra prayātā gacchanti
brahma brahmavido janāḥ (8.24)

agnir = agniḥ — summer season; jyotir = jyotiḥ — bright atmosphere; ahaḥ — daytime; śuklaḥ — bright moonlight; saṇmāsā — six months; uttarāyaṇam — the time when the sun appears to move north; tatra — at that time; prayātā — departing; gacchanti — they go; brahma — to the spiritual location; brahmavido = brahmavidaḥ — knowers of the spiritual dimension; janāḥ — people

The summer season, the bright atmosphere, the daytime, the bright moonlight, the six months when the sun appears to move north; if at that time, they depart the body, those people who know the spiritual dimension, go to the spiritual location. (8.24)

Commentary:

As we study this verse, it helps to recall the procedures used by the military and scientific communities to plan a rocket launch in order to rendezvous with an orbiting station or to launch a scientific probe to another planet. For example, the opportunity to travel to Mars via the Hohmann transfer orbit occurs only once every two years. If the launch window is missed, then the rocket must be launched to another destination instead or it must wait until another window opens for travel to Mars. In the same manner, the atmospheric conditions and time of year greatly affect where we will and can go after departure from this body.

This pertains to those who live in the northern hemisphere of the earthly planets. Such people must deal with the characteristics of their location in reference to the equator and the tilting of the earth on its axis in reference to the sun. Even though the influence of the sun upon a yogin is flatly denied by Śrī Paramhansa Yogananda, that influence is there nevertheless, and no limited being can deter it. The performance of yoga cannot completely nullify the solar influence. In fact, a whole discipline in prāṇāyāma entails studying that solar influence and learning how to make the best use of it. The same applies to the influence from the moon. The system of alternate breathing helps to equalize these influences, which are experienced in the yogi's psyche as solarized and lunarized prāṇa or very subtle sun charged or moon—charged mento—emotional energy.

From personal experience, I state conclusively that a yogi's subtle body responds to the increase or decrease of solar and lunar energy in the atmosphere. One who remembers his subtle night activities which occur when his gross body sleeps, would know of the times when he is able to astral—project easily to countries in the tropics or to those in cold regions, all depending on the time of year and predominance of solar or lunar energies. At other times, one may try to astral—project to certain places and find that one cannot move one's subtle body there because of the repelling force of the solar or lunar influences.

As dust particles sometimes travel all the way from the Sahara desert in Africa to the United States or Canada, so the subtle bodies of human beings and animals sometimes move across the Atlantic or Pacific Oceans at night when the solar or lunar forces move such bodies by the respective influences. Even so, most people are not conscious of the movements of their subtle forms during the sleeping actions of their gross bodies.

The same type of influence is manifested when one tries to leave this planet to go to other dimensions. There are forces which keep one hog—tied to a particular world. These restrictive energies cannot be lifted by wishful thinking. A person cannot go to heaven merely by wishing for it. He must first erase the influences which keep him zone—bound. For that, the definite method is yoga practice. Śrī Paramhansa Yogananda surmises that this summer season, the daytime, the bright moonlight and the six months, pertain to the raising of the Kuṇḍalinī chakra. This is a fact and we agree with him that unless one has raised the Kuṇḍalinī chakra, one cannot be successful at yoga practice. One must complete Kuṇḍalinī yoga as well as celibacy and purity of psyche yoga before one can advance to kriyā yoga in earnest and in that sense, he is correct.

Guru Paramhansaji is incorrect however in suggesting that with the mastery of these aspects, one can master everything in terms of solar and lunar nullification. A limited being, even if he is an accomplished yogi, cannot master everything in terms of solar and lunar influences. He too must cooperate with such influences and use the positive supports while avoiding the setbacks. These powers, the sun and moon, are not just physical aspects as Śrī Paramhansaji seems to suggest. They exert astral, psychic and supernatural influences as well.

Even if we bypass their physical limitations, still we will be stuck with their psychic and supernatural impositions. Therefore this verse is no joking matter nor is it an analogy about the Kuṇḍalinī chakra. Verses that pertain to the awakening of the Kuṇḍalinī chakra were stated in Chapter Four. In addition, in his instruction to Śrī Uddhava, Śrī Krishna deals with the Kuṇḍalinī chakra in detail. Those instructions are in the Eleventh Canto of the Śrīmad Bhāgavatam (Bhāgavat Purāṇa).

As kriyā yogis we should abandon any ideas about ultimate supremacy. Even in the liberated states we will remain as limited beings, though not as limited as we are at present. Even then we will have to reckon with greater powers and their limiting influences.

The summer season here means that season in the northern hemisphere. If the yogi lives in the Southern Hemisphere, say Bolivia for instance, the summer season would be at another time of the year. If he lives near the equator, it would not be significant in the same way. The influence of the sun and moon on these respective places varies according to his location.

The bright atmosphere in the northern hemisphere is the time of sun's increased influence in that region. In other worlds, the subtle energies coming from the sun at that time are greater and do facilitate the movement of pranic energies in the psyche of the yogi.

However as Śrī Krishna stated, only those people who know of the spiritual dimension (brahmavido) go to the spiritual location (brahma). Others, who leave their bodies at such time, may take advantage of the natural atmosphere but they will not make proper use of the supernatural or psychic skies. Their subtle bodies are not energised sufficiently to perceive the higher frequencies of the supernatural and spiritual dimensions. Due to their determined focus on this physical world, they will again go down into a man's body for taking rebirth as the son or daughter of his mate or wife. Such is the life.

Some yogis, the very advanced ones and the supernatural beings who took a physical body, may transcend these conditions and reach the spiritual dimensions even at such unfavorable times, but others will not be able to do so. Even a person as great as Bhīṣma who was a mahāyogī of repute, did not chance leaving his body at such an unfavorable time. We hear in the *Mahābhārata* that he deliberately delayed the death of his physical form so that he would leave during the six months when the sun appears to move to the northern part of the sky. This definite system is watched carefully by yogis who understand the natural and supernatural atmospheric influences and who know that a limited being remains under certain restrictions imposed by the all—surrounding realities.

धूमो रात्रिस्तथा कृष्णः
षण्मासा दक्षिणायनम् ।
तत्र चान्द्रमसं ज्योतिर्
योगी प्राप्य निवर्तते ॥८.२५॥
dhūmo rātristathā kṛṣṇaḥ
ṣaṇmāsā dakṣiṇāyanam
tatra cāndramasaṁ jyotir
yogī prāpya nivartate (8.25)

dhūmo = dhūmaḥ — smoky, misty or hazy season; rātris — night time; tathā — as well as; kṛṣṇaḥ — the dark moon time; saṇmāsā — six months; dakṣiṇāyanam — the time when the sun appears to move south; tatra — at that time; cāndramasam — moon; jyotir = jyotiḥ — light; yogī — yogi; prāpya — attaining; nivartate — is born again

The smoky, misty or hazy season, as well as in the night—time, the dark—moon time, the six months when the sun appears to move south; if the yogi departs at that time, he attains moonlight, after which he is born again. (8.25)

Commentary:

If a yogi leaves his body during the smoky, misty or hazy season, as well as in the night time, or during the dark moon time, or the six months when the sun appears to move away from the location in which he resides, then his spirit will, more than likely, head for the moonlight. This means that he will be causelessly attached to the astral dimension of the moon planet or he may stay in the moonlight as it shines on this earthly place or through space. From there he will again come back to the earth, because it so happens that the force of the moonlight is absorbed by the seas and vegetation of this earth.

The influence of the moon is felt by a neophyte yogi when he does prāṇāyāma. Either bhastrika rapid breathing or alternate anuloma—pratiloma breathing will make it evident to a yogi that the moon's energy is a negative force, which will keep him zone—bound. When however the moon energy is surcharged by sun force, it becomes a positive force for the yogi. The influences of the moon can be understood by keeping track of the tides of the Atlantic or Pacific Ocean. These large bodies of water are obedient to the influences of the moon and it is not just the natural world which is affected. It is the supernatural as well, because the moon has a supernatural counterpart.

The question is: Should a yogi plan his death in such a way to leave his body in the six months when the sun's energy prevails the most? The answer is no. A yogi should not plan as Bhīṣma did, but if a yogi finds that the time of the death of his body can be adjusted, then he may do that. It all depends on whether one has that siddhi power when it is time to leave the physical body. If one has that much practice whereby one can control departure from the body, then surely one should leave at a favorable time but one should not use artificial means to do this. It has to be natural means controlled by a complete and successful yoga practice. At the same time, a yogi should not be concerned if he is not that successful. The main thing is to develop a habitual practice before one is circumstantially forced to leave the body. We are limited beings. We should be realistic with ourselves and not assume a false absoluteness.

Ultimately, everything is in the hands of providence. We should do our best, endeavor as much as we can and watch to see how providence handles the rest.

शुक्लकृष्णे गती ह्येते
जगतः शाश्वते मते ।
एकया यात्यनावृत्तिम्
अन्ययावर्तते पुनः ॥८.२६॥
śuklakṛṣṇe gatī hyete
jagataḥ śāśvate mate
ekayā yātyanāvṛttim
anyayāvartate punaḥ (8.26)

śuklakṛṣṇe — light and dark; gatī — two paths; hyete = hy (hi) — indeed + ete — these two; jagataḥ — of the universe; śāśvate — perpetual; mate — is considered; ekayā — by one; yāty = yāti — goes away; anāvṛttim — not return; anyayāvartate = anyayā — by other + āvartate — comes back; punaḥ = punar — again

The light and the dark times are two paths which are considered to be perpetually available for the universe. It is considered so by the authorities. By one, a person goes away not to return; by the other he comes back again. (8.26)

Commentary:

The word jagatah means the universe and does not pertain to just one person's body. This is not an analogy of the personal Kuṇḍalinī system in the body of a yogi. It pertains to certain natural and supernatural laws, having to do with planetary influences which we may or may not be able to nullify.

The kuṇḍalinī system is important and without it one cannot utilize the supernatural systems in any meaningful way. Therefore undoubtedly as Śrī Paramhansaji stated, the raising of the Kuṇḍalinī is a central issue. However its actuation does not nullify the limitedness of the yogi or the impositions of the natural and supernatural laws of nature. The yogi has to learn to take advantage when there is an oppurtuny and to be satisfied when he is not permitted an outlet.

By one allowance, by the path of light if enters into it, he would not return and by another imposition, by the path of darkness, he certainly will reenter to take another body and try again. So much of this depends on supernatural agency, but the yogi should be prepared for opportunities. We should not be resentful because we are limited. We should not superimpose on ourselves an idea that by yoga we will become unlimited. These attitudes are unnecessary. We should merely prepare ourselves to take the advantages that nature and God may offer at any given time.

नैते सृती पार्थ जानन्
योगी मुह्यति कश्चन ।
तस्मात्सर्वेषु कालेषु
योगयुक्तो भवार्जुन ॥८.२७॥
naite sṛtī pārtha jānan
yogī muhyati kaścana
tasmātsarveṣu kāleṣu
yogayukto bhavārjuna (8.27)

naite = na — not + ete — these two; sṛtī — two paths; pārtha — O son of Pṛthā; jānan — knowing; yogī — yogi; muhyati — is confused; kaścana — at all; tasmāt — therefore; sarveṣu — in all; kāleṣu — in times; yogayukto = yogayuktaḥ — disciplined in yoga practice; bhavārjuna = bhava — be + arjuna — Arjuna

Knowing these two paths, O son of Pṛthā, the yogi is not confused at all. Therefore at all times, be disciplined in yoga practice, O Arjuna. (8.27)

Commentary:

Understanding how the natural and supernatural mundane energy operates and how he can cannot utilize it, according to the time and place, according to his ability and according to the opportunities or barricades, the yogi is not confused about anything. He accepts his limited autonomy and is agreeable with whatever position he is placed in by reality.

Thus at all times, a yogi should maintain yoga practice, so that if perchance he gets the opportunity to take the path of no return, he can make good use of it.

वेदेषु यज्ञेषु तपःसु चैव
दानेषु यत्पुण्यफलं प्रदिष्टम् ।
अत्येति तत्सर्वमिदं विदित्वा
योगी परं स्थानमुपैति चाद्यम् ॥८.२८॥

vedeṣu yajñeṣu tapaḥsu caiva
dāneṣu yatpuṇyaphalaṁ pradiṣṭam
atyeti tatsarvamidaṁ viditvā
yogī paraṁ sthānamupaiti cādyam (8.28)

vedeṣu — from study of the Vedas; yajñeṣu — from religious ceremonies and disciplines; tapaḥsu — from austerities; caiva — and indeed; dāneṣu — from scripturally—recommended acts of charity; yat = yad — which; puṇyaphalam — good result; pradiṣṭam — described; atyeti — goes beyond; tat – this; sarvam — all; idam — this; viditvā — having known; yogī — yogi; param — supreme; sthānam — state; upaiti — goes; cadyam = ca — and + adyam — primal

The yogi, having known all this, goes beyond the good results which are derived from study of the Veda, beyond religious ceremonies and disciplines, beyond austerities and beyond offering scripturally—recommended gifts in charity. He goes to the Supreme Primal State.

Commentary:

The yogi advances beyond the state of mind and the formulation of attitude which focuses the psychology on achieving good results in mundane existence. This is first attained by mastering Kuṇḍalinī yoga, which causes the life force to ascend from its ancient and primitive habitat, the cave of the mūlāldhāra chakra which is at the base of the spinal column. Permanently moving the kuṇḍalinī out of that place is a feat for a neophyte. Once he achieves that he gets a taste of living without expecting good results.

A yogi on such a path cares less about good results in the social field, because in his mind, he will not return to this world. He does not have to protect his future mundane interests by being kind to anyone in the conventional sense. Normally he would have to return and face the various resentments which accrue from non—sentimental actions. We see this in the case of Arjuna where he wanted to observe the laws of etiquette and be kind, so as to avoid social repercussions. Śrī Krishna urged Arjuna to abandon that emotional stance and to act with indifference, as a soldier in callous disregard for relatives and friends. Irregardless of future consequences, Arjuna was to fight boldly and relate only to the Supervising Universal Lord.

Knowing about good results (punyaphalam) derived from study of the Veda and other scriptures, and those results derived from religious ceremonies and disciplines, as well as those from austerities and the offering of scripturally recommended charity, the yogi decides not to act on the basis of getting those results. In a nonchalant detached way he acts but without leaving an impression on the subtle material nature for reaping benefits in the future. Thus he becomes freed from hopes, hankerings and aspirations.

And then somehow, yes somehow, by the grace of providence, with the blessings of the very material nature which kept him bound for so long, there is an opening in time: All natural and supernatural barricades disappear. The yogi goes to the Supreme Primal State, by virtue of his preparation for the opportunity through a consistent practice.

CHAPTER 9

The Devotional Attitude*

श्रीभगवानुवाच
इदं तु ते गुह्यतमं
प्रवक्ष्याम्यनसूयवे ।
ज्ञानं विज्ञानसहितं
यज्ज्ञात्वा मोक्ष्यसेऽशुभात् ॥९.१॥
śrībhagavānuvāca
idaṁ tu te guhyatamaṁ
pravakṣyāmyanasūyave
jñānaṁ vijñānasahitaṁ
yajjñātvā mokṣyase'śubhāt (9.1)

śrībhagavān — the Blessed Lord; uvāca — said; idam — this; tu — but; te — to you; guhyatamam — most secret; pravakṣyāmy = pravakṣyāmi — I will explain; anasūyave — to one who is not cynical; jñānam — knowledge; vijñānasahitaṁ = vijñāna — experienced + sahitam — with; yaj = yad — which; jñātvā — having known; mokṣyase — you will be freed; 'śubhāt = aśubhāt — from impurity

The Blessed Lord said: But I will explain to you who are not cynical, the most secret truths, the knowledge with the experience,which having known, you will be freed from impurities. (9.1)

Commentary:

Following the tone of the last seven chapters, Two through Eight, we can assume that Śrī Krishna will now tell us more about Himself. He covered elementary yoga. He covered advanced practice. He introduced the more advanced stages of the psyche—purified yogi, turning his cultivated mystic perception to the primal causes and to the Supreme Person as well. Thus naturally the next explanation covers the Supreme Person.

Citing that Arjuna was not cynical, Śrī Krishna now He would explain the most secret truths, the knowledge along with the experience, which having known, Arjuna would be freed from even more impurities.

This is easy to understand for anyone who has practiced kriyā yoga to proficiency. As soon as one purifies a sector of the psyche, one discovers another region which needs to be fixed. There are so many impurities that the kriyā yogi has an on—going task of self—purification. When cleaning, one first notices the very large and obvious blemishes. As soon as those are removed, smaller and yet smaller ones come into focus.

**The Mahābhārata contains no chapter headings. This title was assigned by the translator on the basis of verse 26 of this chapter.*

It is just like the senses of the psyche. Such senses find the minutest discrepancies in purely mundane phenomena. It becomes very disturbed until such blemishes are corrected. Hence, researchers spend years upon years in laboratories trying to invent more and more perfect materials to satisfy the nit—picking senses. We kriyā yogis learn a valuable lesson from the psyche of how to be fussy about psychic purity. As soon as we learn this lesson sufficiently, we become sensitive about spiritual development, just as we are about sensual forms and shapes.

A kriyā yogi, if he is at all cynical to the *Bhagavad Gītā* or to providence, will by that attitude curtail his advancement. He will advance if he practices but his progress will be slow. As soon as he can dismiss the cynical attitude, he will progress rapidly. There are many neophyte yogis who either do not understand the *Bhagavad Gītā* or who understand it all too well and therefore do not like Śrī Krishna's forcing Arjuna to take the path of no return. That course appears to be reckless and callous to human relationships. Such neophyte practitioners will be forestalled in progression.

Another type of neophyte yogi hates the idea of earning a waiver from cultural activities. Such persons also will move very slowly on the path because they fail to absorb the grace of material nature, a grace without which one cannot become liberated. One must learn to appreciate the motherly protection offered by material nature, even though at times, its potency deters spiritual practice. All in all one must be appreciative of any type of destiny, good or bad, favorable or unfavorable.

Śrī Bābāji Mahasaya stated this:

"A kriyā yogi is like an orphan, an infant without mother or father, just like Skanda after he returned from the world tour of pilgrimages and found out to his dismay that his parents had, in a sense, disowned him by giving the entire heritage, wives, property, services and all to Ganesha.

"However such an orphan should not be resentful. He should instead focus his mind on the objective. Realizing that no one owes him anything, he should carry on in this life as usual with all appreciations even to those parents or people who abandoned him. Moving along as a free spirit, he will in due course of time take the path of no return. That is a true yogi who has my blessings.

"A kriyā yogi always gets the blessings of Śrī Krishna, Śrī Balarāma and Śrī Mahādeva, as well as that of Śrī Nārada Muni and the Devata Brahmā. If on any occasion, he cannot perceive this fortune, then at least he should know that mahāyogīns do assist him. These mahāyogīns give him many details of the yoga practice. He should never despair. Let him continue the practice until he attains perfection. Let him persevere."

Jñānam vijñānamsahitam means the knowledge with (sahitam) the experience. As kriyā yogins we do not wait until the time of death to get the experience. Honestly speaking we want the experience now in this material life, so that later at the time of death, we are well versed in the geography of the hereafter.

राजविद्या राजगुह्यं
पवित्रमिदमुत्तमम् ।
प्रत्यक्षावगमं धर्म्यं
सुसुखं कर्तुमव्ययम् ॥९.२॥
rājavidyā rājaguhyaṁ
pavitramidamuttamam
pratyakṣāvagamaṁ dharmyaṁ
susukhaṁ kartumavyayam (9.2)

rājavidyā — ultimate information; rājaguhyam — greatest secret; pavitram — purifier of consciousness; idam — this; uttamam — transcendental; pratyakṣa — by direct experience; avagamam — understood; dharmyam — the principle of religion; su— sukham — very happy; kartum — to execute; avyayam — everlasting.

This is the ultimate information, the greatest secret, the purifier of consciousness. It is plain to see, righteous, easy to practice and thoroughly consistent. (9.2)

Commentary:

Again Śrī Krishna brings up the idea of pavitram, which is purification of the psyche. This is in the advanced stages. In the neophyte stages, He presented it. Now again, even in the advanced levels, He mentions it. Whatever the neophyte purified, which brought him to the advanced levels, now serves to show him the more subtle impurities. He removed one hurdle and found another. He cleared one part of his psyche to see another muddled area. Śrī Krishna said that whatever He would describe in this chapter, would be plain to see, easy to practice and thoroughly consistent for the yogi devotee who takes this information and puts it to use.

अश्रद्दधानाः पुरुषा
धर्मस्यास्य परंतप ।
अप्राप्य मां निवर्तन्ते
मृत्युसंसारवर्त्मनि ॥९.३॥
aśraddadhānāḥ puruṣā
dharmasyāsya paraṁtapa
aprāpya māṁ nivartante
mṛtyusaṁsāravartmani (9.3)

aśraddadhānāḥ — having no faith; puruṣā — people; dharmasyāsya = dharmasya — of the righteous behavior + asya — of this; paraṁtapa — stern subduer of the enemy; aprāpya — not attaining; mām — to Me; nivartante — they are born again; mṛtyusaṁsāravartmani = mṛtyu — death + saṁsāra — cyclic rebirth + vartmani — in the course

People who have no faith in this righteous behavior, who have not attained Me, are born again in the cyclic course of death and rebirth, O stern subduer of the enemy. (9.3)

Commentary:

This is not a condemnation of such people but rather an explanation of their condition as Śrī Krishna sees it. And who are these people? Are any of them devotees of Śrī Krishna? Or are they all non—believers who reject Him accept other powerful figures in human history or another authority they conceive as the Supreme?

Certainly, some are devotees. Someone may have faith in his righteous behavior but may not have attained Śrī Krishna in the advanced way described in previous chapters. Such a person, the neophyte who has not mastered the advanced practice, would be born again in the cyclic course of death and rebirth. This applies to most of us, including neophyte yogis.

मया ततमिदं सर्वं
जगदव्यक्तमूर्तिना ।
मत्स्थानि सर्वभूतानि
न चाहं तेष्ववस्थितः ॥९.४॥
mayā tatamidaṁ sarvaṁ
jagadavyaktamūrtinā
matsthāni sarvabhūtāni
na cāhaṁ teṣvavasthitaḥ (9.4)

mayā — by Me; tatam — pervaded; idam — this; sarvam — all; jagad = jagat — world; avyaktamūrtinā = avyakta — invisible + mūrtinā — by form; matsthāni — standing on Me, surviving on Me; sarvabhūtāni — all beings; na — not; cāham = ca — and + aham — I; teṣv = teṣu — in them; avasthitaḥ — standing on, surviving on

This world is pervaded by My invisible form. All beings survive on My energy but I am not surviving on theirs. (9.4)

Commentary:

Śrī Krishna will now give a course in the higher realizations attained by the great yogins. This, for us, is mere information. We should have faith in it. However we should not treat this information with the same weight as experience. The experience is mystic vision, attained only after we quieted the disturbing sensuality and converted our imagination into actual mystic vision using supernatural eyes through which we see beyond the limitations of this cloudy psychological perception.

Within such mystic vision we see that this world is pervaded by Śrī Krishna's invisible form and that all beings survive on the energy radiated from Śrī Krishna; but Śrī Krishna Himself does not survive by taking energy from anyone.

न च मत्स्थानि भूतानि
पश्य मे योगमैश्वरम् ।
भूतभृन्न च भूतस्थो
ममात्मा भूतभावनः ॥९.५॥
na ca matsthāni bhūtāni
paśya me yogamaiśvaram
bhūtabhṛnna ca bhūtastho
mamātmā bhūtabhāvanaḥ (9.5)

na — not; ca — and; matsthāni — standing on Me, surviving on Me; bhūtāni — beings; paśya — behold; me — My; yogam = yoga – psychological power; aiśvaram — supremacy; bhūtabhṛn = bhūtabhṛt — sustaining beings; na — not; ca — and; bhūtastho = bhūtasthaḥ — existing on the beings; mamātmā = mama — My + ātmā — self; bhūtabhāvanaḥ — causing beings to be

And the created beings are not existing on Me. Behold My psychological supremacy. While sustaining the beings and not existing on them, I Myself cause them to be. (9.5)

Commentary:

Śrī Krishna declared in the previous verse that the created beings survive on His power. Now He states the contrary, that they do not exist on Him. From one perspective the beings survive on His energy, and from another view they are not being sustained by Him either. What does this mean?

Supernatural insight is required to perceive this. To illustrate, one can look at the sun. Life on earth is sustained by the sun's energy; yet, we do not physically exist on the sun. Likewise, all beings survive on Sri Krishna's invisible energy, but do not exist directly on Him.

Śrī Krishna says paśya me yogam aiśvaram which means behold (paśya) My (me) psychological power (yoga) and supremacy (aiśvaram). He claims that while He sustains the beings, and while He does not exist on them or depend on them, still He causes them to be. In another sense, they do not depend on Him, because as He previously described, they are more reliant on material nature than anything else.

Some great yogins as well as great philosophers deny this statement of Śrī Krishna, which suggests that there is a Supreme Being, a Supreme Individual Who causes the world but Who is also ever detached from it, Who does not allow the world to feed back into His nature. They say that it is not possible for any individual to be in such an absolute position in reference to the other multiple existences. However Śrī Krishna claims this supremacy and a simultaneous immune detachment. Disproving Him is quite a task for any limited being.

यथाकाशस्थितो नित्यं
वायुः सर्वत्रगो महान् ।
तथा सर्वाणि भूतानि
मत्स्थानीत्युपधारय ॥९.६॥
yathākāśasthito nityaṁ
vāyuḥ sarvatrago mahān
tathā sarvāṇi bhūtāni
matsthānītyupadhāraya (9.6)

yathākāśasthito = yathākāśasthitaḥ = yathā — as + ākāśa — space + sthitaḥ — situated; nityam — always; vāyuḥ — wind; sarvatrago = sarvatragaḥ — everywhere going, pervasive; mahān — powerful; tathā — so; sarvāṇi — all; bhūtāni — beings; matsthānīty (matsthānīti) = matsthānī — exist under Me + iti — thus; upadhāraya — consider thoroughly

As the powerful wind is always situated in space and is pervasive, so all beings exist under My influence. Consider this thoroughly. (9.6)

Commentary:

Sri Krishna explained His influence by comparing it to the pervasive wind which inhabits space. Similarly, scientists refer to dark matter and dark energy in this way. It is estimated that as much as three quarters of all energy in the universe is dark energy, undetectable by emissions, evident by its gravitational effects and diffusely spread through space, including Earth. The entire universe exists under the influence of this dark energy; likewise, all beings exist under the pervasive influence of the Supreme Person

सर्वभूतानि कौन्तेय
प्रकृतिं यान्ति मामिकाम् ।
कल्पक्षये पुनस्तानि
कल्पादौ विसृजाम्यहम् ॥९.७॥
sarvabhūtāni kaunteya
prakṛtiṁ yānti māmikām
kalpakṣaye punastāni
kalpādau visṛjāmyaham (9.7)

sarvabhūtāni — all beings; kaunteya — son of Kuntī; prakṛtim — material nature; yānti — retrogress into; māmikām — my own; kalpakṣaye — at the end of a day of Brahma; punas = punar — again; tāni — they; kalpādau — at the beginning of a day of Brahma; visṛjāmy = visṛjāmi — I produce; aham — I

O son of Kuntī, all beings retrogress into My own material nature at the end of Brahmā's day. I produce them again at the beginning of Brahmā's next day. (9.7)

Commentary:

The storage place for us during the down—time of this mundane creation is given as material nature (prakṛtim). This applies to the non—liberated entities and even to some of the liberated ones. This is the time when the universe is shut down for conscious existential purposes. If Śrī Krishna produces the beings again at the start of Brahmā's day, it means that they go into a sort of hibernation, where they are not objectively aware as we are now. This is not hard to believe. In normal experience, we endure phases of unconsciousness from time to time.

A chemical like chloroform can put us into a state of unconsciousness very easily. Substances like chloroform have subtle counterparts which affect the psychological sensing equipments in our subtle bodies. Hence if those equipments are put out of commission, we endure phases of unconsciousness accordingly. This happens because the limited spirit has no direct way of perceiving the subtle or gross material existence. He or she depends on the psychological equipments produced by the Supreme Being for use in various forms of life in various dimensions.

The retrogression of the beings (yānti) into material nature does not signify full reliance on material nature but it does indicate dependence on that energy for the time being. It also means that the primary psychological makeup of the personalities includes in part, the subtle material nature, fashioned into psychic sensing mechanisms.

The production of the beings at the beginning ofBrahmā's day was not a sudden awakening for most. It is something gradual. In fact, even though Śrī Krishna mentioned such a sudden starting point of Brahmā's day, it might be millions of years before a particular being becomes aware of himself in the creation. Certainly, the supernatural people like Brahmā are aware near the onset but not others. Once we are released from the closed psychological darkness and slumber of Brahmā's night, we first encounter a sort of twilight. Full self—consciousness comes later on as psychic equipments are made available to us.

The condition of Brahmā's mind heavily influences whether a host of the beings come into objective awareness or not. Thus we see that on this planet, there were prehistoric creatures with monstrous bodies. Now they are no longer here. Time displaced them with human beings and more refined life forms. Much of it depends on the ideas in the mind of Brahmā at a particular time.

There are trillions and trillions of possible life forms and trillions and trillions of dimensions for living. The physical world as we know it, is not everything. In fact it is a very minute portion of the habitat for the beings. Everything hinges on supernatural power.

Some modern scientists are dismayed by not finding perceptible physical life forms on any nearby planets. They have researched this with satellites and with a bevy of reliable electronic probes. A mystic investigation carried out by developing the power of the subtle body through kriyā yoga practice reveals many habited dimensions adjacent and parallel to our physical zone. Unfortunately, these cannot be appreciated by our physical bodies.

Modern scientists are thinking of sending missions into space to find life on planets in other galaxies or in other star systems but such a venture is a huge mistake and a great waste of curiosity. For one thing, even if a scientist makes such research there is no guarantee for him that he will again take his next body as a human being on this planet. Suppose he takes an animal form, then he will not reap the benefits of the research. Or suppose he slips into another dimension at the time of death, then he might end up in a world nearby that has no advanced scientific civilization like the one he prefers. Thus the whole endeavor for space travel is more or less just whimsical endeavor because there are too many variables which indicate that a living being cannot control where and when he will take birth. Yoga practice is therefore much better than scientific research.

As a side note, those who use hallucinogenic drugs to probe into other dimensions, had better be careful about it. They do not know if they will take animal forms here or there in the next transmigration. If the Supreme Being disapproves of these methods of drug research into the frequencies of consciousness, then He might act supernaturally in such a way as to cause them to enter a species in which their human initiatives are suspended for the time being.

प्रकृतिं स्वामवष्टभ्य
विसृजामि पुनः पुनः ।
भूतग्राममिमं कृत्स्नम्
अवशं प्रकृतेर्वशात् ॥९.८॥
prakṛtiṁ svāmavaṣṭabhya
visṛjāmi punaḥ punaḥ
bhūtagrāmamimaṁ kṛtsnam
avaśaṁ prakṛtervaśāt (9.8)

prakṛtim — material nature; svām — own; avaṣṭabhya — supported on, founded on; visṛjāmi — I produce; punaḥ punaḥ — repeated, again and again; bhūtagrāmam — the multitude of beings; imam — this; kṛtsnam — whole; avaśam — powerless; prakṛter = prakṛteḥ — of material nature; vaśāt — in respect to the potency

On the foundation of material nature, I repeatedly produce this whole multitude of beings, which is powerless in respect to the potency of material nature. (9.8)

Commentary:

This statement, take it or leave it, is undoubtedly true as proven repeatedly by the manipulations of our consciousness through adjustments in material nature, adjustments which are necessitated by natural or supernatural forces, by personal or impersonal agencies.

Many teachers of the Krishna Conscious path in disciplic succession, portrayed Śrī Krishna as the concerned and loving eternal father, Who is eager to free all limited entities who submit as His eternal servants. In truth, this statement reveals another aspect which runs contrary to what these preachers advocate. It may be that such preachers prey upon our insecurities as fallible and relative living beings in this world, powerless (avaśaṁ) in respect to the potency of material nature. We are powerless in that presently our objective awareness hinges on a relationship with material nature. So long as that reliance exists, we will remain as helpless beings, continually manifested by material nature into objective consciousness or individuality and then demanifested into subjective awareness of suspended individuality.

The amazing thing is that here we have a person who used a material body and who stood on a chariot as its driver for Prince Arjuna, telling us that He produced and now regulates our objective and subjective sense of individuality on a cosmic scale. Such a thing is hard to believe. We can, however, just imagine the power of such a person, if at all we are to accept what He says.

If we are honest about it, we can easily accept that we are powerless in the liaison we have with material nature but it is harder to conceive of the power which Śrī Krishna claims to wield over both material nature and ourselves.

Most people are scared of death and try to avoid it because they instinctively understand that death signifies their lack of control over awareness. Hence it is clear that we are helpless in respect to the potency of material nature.

Merely by believing in a Supreme God and proclaiming oneself as His devotee or as a devotee of His devotee, does not remove the fear of death. It does not remove our insecurity about leaving the present body. Our categorical situation as insecure starved spiritual beings still remains. It is only by yoga practice that one can stretch into his highest spiritual categorization to reach potential. Otherwise one keeps coming back into this world in the same state of helplessness.

The plain fact is this: God, whether He be Śrī Krishna or someone else or even if God is merely the sum total reality, has us in a condition of helplessness. He, the Supreme Being, or That, the Supreme Reality, is not that concerned; otherwise we would never be in this condition in the first place. Alternately, maybe the concern is present right now but we are not in a position to take advantage of it. Or we lack the spiritual composition which readily responds to it.

न च मां तानि कर्माणि
निबध्नन्ति धनंजय ।
उदासीनवदासीनम्
असक्तं तेषु कर्मसु ॥९.९॥
na ca māṁ tāni karmāṇi
nibadhnanti dhanaṁjaya
udāsīnavadāsīnam
asaktaṁ teṣu karmasu (9.9)

na — not; ca — and; mām — Me; tāni — these; karmāṇi — cultural acts; nibadhnanti — they bind; dhanaṁjaya — conqueror of rich countries; udāsīnavad = udāsīnavat — indifferently; āsīnam — sitting, being situated; asaktam — unattached; teṣu — in these; karmasu — in cultural actions

And these cultural activities do not bind Me, O conqueror of rich countries. Since I am situated indifferently, I remain unattached to the activities. (9.9)

Commentary:

The cosmic operation is, for Krishna, just a cultural activity, just as setting up a large factory which employs thousands of employees is merely an enterprise for a wealthy human being. To Śrī Krishna, it is a side feature of His personal life. So what is His personal life? Where does He live? What sorts of beings reside in His world?

He portrays that He produces this world and is detached from it so much so that it is just something casual, something by—the—way, something trivial, but a necessary contribution of His to the spiritually poverty—stricken beings like you and me. What a portrayal!

मयाध्यक्षेण प्रकृतिः
सूयते सचराचरम् ।
हेतुनानेन कौन्तेय
जगद्विपरिवर्तते ॥९.१०॥
mayādhyakṣeṇa prakṛtiḥ
sūyate sacarācaram
hetunānena kaunteya
jagadviparivartate (9.10)

mayādhyakṣeṇa = mayā — with Me + adhyakṣeṇa — as supervisor; prakṛtiḥ — material nature; sūyate — produces; sacarācaram — moving and non—moving things; hetunānena = hetunā — by cause of + anena — by this; kaunteya — son of Kuntī; jagad = jagat — world; viparivartate — operates

With Me as the supervisor, material nature produces moving and nonmoving things. By this cause, O son of Kuntī, the universe operates. (9.10)

Commentary:

As the Supervisor, the adhyakṣeṇa, the person viewing it from a distance but whose view affects it, Śrī Krishna said that material nature produces the moving and nonmoving things. There was a sannyasi named Kīrtanānanda Swami Śrīla Bhaktipāda. Titled as Śrīla Bhaktipāda in the tradition of his teacher, Śrīla Prabhupāda, he used to quote this verse of the *Bhagavad Gītā* regularly to explain that Śrī Krishna, his God, was ruling over everything in material nature and therefore everything would go well for all persons who surrendered to him, his spiritual master and their God. Later on that same Swami was imprisoned for many years.

Exactly what happened is still not clear, but the lesson learned is that Śrī Krishna conducts His supervisory role for a broader purpose than protecting His devotees. If we hear the *Gītā* as it was spoken to Arjuna and not as we want to hear it, we know that Śrī Krishna is very detached not only from material nature but from the living beings glued to that energy. Krishna already said that we were helpless in nature's clutches. He did not say that only the non—devotees are helpless. His statement pertains to all beings, believers and non—believers.

A devotee should not assume that Krishna will or does operate this system just for the benefit and prosperity of devotees. Such an idea is a perversity of mundane consciousness and an attempt to hijack the *Gītā* for convenience sake and for attracting naïve followers.

Repeatedly in the Bhāgavat Purāṇa and in the *Mahābhārata*, the book from which the *Bhagavad Gītā* was extracted, we see the ruination of devotees of Krishna, of believers in God. Some say these are special arrangements of Śrī Krishna. However, what does that have to do with the mistakes made by devotees? What does that have to do with reactions brought on by material nature in its attempt to balance its laws of cause and effect? For sentimental people, it is easy to discuss this as Krishna's arrangement, or an unfavorable byproduct of material nature's assault, but for kriyā yogis, these explanations are false.

If indeed the universe operates under Śrī Krishna's supervision, then His interaction is common. Under His supervision, as stated in this verse, material nature produces the objects and circumstances directly.The question becomes how the individual respects these arrangements. because as Śrī Krishna stated in this verse, material nature is producing the stuffs and circumstances directly. That is how the universe operates

अवजानन्ति मां मूढा
मानुषीं तनुमाश्रितम् ।
परं भावमजानन्तो
मम भूतमहेश्वरम् ॥९.११॥
avajānanti māṁ mūḍhā
mānuṣīṁ tanumāśritam
paraṁ bhāvamajānanto
mama bhūtamaheśvaram (9.11)

avajānanti — they hold a low opinion; mām — Me; mūḍhā — the foolish people; mānuṣīm — human; tanum — body; āśritam — having assumed; param — higher; bhāvam — being; ajānanto = ajānantaḥ — not knowing; mama — of Me; bhūtamaheśvaram = bhūta — being + maheśvaram — Almighty God

The foolish people, not knowing My higher existence as the Almighty God of the beings, hold a low opinion of Me as having a human body. (9.11)

Commentary:

Great controversy transpired because Śrī Krishna, in a human body (mānuṣīṁ tanum), declared Himself as the Almighty God (maheśvaram). Some people feel that the Almighty God would not take on a human form which is limited and subjected to death. On the other hand, there are those devotees who forcefully deny that Śrī Krishna had a material body. Their view is that His form is always transcendental and cannot be physical at any time. They do not accept that Śrī Krishna took a flesh and blood form.

Here however, a reader should carefully study the Sanskrit and pay particular attention to the words mānuṣīm, tanum and āśritam.

Śrī Krishna tactfully suggests that as human beings we should not form the conclusion that His birth is like ours or that because He took a human body as the son of Devakī and Vasudeva, He is not the Almighty God. The Almighty God can take such a body and still be that Supreme Being. One should not hold a low opinion of Śrī Krishna merely because He took a human body. The same principle applies to the great yogins who came down into human forms and who seemingly perfected themselves through the use of a human form.

We as kriyā yogins must see that they are higher beings, manifested to set an example for us and to carve out an escape route for our advantage. We have to understand their higher being (param bhāvam). It is not that all the living entities who take these lower forms are lower. Some are much higher than we are. Their assumption of a lowly state does not condemn them to that status. They resume their existential superiority as soon as their purposes are served in this world.

मोघाशा मोघकर्माणो
मोघज्ञाना विचेतसः ।
राक्षसीमासुरीं चैव
प्रकृतिं मोहिनीं श्रिताः ॥९.१२॥
moghāśā moghakarmāṇo
moghajñānā vicetasaḥ
rākṣasīmāsurīṁ caiva
prakṛtiṁ mohinīṁ śritāḥ (9.12)

moghāśā — people with vain hopes; moghakarmāṇo = moghakarmāṇaḥ — people with purposeless actions; moghajñānā — people with incorrect information; vicetasaḥ — without discrimination; rākṣasīm — wicked; āsurīm — devilish; caiva — and indeed; prakṛtim — mode of material nature; mohinīm — deluding feature; śritāḥ — relying on

Persons with vain hopes, purposeless actions, and incorrect information, who lack discrimination, being wicked and devilish, rely on the deluding feature of material nature. (9.12)

Commentary:

Prakṛtim mohitam is generally known as maya which is the deluding feature of material nature. This feature keeps many living entities spellbound. It gives information and reveals much but its insight is devilish and incorrect. By expanding vain hopes in the mind of a living entity, the deluding feature causes the living being to work strenuously for something that will not be. As such it sponsors certain frustrations time after time and brings on depression and a demeaning mentality.

A person can break out of this influence, but he must first take advice from those who are already resistant to it. Gradually by practice in changing habits, one can be freed.

महात्मानस्तु मां पार्थ
दैवीं प्रकृतिमाश्रिताः ।
भजन्त्यनन्यमनसो
ज्ञात्वा भूतादिमव्ययम् ॥९.१३॥
mahātmānastu māṁ pārtha
daivīṁ prakṛtimāśritāḥ
bhajantyananyamanaso
jñātvā bhūtādimavyayam (9.13)

mahātmānaḥ — great souls; tu — but; mām — Me; pārtha — son of Pṛthā; daivīm — supernatural; prakṛtim — material energy; āśritāḥ — being reliant; bhajanty = bhajanti — they worship; ananyamanaso = ananyamanasaḥ — persons whose minds do not deviate; jñātvā — knowing; bhūtādim — originator of beings; avyayam — constant factor

But great souls, being reliant on the supernatural level of material nature, worship Me, without deviation, knowing Me as the originator of beings, the constant factor. (9.13)

Commentary:

The supernatural level of material nature, daivim prakṛtim, is known to advanced yogis as the chidakasha. In normal perception we perceive through the akasha or atmosphere. The fish, for instance, use the watery domain as their atmosphere or medium for perception. Their eyes, or other senses are adapted to that medium for perceiving. Presently for seeing through the gross atmosphere, we only require the use of our passionate energy.

For seeing through the chidakasha, the supernatural air, we have to shift over to the mode of goodness completely. This is known as the sattva guṇa energy.

No matter what we perceive in this world through gross sense perception, it is filtered through the akasha passionate gases. It is not supernatural. Certainly it is not spiritual, even though it is an indication of the spirituality which supports it.

It is very hard for anyone to understand supernatural perception. This is because the physical vision is very strong and magnetic. Once a living being develops the physical vision, his tendency is to reject anything else. He becomes reluctant to desire anything else. By this reluctance, he remains restricted to physical vision and to imagination, which is an inverted vision.

When by yoga procedures, the living entity ceases to imagine in the akasha energy, then the imagination organ develops the ability to perceive the supernatural level. Just as a healthy living entity sees physical objects clearly, so a yogi sees through the chidakasha supernatural sky when his imagination stops endeavoring with the impressions of the gross and subtle mundane sense objects.

The use of psychedelic and narcotic drugs affects the psyche in such a way as to enlarge the range of vision into the subtle material energy but it does not help in penetrating the supernatural level. Only yoga facilitates this. That is the monopoly or specialty of yoga practice. That is why it is so necessary.

Sometimes suddenly without any yoga practice, a person sees into the supernatural sky, but that is infrequent. For regular supernatural perception, yoga is necessary.

It is hard to understand the chidakasha, but it may be comprehended in this way: When one opens the physical eyelids, one sees into the akasha, the normal atmosphere. Similarly if one leaves his material body and takes refuge in his subtle form only, the subtle eyes of that body will see clearly through the subtle world, according to the particular dimension. This subtle vision comes through two eyes just as physical vision does. We experienced this already when we perceived objects in dreams. When, however, a yogi closes his physical eyelids and sees clearly through one eye of perception in the center of the head, then he is using the chidakasha. Such perception is very clear. It is not an imagination but it uses the tool of imagination as the seeing eye.

When the tool of imagination works within itself, it is imagination. When it is focused to penetrate the speckled dark consciousness that surrounds the living entity when his eyes are closed, then it functions as the one supernatural seeing eye.

Readers are asked to be patient with these explanations since it is very hard to explain something that is outside our usual physical and subtle references. One thing is certain: Just as a human being did not create his physical eyes, just as they were formed naturally in the womb of his mother's body, so one does not create the single supernatural eye. It is created under certain conditions naturally. These conditions occur by the higher yoga practice of pratyāhār sense withdrawal, dhāraṇa concentration, dhyāna contemplation and samādhi trance states. If that vision could be created without austerities, no one would bother with yoga practice. The yogi sets the condition for the development of that supernatural vision. He does not create it. It develops just as, for a human embryo, physical eyes are formed naturally in the womb of the mother.

How does a yogi know that he has this supernatural perception? He knows when during meditation, suddenly and causelessly, he finds that the darkness in the head suddenly clears or parts away and he sees clearly into and through another atmosphere even while the physical eyelids are closed. This is a steady vision and not a shifting or color—spiraled vision caused by a hallucinogenic or narcotic drug. It occurs of its own accord when by chance a yogi experiences it for a second or for a minute or for hours on end. Otherwise a person can be as religious as his or her heart desires and still be restricted to just physical vision and haphazard subtle perception.

One has to master Kuṇḍalinī yoga, celibacy yoga, and also purity of psyche yoga before one can develop that vision consistently. One's imagination must cease its internal gyrations before one can develop that vision, just as Śrī Patañjali attested in his *Yoga Sūtras* about stopping the vrittis (mental movements within the buddhi organ).

Reliance on the supernatural level of material nature does not come easily for a limited being, what to speak of a purely spiritual reliance. Hence it is a wonder that some spiritual masters portray the shift to the spiritual level to be as easy as chanting a mahāmantra like,

Hare Kṛṣṇa Hare Kṛṣṇa, Kṛṣṇa Kṛṣṇa Hare Hare
Hare Rāma Hare Rāma, Rāma Rāma Hare Hare

From the mouth of Śrī Krishna, the main person addressed in that mantra, the kriyā yoga process is professed. As He said, the great souls, being reliant on the supernatural level of material nature, worship Him without deviation, knowing Him as the originator of the beings, the constant factor, Who is in the background of manifested matter.

सततं कीर्तयन्तो मां
यतन्तश्च दृढव्रताः ।
नमस्यन्तश्च मां भक्त्या
नित्ययुक्ता उपासते ॥९.१४॥
satataṁ kīrtayanto māṁ
yatantaśca dṛḍhavratāḥ
namasyantaśca māṁ bhaktyā
nityayuktā upāsate (9.14)

satatam — always; kīrtayanto = kīrtayantaḥ — glorifying; mām — Me; yatantaśca = yatantaḥ — endeavoring + ca — and; dṛḍhavratāḥ = dṛḍha – firm + vratāḥ — vows; namasyantaśca = namasyantaḥ — paying respects to + ca — and; mām — Me; bhaktyā — with devotion; nityayuktā = nitya – always + yuktā — disciplined; upāsate — worship

Always glorifying Me, endeavoring with firm vows, paying respect to Me with devotion, being always disciplined, they worship Me. (9.14)

Commentary:

Nowadays kīrtayanto, the system of glorifying Śrī Krishna, is a very big issue being put forward as the only process for salvation. In the time of Śrī Krishna it was a part of the process. It was stressed by the great souls who achieved the psychological purification which brought them into supernatural perception.

Firm vows are also stressed nowadays especially in relation to fasts on Ekādaśī days, chanting a set number of rounds of a mahāmantra each day, fasting on festival days, especially on Janmāṣṭmī, eating only food which is offered to the Deity form of Śrī Krishna or alternately one of His recognized incarnations, offering worship to a spiritual master in the disciplic succession, regardless of whether he mastered yoga, and agreeing to hear lectures.

This system is not exactly what Śrī Krishna spoke of in this verse. The vows He discussed concern mostly the yoga disciplines and systems of penance which support it. These may or may not include some of the vows advocated by modern devotee—leaders.

Paying respect to Śrī Krishna is now seen as only paying respect to Śrī Krishna's Deity Form in the temple. This form is considered the be all and end all of Śrī Krishna, as the Supreme Personality of Godhead in His spiritual Form. That is a bit different from the yoga system which allows the devotee to worship that same form and to aspire simultaneously to see the actual spiritual Form of the Lord which is not a marble, brass, or painted rendition. Following in the footsteps of Dhruva, Nārada and others, the yogi devotee worships the Deity Form but does not stop there. He meditates deeply in order to reach the Lord on other sides of existence. He does not accept the premise that the Deity Form is the ultimate Divine Form. He is not satisfied worshipping in that way and seeks to reach Krishna through mystic yoga.

ज्ञानयज्ञेन चाप्यन्ये
यजन्तो मामुपासते ।
एकत्वेन पृथक्त्वेन
बहुधा विश्वतोमुखम् ॥९.१५॥

jñānayajñena cāpyanye
yajanto māmupāsate
ekatvena pṛthaktvena
bahudhā viśvatomukham (9.15)

jñānayajñena = jñāna — concept + yajñena — by discipline; cāpy (capi) = ca — and + api — also; anye — others; yajanto = yajantaḥ — performing regulated worship; mām — Me; upāsate — they worship; ekatvena — with the singular basis; pṛthaktvena — as variety; bahudhā — variously shown; viśvatomukham — facing all levels

By the discipline of concepts, others do perform regulated worship of Me as the Singular Basis and as the Variety, facing all levels of reality simultaneously. (9.15)

Commentary:

Both yogis and non—yogis follow the method of this verse which is the discipline of concepts (jñānayajñena). However the yogis advance further than the concepts by their supernatural and spiritual experiences which free them from relting on concepts only. It is like a man who desires to go to a faraway country but only has a map given to him by someone who went there. The man with the map has only a concept. He may misinterpret the information because his mental references are not broad enough to correlate some symbols and signs to their true representation. When, however, that man reaches the faraway place, he drops his dependence on the map and can see the country firsthand.

In the yoga system, we gradually free ourselves from the concepts about the other sides of existence when we go to those extraterrestrial places and experience firsthand.

Some non—yogis also become freed by revelations and by sudden bestowals of overwhelming graces which flood out their limited perception, replacing it with mystic vision, once and for all. But such experiences are few and far between. The vast majority of non—yogis do not have such experiences; they are left with concepts only. They, of necessity, become dogmatic, clinging to an institution and systematically harassing themselves, their fellows and the public, while expressing the frustration they feel because of not being able to convert concepts into reality.

However, Śrī Krishna does recognize them as devotees so long as they maintain the discipline of concepts by using sharp discrimination and constantly consulting more elevated souls and scriptures written by such people and provided they perform regulated worship of Him as the Singular Basis and as the Variety, facing all levels of reality simultaneously. Such devotees use an Icon Deity Form of Śrī Krishna and are Krishna conscious as Śrī Krishna instructed in the *Bhagavad Gītā*, especially in the next chapter (Chapter Ten).

The whole scope of the modern movement of Krishna Consciousness, introduced by His Divine Grace A.C. Bhaktivedanta Swami Prabhupada, is described in this verse 15 of Chapter Nine. Some of his followers may regard this remark as a slight on that great teacher of Krishna Consciousness. They are attached to their concepts of Krishna's pastimes and think their ideas of pure devotion to Krishna are free from errors and misconceptions. In that consideration, they are incorrect. Without yoga, it is less likely that they will have an accurate conception, and even an accurate one is not the experience. We stress the experience here. Anything else is only notional.

अहं क्रतुरहं यज्ञः
स्वधाहमहमौषधम् ।
मन्त्रोऽहमहमेवाज्यम्
अहमग्निरहं हुतम् ॥९.१६॥
ahaṁ kraturahaṁ yajñaḥ
svadhāhamahamauṣadham
mantro'hamahamevājyam
ahamagniraham hutam (9.16)

aham — I; kratur — Vedic ritual; aham — I; yajñaḥ — sacrificial ceremony; svadhāham = svadhā — sanctified offering + aham — I; auṣadham — medicinal herb; mantro = mantraḥ — sacred sound; 'ham = aham — I; evājyam = eva — indeed + ājyam — ghee; aham — I; agnir = agniḥ — fire; aham — I; hutam — oblation

I am represented as the Vedic ritual. I may also be seen as the sacrificial ceremony or as the sanctified offering. I may be regarded as the medicinal herb. I may be seen as the ghee, fire or oblation given. (9.16)

Commentary:

No matter what a devotee of Śrī Krishna advocates, if he lacks the mystic, supernatural and spiritual experience, it means that he only has a concept. Such an idea will invariably be incorrect. This is because the system of conceptualization itself entails a certain degree of misconception. The devotee must gain direct experience using a supernatural and spiritual form. He must see through his own supernatural or spiritual eyes, not the eyes of his guru or the eyes of the scriptures. He himself must develop that sort of vision just as he had developed physical perception by taking a body through earthly parents. It must be that direct.

In this verse 16, some basis of Krishna consciousness is given. In Chapter Ten, a full course will be described. That course is neglected by those devotees who feel that it is elementary. They claim to have moved on to the higher discourse of Krishna consciousness which relates to the feelings of devotion (bhakti) to Śrī Krishna, by dwelling on the pastimes of the Lord, especially of the cowherd community of Vṛndāvana. However even in such considerations, there must be conceptions. Subsequently there must be errors in understanding due to the impurities of the devotees who consider those pastimes.

Let us not forget one thing: This same Śrī Krishna Who spoke the *Bhagavad Gītā* to Arjuna is the same Śrī Krishna Who in childhood, lived with the inhabitants of Vṛndāvana. He did not, during the discourse of the *Gītā*, point us to those pastimes. We should consider why Śrī Krishna did not tell Arjuna to merely chant *Hare Krishna* and be happy and not to worry about the Kuru conflict at all. Why did He not tell Arjuna to dwell on the Vṛndāvana līlā (pastimes)? Why did Śrī Krishna not advocate these as they are advocated by many teachers in the Krishna conscious societies?

The Krishna conscious course as it is taught here by Śrī Krishna and introduced now in this verse 16 of Chapter Nine is of interest to us as kriyā yogis. We should not see it as something basic or something for those who have no devotion. It is important to us, as part of the curriculum of kriyā yoga.

In that way, we can see Śrī Krishna as being represented in the Vedic ritualistic ceremonies. He is represented therein as the ritual itself, as the ceremony at large, as the sanctified offering, as the medicinal herb used, as the sacred sound uttered, the ghee, the fire and the oblation. All this should be perceived as Śrī Krishna Himself intermingled with formal religious ceremonies of Vedic origin.

पिताहमस्य जगतो
माता धाता पितामहः ।
वेद्यं पवित्रमोंकार
ऋक्साम यजुरेव च ॥९.१७॥
pitāhamasya jagato
mātā dhātā pitāmahaḥ
vedyaṁ pavitramoṁkāra
ṛksāma yajureva ca (9.17)

pitāham = pitā — father + aham — I; asya — of this; jagato = jagataḥ — of the universe; mātā — mother; dhātā — creator; pitāmahaḥ — grandfather; vedyam — subject to be known; pavitram — purifier; oṁkāra — sacred syllable Om; ṛk — Rig Veda; sāma — Sāma Veda; yajur — Yajur Veda; eva — indeed; ca — and

I am the father of this universe, the mother, the creator, the grandfather, the subject of education, the purifier, the sacred syllable Om, the *Rig*, Sama, and Yajur Vedas. (9.17)

Commentary:

The sketch of Krishna consciousness as Lord Krishna taught it to Arjuna is given in these verses, 16 through 19. Studying these carefully and then taking the full course given in Chapter Ten, we clearly see the difference between this curriculum and the one toted by modern teachers who define Krishna consciousness in terms of Krishna's relationship with the gopis and cowherd boys. Their relationship is a more advanced stage of Krishna consciousness that unfortunately gives impure persons the belief that they are capable of pure sentiments.

This curriculum is more basic and practical in terms of our present condition in close affiliation to material nature. It was given to Arjuna who was the dear friend of Śrī Krishna. As such it is good for us, the kriyā yogis. We will hear directly from Śrī Krishna on how to develop a Krishna conscious outlook from the ground up.

The father, the mother, the inventor, the grandfather of our bodies, the subject of education — these are common factors in daily experience. The Vedic ritual and its sacrificial procedures, the sacred syllable *Om*, the *Ṛg, Sāma*, and *Yajur Vedas* are not familiar to those of us who use Western bodies but are familiar to some who took birth in the Eastern setting.

गतिर्भर्ता प्रभुः साक्षी
निवासः शरणं सुहृत् ।
प्रभवः प्रलयः स्थानं
निधानं बीजमव्ययम् ॥९.१८॥
gatirbhartā prabhuḥ sākṣī
nivāsaḥ śaraṇaṁ suhṛt
prabhavaḥ pralayaḥ sthānaṁ
nidhānaṁ bījamavyayam (9.18)

gatir = gatiḥ — objective; bhartā — supporter; prabhuḥ — master; sākṣī — observer; nivāsaḥ — existential residence; śaraṇaṁ — shelter; suhṛt — friend; prabhavaḥ — origin; pralayaḥ — cause of universal disintegration; sthānam — foundation; nidhānam — reservoir of energies; bījam — case; avyayam — non—deteriorating

I am the objective, the supporter, the master, the observer, the existential residence, the shelter, the friend, the origin, the cause of universal disintegration, the foundation, the reservoir of energies, and the non—deteriorating cause. (9.18)

Commentary:

The objective, whatever it may be, the supporter of the objective, the master of a group, the observer looking and analyzing what he sees, the existential residence of the spirit any his psychic equipments, the shelter for whoever, the friend of a person, the origin of whatever — these are items with which we commonly identify. Conversely, the cause of the universal disintegration, the foundation, the reservoir of energies and the non—deteriorating cause are abstract principles which presently are beyond our reach.

Kriyā yoga, however, equips us with the increased sense perception through which we can perceive these.

तपाम्यहमहं वर्षं
निगृह्णाम्युत्सृजामि च ।
अमृतं चैव मृत्युश्च
सदसच्चाहमर्जुन ॥९.१९॥
tapāmyahamahaṁ varṣaṁ
nigṛhṇāmyutsṛjāmi ca
amṛtaṁ caiva mṛtyuśca
sadasaccāhamarjuna (9.19)

tapāmy (tapāmi)— I produce heat; aham — I; aham — I; varṣam — rainfall; nigṛhṇāmy = nigṛhṇāmi — I withhold; utsṛjāmi — I release; ca — and; amṛtam — relatively—long life span of the celestial bodies; caiva — and indeed; mṛtyus— quick death of earthly bodies; ca — and; sad = sat — eternal life; asac = asat — short—term existence; cāham = ca — and + aham — I; arjuna — Arjuna

I produce heat. I withhold and release rainfall. I arrange the relatively—long life span of celestial bodies and the quick death of the earthly ones, as well as the short—term existence and eternal life. (9.19)

Commentary:

The problem with the practical aspect of this layout of Krishna consciousness is proving it. What is the proof that Śrī Krishna arranges all this? How come our sense perception does not trace any of this to Him? At present, Śrī Krishna is not even before us in a living human body, the way He was for Arjuna.

In considering this, we have to save ourselves from the habit of relying solely on imagination and belief. Belief as a mechanism for conviction is trite with error and misconception. As kriyā yogis, people seeking realism, we want to avoid belief which ruins clarity and produces addictive biases for the avoidance of truth.

Taking what Śrī Krishna said for granted, and hoping that it is not a put—on, like the claims of so many human personalities mythicized in history, we may regard Him as the producer of life—sustaining heat, as the creator of temporary life and quick death, and as the creator of eternal life.

Eternal life is hard to understand since we do not have eternal memories, for even if we are indeed eternal beings, still without eternal memories, that span of time eludes us. The long span of celestial life may be investigated by developed mystic perception. Through that we can experience subtle forms objectively and make observations about their enduring qualities.

Items like heat and rainfall cannot be easily investigated. Heat for instance, must have originated physically from the cosmic explosions which produced our sun It would not be easy to investigate the origin of the sun to discover Śrī Krishna or someone else as its source. Thus we may take what Śrī Krishna said for granted.

Rainfall can be traced by a mediocre yogi, to astral beings, persons using subtle bodies, who collect psychic vibrations which exude in the astral atmosphere over the earth and then convert those into electromagnetic force to produce rainfall. This can be done by a yogi. However, tracing such astral beings to Śrī Krishna is not an easy matter.

त्रैविद्या मां सोमपाः पूतपापा
यज्ञैरिष्ट्वा स्वर्गतिं प्रार्थयन्ते।
ते पुण्यमासाद्य सुरेन्द्रलोकम्
अश्नन्ति दिव्यान्दिवि देवभोगान् ॥९.२०॥

traividyā māṁ somapāḥ pūtapāpā
yajñairiṣṭvā svargatiṁ prārthayante
te puṇyamāsādya surendralokam
aśnanti divyāndivi devabhogān
(9.20)

traividyā — knowers of the three Vedas; mām — Me; somapāḥ — soma drinkers; pūta — reformed; pāpā — bad tendencies; yajñaiḥ — with sacrificial procedures; iṣṭvā — worshiping; svargatim — path of heaven; prārthayante — they desire; te — they; puṇyam — merit based; āsādya — attaining; surendra — king of the angelic people; lokam — world; aśnanti — they enjoy; divyān — angelic; divi — in the astral region; devabhogān — celestial delights

The knowers of the three *Vedas*, the soma drinkers, and those who are reformed of bad tendencies, worship Me with sacrificial procedures. They desire to be transferred to heaven. Attaining the merit—based world of Surendra, the king of the angelic people, they enjoy celestial delights in the astral region. (9.20)

Commentary:

There is some contention that the soma drinkers took a sanctified beverage in religious ceremonies. Some say that this was a drink which was made from hallucinogenic mushrooms. Apart from the contention it is certain that those who took the soma beverage were able to see and converse with beings in the subtle world, particularly with the devas or supernatural rulers who govern various dimensions in the astral kingdoms. There was another method of communicating with these devas however, that of yoga austerities through which the yogi left his physical body and journeyed with his subtle form into the subtle dimensions, being transferred there by effective yoga austerities. Arjuna did this and so did Śrī Krishna. A modern yogi, if he is serious enough, and if he performs sufficient austerities can also achieve this. Surendra was known to Arjuna personally. The *Mahābhārata* states that by yoga kriyās taught to Arjuna by Yudhiṣṭhira and Krishna Dvaipāyana Vyāsadeva, Arjuna transferred his consciousness into his energized subtle body and journeyed to the Swārga Loka world of this Surendra.

In this verse, Śrī Krishna singled out the knower of the three *Vedas*, the soma drinkers, and those who are reformed of bad tendencies saying that they worship Him with sacrificial procedures. This implies that some devotees of Krishna are not knowers of the three *Vedas* and are not soma drinkers and are not reformed of bad tendencies.

After enjoying the celestial delights in astral forms, those who qualified for the astral elevation return to the earth again, as we hear in the next verse.

ते तं भुक्त्वा स्वर्गलोकं विशालं
क्षीणे पुण्ये मर्त्यलोकं विशन्ति ।
एवं त्रयीधर्ममनुप्रपन्ना
गतागतं कामकामा लभन्ते ॥९.२१॥

te taṁ bhuktvā svargalokaṁ viśālaṁ
kṣīṇe puṇye martyalokaṁ viśanti
evaṁ trayīdharmam anuprapannā
gatāgataṁ kāmakāmā labhante (9.21)

te — they; tam — it; bhuktvā — having enjoyed; svarga — angelic paradise; lokam — world; viśālam — multi-dimensional; kṣīṇe — in being exhausted; puṇye — in pious merit; martyalokam — world of short-life duration; viśanti — they enter; evam — thus; trayī — three Vedas; dharmam — injunctions for righteous life style; anuprapannā — adhering to; gatāgatam — going away and coming back; kāmakāmā — those who aspire for pleasures and luxuries; labhante — they get the opportunity

Having enjoyed the multi—dimensional, angelic paradise world, exhausting their pious merits, they enter the world of short—life duration. Thus adhering to the tri—part Vedic injunctions for righteous life style, those who aspire for pleasures and luxuries get the opportunity to go to heaven and come back to the earth again. (9.21)

Commentary:

There is a difference between the deva people and the qualified visitors from the earth. The deva persons are permanent residents of the multi—dimensional astral world. The earthly people who go there, remain only so long as they are supported by the force of pious credits developed while living a righteous lifestyle on the earth. It means therefore that the earthly visitors are always prone to leaving the astral paradises, places which are dreamed of as being heaven, the kingdom of God.

The tri-part Vedic injunctions dictate what materials to use for what purpose and also apply to other religions which may, unknowingly, be observant of the ancient Vedic stipulations. It is attested by Christians and Muslims that Lord Jesus Christ and the Prophet Mohammed facilitate such an astral place. However even in such religions, the accumulation of pious credit is limited by a human being's short lifespan. As such the force of his acquired piety soon peters out, causing him to return to the earthly environment after a short time.

अनन्याश्चिन्तयन्तो मां
ये जनाः पर्युपासते ।
तेषां नित्याभियुक्तानां
योगक्षेमं वहाम्यहम् ॥९.२२॥

ananyāścintayanto māṁ
ye janāḥ paryupāsate
teṣāṁ nityābhiyuktānāṁ
yogakṣemaṁ vahāmyaham (9.22)

ananyāś — to no other person; cintayanto = cintayantaḥ — keeping the mind attuned to; mām — Me; ye — who; janāḥ — people; paryupāsate — they worship; teṣām — concerning them; nityābhiyuktānāṁ = nitya — always + abhiyuktānām — of those who cultivate yoga disciplines; yogakṣemam — welfare; vahāmy = vahāmi — I tend to; aham — I

I tend to the welfare of the persons who worship Me and no other person, who keep their minds attuned to Me, and who always cultivate the yoga disciplines. (9.22)

Commentary:

All these saviors of humanity, persons like Śrī Krishna, Śrī Rāma, Lord Jesus Christ the Son of God, and some others of repute who left their impact on human history, have stated similarly that those who accept them will be rescued or saved, provided certain disciplines are followed.

Śrī Krishna requires one to focus on Him alone, as a requirement for getting the protection He offers. In this verse also, yoga disciplines are required, unlike the proposals put forward by many teachers of modern Krishna conscious religions.

What Śrī Krishna meant by tending to the welfare (yogakṣemam) of these advanced devotees may be understood by studying His relationship with Arjuna. Śrī Krishna, in protecting Arjuna, did not allow the warrior to do whatever he wanted. Instead Arjuna was guided according to Krishna's expertise. Arjuna felt pained initially in trying to follow Śrī Krishna's suggestions to fight at Kurukṣetra. It was not clear who Arjuna was to fight for or for what cause. During the discourse Śrī Krishna revealed that He was the One behind the confrontation. He ordered the violence to transpire.

Thus when Śrī Krishna said that He would tend to the welfare of the advanced devotees, that might be a very stern relationship in some cases, and the devotee may find it hard to comply with Śrī Krishna's sense of timing and His biases towards the limited beings who oppose His supernatural will.

येऽप्यन्यदेवता भक्ता
यजन्ते श्रद्धयान्विताः ।
तेऽपि मामेव कौन्तेय
यजन्त्यविधिपूर्वकम् ॥९.२३॥

ye'pyanyadevatā bhaktā
yajante śraddhayānvitāḥ
te'pi māmeva kaunteya
yajantyavidhipūrvakam (9.23)

ye — who; 'py = api — even; anyadevatābhaktā = anya — other + devatā — supernatural rulers + bhaktā — worshipping; yajante — they do prescribed ceremonies and disciplines; śraddhayānvitāḥ = śraddhayā — with faith + anvitāḥ — with; te — they; 'pi = api — also; mām — Me; eva — indeed; kaunteya — son of Kuntī; yajanty = yajanti — they do prescribed ceremonies and disciplines; avidhipūrvakam — not by the recommendation

Those who, with religious ceremonies, disciplines and faith, devotedly worship other supernatural rulers, indirectly petition Me, O son of Kuntī, although they do not perform the ceremonies and disciplines by My recommendation. (9.23)

Commentary:

Śrī Krishna dissected the resistance of others to Himself. He explains how we may approach others besides Himself. He admits that there are others who hail as Supreme Beings, who are seen as Supreme God, and who are worshipped faithfully and devoutly by other human beings. By this, He says, worshippers indirectly worship and petition Him, since He is the ultimate authority.

A yogi may research this by checking on his source origin as a personality. If in reaching back, one does not find Śrī Krishna as the immediate person source, then one may check to identify who exactly is the immediate person source of oneself. One may have to penetrate various personalities to get back far enough to find Śrī Krishna or some other primal being. Such research is comparable to penetrating the outer layers of a plant bulb with a needle to find the core. or to being a twig on a large tree and trying to reach back and discover the central portion of it. It is starting at the rim of a wheel and reaching in to find the spoke and axle.

If existentially, one is situated far away from the core personalities, from the Axis Supreme, then it is hardly likely that one will reach back far enough to discover the Supreme Person. Still, Śrī Krishna claimed Himself as the Supreme Person. Others feel He is Lord Shiva. Others recognize Him as the Father of Jesus Christ, and even others have varying views. Some feel that the Supreme is not a person.

That other devotees can worship other beings as the Supreme while ignoring the recommendation of Śrī Krishna, speaks for the vastness of this existence and the reality of the supernatural sensing mechanisms attuned by various charismatic super—people.

If Śrī Krishna is indeed the Core Personality of the existences, then how is it possible that He could be ignored by any other person? It is either that He over—estimated Himself or that it is not possible for everyone to penetrate the complex connections of the source personalities. Thus people will, of necessity, mistake God for this or that powerful personality who is not the Supreme Being, but who is charismatic enough to masquerade as such.

अहं हि सर्वयज्ञानां
भोक्ता च प्रभुरेव च ।
न तु मामभिजानन्ति
तत्त्वेनातश्च्यवन्ति ते ॥९.२४॥
ahaṁ hi sarvayajñānāṁ
bhoktā ca prabhureva ca
na tu māmabhijānanti
tattvenātaścyavanti te (9.24)

aham — I; hi — truly; sarvayajñānām = sarva — all + yajñānām — of religious ceremonies and disciplines; bhoktā — the person who appreciates; ca — and; prabhur = prabhuḥ — master; eva — indeed; ca — and; na — not; tu — but; mām — Me; abhijānanti — they recognize; tattvenātaś = tattvena — by reality + ataḥ — hence; cyavanti — they deviate form the path of virtue; te — they

Indeed I am the Master of all religious ceremonies and disciplines and I am the person Who should appreciate such procedures. But they do not recognize Me; hence they deviate from the path of virtue. (9.24)

__Commentary:__

Śrī Krishna presents Himself as the personal standardization of the religious ceremonies and disciplines, as the Person who ultimately should experience the efforts and offerings made by all living beings. The bhoktā is the person who evaluates and experiences something, like a milk checker at a dairy farm. If the cows chew the wrong grasses and grains and if they feel insecure emotionally, the taste of their milk and the percentage of fat in it will be affected. The checker, by looking at the milk, by pouring a little of it, states whether it is of the highest quality. Śrī Krishna thus puts Himself forward as the ultimate authority.

Because we do not recognize Him as the Final Sampler or Approver, we deviate from the path of virtue and use others as the reference. These others, Krishna indicated, do not have the sense to detect the consistent and unerring path of virtue.

These are tremendous statements made by Śrī Krishna because in instances of so many human beings, we naturally and effortlessly neglect Śrī Krishna. In fact, for most human beings, it is unnatural for them to consult Śrī Krishna to gage and authorize what they do. Śrīla Bhaktivedanta Swami, His Divine Grace, as he arranged to be called, gave his view that Krishna consciousness was not a super—imposition on the mind of the living being. He advocated it as the real consciousness, while dismissing everything else as conditioning. Actually, in our daily lives we experience mundane existence as the reality and everything else as the superimposition.

In fact in kriyā yoga, one quickly discovers that if he wants to slip out of this dimension, he will have to endeavor considerably since it is unnatural for any of us to effectively transcend this reality. This realization spurs determination to perform the yoga austerities which cause us to switch from lower frequencies to higher ones.

यान्ति देवव्रता देवान्
पितॄन्यान्ति पितृव्रताः ।
भूतानि यान्ति भूतेज्या
यान्ति मद्याजिनोऽपि माम् ॥९.२५॥
yānti devavratā devān
pitṝnyānti pitṛvratāḥ
bhūtāni yānti bhūtejyā
yānti madyājino'pi mām (9.25)

yānti — they go; devavratā — those who satisfy the supernatural rulers; devān — supernatural rulers; pitṝn — pious ancestors who exist as departed spirits; yānti — go; pitṛvratāḥ — those who satisfy the pious ancestors; bhūtāni — the ghostly spirits; yānti — go; bhūtejyā — those who satisfy the ghosts; yānti — they go; madyājino = madyājinaḥ — those who satisfy Me; 'pi = api — surely; mām — Me

Those who satisfy the supernatural rulers, go to those authorities. Those who satisfy the pious ancestors, associate with such departed spirits. Those who try to satisfy the ghosts, go to those beings. Those who try to satisfy Me, surely approach Me. (9.25)

Commentary:

The system of worship is based on attraction to specific persons and things. Based on desires which somehow overpower a person, endeavors are made to achieve certain ends. For most human beings this is done instinctively, and then it is rationalized into the conscious mind. This automatic rationalization into the conscious mind is the root cause of conditioning in material existence. The kriyā yoga process in its median phase aims at eradicating this rationalisation mechanism. This is done in the 5th stage of yoga, the pratyāhār sense withdrawal stage, while referencing to the 3rd and 4th stages of haţha yoga and prāṇāyāma.

The mahāyogī Śrī Gorakshnath was the one who elevated the importance of haţha yoga. In an era after the time of Śrī Krishna and Arjuna, haţha yoga suffered a lapse. Later, great yogins like Śrīla Gorakshnath revived it. Because young boys who took to yoga were diverted from householder life, a resistance to yoga developed in India. A sourness and resentment to it manifested. Thus even the Vaishnava teachers pronounced it as undesirable. They echoed the fears of females who were left without male protectors when the young men desisted from householder life and took up yoga practice, avoiding cultural activities.

As we hear in the *Gītā*, Śrī Krishna did not advocate avoidance of cultural acts. He Himself performed cultural acts by His own absolute sense of duty and specially manifested to enforce such performance in the life of Arjuna. In fact, the *Gītā* demonstrates this requirement for young people to complete cultural tasks even if they are attracted to yoga.

Developments in India culminated to the point where Lord Śrī Caitanya Mahāprabhu practically outlawed yoga practice and where those authorities in His disciplic succession turned their backs against it and took steps to erase it from the *Gītā*. However yoga is part of Krishna consciousness. Without it one cannot effectively bring on the psychological purification described in the *Gītā*. As such those who worship Śrī Krishna, but who do not perform yoga, will not get the purification derived from yoga.

The demigod worshippers of today, even the devotees of Krishna, are not purified on the psychological level when they worship the Krishna Mūrti and the acharyas who come down in the disciplic succession from Śrī Krishna. These people do not realize that Śrī Krishna cannot be reached by an impure psyche. If they read this, they will be appalled that I dared to suggest it. They may conclude that I am offensive to them and to persons like Śrīla Bhaktivedanta Swami, who in my view is one of those supernatural rulers, came down to institute and enforce his own authority under the cover of Krishna worship.

A person should not take an abrupt move and just begin worshipping Śrī Krishna as suggested in this verse. That is hardly possible since the psychological purification, described in Chapter Five verse 11 and Chapter Six verse 12, cannot be attained overnight. In fact one only worships Śrī Krishna effectively after one's psychology is purified and one has mastered the samādhi process of yoga. Otherwise the worship performed will be a rehearsal or a cultivation of the worship habit. Such a preparation has value but still it is not the actual pure worship.

Those who try to satisfy Śrī Krishna will surely approach Him but that does not mean that a person with an impure psychology can actually satisfy Him. Arjuna could not do so when his psychology was impure as we heard in Chapter One and in the early part of Chapter Two. In fact, in that stage Arjuna was opposed to Krishna, point for point. He refused to follow Krishna's suggestions, thinking that these were counterproductive and hostile to human existence and basic etiquette.

Arjuna did not, as some modern teachers suggest to us, gloss over Krishna's instructions by accepting them superficially with a belief posture that whatever Krishna wants is blissful and happy. Instead Arjuna challenged Krishna in a straightforward and polite way, quoting scriptures against Krishna. Arjuna was concerned because Krishna's instructions went against the grain and had a reckless content to them. They disregarded basic human relations and were poised to uproot the Kuru family tradition.

Hardly any of Krishna's devotees on this planet are actually going to Krishna because they do not have the psychological purity of intent required. They cannot be going to the same Krishna who spoke to Arjuna unless Krishna has since changed His posture, a proposal that is ridiculous. Most devotees are in fact going to other supernatural rulers and their counterparts, persons like Śrīla Bhaktivedanta Swami, His Divine Grace as he credited himself.

It was Śrī Gorakshnath's advent into this world which caused, as a by—product, the discouragement of yoga practice among the Vaishnavas. By the time Śrī Bābāji Mahasaya began to teach Śrī Lahiri Mahasaya, the discouragement was so rooted, that Śrī Bābāji's efforts to make yogis take householder life, hardly convinced the Vaishnava leaders to include yoga in their practice as the vital and central part of devotional disciplines.

Thus today one must fight for the right to do kriyā yoga even though so much of the *Gītā* concerns just that, as we heard so far up to this Chapter Nine. Gorakshnath, like Śrī Skanda Kumāra, another mahāyogī and figurehead of living entities, emerged initially from the celibate energies in Lord Shiva's body. It is natural for him to be unresponsive to the householder ashram and to women who are the founders of domestic life. On the other hand, Śrī Bābāji Mahasaya came from a part of Lord Shiva which has both the nurturing powers and the celibate energies. He introduced kriyā yoga for householders, something which was practiced by Śrīla Vyāsadeva and which he unsuccessfully told Shuka to take up in earnest.

The struggle continues because the origins of various entities are in conflict, and one part of Lord Shiva's nature might be opposed to another perpetually. I, myself, am here to promote the householder life for kriyā yogis with effective celibate practices. I am not oppose to a celibate life but I am against such a life for those persons who do not have the waiver from the Supreme Being, from Śrī Krishna. For them, I pioneered a method of celibate practice under the guidance of Lord Shiva, Śrī Bābāji Mahasaya, Śrīla Yogeshwarananda Yogiraja, Śrīla Agastya Muni, the originator of complex kriyās for those of us who use crude physical forms, and Śrī Hanumānji, who graciously showed me some of the kriyās he used to change the half—man half—monkey body he used. There are others who influenced me and their names are mentioned in other books which I wrote or am presently composing.

A male who thinks that he can sidestep all females, is making a very serious mistake. Yes, Skanda Kumāra did that. The four Kumaras did that. Others did that. But that does not mean that you will do it. Most of you will not be doing any such thing. It is not within your scope existentially.

पत्रं पुष्पं फलं तोयं
यो मे भक्त्या प्रयच्छति ।
तदहं भक्त्युपहृतम्
अश्नामि प्रयतात्मनः ॥९.२६॥
patraṁ puṣpaṁ phalaṁ toyaṁ
yo me bhaktyā prayacchati
tadahaṁ bhaktyupahṛtam
aśnāmi prayatātmanaḥ (9.26)

patram — leaf; puṣpam — flowers; phalam — fruit; toyam — water; yo = yaḥ — who; me — Me; bhaktyā — with devotion; prayacchati — he offers; tad — that; aham — I; bhaktyupahṛtam = bhakty (bhakti) — devotional + upahṛtam — given; aśnāmi — I accept; prayatātmanaḥ = prayata — disciplined, purified + ātmanaḥ — from the person

I do accept that given devotion from a disciplined, purified person who offers Me a leaf, flower, fruit or water with a devotional attitude. (9.26)

Commentary:

Some who attempt to satisfy the suggestion in this verse have the bhaktyā, the given devotion, but they do not have the discipline and resultant psychological purification. Following the lead of their authorities, they polish off their services to Śrī Krishna as being exactly what Śrī Krishna requires in this verse. In that, they foil their attempts to satisfy Śrī Krishna. Others cull choice statements from these scriptures and from Bengali scriptures in which the yogic disciplines are not a requirement for being an advanced devotee.

Until a person achieves both the devotional and the psychological purification as described in Chapter Five verse 11 and Chapter Six verse 12, his offerings of a leaf, a flower, a fruit or some water would not be accepted by Śrī Krishna.

This, however, does not mean that such offerings cannot be made to the Krishna Mūrti or the Krishna idol. It can be done, but the devotee should know that he is practicing only. When his psychological purification is effected, his devotion would be pure and his offerings would then be fully approved.

In the system introduced by Śrīla Bhaktivedanta Swami, His Divine Grace as he preferred to be called, there is a beginner stage for the devotee which is the neophyte level of the motions of serving Śrī Krishna. He knows that he is not pure but performs routine devotional service, sadhanā bhakti. At that level, the training stage, the devotee understands that he is going through a transitory period, under the direction of a Swami, who is supposed to be a pure devotee of Śrī Krishna.

By such service to the pure devotee, the neophyte should gradually move into the pure stage. However this system is not the kriyā yoga path. In kriyā yoga one gets purity by following the stipulation in verse 11 of Chapter Five and verse 12 of Chapter Six, that of kriyā yoga practice and supervised cultural involvements which contribute to the duties of the Supreme Being by acting as a small—time agent of His.

This verse calls to mind the time when Śrī Krishna discussed the background behind His advent as the son of Devakī and Vasudeva. He cited His parents' previous austerity for purification. In a previous era, they performed the yoga tapasya to effect such purity. It was not their devotion alone but the purity energy which was the content of such devotion. This is described in the Śrīmad Bhagavata Purāṇa.

यत्करोषि यदश्नासि
यज्जुहोषि ददासि यत् ।
यत्तपस्यसि कौन्तेय
तत्कुरुष्व मदर्पणम् ॥९.२७॥
yatkaroṣi yadaśnāsi
yajjuhoṣi dadāsi yat
yattapasyasi kaunteya
tatkuruṣva madarpaṇam (9.27)

yat = yad — what; karoṣi — you do; yad — what; aśnāsi — you eat; yaj = yad — what; juhoṣi — you present ceremonially; dadāsi — you gave away; yat = yad — what; yat = yad — what; tapasyasi — you perform as a discipline; kaunteya — son of Kuntī; tat = tad — that; kuruṣva — do; madarpaṇam — offering to Me

Whatever you do, whatever you eat, whatever you present ceremonially, whatever you give away, whatever you perform as a discipline, O son of Kuntī, do that as an offering to Me. (9.27)

Commentary:

This *Gītā* verse is widely abused by devotees of Krishna who do not have the required psychological purity. They feel that whatever they do, whatever they eat, whatever they present ceremonially, whatever they give away and whatever they perform as a discipline should be done as an offering to Śrī Krishna and should be regarded as being approved. Encouraged by their leaders, these devotees indulge in a dangerous miscalculation which often leads to their degradation.

The mistake occurs because many devotees unconsciously select from the *Gītā* only the highlighted verses which are shown to them by authorities. Not being able to distinguish what is meant for Arjuna alone and for devotees on par with him, they select those verses which supplement their existential insecurities. They do themselves a disfavor by believing that those verses apply to their situations.

Kaunteya means O son of Kunti. What I will tell you is this: This verse applies to Arjuna only and not to others unless they have the required psychological purity and devotion. Let us suppose that a devotee has that purity but did not do the yoga kriyās and cultural services mentioned in *Bhagavad Gītā* verses 5.11 and 6.12. Then it means that even without a current yoga practice, he is covered in this verse. Of course, his purity must be validated as it is described throughout the *Gītā*. One does not get purity simply through the disciplic succession from Śrī Krishna. He must have it independently. Thus a person may have that purity without having performed yoga in this present lifetime. It is possible. It cannot be denied.

However his possession of it does not transfer to his disciples unless they successfully perform the austerities and take up cultural duties, just as Arjuna was circumstantially forced to do when Śrī Krishna applied this *Bhagavad Gītā* pressure upon him. Usually it cannot be done.

शुभाशुभफलैरेवं
मोक्ष्यसे कर्मबन्धनैः ।
संन्यासयोगयुक्तात्मा
विमुक्तो मामुपैष्यसि ॥९.२८॥
śubhāśubhaphalairevaṁ
mokṣyase karmabandhanaiḥ
saṁnyāsayogayuktātmā
vimukto māmupaiṣyasi (9.28)

śubhāśubha — good and bad; phalair (phalaiḥ) — with consequences; evam — thus; mokṣyase — you will be liberated; karmabandhanaiḥ — from the implications of action; saṁnyāsa — renunciation; yoga — yoga; yukta — disciplined; ātmā — self; vimukto = vimuktaḥ — liberated; mām — Me; upaiṣyasi — you will attain

Thus you will be liberated from good and bad consequences and from the implications that come from action. Being liberated by the discipline of yoga as it was applied to renunciation, you will come to Me. (9.28)

Commentary:

The first part of this verse, the part about being liberated from consequences and their implications, is loved by modern devotees of Śrī Krishna. However on a closer view of the conditions for these guarantees, it is obvious that this applies specifically to Arjuna and to people like Arjuna who are that close to Śrī Krishna and who are that disciplined in yoga and in cultural performance.

Ignoring the stipulations about samnyāsa yoga yuktātmā, being liberated by the discipline of yoga applied to renunciation, modern devotees of Krishna seize this guarantee, flashing it on human society to assure themselves and others that whatever they do is alright with Śrī Krishna, and that no matter what they do, provided it is authorized by their leader, it will free them from good or bad consequences.

Of course this bolsters only their sense of insecurity because they are not covered in the guarantee. For yogis, these statements have meaning because it tells us how we can go to Śrī Krishna, under what conditions and by what stipulations. This business—like attitude of Śrī Krishna in clearly laying out His protection plan, is a service to us as yogis, so that we harbor no misconceptions and indulge in no fantasies about spiritual development.

We admire Arjuna for his closeness to Śrī Krishna and for the fact that he did qualify even though he was a warrior by caste and occupation, but we hold ourselves on par with him. We have much to do to qualify for these guarantees.

समोऽहं सर्वभूतेषु
न मे द्वेष्योऽस्ति न प्रियः ।
ये भजन्ति तु मां भक्त्या
मयि ते तेषु चाप्यहम् ॥९.२९॥

samo = samaḥ — equally disposed; 'ham = aham — I; sarvabhūteṣu — to all beings; na — not; me — of Me; dveṣyo = dveṣyaḥ — shunned; 'sti = asti — is; na — not; priyaḥ — especially dear; ye — who; bhajanti — they worship; tu — but;

samo'haṁ sarvabhūteṣu
na me dveṣyo'sti na priyaḥ
ye bhajanti tu māṁ bhaktyā
mayi te teṣu cāpyaham (9.29)

mām — Me; bhaktyā — with devotion; mayi — in Me; te — they; teṣu — in them; cāpy = cāpi — and too; aham — I

I am equally disposed to all beings. No one is shunned by Me nor is anyone especially dear to Me. But those who worship Me with devotion are My favorite and I am special to them too. (9.29)

Commentary:

Recently this verse was interpreted frankly in terms of a dividing line between the devotees of Śrī Krishna and the non—devotees. In some spiritual groups, to be a devotee of Śrī Krishna, one must be attracted to Krishna above all other divine persons and be a disciple of a certain spiritual master. Others who are attracted to Krishna and who take other spiritual masters are considered to be bogus or illegitimate. The idea was that devotees in this verse meant only a certain spiritual master and his followers. Such a narrow categorization only reinforces the insecurity of a certain spiritual master and his loyal disciples. It does not in anyway explain this verse.

Leaving all that aside, we may look at this verse in the way a lawyer regards a law before entering a courtroom where he will be counseled by a judge. This is one of the trickiest verses to understand. By a casual reading, one gets the idea that there is a double standard. Discovering that double standard, which in fact does not exist, a devotee is misled in his understanding and feels that since he is a devotee, he is the Lord's favorite (priyah), and that others not in his sect who do not accept his spiritual master, are regarded by Śrī Krishna in more nonchalant way. Actually everyone, the devotees and the non—devotees, are treated impartially by Śrī Krishna.

This is shown clearly in Śrī Krishna's relationship with Arjuna. Even though Arjuna was in direct touch with Śrī Krishna and traveled extensively with Śrī Krishna to help in His self—appointed world—saving missions, still, Arjuna risked being cast aside by Śrī Krishna if he did not perform at Kurukṣetra in the dangerous and emotionally—unpalatable task of killing or hurting relatives on a warfield.

Śrī Krishna never said anything like this: "Arjuna, I understand how you feel about this killing business. You are My buddy, an eternal and great friend of Mine. You are excused from this mission. Your refusal to cooperate is alright with Me. Never mind it, you are My loving devotee. Whatever you want will be fulfilled by Me."

This verse states basically that no living being is shunned completely by Śrī Krishna nor is anyone especially dear to Him to the extent that such a person could disagree with Śrī Krishna and still remain in good standing. Sooner or later, the disagreement would have to be settled in Krishna's favor. This applies to devotees and non—devotees. Everyone, devotees included, pure devotees even, must be careful in their relationship with Śrī Krishna, especially in taking Him seriously as the Supreme Personality of Godhead. The term Supreme Personality of Godhead was developed more or less by Śrīla Bhaktisiddhānta Sarasvatī, a devotee spiritual master of the Gauḍīya Math Sampradāya, and it was popularised by His disciple, Śrīla Bhaktivedanta Swami, one of the most charismatic figures in the history of Krishna consciousness.

The undertone of this verse implies that because everyone has his or her own individuality which is harnessed to a set of psychological equipments for perceiving reality, it is likely that someone will develop a contrary view that conflicts with that of Śrī Krishna.

Since they try to focus only on a positive relationship to Krishna, many modern leaders do not discuss these issues. Their avoidance does nothing to remove it. As kriyā yogis we face it completely, so we can understand the unpalatable parts of the relationship we want to have with Śrī Krishna.

So long as we worship Śrī Krishna with the devotion which comes from our yogicly-purified or otherwise—purified psyche, and so long as we do as He suggests, then we are His favorite and He is special to us too; but as soon as we find ourselves in a hard way, unwilling to carry out His instruction, then we will be put into an indifferent and somewhat caustic relationship with Him.

अपि चेत्सुदुराचारो
भजते मामनन्यभाक् ।
साधुरेव स मन्तव्यः
सम्यग्व्यवसितो हि सः ॥९.३०॥
api cetsudurācāro
bhajate māmananyabhāk
sādhureva sa mantavyaḥ
samyagvyavasito hi saḥ (9.30)

api — also; cet = ced — if; sudurācāro = sudurācāraḥ — wicked person; bhajate — worships; mām — Me; ananyabhāk — without being devoted to another; sādhur = sādhuḥ — saintly; eva — indeed; sa = sah — he; mantavyaḥ — should be considered; samyag = samyac — correctly; vyavasito = vyavasitaḥ — decided; hi — indeed; saḥ — he

If a wicked person worships Me without being devoted to any other authority, he is considered saintly, for he decided correctly. (9.30)

Commentary:

A wicked person may still be committed to criminal acts at the time when he decides to worship Śrī Krishna. Only his decision to approach Śrī Krishna should be credited as a saintly action. Such a person might return to criminal acts, or from then on, he might take up a disciplined moral life. Regardless, his one act of devotedly approaching Krishna gives him a saintly credit.

क्षिप्रं भवति धर्मात्मा
शश्वच्छान्तिं निगच्छति ।
कौन्तेय प्रतिजानीहि
न मे भक्तः प्रणश्यति ॥९.३१॥
kṣipraṁ bhavati dharmātmā
śaśvacchāntiṁ nigacchati
kaunteya pratijānīhi
na me bhaktaḥ praṇaśyati (9.31)

kṣipram — quickly; bhavati — he becomes; dharmātmā — a person whose character is virtuous; śaśvacchāntim = śaśvac (śaśvat) — eternal + chāntim (śāntim) — spiritual peace; nigacchati — he experiences; kaunteya — son of Kuntī; pratijānīhi — take note!; na — not; me — of Mine; bhaktaḥ — devotees; praṇaśyati — is ruined permanently

He quickly becomes a person whose character is virtuous. He experiences the eternal spiritual peace. O son of Kuntī, take note of it! No devotee of Mine is ruined permanently. (9.31)

Commentary:

This verse builds on the previous verse. If the wicked person approaches Śrī Krishna undistractedly, once and for all, then he quickly becomes someone whose character is virtuous. This happens by the sustaining force of Krishna's antiseptic association. That person eventually experiences the eternal spiritual peace derived from a close relationship with Śrī Krishna.

In addition, Śrī Krishna acknowledged the person who comes to Him like this but then returns to a criminal life. Because the person went undistractedly to Krishna just once, that person cannot be permanently ruined because Śrī Krishna takes note of the undistracted approach and takes responsibility to rehabilitate that person into His full association.

मां हि पार्थ व्यपाश्रित्य
येऽपि स्युः पापयोनयः ।
स्त्रियो वैश्यास्तथा शूद्रास्
तेऽपि यान्ति परां गतिम् ॥९.३२॥
māṁ hi pārtha vyapāśritya
ye'pi syuḥ pāpayonayaḥ
striyo vaiśyāstathā śūdrās
te'pi yānti parāṁ gatim (9.32)

mām — Me; hi — indeed; pārtha — son of Pṛthā; vyapāśritya — by relying on; ye — who; 'pi = api — also; syuḥ — they should be; pāpayonayaḥ — persons from sinful parentage; striyo = striyaḥ — women; vaiśyāḥ — businessmen; tathā — even; śūdrās — laborers; te — they; 'pi = api — also; yānti — they move towards; parām — supreme; gatim — goal

O son of Pṛthā, by relying on Me, even persons from sinful parentage, women, businessmen, and laborers, do move towards the supreme goal. (9.32)

Commentary:

By relying on Śrī Krishna one will indeed move towards the supreme goal, there is no guarantee that one can achieve this in a single life. Furthermore, just because one agrees to follow a particular devotee spiritual master, one does not instantly gain a virtuous character.

This verse applies to persons from families of ill—repute, families of low caste or low social status, females who are disinclined to sensual restrictions and strict regulations, businessmen whose minds remain glued to financial concerns and even laborers who lack the capacity for management and care very little about the direction of human society. This provides hope to all those who might rely on Krishna in part, but does not guarantee a quick adjustment in character to make them saintly in all their future actions. Only those who take the full course and remain permanently under Krishna's direction, will quickly acquire the virtuous character.

किं पुनर्ब्राह्मणाः पुण्या
भक्ता राजर्षयस्तथा ।
अनित्यमसुखं लोकम्
इमं प्राप्य भजस्व माम् ॥९.३३॥
kiṁ punarbrāhmaṇāḥ puṇyā
bhaktā rājarṣayastathā
anityamasukhaṁ lokam
imaṁ prāpya bhajasva mām (9.33)

kim — how; punar — more again, more accessible; brāhmaṇāḥ — brahmins; puṇyā — piously—inclined; bhaktā — devoted; rājarṣayaḥ — yogi kings; tathā — also; anityam — temporary; asukham — miserable; lokam — world; imam — this; prāpya — having acquired; bhajasva — devote yourself; mām — Me

How much more accessible then, is it for the piously—inclined brahmins and yogi kings? Having acquired an opportunity in this temporary, miserable world, you should devote yourself to Me. (9.33)

Commentary:

Spiritual knowledge of the theory of yoga practice, as well as the description of the resulting experiences and the geographic information of other dimensions, was taught initially to brahmins and to the rulers. The path of the rulers is karma yoga which Śrī Krishna taught Arjuna in this *Bhagavad Gītā*. The path of jñāna yoga was taught to the brahmins who did not have the rulership responsibilities.

Generally speaking, others were excluded. This is why, in the previous verse, those of sinful parentage, women, businessmen and laborers, were mentioned in a derogative way. Vedic culture, in the time of Lord Krishna, was prejudiced, such that only the two highest castes were introduced to certain disciplines. There were four castes generally and a fifth class in such disrepute that it did not merit a rating. That fifth class was regarded as outcast in the previous verse. Śrī Krishna lists them as being of sinful parentage (pāpayonayah). The four castes were the brahmin educators, the ruling class, the business people and the laboring class.

In Vedic culture, women were regarded as a class all by themselves depending on which family they were born into and the caste privileges exercised by the family they entered by marriage. Thus, since their status was reliant on connection, Śrī Krishna listed them in verse 32 in the derogative category.

Some commentators seeking to remove the derogative connotations in verse 32, have stated that this is not a prejudiced listing. However the plain truth is just that. Most importantly, it reflects the social conditions which endured in that time. Like it or not, that was the situation. There is enough evidence of this in the Vedic histories to show that women were rated by family affiliation and especially by their status after marriage.

Śrī Krishna, in a stark admission of the disparities of existence, questions Arjuna about the accessibility of the eternal spiritual peace in relationship to Himself as explained in verse 31 above. He asks Arjuna about the accomplishments of the piously—inclined brahmins and the yogi kings. He warns that having acquired an opportunity in this temporary miserable world, Arjuna would be wise to devote himself to Śrī Krishna.

This, as its tone proclaims, is a sort of ultimatum for Arjuna to surrender completely to Krishna's plan to bring war upon the uncooperative Kurus.

मन्मना भव मद्भक्तो
मद्याजी मां नमस्कुरु ।
मामेवैष्यसि युक्त्वैवम्
आत्मानं मत्परायणः ॥९.३४॥
manmanā bhava madbhakto
madyājī māṁ namaskuru
māmevaiṣyasi yuktvaivam
ātmānaṁ matparāyaṇaḥ (9.34)

manmanā — one whose mind is fixed on Me; bhava — be; madbhakto = madbhaktaḥ — being devoted to Me; madyājī — performing ceremonial worship of Me; mām — to Me; namaskuru — make obeisance; mām — Me; evaiṣyasi = eva — indeed + esyasi — you will come; yuktvaivam = yuktva — disciplined + evam — thus; ātmānam — self; matparāyaṇaḥ — with Me as the Supreme Objective

With the mind fixed on Me, being devoted to me, performing ceremonial worship to Me, make obeisance to Me. Being thus disciplined, with Me as the Supreme Objective, you will come to Me. (9.34)

Commentary:

This excludes everyone but Śrī Krishna. There is no indication of a liaison between us and Krishna. Of course, this instruction is given to Arjuna alone. It does not necessarily apply to others, except that, many spiritual masters, who come in disciplic succession, use these verses to justify themselves as indispensable agents of Krishna.

Even though yoga is not mentioned directly in this verse, it is contextually implied based on what was said before in these eight chapters from Chapter Two through this Chapter Nine. Therefore, this verse summarizes the requirements for attaining the Supreme Objective, Sri Krishna. One's mind must be fixed on Krishna. The psyche should be purified through yoga practice. One should be devoted to Krishna. One must perform ceremonial worship to Krishna with the added clarity of mystic perception attained through steady yoga practice. Finally, one must make the proper obeisances after receiving the proper realization from the supernatural and spiritual revelations received by one's expertise in yoga. Without these yogically-inspired achievements, one's services will be flawed at best and will not be fully accepted by Krishna.

CHAPTER 10

A Fraction of Krishna's Splendor*

श्रीभगवानुवाच
भूय एव महाबाहो
शृणु मे परमं वचः ।
यत्तेऽहं प्रीयमाणाय
वक्ष्यामि हितकाम्यया ॥ १०.१ ॥
śrībhagavānuvāca
bhūya eva mahābāho
śṛṇu me paramaṁ vacaḥ
yatte'haṁ prīyamāṇāya
vakṣyāmi hitakāmyayā (10.1)

śrī bhagavān — the Blessed Lord; uvāca — said; bhūya — again; eva — indeed; mahābāho — O powerful man; śṛṇu — hear; me — from Me; paramam — supreme; vacaḥ — information; yat = yad — which; te — to you; 'ham = aham — I; prīyamāṇāya — to one who is beloved; vakṣyāmi — I will explain; hitakāmyayā — desiring your welfare

The Blessed Lord said: Again, O powerful man, hear from Me of the supreme information. Desiring your welfare, I will explain it, O beloved one. (10.1)

Commentary:

At the beginning of Chapter Nine, Lord Krishna said that he would explain the most secret truths, the knowledge with the experience, which having known, Arjuna would be freed from impurities. Now again (bhūya), Śrī Krishna explains more of that information, but on the basis of Arjuna's non—cynical attitude (anasūyave B.G. 9.1) and Śrī Krishna's desire for Arjuna's welfare. Arjuna was so dear that Śrī Krishna personally cultivated him. In fact Arjuna is addressed by Śrī Krishna as one who is beloved of Krishna (prīyamāṇāya). Are we in such a position in reference to Śrī Krishna?

From the point of view of the entire *Gītā* discourse, all eighteen chapters, this verse shows clearly that Śrī Krishna did not want to discard Arjuna as His confidential assistant in the mean business of punishing the limited entities who opposed the supreme will. Krishna wanted to keep Arjuna in that position no matter what, even if Arjuna disagreed. Thus Krishna took extra care to explain many details about the relationship between Himself and the living entities.

**The Mahābhārata contains no chapter headings. This title was assigned by the translator on the basis of verse 41 of this chapter.*

न मे विदुः सुरगणाः
प्रभवं न महर्षयः
अहमादिर्हि देवानां
महर्षीणां च सर्वशः ॥१०.२॥
na me viduḥ suragaṇāḥ
prabhavaṁ na maharṣayaḥ
ahamādirhi devānāṁ
maharṣīṇāṁ ca sarvaśaḥ (10.2)

na — not; me — of Me; viduḥ — they know; suragaṇāḥ — the supernatural rulers; prabhavam — the origin; na — nor; maharṣayaḥ — great yogi sages; aham — I; ādir = ādiḥ — source; hi — in fact; devānām — of the supernatural rulers; mahārṣīnām — of the great yogi sages; ca — and; sarvaśaḥ — in all respects

The supernatural rulers do not know My origin, nor do the great yogi sages. In all respects, I am the source of the supernatural rulers and the great yogi sages. (10.2)

Commentary:

At this point, Lord Krishna emphatically addresses Arjuna's doubts as to whether Krishna was the Supreme Divine Person, rather than a divine person among the many divinities which the Vedic culture accommodates. This statement establishes Lord Krishna as greater than Lord Shiva, Lord Brahmā and Lord Nārāyaṇa, figures of repute in the time of Śrī Krishna. After all, Śrī Krishna was physically present. Therefore His claims of supremacy were not easy to accept.

Arjuna, like Śrī Krishna, had worshipped Lord Shiva and had perfected the yoga austerities which enable a person using a physical body to see into the supernatural dimension where Lord Shiva and his wife Gauri lived. Therefore, Śrī Krishna intended to show that even though Arjuna successfully petitioned and received weapons from Lord Shiva, and even though Lord Krishna as the initiated disciple of the mahāyogīn Upamanyu, also successfully reached Lord Shiva and Goddess Gauri through yoga tapasya, still Krishna Himself was the senior most Divinity.

Hearing this statement of supremacy, Arjuna was to shift his confidence completely to Śrī Krishna. Śrī Krishna tactfully hinted this in chapter 9, verse 30, when He spoke of His antiseptic influence on persons who worship Him without being devoted to any other authority (ananyabhāk).

To address concerns that not all supernatural rulers subscribed to Śrī Krishna's declarations about Himself, Krishna stated that the supernatural rulers do not know His origin nor do the great yogi sages. Thus how could they acclaim Him? The wording is technical. Śrī Krishna first spoke of the rajarshis, the yogi kings, now He speaks of the maharshis, who are the brahmin rishi yogis. These were the highest human beings at the time of Krishna and Arjuna.

यो मामजमनादिं च
वेत्ति लोकमहेश्वरम् ।
असंमूढः स मर्त्येषु
सर्वपापैः प्रमुच्यते ॥१०.३॥
yo māmajamanādiṁ ca
vetti lokamaheśvaram
asaṁmūḍhaḥ sa martyeṣu
sarvapāpaiḥ pramucyate (10.3)

yo = yaḥ — who; mām — Me; ajam — birthless; anādim — beginningless; ca — and; vetti — knows; lokamaheśvaram — Almighty God of the world; asaṁmūḍhaḥ — unconfused, perceptive; sa = saḥ — he; martyeṣu — of those who use perishable bodies; sarvapāpaiḥ — from all faults; pramucyate — is freed

Of those who use perishable bodies, the one who regards Me as birthless and beginningless and who knows that I am the Almighty God of the world, is the perceptive person. He is freed from all faults. (10.3)

Commentary:

Transitioning from the supernatural people who do not use perishable bodies, Śrī Krishna addressed those with short life-spans, stating that those who regard Him as birthless and beginningless, and who know that He is the Almighty God, despite His advent in a material form, is the perceptive person. That person, He said, is freed from all faults.

Obviously, seeing such a thing directly is not ordinary. The question is: Who directly sees this? Many who believe this preach it have convinced themselves that their intellectual grasp constitutes true vision of it. Actually, how many perceive this with supernatural and spiritual vision?

बुद्धिर्ज्ञानमसंमोहः
क्षमा सत्यं दमः शमः ।
सुखं दुःखं भवोऽभावो
भयं चाभयमेव च ॥ १०.४॥
buddhirjñānamasaṁmohaḥ
kṣamā satyaṁ damaḥ śamaḥ
sukhaṁ duḥkhaṁ bhavo'bhāvo
bhayaṁ cābhayameva ca (10.4)

buddhir = buddhiḥ — intelligence; jñānam — knowledge; asaṁmohaḥ — non—confusion, sanity; kṣamā — patience; satyam — truthfulness; damaḥ — self-control; śamaḥ — tranquility; sukham — pleasure; duḥkham — pain; bhavo = bhavaḥ — existence; 'bhāvo = abhāvaḥ — non—existence; bhayam — fear; cābhayam = ca — and + abhayam — fearlessness; eva — indeed; ca — and;

Intelligence, knowledge, sanity, patience, truthfulness, self—control, tranquility, pleasure, pain, existence, non—existence, fear, fearlessness... (10.4)

Commentary:

These and the qualities listed in the next verse are segments of energy in the psychology of a living being. These not only concern the human beings; they also inhabit the psyche of every other type of creature, even the microscopic ones. The human being is special, since he possesses the facilities for sorting these psychological segments. The other life forms cannot differentiate the segmentations.

अहिंसा समता तुष्टिस्
तपो दानं यशोऽयशः ।
भवन्ति भावा भूतानां
मत्त एव पृथग्विधाः ॥ १०.५॥
ahiṁsā samatā tuṣṭis
tapo dānaṁ yaśo'yaśaḥ
bhavanti bhāvā bhūtānāṁ
matta eva pṛthagvidhāḥ (10..5)

ahiṁsā — non—violence; samatā — impartiality; tuṣṭiḥ — contentment; tapo = tapaḥ — austerity; dānam — charity; yaśo = yaśaḥ — fame; 'yaśaḥ = ayaśaḥ — infamy; bhavanti — are; bhāvā — existential conditions; bhūtānām — of the beings; matta — from Me; eva — alone; pṛthagvidhāḥ — multiple

...non—violence, impartiality, contentment, austerity, charity, fame and infamy, are multiple existential conditions, which are derived from Me alone. (10.5)

Commentary:

The difference between static mundane energy and the active type is the exhibition of these qualities. Exactly how the static power becomes capable of exhibiting these qualities is not described, but Śrī Krishna claimed to have imparted or have caused, from Himself, the exhibition. Śrīla Yogeshwarananda, a great modern yogin, concluded through his own research of the causal plane that by the proximity of the Supreme Spirit or parambrahman, subtle and gross matter began to exhibit these qualities. The yogin attributed it to the Supreme Spirit which he sensed to be a vast infinite reality which is near to matter and which causes changes by proximity only.

What should we believe? Who should we believe? It all depends on our individual natures. One person will be inclined to accept what Śrī Krishna said. Another will vouch for what Śrīla Yogeshwarananda and others like him testified. Yet another will be doubtful of either view. A kriyā yogi is more inclined to research the reality.

In my own experience from this life as well as what I can recall consciously and intuitively from past lives, the Cause of all causes is both a Personality and a primal energy combined. That personality also happens to be a multi—personality who is split into several million personalities. How He does this is a mystery. At the same time, there is a primal energy which splits up. It is not that these personal and energetic realities split up at a particular point in time. I found that they were split before I could perceive them. I know however that after I emerged from one of the personalities, others emerged from me. Thus I deduced a time medium or a regulated splitting action.

The phenomena of these origins can be understood by observing what happens when a woman becomes pregnant. At that time there is an entity in her body whose psyche draws nutrients from her uterus. Later on, the entity comes out in an individual body. The woman is there. The entity is there. It seems to be a split off but we know for sure that actually there is no division, for if the child was part of her body eternally, it would not come out in its own developed form.

However, we observe an existential dependence between the child and the mother, or in other words, it seems that the entity using the child form is psychologically dependent on the entity functioning as the mother. Thus we see something else. We see an emotional connection in the personalities. This may prove to be a temporary or circumstantial dependence. This may be on—going. We admit that while in the belly of the mother's form, the embryo was completely dependent on the mother's energies, not the mother's personality.

This is complex. My point is that there is a Personal Source and there is an Energy Source. None of this is impersonal even though some commentators use the term impersonal. No one can actually prove that anything is impersonal because we cannot be sure at anytime as to whether there is a natural or supernatural owner in real terms. We cannot be sure of the absence of a remote controller who exists in a parallel dimension unseen.

Jesus Christ, Lord that He is, tried to explain this by speaking of the property—owner who owned a large estate which had to be tended by several hired managers. Once, the owner went away. He left after subdividing the estate and assigning management to various supervisors. After some time, the managers forgot him. The point is that even though something appears to be impersonal and even though one might fail to locate the proprietor, he still exists somewhere.

Accordingly, it is believed that Jesus was a special son of God sent to check up on some managing leaders on this planet. However such managers had all but forgotten that there was a planetary owner. For one thing they had transpired into various bodies for a very, very long time. In each body, they could not even remember their former identity, even though the instinct for management remained intact. They did not recognize Jesus as a special son of the manager. They felt that his discourse was a tactic to undermine and supersede their power, which was, of course, the very idea. One requires a sense or an instinct to understand this because the Supreme Proprietor is reluctant to prove Himself to anybody.

Like it or not, personality can be found everywhere in the mundane, psychic, supernatural and spiritual spheres. It cannot be avoided. Even though from this physical place, yogis like Śrīla Yogeshwarananda reached the causal plane, they found that they had to secure their own existence space because others were already residing there, living in casual forms without any subtle or grossly manifested body. Thus everywhere we turn, we will find personalities and materials of some sort, even if they are subtle, supersubtle or spiritual. The segmentation of the cultural personalities also does not make the matter simpler. It does not erase territorial rights and aspects of that nature. Even though the cultural personalities we encounter on a physical planet are for the most part, collages of physical energy, appearing as one homogeneous somebody but being in actuality a circumstantial existential mix-up, still we have to deal with personal rights. It is the same everywhere else we turn.

When I go to parallel worlds as I regularly do in astral travels, I encounter territorial rights in each of these places. It cannot be avoided. No amount of belief in an impersonal force can erase it. It is there, facing us from every dimension.

Few realize that this list in verses 4 and 5 comprises the various segments of the cultural personality. These are the intelligence organ in the subtle body, the knowledge acquired in the subtle and gross forms, the sanity in the inherent nature of the individual, the patience he or she or it has, the truthfulness he or she or it is demonstrates, the self control, the tranquility, the pleasure and pain the form can endure, the existence of itself as it feels to be, the non—existence or blank aspect of itself as it does not register in other domains, the fear of its relative position, the fearlessness it feels because it is boosted by the overall reality, the non—violence it is capable of, its impartiality, its contentment as an instinct, its austerity, its charity, and its fame and infamy.

महर्षयः सप्त पूर्वे
चत्वारो मनवस्तथा ।
मद्भावा मानसा जाता
येषां लोक इमाः प्रजाः ॥१०.६॥
maharṣayaḥ sapta pūrve
catvāro manavastathā
madbhāvā mānasā jātā
yeṣāṁ loka imāḥ prajāḥ (10.6)

mahārṣayaḥ — great yogi sages; sapta — seven; pūrve — in ancient times, of old; catvāro = catvāraḥ — four celibate boys; manavaḥ — primal sexually—disciplined procreators; tathā — also; madbhāvā — coming from Me; mānasā — mentally; jātā — produced; yeṣāṁ — of whom; loka — universe; imāḥ — these; prajāḥ — creatures

The seven great yogi sages of old, the four celibate boys, and also the primal sexually—disciplined procreators come from Me, being produced mentally. From them, the creatures of this universe evolved. (10.6)

Commentary:

According to the *Puranas*, these persons were produced of Brahmā, the Creator sub-God of this world. That Brahmā was supposed to have come from the body of a super person with a gigantic supernatural form, who is known as Garbhodakaśāyī Viṣṇu. Śrī Krishna must have startled Arjuna and everyone else who was listening to the discourse, by declaring Himself as the parent of the seven great yogi sages of old, the four celibate boys and the primal sexually disciplined procreators.

The seven great yogi sages are given by the late Vaishnava authority, Śrīla Śrīdhara Deva Goswami, as Marīci, Atri, Aṅgirā, Pulastya, Pulaha, Kratu and Vasiṣṭha. He gives the four celibate boys as Sanaka, Sanandan, Sanat-Kumāra and Sanātana. There are supposed to be fourteen of the primal sexually disciplined procreators who are popularly known as Manus. A rough equivalent of the Manus are the Adams in the Christian description of creation. In Christianity there was supposed to be an Adam and Eve who were miraculously produced by God as living adult forms and who by sexual linkage produced human babies. Similarly Manu and Shatarupa produced the human species in the Vedic version.

At first glance, much of the evidence of anthropology seems to throw aside these religious versions of creation, since the record of fossils suggests a progression from ape to prehistoric man to modern man. In reality, the track of anthropology lends even more credence to the religious version, since it does not explain the supernatural force which caused the radical departure from primitive forms. Let us suppose that the theory of the anthropologists is correct. That would mean that the human forms we now use, gradually, over hundreds of thousands of years, evolved from primitive prehistoric forms, all coming out of Africa. Originally Africa had the climate to permit the development of such forms. Even the forces which cause the changes in the looks and functions of these forms cannot be explained as merely being climactic and environmental pressures.

The problem with the anthropologist view is that it does not entertain the supernatural influences. Actually the argument between those who believe in a God as the creator and those who accept the fossil evidence and who believe in nature as the creator, should be reconciled in recognition of both God and nature. Both are involved in the creative milieu.

As soon as conditions are suitable on any planet at any time, in any dimension, the living entities take the initiative. They have the capacity to exploit. It is irrelevant really as to how the human forms came about. Nobody is asking how the dinosaurs came about because we hardly recognize that spirits also used dinosaur bodies and sought opportunities just the same. Where are those spirits who used those dinosaur forms? Have they all transmigrated into other species? Or have they gone somewhere else in the universe where a planet was ready for their habitation?

The mystery of the creation of gross forms for human beings and other creatures is solved before our eyes in the formation of human embryos in the body of a woman. Śrīla Yogeshwarananda, that great yogin, did his mystic time-transfer into the past and saw that the primal sexually-disciplined procreators were produced out of matter naturally, just the way babies are produced in a womb by ingestion of the nutrients in a woman's form.

It is not hard to understand this. One does not have to believe in God to see this. After all, it is natural, because a man and a woman, as sexual partners, do not have to believe in a Christian or a Hindu God to produce children. It happens by a more natural agency which has little to do with theism or atheism.

For the yogi, these things must be considered. He must see that in his course of practice, he must develop the mystic vision to see the causes of the creation. Śrī Krishna's grand claims are alright for the time being, until we can find out exactly what happened to produce these forms. On the other hand, there is no reason to doubt Śrī Krishna, to think that what He claims borders on the ridiculous. The fossil evidence of the anthropologists, while carefully and meticulously presented, lacks an explanation of the supernatural factor. Presently without the mystic means, we can neither prove nor disprove what Śrī Krishna claimed. One thing is certain: There is a background which remains hidden. It cannot be figured out through the discovery of fossils. That background does not leave fossil prints because it is psychological. Someone may dig up the fossil of a great scientist one hundred thousand years from now, but that skeleton will never explain the genius of that personality. This is what I mean by psychological.

Anthropology has value, undoubtedly. Only a religious bigot will neglect the study of it, but that does not mean that it shows the completion. It clearly reveals what nature selected to show us about what happened physically. Nature is very shrewd, however, just as the modern newscasters show us their preference in carefully edited films. It is not only the human beings who have biases. Nature does also. By leaving the record of fossils, she shows us the limitations we encountered when trying to develop these gross bodies. Thus she is to be respected.

One should not, as a yogi, ignore the evidence of anthropology because we know very well how dependent we are on material nature, especially on gross evolution. All the same, we should not take anthropology as the complete explanation. We have to pry into the mystic side, because it is our only recourse to research the supernatural part of this vast creation.

When Śrī Krishna says that He is this or He is that, we should not reject Him. Nor should we run off and flag down every man with Krishna consciousness as some preachers request us to do. There is no statement in the *Gītā* which says that we should do this. In Chapter Eighteen, Śrī Krishna spoke of telling the *Gītā* to a select few. We will study the verse. He does not say, as modern teachers do, that we should proselytize every human being everywhere.

A yogi's concern is to find the ultimate cause and to see it for himself, not just to believe it because his guru says it, or because Śrī Krishna or some other divinity proclaimed it.

Actually this writer could care less whether the Hindu God, the Christian God or some other God is proven conclusively as the Supreme Person. It is irrelevant because no matter Who that Person may be, it will still be reduced to our compliance with Him. The difficulty of that compliance will remain. There will be disagreement with that God no matter Who He is. Only a person with a childish mind goes on imagining a happy relationship with a favorite God. The real relationship with such a Person is apart from the imagined devotion and affection conceived when one's psychology exists in an impure state, which will be rejected by the divinity.

Modern religious leaders take great advantage of the petty-minded persons who cherish some God whom they feel is supreme, and who, to their view, has to be the Ultimate Personality. Imagining such a thing, they hold in a part of their mind, the image of that God and themselves in contrast to the whole world, but such considerations are for small-minded persons. For the purpose of kriyā yoga, one needs to leave all that aside.

एतां विभूतिं योगं च
मम यो वेत्ति तत्त्वतः ।
सोऽविकम्पेन योगेन
युज्यते नात्र संशयः ॥१०.७॥
etāṁ vibhūtiṁ yogaṁ ca
mama yo vetti tattvataḥ
so'vikampena yogena
yujyate nātra saṁśayaḥ (10.7)

etām — this; vibhūtim — divine glory; yogam — yoga, extensive mystic discipline; ca — and; mama — of My; yo = yaḥ — who; vetti — experience; tattvataḥ — in reality; so = saḥ — he; 'vikampena = avikampena — by consistent; yogena — by yoga practice; yujyate — is harmonized with; nātra = na — not + atra — here; saṁśayaḥ — doubt

Whosoever experiences in reality, this divine glory and extensive mystic discipline of Mine, becomes harmonized with Me by consistent yoga practice. There is no doubt about this. (10.7)

Commentary:

Avikampena means unwavering, consistent and steady. This consistency activates the divine realization described, knowing the divine nature of Śrī Krishna by upgrading oneself to a level where it can be perceived and then remaining focused there. This is done by yoga practice, yogena. It is very clear.

Being harmonized with Śrī Krishna does not mean to be one with Him or to merge with Him, but rather to reach a level where He is perceived distinctly and where one experiences their own with a divine nature without mundane attributes. It is harmonizing with Krishna, not a unity with Him in terms of becoming Him or anything like that. It is attained through consistent yoga practice that is ongoing and steady (avikampena yogena).

Not all the kriyā yogis will experience this. It all depends on whether or not one gets this sort of revelation in visions and meditations. One yogi may experience the supreme reality in that personal way, or he might perceive another deity when having the visions. Śrī Krishna does not state anywhere in the *Gītā* that all the yogis will perceive this. There is no point in stating that every successful transcendentalist has to be Krishna conscious in this personal way described by the Lord, nor should all neophyte yogis expect to have this experience. Instead a yogi should practice, and keep track of his own experiences, noting well how he is causelessly drawn into certain mystic and spiritual experiences which are peculiar to him.

अहं सर्वस्य प्रभवो
मत्तः सर्वं प्रवर्तते ।
इति मत्वा भजन्ते मां
बुधा भावसमन्विताः ॥१०.८॥
ahaṁ sarvasya prabhavo
mattaḥ sarvaṁ pravartate
iti matvā bhajante māṁ
budhā bhāvasamanvitāḥ (10.8)

aham — I; sarvasya — of all; prabhavo = prabhavaḥ — originator; mattaḥ — from Me; sarvam — everything; pravartate — proceeds; iti — thus, in this way; matvā — having thought; bhajante — they worship; mām — Me; budhā — intelligent person; bhāvasamanvitāḥ = bhāva — states of being, meditative ability + samanvitāḥ — endowed with

I am the originator of all. From Me, everything proceeds. Thinking of Me in this way, the intelligent persons, who are endowed with meditative ability, worship Me. (10.8)

Commentary:

This is a meditative process, one of mystic vision through introspection in the perfectional stages of practice, which comes from mastery of the two last stages of yoga namely, dhyāna contemplation and samādhi trance stages. This is keynoted by the term bhāva samanvitāh.

Matvā means thinking and considering. This is not the kind of thinking that comes from just hearing and then conceptualizing. This is a deep kind of thinking occurring after one masters the pratyāhār sense withdrawal procedure and also performs prāṇāyāma to quell the disturbing sensuality which is produced from turbulent and sensually—agitating subtle energy (prāṇa).

Śrī Krishna claims Himself as the originator of all (aham sarvasya prabhavah). To realize this and to worship Him as described, one must do much more than hear of this in the *Gītā* or from an authority in the disciplic succession. If the authority in disciplic succession did not master all the stages of yoga and did not practice trance consciousness in isolation, then what he says cannot be meaningful in terms of this verse. He will not be able to transmit this to a disciple because he does not have it as part of his own experience. If he has also heard from a spiritual master who was not a masterful yogi, then he cannot relay this experience because neither he nor his predecessor has the qualification.

One must hear this from an authority who practiced the discipline to this extent and that is not all. One must hear from him and then one must practice personally. Then one can have the experience of Śrī Krishna and can verify what Śrī Krishna said. Otherwise it is all belief, based on being convinced by another person. Such a belief is good but it is not the experience described in this verse.

मच्चित्ता मद्गतप्राणा
बोधयन्तः परस्परम् ।
कथयन्तश्च मां नित्यं
तुष्यन्ति च रमन्ति च ॥ १०.९॥
maccittā madgataprāṇā
bodhayantaḥ parasparam
kathayantaśca māṁ nityaṁ
tuṣyanti ca ramanti ca (10.9)

maccittā — those who think of Me; madgataprāṇā — those who concentrate the life energy onto Me; bodhayantaḥ — enlighten; parasparam — one another; kathayantaśca = kathayantaḥ — speaking of + ca — and; mām — of Me; nityam — constantly; tuṣyanti — they are content; ca — and; ramanti — they are happy; ca — and

Those who think of Me, who concentrate the life energy on Me, who enlighten one another and speak of Me constantly, are content and happy. (10.9)

<u>Commentary:</u>

Madgataprāṇā verified that this is a yogic process and that the person must be masterful at prāṇāyāma yoga, the yoga which gives mastery over prāṇa. One cannot fully concentrate the prāṇa on Śrī Krishna merely by thinking of Śrī Krishna's pastimes. Those who do not understand how the psyche operates, thinks this is possible. Only a person who mastered prāṇāyāma yoga can successfully concentrate his life force on Śrī Krishna in full.

Not doing yoga, not knowing anything about the perfection of it, seeing it as unnecessary, thinking of Śrī Krishna as he learned about Him from a spiritual master in the authorized disciplic succession, reading about Him in Śrīmad Bhāgavatam, trying one's best to control one's life by services to the temple of Krishna and to His missionary devotees, taking the time to attend lectures about Krishna, talking with devotees about Him, sharing views and realizations, speaking of Him constantly, will also bring on a contentment and happiness. Still, that is not the same happiness experienced by a devotee who perfected the yoga practice.

As a kriyā yogi, one must be determined to take the full course of yoga, all eight stages. That will improve the quality of the relationship with Krishna and qualify one for these guarantees in the *Gītā*. Do not be deterred by those who say that yoga is irrelevant in the Age of Kali, and that only chanting of the Holy Name has any meaning. Chanting of the Holy Name does have meaning. Thus when one gets his psyche purified by yoga practice, his chanting has all the more value indeed.

तेषां सततयुक्तानां
भजतां प्रीतिपूर्वकम् ।
ददामि बुद्धियोगं तं
येन मामुपयान्ति ते ॥ १०.१० ॥
teṣāṁ satatayuktānāṁ
bhajatāṁ prītipūrvakam
dadāmi buddhiyogaṁ taṁ
yena māmupayānti te (10.10)

teṣām — of these; satatayuktānām = satata — constantly + yuktānām — of the disciplined; bhajatām — of the worshippers; prītipūrvakam — with affection; dadāmi — I give; buddhiyogam — technique of insight yoga, application of yoga to the use of intelligence; tam — it; yena — by which; mām — Me; upayānti — they draw near; te — they

Of those who are constantly disciplined, who worship with affection, I give the technique by which they draw near to Me. (10.10)

Commentary:

Buddhi yoga is mastered after one perfects the pratyāhār sensual energy withdrawal practices. These are mostly mystic processes. Buddhi yoga is practiced after the yogi realizes the value of haţha yoga, a system of postures and prāṇāyāma yoga that facilitates study on how prāṇa courses through the subtle body.

Buddhi yoga is a part of kriyā yoga. It means just what it says, namely buddhi or the intellect organ of the subtle body under the discipline of yoga austerities. In buddhi yoga, one begins to sort the difference between the life force in the spine of the body and the intellect which is an organ housed in the head of the subtle form. That organ is not the mind but it is contained or housed in the mind which is a subtle compartment surrounding the head of the subtle form. The buddhi is a system of subtle lights which flicker in the subtle world and which operate as subtle sensing mechanisms.

Śrī Krishna said in this verse, that those who are His devotees, who are affectionate to Him and who are constantly disciplined in behavior and in their yoga practice, are given by Him, the technique of insight yoga, through which they draw very close to Him.

Actually this does not mean that one can get that close to Śrī Krishna by other means because the other means do not open the visionary powers of the intellect organ, through which one can see in the sky of consciousness, the chidakasha (chit—akasha). It is in that sky of consciousness that one perceives the supernatural and spiritual forms of the divinities.

It is amazing that these statements of Śrī Krishna which apply to kriyā yoga only, and to advanced kriyā yoga at that, are used by those authorities in the disciplic succession who do no yoga, who are adverse to it, and who slander it, because the system of bhakti that they follow, the system of devotional service they advocate, is an entirely different system which does not include these techniques.

तेषामेवानुकम्पार्थम्
अहमज्ञानजं तमः ।
नाशयाम्यात्मभावस्थो
ज्ञानदीपेन भास्वता ॥ १०.११ ॥
teṣāmevānukampārtham
ahamajñānajaṁ tamaḥ
nāśayāmyātmabhāvastho
jñānadīpena bhāsvatā (10.11)

teṣām — of them; evānukampārtham = eva — indeed + anukampā — assistance + artham — interest; aham — I; ajñānajam — ignorance produced; tamaḥ — stupefying influence of material nature; nāśayāmy = nāśayāmi — I caused to be banished; ātmabhāvastho = ātmabhāvasthaḥ — situated in the self; jñānadīpena = jñāna — knowledge, realized + dīpena — with light, with insight (jñānadīpena — with realized insight); bhāsvatā — clear, shining, clarity of consciousness

In the interest of assisting them, I Who am situated within their beings, cause the ignorance, produced by the stupefying influence of material nature to be banished by their clear realized insight. (10.11)

Commentary:

This purely results from a firm kriyā yoga practice, when the intellect organ in the head of the subtle body is perceived by the yogi and when he has controlled his imagination orb to such a degree that it functions as an eye, as a seeing instrument to perceive the objects in the sky of consciousness. Just as when a human being opens his eyelids, he automatically sees anything before him in the sky of mundane energy in the particular dimension that his body is attuned to, so when the advanced yogi closes his physical eyes, he may see through one opening which is created out of his imagination orb in the intellect of the subtle form.

At first one must master Kuṇḍalinī yoga which is accelerated by firing up the bhasvara agni power which is a combination of air, subtle air and hormones in the gross body. These are energized by prāṇāyāma practice, particularly by bhastrika rapid breathing and by alternate breathing. Once the bhasvara agni is properly kindled, it reaches up the spine and enters the brain of the subtle form. It increases the brilliance of the intellect organ.

The ignorance which Śrī Krishna causes to be banished is the darkness inside the head of the subtle form which normally remains there and disallows any perception of objects in the sky of consciousness (the chidakasha). When this darkness is lifted, the yogi sees even if his physical eyes are closed. Then the darkness inside the head is dissipated, replaced by a clear sky in which there are supernatural and spiritual objects. The yogi then begins to see what he never saw before and what others can only conceptualize or imagine according to hints given by Śrī Krishna and others like Him. This is an individual accomplishment. Each person must attain this individually by his own efforts at yoga austerities and by the grace bestowed by Śrī Krishna and other divinities.

अर्जुन उवाच
परं ब्रह्म परं धाम
पवित्रं परमं भवान् ।
पुरुषं शाश्वतं दिव्यम्
आदिदेवमजं विभुम् ॥ १०.१२ ॥
arjuna uvāca
paraṁ brahma paraṁ dhāma
pavitraṁ paramaṁ bhavān
puruṣaṁ śāśvataṁ divyam
ādidevamajaṁ vibhum (10.12)

arjuna — Arjuna; uvāca — said; param — supreme; brahma — spiritual reality; param — supreme; dhāma — refuge; pavitram — reformer; paramam — supreme; bhavān — You, O Lord; puruṣam — person; śāśvatam — eternal; divyam — divine; ādidevam — Primal God; ajam — birthless; vibhum — one whose influence spreads everywhere

Arjuna said: Hail to You Who are the Supreme Reality, the Supreme Refuge, the Supreme Reformer, O Lord. You are the eternal divine Person, the Primal God Who is birthless, and Whose influence spreads everywhere. (10.12)

Commentary:

Arjuna said this both as a devotee who loved Krishna and did service for Him, and as a great yogi who understood by practice most of what Śrī Krishna described to Him. Arjuna's austerities in yoga are described in the *Mahābhārata* literature which is a history of the activities of the five Pandavas brothers, Arjuna being the third elder.

The *Mahābhārata* describes Arjuna's success in the yoga kriyās which were taught to him by Śrī Yudhiṣṭhira, the eldest Pandava. Yudhiṣṭhira was taught these by Śrīla Vyāsadeva, the writer of the *Mahābhārata* literature and the actual grandfather of the Pandavas. These people were successful kriyā yogis. Arjuna's listening to the *Gītā* is a world apart from modern devotees who listen but who did not perform kriyā yoga. Such devotees cannot really understand the *Gītā*, because they lack the technical knowledge required to fathom the yoga terms. Yes, we see that many authorities in disciplic succession, know very little about yoga. Still they bravely write commentaries and take steps to get their books standardized as authoritative *Bhagavad Gītās*.

As a kriyā yogi, Arjuna could really say as he did:

"Hail to You, Śrī Krishna, Who are the Supreme Reality, the Supreme Refuge, the Supreme Reformer, O Lord. You, Śrī Krishna, are the eternal divine Person, the Primal God Who is birthless and Whose influence spreads everywhere."

आहुस्त्वामृषयः सर्वे
देवर्षिर्नारदस्तथा ।
असितो देवलो व्यासः
स्वयं चैव ब्रवीषि मे ॥ १०.१३ ॥
āhustvāmṛṣayaḥ sarve
devarṣirnāradastathā
asito devalo vyāsaḥ
svayaṁ caiva bravīṣi me (10.13)

āhuḥ — they declare; tvām — You; ṛṣayaḥ — yogi sage; sarve — all; devarṣir = devarṣiḥ — supernatural yogi sage; nāradaḥ — Narada; tathā — as well as; asito devalo —Asita Devala; vyāsaḥ — Vyāsa; svayam — your own self; caiva = ca — and + eva — indeed; bravīṣi — You state; me — to Me

All the yogi sages, as well as the supernatural yogi sage Narada, Asita Devala, and Vyasa declare this of You. And You Yourself state this to me. (10.13)

Commentary:

Nārada, Asita Devala and Vyāsa are not just devotees of Śrī Krishna but rather they are yogi devotees, with stress on their yoga expertise. These were masters of kriyā yoga in that very life. They were not devotees who merely claimed that since they did yoga in their previous lives, they did not have to do it again, or that since they were following the path of Krishna consciousness, it indicated that they perfected yoga in previous lives.

My point in this commentary is that one has to be a yogi. If indeed one senses that one did yoga in the past, then one must again do it all over again, even if only to review it and to be accelerated in the path. Only by that, will one get the clarifying insight of buddhi yoga which is yielded by a firm practice. The yogi sage Vyāsa, as well as the supernatural yogi sages, Nārada and Asita Devala, had records of current kriyā yoga practice. Śrī Krishna Himself, Lord that He puts Himself forward to be, had record of kriyā yoga practice, such that Śrī Krishna took lessons from Upamanyu Rishi for about five months, attained samādhi, saw through the chidakasha, the sky of consciousness, and saw the supernatural forms of Lord Shiva and His wife Umā.

Incidentally one person named Devala Rishi, who is not the Asita Devala mentioned in this verse, was the official spiritual master of the five Pandavas brothers. He was a masterful kriyā yogi. Additionally, the technique which Arjuna used for going to the Svārgaloka heavenly world to get celestial weapons and supernatural assistance, was given by Śrīla Vyāsadeva to Yudhiṣṭhira. This gives us some idea of how advanced Yudhiṣṭhira was in the kriyā art.

सर्वमेतदृतं मन्ये
यन्मां वदसि केशव ।
न हि ते भगवन्व्यक्तिं
विदुर्देवा न दानवाः ॥१०.१४॥
sarvametadṛtaṁ manye
yanmāṁ vadasi keśava
na hi te bhagavanvyaktiṁ
vidurdevā na dānavāḥ (10.14)

sarvam — all; etad — this; ṛtam — true; manye — I believe; yan = yad — which; mām — me; vadasi — you say; keśava — O Keśava; na — not; hi — indeed; te — to you; bhagavan — O Blessed Lord; vyaktim — form; vidur = viduḥ — they know; devā — the supernatural rulers; na — nor; dānavāḥ — descendants of Danu, enemies of the supernatural rulers

All that You say to me is true. I believe it, O Keśava. Indeed it is not possible to understand You, O Bhagavan, Blessed Lord. Neither the supernatural rulers nor their enemies, the descendants of Danu, can know Your form. (10.14)

Commentary:

According to the *Mahābhārata*, Arjuna's material body entered samādhi somewhere in the Himalayan mountains. From there, Arjuna's pranically—energized subtle form entered the celestial regions, going to the place where Indra demigod presides. At that celestial place, he was asked to fight some descendants of Danu, who though related to the supernatural rulers, usually act as their political opponents. This story was told by Arjuna to Yudhiṣṭhira after Arjuna recovered his material body which was in trance, and after Arjuna rejoined the brothers in preparation for the civil war. The story is as follows.

When Śrī Arjuna, after performing austerities and entering samādhi, went to the heavenly planets, he was greeted there as a celebrity. Indra, the ruler of that place, greeted him warmly and afforded Arjuna an important seat. After sometime, Arjuna was trained in mystic combat and in using very advanced supernatural weapons. These weapons, which might be compared to modern atomic and nuclear weapons, operate in such a way as to demolish subtle objects either on a grand or local scale.

From our perspective we can say that Arjuna was trained in supernatural warfare. The importance of such subtle combat is this: Whatever takes place on the gross level is an after-product of what transpires on the subtle plane. There are many species of life. Within each, there are many races and many family groupings. All these vie for a position in the subtle and gross material dimensions. Hence there is a need for protection so as not to be displaced by others. Arjuna was involved in that protection business on this planet, but to win in the civil struggle of the Kuru family, he was required to first win the subtle struggle between the ruling supernaturals and their opponents.

When the time came to pay his teacher's fee on the heavenly planet, Arjuna was asked to use his military expertise to vanquish the Dānavas, who previously had defeated the legitimate rulers of that heavenly place, and who had occupied some celestial cities.

For the battle, Arjuna was given the chariot of the celestial king and the King's charioteer, a driver named Matali. This chariot, being a subtle conveyance, flew through the sky without an engine. It was drawn by 100,000 horses. Arjuna mounted it with the celestial persons.

After traveling for a time in subtle space, Matali reached the city of the Dānavas, the opponents whom Arjuna was to vanquish. Those people heard the chariot beforehand. They became very distressed to think that Indra, whom they defeated had returned for combat. They did not understand that even though the chariot was Indra's, the warrior was a different man. Immediately after, they closed the celestial palace city and prepared defense. Arjuna, seeing this, blew his conch to signal that he came for a confrontation.

Many warriors came out of the city dressed in armor with comparable weapons of various sorts. They surrounded Arjuna and attacked. Arjuna began displacing hundreds of them from that dimension. He had superior skill and superior weapons which were specifically created for this task. Arjuna found, however, that there were so many opponents that he could not displace them all. They kept coming one after the other in droves and hurling various types of weapons. At last he became disheartened. His initial enthusiasm waned. He became discouraged and fearful for his own life. Seeing his condition, Matali the charioteer, displayed even more courage and maneuvered the chariot in such a skillful way that Arjuna repossessed his morale.

In the meantime, some of the superior Dānavas came out of the city. They used magical weapons to curb Arjuna. They created darkness. They created all sorts of frightening phenomena, some of which affected the horses of Arjuna's chariot. The creatures were stunned. Even Matali, who was experienced in sorcery, became visibly frightened. He stumbled. The golden goad which he used to signal the horses fell from his hand. He said to Arjuna, "Where are you? I cannot see anything."

Arjuna became fearful again but Matali remembered previous battles which were similar and described these, stating that perhaps Brahmā, the creator of the worlds, might have desired that those places be destroyed completely, and so may have empowered the Dānavas for victory.

Hearing this and being confident of his own prowess, Arjuna took courage and decided to win that battle. He said to Matali, "Now look at what I will do. Have no fear. Just hold the position, charioteer."

In the meantime the Dānavas felt that they had won the battle and that Arjuna was finished. But again they saw Arjuna regroup and attack. This time the Dānavas hid in subtle darkness. They saw Arjuna but he could not view them. They attacked him but he could not respond since he could not perceive them. However, using some mystic techniques, Arjuna perceived them. He killed many. The survivors retreated into their city. Soon after, many who were killed by Arjuna, miraculously regained their bodies and flew upwards and were airborne. Arjuna became baffled by this. Matali, familiar with sorcery, told Arjuna to use the thunderbolt weapon. With this, Arjuna killed the subtle bodies of those resurrected Dānavas. Their souls were shifted into other dimensions.

In this verse of Chapter Ten, Arjuna mentioned the descendants of Danu because both they and the supernatural rulers are expert at sorcery, magical mystic acts which affect both the subtle and gross manifestations. These people are in a position to ease or strain us. By mystic perception, they can know just about everything, but Arjuna declared that they could not know the form of Sri Krishna.

This is not a repeat of something Arjuna heard but it is based on Arjuna's direct observation about the supernatural power of the devas and their opponents. Arjuna himself by the austerities performed, outpaced the mystic capacity of the devas. Thus he knew that since he could not investigate Śrī Krishna's form, neither could they.

स्वयमेवात्मनात्मानं
वेत्थ त्वं पुरुषोत्तम ।
भूतभावन भूतेश
देवदेव जगत्पते ॥१०.१५॥

svayam — yourself; evātmanā = eva — indeed + ātmanā — by yourself; 'tmānam = ātmānam — yourself; vettha — you know; tvam — you; puruṣottama — Supreme Person; bhūtabhāvana — one who sustains the

svayamevātmanātmānaṁ
vettha tvaṁ puruṣottama
bhūtabhāvana bhūteśa
devadeva jagatpate (10.15)

existence of all others; bhūteśa — Lord of created beings; devadeva — God of the gods; jagatpate — Lord of the universe

You alone know Yourself, O Supreme Person, O maintainer of the creatures, O Lord of the created beings, O God of gods, O Lord of the universe. (10.15)

Commentary:

In a firm and bold declaration, Arjuna stated that Lord Krishna alone knows Himself. This verse is rarely quoted by preachers of the *Gītā* but is an important verse. Arjuna declared in easy Sanskrit that only Śrī Krishna can know Himself. No one else has the means to check Krishna, because He is beyond their sensual and investigative processes. The first line reads: svayam eva ātmanā ātmānam. This could be pronounced easily in English as: svai am ey va aatmanaa aatmaanam. Taken literally, the translation is svayam——yourself, eva——alone, indeed, ātmanā——by yourself, ātmānam——yourself. The first two words of the second line of this verse, vettha tvam, mean you know.

Despite what we have heard about Krishna, for or against what He claimed in the *Gītā*, despite what is written about Him in the *Puranas* and the *Mahābhārata*, here Arjuna, the yogicly-achieved warrior, makes his own statement. As kriyā yogis following behind Arjuna, we can accept what he stated at face value; only Śrī Krishna can know Śrī Krishna and Krishna is the Supreme Person, the Maintainer of the creatures, the Lord of the universe.

For the time being we cannot verify this because we lack the means. Kriyā yoga gives us ability to verify some but not all of it. It would be left to Śrī Krishna to reveal Himself to each individual as He would soon expose Himself to Arjuna. If we accept no one else, it seems to me, that we can accept Arjuna, if only because of his simplicity of approach, his lack of motivation to dominate us as a guru and his yogic accomplishment which caused him to come within range of Lord Shiva and Goddess Umā.

I feel we can accept what Arjuna says and then move on from there to perfect the practice, so that each of us can see directly, by the grace of Arjuna and Śrī Krishna. By the grace of Arjuna, by the energy he left in this verse, we can be successful in kriyā yoga, certainly!

वक्तुमर्हस्यशेषेण
दिव्या ह्यात्मविभूतयः ।
याभिर्विभूतिभिर्लोकान्
इमांस्त्वं व्याप्य तिष्ठसि ॥१०.१६॥
vaktumarhasyaśeṣeṇa
divyā hyātmavibhūtayaḥ
yābhirvibhūtibhirlokān
imāṁstvaṁ vyāpya tiṣṭhasi (10.16)

vaktum — to describe; arhasy = arhasi — you can; aśeṣeṇa — without deleting anything, thoroughly; divyā — supernatural; hy = hi — in truth; ātmavibhūtayaḥ — wondrous manifestations of Yourself; yābhir = yābhiḥ — by which; vibhūtibhir = vibhūtibhiḥ — wondrous manifestations; lokān — worlds; imāṁs — these; tvam — you; vyāpya — pervading; tiṣṭhasi — you are situated

Please describe thoroughly, Your supernatural wondrous manifestations by which You pervade these worlds and are situated in them. (10.16)

Commentary:

This is a verse of blessing from Arjuna to us, the yogis who honestly want to know about these things and who would like to see some of this, at least enough to remove the misgivings in our nature about these declarations. Arjuna petitioned for himself and for us.

Let Śrī Krishna give details about the mystery of His mystic glory, of how He pervades these worlds and is situated in them. We cannot see the whole reality but we may view a part of it. Our developed perception, even if limited in the most advanced stage, would give us a view of these wondrous manifestations.

कथं विद्यामहं योगिंस्
त्वां सदा परिचिन्तयन् ।
केषु केषु च भावेषु
चिन्त्योऽसि भगवन्मया ॥१०.१७॥
kathaṁ vidyāmahaṁ yogiṁs
tvāṁ sadā paricintayan
keṣu keṣu ca bhāveṣu
cintyo'si bhagavanmayā (10.17)

katham — how; vidyām yogiṁs I will know; aham — I; yogiṁs = yogin — O mystic master; tvām — You; sadā — constantly; paricintayan — meditating; keṣukeṣu — in what, in what; ca — and; bhāveṣu — in aspects of existence; cintyo = cintyah — to be considered; 'si = asi — You are; bhagavan yogiṁs Blessed Lord; mayā — by me

How will I know You, Mystic Master, O Yogi? Is it by constantly meditating? In what aspects of existence are You to be considered by Me, O Blessed Lord? (10.17)

Commentary:

One thing that many devotees fail to realize is this: Śrī Krishna is a yogi, a practicing yogi. He is not hostile to yoga practice unless it is done with demonic intentions. Śrī Krishna performed yoga practice, just as he entered householder life, fought battles, ruled a kingdom and so on. When Arjuna addressed Krishna as a yogin, it is not a superficial honorary title. It is because Śrī Krishna mastered the austerities.

Arjuna appealed for clarification on the method of knowing Śrī Krishna's glories. Is it by meditation that we can get direct vision of Krishna's mysteries? How should we research His glories? In what aspects of existence can He be known?

विस्तरेणात्मनो योगं
विभूतिं च जनार्दन ।
भूयः कथय तृप्तिर्हि
शृण्वतो नास्ति मेऽमृतम् ॥१०.१८॥
vistareṇātmano yogaṁ
vibhūtiṁ ca janārdana
bhūyaḥ kathaya tṛptirhi
śṛṇvato nāsti me'mṛtam (10.18)

vistareṇātmano (vistareṇātmanaḥ) = vistareṇa — with detail + ātmanaḥ — of Yourself; yogam — yoga, self—disciplinary methods and the resultant mystic power; vibhūtim — splendrous form; ca — and; janārdana — O motivator of the people; bhūyaḥ — more; kathaya — explain; tṛptir = tṛptiḥ — final satisfaction; hi — indeed; śṛṇvato = śṛṇvataḥ — of hearing; nāsti = na —not + asti — is; me — of me; 'mṛtam = amṛgtam — sweetness

Explain in more detail about Your self—disciplinary methods and the resultant mystic power and of Your splendrous form, O motivator of the people. There is no final satisfaction for me in hearing Your sweet words. (10.18)

Commentary:

How admirable is this statement of Arjuna's to Śrī Krishna! What are Śrī Krishna's yoga processes? What does He do when He performs yoga? What practice would give us direct insight into His glories?

Arjuna declared that, for him, there was no final satisfaction in hearing Śrī Krishna's sweet words.

श्रीभगवानुवाच
हन्त ते कथयिष्यामि
दिव्या ह्यात्मविभूतयः ।
प्राधान्यतः कुरुश्रेष्ठ
नास्त्यन्तो विस्तरस्य मे ॥१०.१९॥
śrībhagavānuvāca
hanta te kathayiṣyāmi
divyā hyātmavibhūtayaḥ
prādhānyataḥ kuruśreṣṭha
nāstyanto vistarasya me (10.19)

śrībhagavān — the Blessed Lord; uvāca — said; hanta — listen; te — to you; kathayiṣyāmi — I will talk of; divyā — supernaturally; hy = hi — truly; ātmavibhūtayaḥ — own wondrous forms; prādhānyataḥ — most prominent; kuruśreṣṭha — O best of the Kuru clan; nāsty (nāsti) = na — not + asti — is; anto = antaḥ — limit; vistarasya — to the influence; me — My

The Blessed Lord said: Listen, I will talk to you of the most prominent of my supernatural manifestations, O best of the Kuru clan, for there is no limit to My influence. (10.19)

Commentary:

Despite the excitement felt and displayed by Arjuna, Śrī Krishna in His usual cool—headed mood, said He would describe the most prominent of His supernatural manifestations, since there was no limit to His influence in the subtle and gross mundane creations. It would be sufficient to give Arjuna an idea of how to confirm Krishna's supernatural radiance.

अहमात्मा गुडाकेश
सर्वभूताशयस्थितः ।
अहमादिश्च मध्यं च
भूतानामन्त एव च ॥१०.२०॥
ahamātmā guḍākeśa
sarvabhūtāśayasthitaḥ
ahamādiśca madhyaṁ ca
bhūtānāmanta eva ca (10.20)

aham — I; ātmā — self; guḍākeśa — sleep—regulator; sarvabhūtāśayasthitaḥ = sarva — all + bhūta — beings + āśaya — mystic resting place + sthitaḥ — situated in; aham — I; ādiśca = ādiḥ — beginning + ca — and; madhyam — middle; ca — and; bhūtānām — of the beings; anta — end; eva — indeed; ca — and

O sleep regulator, I am the person Who is situated in the mystic resting place of all beings. I am responsible for the beginning, middle, and end of all beings. (10.20)

Commentary:

There is a resting place in each being, otherwise each being could not sleep and rise as if properly rested. That location exists. Where is it? We are usually unconscious or semi—conscious when resting. We cannot determine the psychological location of the resting place. We are like men who are taken to a room blind—folded and who are released from that room in the same sightless condition. How would we ever know where the room is located?

In the yoga process, one learns how to enter samādhi trance states, wherein one consciously exits from this dimension and enters into other psychological niches. One such entry is into the resting place within one's being. In samādhi one enters that place with a minute objectivity, so that one can know where it is located and see who else resides in it.

Śrī Krishna claims that He resides in there always.

Arjuna was addressed by Śrī Krishna as guḍākeśa, the sleep regulator, because Arjuna had once conquered sleep when he did yoga austerities. Arjuna was known to have a relatively greater control over the sleeping impulse in the psyche. This sleeping impulse is controlled by the life force. Thus by mastering the 4th stage of yoga, prāṇāyāma, one gains some mastery over the sleeping tendency of the life force.

Śrī Krishna presented Himself as being responsible for the beginning, middle, and end of all beings. This is because what we understand as our being or our psychology, both individually and collectively, is an aggregate of various parts. It is not just one subtle item. Śrī Krishna regarded Himself as the person under whose supervision, these beings are formulated, maintained and demolished. The being of a person consists of his spirit, his sense of I—ness, his mind, his intellect organ in the subtle body, and his life force, with or without a material gross body.

आदित्यानामहं विष्णुर्
ज्योतिषां रविरंशुमान् ।
मरीचिर्मरुतामस्मि
नक्षत्राणामहं शशी ॥ १०.२१ ॥
ādityānāmahaṁ viṣṇur
jyotiṣāṁ raviraṁśumān
marīcirmarutāmasmi
nakṣatrāṇāmahaṁ śaśī (10.21)

ādityānām — of the Adityas; aham — I; viṣṇur = viṣṇuḥ — Vishnu; jyotiṣām — of lights; ravir = raviḥ — the sun; aṁśumān — radiant; marīcir = marīciḥ — Marici; marutām — of the thunderstormers; asmi — I am; nakṣatrāṇām — of the stars; aham — I; śaśī — the moon

Of the Ādityas, I am Vishnu. Of lights, I am represented by the radiant sun. Of the thunderstormers, I am represented by Marīci. Of the stars, I am signified by the moon. (10.21)

Commentary:

The rest of this chapter concerns the preliminary course in Krishna consciousness, the original lessons taught by Śrī Krishna to Arjuna. Nowadays many teachers of Krishna consciousness make certain that they become known as originators of this teaching but here we see that Śrī Krishna Himself taught the course to Arjuna. We can learn it directly from Śrī Krishna in these verses. By studying this, we can adhere to and be self—indoctrinated in Krishna consciousness.

Even though the modern teachers seem to think that a person cannot be Krishna conscious unless he keeps their association or joins their society, toeing their line, here we get the idea from Śrī Krishna that we can train ourselves in Krishna consciousness by attributing major personalities and objects to Him.

As a disciple in the society established by Śrīla A.C. Bhaktivedanta Swami Prabhupāda, I was instructed by one of his sannyasi disciples named Kīrtanānanda Swami, to always remember Śrī Krishna and never to forget Him. This was an instruction which he gave to all others who came in contact with him. Their system was to indoctrinate themselves and all others to be Krishna conscious along the lines given in these verses. However they did not mention at any stage that the course was given in detail in the *Gītā*. Instead the impression was conveyed that it came down from Swami Bhaktivedanta, that powerhouse of the Krishna consciousness society.

For the purposes of yoga, we do not want to impress anyone with that sort of idea. For kriyā yoga, one must understand that this system of elementary Krishna consciousness was taught directly by Śrī Krishna. One should make a careful study of these verses in Chapter Ten to see how to indoctrinate oneself, so that the tendency for associative thinking is diverted from social consciousness to this Krishna consciousness.

For the purposes of yoga, this is only elementary Krishna consciousness and nothing else. The advanced level is different. The elementary course is necessary initially. When one masters the pratyāhār sense withdrawal and the other higher stages of yoga, this system becomes for the most part, unnecessary, because then one will have direct mystic and spiritual perception and would not need to rely on associative thinking.

To study this elementary Krishna consciousness and to learn how to implement it as a habit, one must take each example given by Śrī Krishna and get as much information as possible on it and see exactly what Śrī Krishna is trying to teach in each case.

For example: The Ādityas were sons of Aditī. They are listed in Canto 6, Chapter Six, verses 38 and 39 of the Śrīmad Bhāgavatam, as Vivasvān, Aryamā, Puṣa, Tvaṣṭā, Savitā, Bhaga, Dhātā, Vidhātā, Varuṇa, Mitra, Śatru and Urukrāma.

The person listed as the example in this verse, named Vishnu, is the same Urukrāma listed in the Śrīmad Bhāgavatam. Two others namely Vivasvān and Aryamā are mentioned elsewhere in the *Gītā*. To understand this teaching of elementary Krishna consciousness, one should know the story of the said Urukrāma or Vishnu. He appeared in a dwarf body and defeated King Bali. Without the use of weapons, He reduced Bali. The story is told in several of the *Puranas*, but specifically in the Bhāgavat and Vishnu *Puranas*. The point is that unless one is familiar with Vedic histories one cannot understand some of the examples. Thus we see that those who took births in Indian families where they were exposed to these stories in infancy, seem to hold a monopoly on understanding many of the examples.

We can understand the examples which are not culturally restricted. The second example of the radiant sun representing Śrī Krishna among the lights, we can understand clearly, perhaps even more so than someone from India who is not so knowledgeable on astronomical data. Recently due to advanced telescopes and satellites, we know for certain that the planets in our solar system are controlled by the sun. It is clear that Śrī Krishna means this elementary Krishna consciousness to be a way of attributing every great thing to Himself, causing us to think of Him, conceive of Him, and associate Him with everything that is spectacular and prominent. This has little to do with spiritual objects. It applies more to the material things which we can plainly see.

In the Vedic history which nowadays is considered to be mostly mythology, Marīci is one of the Marutas or thunderstormers. Modern scientific data indicates that thunderstorms are produced by electromagnetic and chemical energies in the atmosphere. They do not figure in a supernatural factor. Before the days of modern science, the supernatural influences were regarded, even to an absurd degree. This exaggeration of the supernatural factors caused it to become discredited when scientific evidence was later presented.

In the Vedic history, weather is controlled personally. It is not just a matter of electromagnetic and chemical interactions, but this cannot be proven by the scientific methods used today. To understand the Vedic perspective one has to use mystic insight or merely believe the scriptures on faith. Thus for us to understand what Śrī Krishna said from a purely modern stance, it would mean that a hurricane or a tornado is representative of Śrī Krishna in the matter of thunderstorms.

Śrī Krishna wants His devotees to see the moon as being representative of Himself in terms of the stars which shine. This is because to us the moon is the biggest visible object. Modern astronomy clarified that in actuality the stars are much, much bigger objects than the tiny moon which is only a satellite to this planet. To our sense perception, the moon is more predominant in terms of the tides it creates, the moods it induces, and the light it provides.

वेदानां सामवेदोऽस्मि
देवानामस्मि वासवः ।
इन्द्रियाणां मनश्चास्मि
भूतानामस्मि चेतना ॥ १०.२२ ॥
vedānāṁ sāmavedo'smi
devānāmasmi vāsavaḥ
indriyāṇāṁ manaścāsmi
bhūtānāmasmi cetanā (10.22)

vedānām — of the Vedas; sāmavedo = sāmavedaḥ — Sāma Veda; 'smi = asmi — I am; devānām — of the supernatural rulers; asmi — I am; vāsavaḥ — Vāsava Indra; indriyāṇām — of the senses; manaścāsmi = manas — mind + ca — and + asmi — I am; bhūtānām — of the creature forms; asmi — I am; cetanā — consciousness

Of the *Vedas*, I am represented by the Sāma Veda. Of the supernatural rulers, I am represented as Vāsava Indra. Of the senses, I am represented as the mind. In creature forms, I am represented as consciousness. (10.22)

Commentary:

The example of the Sāma Veda can hardly be understood even by many of the commentators who come from India and who give their self—acclaimed authorized commentaries. Many of these people have not read the *Vedas*. They do not take those ancient texts seriously, because to a greater extent, the *Vedas* are not so applicable to the current cultural environment. Thus, in context, the *Vedas* were the most used scripture in India, and the Sāma Veda was the most important and popular one.

The Vedic history states that on the Swārga heavenly planets, King Indra listens to the Sāma Veda. To Arjuna, because he was culturally-aware, every example that Śrī Krishna cited made sense.

Vasava Indra is considered to be an emperor in the heavenly world as the ruler of the small—time lords in that domain. Thus Śrī Krishna presents Indra as His representative.

Both the ancient yoga philosophy and the modern psychology attribute the mind as the regulator and collector of data of the senses. This is easily grasped. Here again the point is made clear that even in the matter of psychology, we can be Krishna conscious by always associating Śrī Krishna with the best, the highest and the most prominent feature.

Śrī Krishna proposed Himself as being representative of consciousness in the creature forms. That consciousness, of course, is the highest force in any material body, a force without which the body is pronounced dead.

रुद्राणां शंकरश्चास्मि
वित्तेशो यक्षरक्षसाम् ।
वसूनां पावकश्चास्मि
मेरुः शिखरिणामहम् ॥ १०.२३ ॥
rudrāṇāṁ śaṁkaraścāsmi
vitteśo yakṣarakṣasām
vasūnāṁ pāvakaścāsmi
meruḥ śikhariṇāmaham (10.23)

rudrāṇām — of the cosmic destroyers; śaṁkaraścāsmi = śaṁkaraḥ — Shankara Shiva + ca — and + asmi — I am; vitteśo = vitteśaḥ — Kubera; yakṣarakṣasām — of the Yakshas and Rakshas; vasūnām — of the Vasus; pāvakaścāsmi = pāvakaḥ — Pavāka + ca — and + asmi — I am; meruḥ — Meru; śikhariṇām — of the mountains; aham — I

Of the cosmic destroyers, I am represented by the Shankara Shiva. Of the Yakshas and Rakshas, I am best represented as Vittesha Kubera. Of the Vasus, I am represented by Pāvaka Agni. Of the mountains, I am represented as Mount Meru. (10.23)

Commentary:

Again throughout this training in elementary Krishna consciousness, a reader should be familiar with Vedic scriptures which include the *Puranas*, the *Mahābhārata* and the

Rāmāyaṇa. Without the familiarity, the meaning of some examples will not be clear. Śrīla Bhaktivedanta Swami, who had an impact on Western society, particularly in the United States and England, taught this elementary Krishna conscious course as well as what he presented as the advanced course which is the learning of Krishna līlā pastimes, which are events from the life of Śrī Krishna as described in the Śrīmad Bhagavata Purāṇa.

I found, however, that his course was haphazardly given to newcomers in his society. For the purposes of kriyā yoga, one does not have to subject oneself to such a society because the elementary course is given here by Śrī Krishna. If one makes the effort, he can learn directly from the *Bhagavad Gītā*. One does not have to join a society and be intimidated by its members, just to learn how to become Krishna conscious.

Vedic literature lists the Rudras as the cosmic destroyers. They are said to be the ones who can make people cry or become very distressed. Even though the physical destruction of the universe is described in the *Puranas*, still there is stress on the supernatural causes of it. The Rudras are said to be the ones who start the fiery explosions which bring on the cosmic destruction. Shankara Shiva is listed here as the foremost of these Rudras. Śrī Krishna wants to be considered as being represented by Shankara.

The example of Vittesha Kuvera also requires some knowledge of the Vedic literature. Arjuna was familiar with the information of these gods of the Vedic pantheon. Thus all the examples were useful to him. Pāvaka Agni is another Vedic figure. Mount Meru is also identified as the highest Himalayan peak, showing that Śrī Krishna wants to be accredited as being the foremost of everything.

पुरोधसां च मुख्यं मां
विद्धि पार्थ बृहस्पतिम् ।
सेनानीनामहं स्कन्दः
सरसामस्मि सागरः ॥१०.२४॥
purodhasāṁ ca mukhyaṁ māṁ
viddhi pārtha bṛhaspatim
senānīnāmahaṁ skandaḥ
sarasāmasmi sāgaraḥ (10.24)

purodhasām — of the family priest; ca — and; mukhyam — chief; mām — me; viddhi — know; pārtha — son of Pṛthā; bṛhaspatim — Bṛhaspati; senānīnām — of the commanders; aham — I; skandaḥ — Skanda; sarasām — of the seas; asmi — I am; sāgaraḥ — the ocean

O son of Pṛthā, know Me as being represented by Brihaspati, the chief of the family priests. Of military commanders, I am represented by Skanda. Of the seas, I am symbolized by the ocean. (10.24)

Commentary:

Bṛhaspati is the chief of the celestial priests in the Swārga heavenly place. Skanda is the military commander of the angelic people. We can readily understand that the ocean is the largest of the seas.

महर्षीणां भृगुरहं
गिरामस्म्येकमक्षरम् ।
यज्ञानां जपयज्ञोऽस्मि
स्थावराणां हिमालयः ॥१०.२५॥
maharṣīṇāṁ bhṛguraham
girāmasmyekamakṣaram
yajñānāṁ japayajño'smi
sthāvarāṇāṁ himālayaḥ (10.25)

maharṣīṇām — of the great yogi sages; bhṛgur = bhṛguḥ — Brigu; aham — I; girām — of spoken words; asmy = asmi — I; ekamakṣaram — one—syllable sound; yajñānām — of the religiously—motivated disciplines; japayajño = japayajñaḥ — the discipline of uttering prayers; 'smi = asmi — I am; sthāvarāṇām — of the stationary objects; himālayaḥ — Himalaya

Of the great yogi sages, Bhrigu is one whom I am best represented by. Of the spoken words, I am represented by the one—syllable sound. Of the religiously—motivated disciplines, I am represented best by the discipline of uttering prayers. Of stationary objects, I am best represented by the Himalayas. (10.25)

Commentary:

Bhṛgu is a great Vaishnava yogi devotee. He is considered to be the foremost Vaishnava ritualist. The famous one-syllable sound in Sanskrit is *Om*, but in other languages *Om* is not even considered. In any language, the most important one-syllable sound would be representative of Śrī Krishna.

The religiously-motivated disciplines for ordinary worship of God centers around the discipline of prayers which aims at calling out to God, petitioning Him and addressing Him in numerous ways. Each religious sect that believes in a Supreme Being, has its particular way of saying prayers. In the Vedic setting the focus is on chanting the name of God. This is called japa. This japa, chanting of the holy names, was stressed by Śrīla Bhaktivedanta Swami as the main process of salvation for this age.

In yoga, however, it is only one of the disciplines we perform. Śrī Krishna wants us to regard japa chanting as being representative of Him, just like the other examples. By the layout of the *Gītā*, we learn that Krishna assigned japa as one of the aspects which represents Him. He does not list it as the only and most important one.

Of the stationary objects, Śrī Krishna is represented by the Himalayas, the highest of the mountain ranges on Earth.

अश्वत्थः सर्ववृक्षाणां
देवर्षीणां च नारदः ।
गन्धर्वाणां चित्ररथः
सिद्धानां कपिलो मुनिः ॥१०.२६॥
aśvatthaḥ sarvavṛkṣāṇāṁ
devarṣīṇāṁ ca nāradaḥ
gandharvāṇāṁ citrarathaḥ
siddhānāṁ kapilo muniḥ (10.26)

aśvatthaḥ — sacred fig tree; sarvavṛkṣāṇāṁ = sarva — all + vṛksāṇām — of trees; devarṣīṇām — of the celestial supernatural yogi sages; ca — and; nāradaḥ — Narada; gandharvāṇām — of the supernatural singers; citrarathaḥ — Citraratha; siddhānām — of the perfected souls; kapilo = kapilaḥ — Kapila; muniḥ — yogi philosopher

Of all trees, I am best represented by the Ashvattha sacred fig tree. Of the supernatural yogi sages, I am represented by Narada. Of the supernatural singers, it is Chitraratha; of the perfected souls, the yogi philosopher Kapila. (10.26)

Commentary:

Generally, the Ashvattha tree is not found on every continent. With the diaspora of Hindus, some of these sacred trees are being planted here and there. The fact remains that the Indian traditional regard for such trees is not transplanted as easily as the trees can be. In other words, the Indian culture will go through dilution and alteration as it is transplanted elsewhere. Even for Hindus abroad, the meaning of the Ashvattha tree as a representation of Śrī Krishna, will lose the significance it had in the time of Arjuna.

A deva rishi is a supernatural sage or a yogi sage. It is a person who practiced or is still practicing yoga and who uses a supernatural body in the astral world. Such a body cannot die except at the end of the universe when all the subtle bodies perish. Right now we are in a subtle body which is enclosed or housed in a gross form. Persons like Nārada no longer take gross bodies. They remain in subtle forms which are regarded as being supernatural because they are highly—energized, far beyond the level of our subtle bodies, the forms we awkwardly use in dreams.

Chitraratha, as the Vedic history states, is the chief of the angelic singers, having the most appealing voice. Śrī Krishna considered this person to be His representative. Kapila, otherwise known as Kapila Muni, the son of Devahūti, and rated as an incarnation of Godhead, is a mahāyogī siddha. He is supreme among the philosopher yogis. His history is narrated in the Śrīmad Bhagavata Purāṇa.

Even though Śrī Kapila Muni was a mahāyogī of repute, the history in the Śrīmad Bhāgavatam focuses on his divinity and his deliverance of his mother, Devahūti. These are fantastic pastimes which bewitch many devotees of Krishna, causing them to think they would be delivered effortlessly by Lord Kapila or by some other Vishnu personality. Such devotees, naive about the means of soul perfection, give little credence to the yoga austerities performed by Srimati Devahūti and her husband Kardama even before Śrī Kapila took birth from Devahūti's body.

The stress is given to Śrī Kapila's philosophy which he explained in detail to Devahūti. Maitreya Muni narrated this to Śrī Vidura, who at the time of listening to the story was an advanced kriyā yogi.

उच्चैःश्रवसमश्वानां
विद्धि माममृतोद्भवम् ।
ऐरावतं गजेन्द्राणां
नराणां च नराधिपम् ॥ १०.२७॥
uccaiḥśravasamaśvānāṁ
viddhi māmamṛtodbhavam
airāvataṁ gajendrāṇāṁ
narāṇāṁ ca narādhipam (10.27)

uccaihśravasam — the supernatural horse Uccaihśrava; aśvānām — of the horses; viddhi — know; mām — me; amṛtodbhavam = amṛta — a sweet celestial sea + udbhavam — born from; airāvatam — Airāvata; gajendrāṇām — of kingly elephants; narāṇām — of men; ca — and; narādhipam — King of men

Of horses, know Me as represented by the supernatural horse Uccaihśrava, which was born of the sweet celestial sea. Of the kingly elephants, know Me as represented by Airāvata, and know Me as the King of men. (10.27)

Commentary:

Uchchaihshravah is mentioned throughout the *Puranas* as a celestial horse of repute. Sometimes it is said that this horse appeared from the stirring of the Ocean of Nectar. Airāvata, a supernatural elephant, also appeared in the same way. This creature serves as the mount of Indra, the ruler of the Swārga heaven. This is significant to those of us who were brought up in India and who were in environments where the *Puranas* were read and the culture was accommodating to the Vedic way of life.

The rest of us, being in tune with other cultures, have a limitation because we cannot get the entire significance of some examples. We can appreciate what Śrī Krishna taught, that whatever or whoever is great, is representative of Him. He is represented by the President of any country, the ruler of men.

आयुधानामहं वज्रं
धेनूनामस्मि कामधुक् ।
प्रजनश्चास्मि कन्दर्पः
सर्पाणामस्मि वासुकिः ॥१०.२८॥
āyudhānāmahaṁ vajraṁ
dhenūnāmasmi kāmadhuk
prajanaścāsmi kandarpaḥ
sarpāṇāmasmi vāsukiḥ (10.28)

āyudhānām — of weapons; aham — I; vajram — supernatural thunderbolt; dhenūnām — of cows; asmi — I am; kāmadhuk — supernatural Kamadhuk cow; prajanaścāsmi = prajanas — begetting + ca — and + asmi — I am; kandarpaḥ — Kandarpa, the god of romance; sarpāṇām — of serpents; asmi — I am; vāsukiḥ — Vāsuki

Of weapons, I am compared to the Vajra supernatural thunderbolt. Of cows, I am represented as the supernatural Kamadhuk. And in the case of begetting, I am represented by Kandarpa, the god of romance. Of serpents, I am represented by Vāsuki. (10.28)

Commentary:

The Vajra thunderbolt is a weapon used by the Indra demigod, who rules the Swārga heavenly place. This is supposed to be a supreme weapon. Even though we never see such a weapon today, some devotees depict it in drawings based on what they read in the *Puranas*. Puranic descriptions give the idea that such a weapon can create lightning. Indra is described as using it to kill opponents in the physical and subtle world.

The application is that any powerful weapon may be viewed as being representative of Śrī Krishna. Thus modern instruments of destruction like missiles which carry the potential for nuclear explosions are representative of Śrī Krishna.

Kāmadhuk is the leader of the supernatural cows and Vāsuki of the supernatural snakes. Apart from the training in elementary Krishna consciousness, we are also being given a basis for a belief in subtle animals and objects. Many of these examples cite subtle persons, animals or objects. It means therefore that on this path, we should at some point perceive subtle things.

Presently, our subtle perception is channeled through the physical body to such a degree that we hardly remember dreams. We are confused as to the difference between the subtle world and imagination. However if we attend to kriyā practice in earnest, our subtle body would shift off from the physical circuits which use it and then we would see into the subtle world more clearly.

In the case of begetting, Śrī Krishna represented Himself through Kandarpa, the demigod of the lusty power through which progeny is generated. The *Puranas* relate that Kandarpa is so charismatic, that he affects even Brahmā, the person who produced his body at the dawn of creation. Such a person that is as influential as Kandarpa is representative of Śrī Krishna.

अनन्तश्चास्मि नागानां
वरुणो यादसामहम् ।
पितृणामर्यमा चास्मि
यमः संयमतामहम् ॥१०.२९॥
anantaścāsmi nāgānāṁ
varuṇo yādasāmaham
pitṝṇāmaryamā cāsmi
yamaḥ saṁyamatāmaham (10.29)

anantaścāsmi = anantaḥ — Ananta + ca — and + asmi — I am; nāgānām — of supernatural snakes; varuṇo = varuṇaḥ — Varuṇa; yādasām — of the aquatics; aham — I; pitṝṇām — of the piously—departed ancestors; aryamā — Aryamā; cāsmi = ca — and + asmi — I am; yamaḥ — Yama; saṁyamatām — of the subduers; aham — I

I am represented by Ananta among the supernatural snakes. I am represented by Varuṇa, among the aquatics. Among the piously—departed spirits, I am represented by Aryamā. Of the subduers, I am represented by Yama. (10.29)

Commentary:

Ananta, Varuṇa, Aryamā and Yama are from the Vedic pantheon. Those of us who are not familiar will not grasp their significance. Ananta, a supernatural snake of repute in the Vedic literature, is rated as an incarnation of Godhead. This creature is depicted in a serpentine body with many heads. He is said to be the bed—couch of Lord Vishnu and is identical with Baladeva, Śrī Krishna's brother. The depiction for the lesson of this elementary Krishna consciousness is that Ananta is the supreme serpent and has divinity. Thus he is representative of Śrī Krishna.

Varuṇa is a supernatural being who presides over the seas, particularly over aquatic wealth. Aryamā presides over departed spirits making sure that they are accommodated in new and appropriate bodies as need be. He supervises their rebirth on earthly planets like this one and facilitates their religious sentiments by giving facility for the worship of God in the spirit world, where these ancestors wait for the opportunity to get infant forms. The place of Aryamā would be termed purgatory in Christian theology.

Yama presides over the death of a human body. His duty is to make sure that persons who acted recklessly or sinfully during their earthly life, are fittingly punished so that ultimately they may be reformed from a criminal mentality. Yama tries to accelerate our learning capability by displaying a personal concern for our reform from anti—social habits. In Christianity, God is presented as the judge of the dead but in the Vedic pantheon, someone else does the task. He is called Yama.

In the history of the kriyā yogis, Yama is a mahāyogī who discovered effective kriyās for realizing his subtle body. He was the spiritual master of Nachiketa of Upanishadic fame. According to the narration, Yama took a crude material body at the time when the first humans began to manifest after an era of cavemen. Yama was the first rishi to consciously separate his subtle form from the physical one. He excelled in the practice and then took the post of judge of the departed souls in order to supervise the final separation of a spirit from a material body. He achieved the position by genius in kriyā practice.

प्रह्लादश्चास्मि दैत्यानां
कालः कलयतामहम् ।
मृगाणां च मृगेन्द्रोऽहं
वैनतेयश्च पक्षिणाम् ॥ १०.३० ॥
prahlādaścāsmi daityānāṁ
kālaḥ kalayatāmaham
mṛgāṇāṁ ca mṛgendro'haṁ
vainateyaśca pakṣiṇām (10.30)

prahlādaścāsmi = prahlādaḥ — Prahlāda + ca — and + asmi — I am; daityānām — of the titan descendants of Diti; kālaḥ — time; kalayatām — of the monitors; aham — I; mṛgāṇām — of the animals; ca — and; mṛgendro = mṛgendraḥ — king of the beasts; 'ham = aham — I; vainateyaśca = vainateyaḥ — son of Vinata + ca — and; pakṣiṇām — of the birds

And I am represented as Prahlāda among the titan descendants of Diti, as time of the monitors, as the king of beasts among the animals, as the son of Vinata among the birds. (10.30)

Commentary:

Prahlāda and Vinata are from the Vedic pantheon. Prahlāda is a reputed devotee of Lord Vishnu. He was rescued from the harassment of his father by the Vishnu personality who appears as Narasingha, a form with the head of a lion and the trunk of a human being. In that birth, Prahlāda appeared in a royal family which did not believe that Lord Vishnu was the Supreme Person. Prahlāda absorbed the Vishnu belief when his mother, being pregnant with his embryo, was counseled by Śrī Nārada Muni.

Prahlāda was the only person in that dynasty who had such a strong belief in Lord Vishnu. Thus Śrī Krishna cites Prahlāda as His representative in that clan. Vinata is a supernatural woman who produced some animal species, one being that of the birds. The son of Vinata mentioned here is Garuḍa who according to the Vedic literature serves as the air-conveyance of Lord Vishnu.

Śrī Krishna represented Himself as time among the factors which monitor existence, and as the lion, the king of the beasts.

पवनः पवतामस्मि
रामः शस्त्रभृतामहम्।
झषाणां मकरश्चास्मि
स्रोतसामस्मि जाह्नवी ॥१०.३१॥
pavanaḥ pavatāmasmi
rāmaḥ śastrabhṛtāmaham
jhaṣāṇāṁ makaraścāsmi
srotasāmasmi jāhnavī (10.31)

pavanaḥ — the wind; pavatām — of the cleansers; asmi — I am; rāmaḥ — Rāma; śastrabhṛtām — of the weapon carriers; aham — I; jhaṣāṇām — of sea monsters; makaraścāsmi = makaraḥ — shark + ca — and + asmi — I am; srotasām — of rivers; asmi — I am; jāhnavī — daughter of Jahnu

Among the cleansers, I am best represented by the wind. Of the weapon carriers, I am best represented by Rāma. Of the sea monsters, I am represented by the shark. Of the rivers, I am represented by Jahnu's daughter. (10.31)

Commentary:

Śrī Rāma and Jahnu's daughter, Jahnavī, are from the Vedic literature. The most famous of the Rāmas is Rāma, the son of Dasharatha of the Rāmāyaṇa fame. There is another famous Rāma who became known as Paraśurāma, the son of Renukā and Jamadagni. Rāma, the son of Dasharatha, is rated as a Godhead personality. Paraśurāma is rated as being empowered. Both of them were foremost warriors, but Rāma proved to be the superior of Paraśurāma.

Jānavī is another name of the Ganges River. Śrī Krishna selected the best of everything to serve as reminders of Himself in this course of elementary Krishna consciousness. He is represented by the wind among the purifiers and the shark among the sea monsters.

सर्गाणामादिरन्तश्च
मध्यं चैवाहमर्जुन ।
अध्यात्मविद्या विद्यानां
वादः प्रवदतामहम् ॥१०.३२॥
sargāṇāmādirantaśca
madhyaṁ caivāhamarjuna
adhyātmavidyā vidyānāṁ
vādaḥ pravadatāmaham (10.32)

sargāṇām — of creations; ādir = ādiḥ — formation; antaśca = antaḥ — ending + ca — and; madhyam — continuation; caivāham = ca — and + eva — indeed + aham — I; arjuna — Arjuna; adhyātmavidyā — knowledge of the Supreme Soul; vidyānām — of sciences; vādaḥ — conclusion; pravadatām — of the logicians; aham — I

Of creations, I am represented by the formation, continuation and ending. O Arjuna, of the sciences, I am knowledge of the Supreme Soul. I am represented by the conclusion of the logicians. (10.32)

Commentary:

Sargāṇām refers to the mundane creations which manifest in the material energy by combination and transmutation. These occur by a supernatural pressure which remains unseen to physical vision. The scientific community is stuck at the point of subtle matter and can go no further to discover the supernatural interference of the spirits and the Supreme Spirit. However in yoga, we are just as eager as the modern scientists to discover the Cause of all causes. We do this by mystic research, using the buddhi organ in the head of the subtle body. We develop prāṇa vision which helps us to see the atomic constituents of matter as well as her nuclear operations.

The scientific community is content to use the buddhi organ for inventing formulas which help them understand the subtle operations of material energy. We use the same intellect for direct mystic perception. There is not much difference between a nuclear physicist and a yogi, except that the yogi uses his intellect for direct perception, rather than to design a computer which can carry out amazingly—detailed calculations.

We, the yogis, reach a stage where we stabilize our intellect organ and then focus it as a seeing eye, while the physicist uses his intellect as a tool for creating precision machines. It is the same subtle organ being used. In the more advanced stages, a yogi outpaces the physicist, since the yogi begins to use the chitta energy in the causal body as seeing-eyes. A physicist, because he cannot go beyond the analytic ability of the intellect organ, cannot go to the causal plane.

There are many successful yogis, who after entering the causal level through samādhi practice, come back into this world to accept glory as spiritual masters of repute and as miracle workers, but some yogis go on and simply disappear out of history. Not all of the yogis are interested in coming back into this world to be adored by the unliberated human beings.

In the elementary Krishna conscious practice, Śrī Krishna desires that a devotee, be he a yogi or not, consider that the formation, continuation and ending of the creations be representative of Him.

Of the sciences, the knowledge of the Supreme Soul is the highest. In kriyā yoga initially, we are concerned with the knowledge of our own souls for self—realization. Later on, following in the footsteps of great mahāyogīs like Markandeya and Śrī Nārada Muni, we do investigation into the Supreme Soul. This, however, is not book knowledge combined with faith or belief in the Supreme Being. This is by direct mystic perception in all soberness with a cleansed psychology.

Modern science has a hard time accommodating the science of the ordinary self and that of the Supreme Self, because these factors are not manifested grossly. The reliance on gross bodies for sense perception causes a limitation in the scientific thinking. However recently, due mostly to ingestion of hallucinogenic drugs, some universities intensified studies on psychology and psychiatry into the field of sciences. Thus there is an effort to bring the self and Supreme Self into the field of investigation.

Some persons feel that Śrīla Bhaktivedanta Swami and others like Śrī Paramhansa Yoganandiji and Swami Vivekananda, as well as others from India, all caused the Western universities to include the self and the Supreme Self in the field of science. However without neglecting these Swamis, we must state that the actual cause of the inclusion of psychology and psychiatry is the intake of hallucinogenic and narcotic drugs by college professors. Hallucinogenic drugs, when taken, affect the subtle body and haphazardly open its psychic perception.

The experience is immediate and requires no austerity. It is very convincing. This caused some professors to influence the faculties of large universities to include psychology and psychiatry as sciences. Śrī Patañjali Maharishi, in his Yoga Sutra, listed herbs as a means of increased subtle perception. Many ascetics in India take potent herbs like marijuana along with certain hallucinogenic mushrooms. Some use opium and its derivatives.

Many of those very same ascetics who took Western bodies, by their intuition of the matter, took herbs again when they took birth in the Western society and were employed as college professors. Hallucinogenic drugs have a way of breaking loose the hold that materialistic culture has over an individual. Thus we see that many Western youths rebelled against their conservative Christian upbringing and joined with Eastern swamis after taking drugs. Some of these swamis unfortunately, being enamoured of themselves and being quick to boast of their empowerment, failed to realize this and neglected to accredit the drugs. Regardless, that does not deny what actually occurred in the 1960s and 1970s in the developed countries.

For instance, Śrīla Bhaktivedanta Swami, our Vaishnava spiritual master, stressed that it was Śrī Krishna and his spiritual master, a certain Bhaktisiddhānta Saraswati, who arranged for his success among American youths. With all due respect to Swami Bhaktivedanta, if we are to accept what he said verbatim, then it would mean that he suggested that the majority of his disciples were influenced by Śrī Krishna and his guru to take LSD, marijuana, peyote mushrooms, psilocybin and such drugs, just so they could disorient themselves from their Western conditioning and join him when he went to the United States in the late 1960s. Most of this is factual, but we do not believe that Śrī Krishna caused it. It occurred by habit of the subtle body. Both their ingestion of hallucinogenic drugs and their subsequent acceptance of his authority and way of thinking were caused by tendencies stored in the subtle bodies. These features were reactivated again in the new life when they took birth in Western civilization. Śrī Krishna has very little to do with this.

When we attribute every act to Śrī Krishna, then His personal actions become confused with the all—pervading energy which is automatically supervising everything.

Śrī Krishna would also like to be remembered when we consider the conclusion of the logicians. In this way, the remembrance of Śrī Krishna could take over the life of a devotee who would recall Śrī Krishna in any and all endeavors.

अक्षराणामकारोऽस्मि
द्वंद्वः सामासिकस्य च ।
अहमेवाक्षयः कालो
धाताहं विश्वतोमुखः ॥१०.३३॥
akṣarāṇāmakāro'smi
dvaṁdvaḥ sāmāsikasya ca
ahamevākṣayaḥ kālo
dhātāhaṁ viśvatomukhaḥ (10.33)

akṣarāṇām — of letters; akāro = akāraḥ — the letter A; 'smi = asmi — I am; dvandvaḥ — two—word compound; sāmāsikasya — of the word combinations; ca — and; aham — I; evākṣayaḥ = eva — indeed + akṣayaḥ — infinite; kālo = kālaḥ — time; dhātāham = dhātā — Dhātā Brahmā + aham — I; viśvatomukhaḥ — one who faces all directions, four—faced

Of letters, I am represented by the letter A. Of the word combinations, I am represented by the two—word compound. I am comparable to infinite time. I am represented by Dhātā, the four—faced Brahmā. (10.33)

Commentary:

The letter A is not the first letter in every alphabet but it is so in Sanskrit, the language in which the *Gītā* was written. The point is that the first letter of any alphabet should be considered as representative of Śrī Krishna. In Sanskrit as well as in English, two—word compounds are used. In Sanskrit, there are many such compounds. Sanskrit has facility for letter changes in compounded words to ease pronunciation of conflicting sounds when words are combined with other words. The two—word compound is the most frequently used compound occurring in the Sanskrit literature.

मृत्युः सर्वहरश्चाहम्
उद्भवश्च भविष्यताम् ।
कीर्तिः श्रीर्वाक्क नारीणां
स्मृतिर्मेधा धृतिः क्षमा ॥ १०.३४
mṛtyuḥ sarvaharaścāham
udbhavaśca bhaviṣyatām
kīrtiḥ śrīrvākca nārīṇāṁ
smṛtirmedhā dhṛtiḥ kṣamā
(10.34)

mṛtyuḥ — death; sarvaharaścāham = sarvaharaḥ — all—devouring + ca — and + aham — I; udbhavaśca = udbhavaḥ — origin + ca — and; bhaviṣyatām — of things which are to be produced; kīrtiḥ — Kīrti, goddess of fame; śrīr = śrīḥ — Shri, goddess of fortune; vāk — Vāk, goddess of speech; ca — and; nārīṇām — of women; smṛtir = smṛtiḥ — Smṛti, goddess of recollection; medhā — Medhā, goddess of counsel; dhṛtiḥ — Dhṛti, goddess of faithfulness; kṣamā — Kṣamā, goddess of patience

I am represented as all—devouring death. I am the foundation of things that are to be produced. And among women, I am represented by Kīrti, the goddess of fame, Śrī, the goddess of fortune, Vāk, the goddess of speech, Smṛti, the goddess of recollection, Medhā, the goddess of counsel, Dhṛti, the goddess of faithfulness and Kṣama, the goddess of patience. (10.34)

Commentary:

Śrī Krishna wants to be regarded when we view the spectre of death, a factor which affects all material manifestation, even the mundane bodies which are used by divine beings like Śrī Krishna. Death consumes all things in the gross and subtle mundane existences. Death of a form causes the entity to shift his attention from one level to another.

Krishna desires to be regarded as the foundation of those things which are yet to be produced. Among women He is represented as the goddess of fame, Śrī, the goddess of speech, Vāk, the goddess of recollection, Smṛti, the goddess of council, Medhā, the goddess of faithfulness, Dhṛti and the goddess of patience, Kşama.

These goddesses are from the Vedic pantheon of deities. In terms of kriyā yoga, we learn from this, that the qualities of fame and oratory, the facets of recollection, good council, faithfulness and patience are sourced in supernatural females. When doing Kuṇḍalinī yoga, one begins to see various deities within the chakras in the subtle body. Sometimes, one of the deities leaves the body and another takes the position. In Kuṇḍalinī yoga, one realizes that what he considered to be himself or his own nature and psychology, is a combination of many energies and personalities.

Fame, fortune, good speech, education, recollection and the other qualities do not necessarily originate with any of us. We may regard these as gifts from supernatural people.

We are not complete. Much of what we are, or what we feel we are, is awarded to us on a continuous or periodic basis.

बृहत्साम तथा साम्नां
गायत्री छन्दसामहम् ।
मासानां मार्गशीर्षोऽहम्
ऋतूनां कुसुमाकरः ॥ १०.३५॥
bṛhatsāma tathā sāmnāṁ
gāyatrī chandasāmaham
māsānāṁ mārgaśīrṣo'ham
ṛtūnāṁ kusumākaraḥ (10.35)

bṛhatsāma — Brihat Sāma Melody; tathā — also; sāmnām — of the Sāma Veda chants; gāyatrī — Gayatri; chandasām — of the poetic hymns; aham — I; māsānām — of months; mārgaśīrṣo = mārgaśīrṣaḥ — November—December lunar month; 'ham = aham — I; ṛtūnām — of seasons; kusumākaraḥ — spring

Of the Sāma Veda chants, the Brhat Sāma melody represents Me. Of the poetic hymns, I am the Gayatri. Of months, I am best represented by the November—December lunar month. Of the seasons, I am best compared to Spring. (10.35)

Commentary:

The Brihat Sāma and Gayatri are Sanskrit poems. The Gayatri is a short poem. These are regarded as sacred in the Vedic system of religion. From the *Puranas*, we get the feeling that when the Sanskrit sound was chanted with exact pronunciation by a qualified mystic priest, certain effects were produced as intended by the priest, but nowadays this hardly happens.

I had a friend who really believed in the Vedic mantras which are mostly one, two or four-line verses. He thought that by chanting certain verses one could do anything. In any case, he was ruined. Nowadays the environment is not responsive to the Vedic chants. There is an effort to revive this but it is a lost cause, because we cannot turn back time. Still many swamis come from India assuring us that they have the ultimate mantras, which will bestow upon us all spiritual things. It is for the most part a farce played out by these swamis.

The Brihat Sāma and the Gayatri are still to be regarded as sacred by kriyā yogis but not for the purpose of using these to get anything. We accept them as sacred. We leave the matter there. Sometimes in the kriyā lineage, one gets a Gayatri mantra. This may be given by the yogi teacher physically or astrally, but such a mantra should not be used to acquire anything. It is mostly used as a Call Prayer and as a contact point with a certain divine personality.

A kriyā yogi should not use a Mahamantra or a Gayatri prayer as a washing machine to cleanse his mind or anything similar. He should wash his mind by prāṇāyāma, which is the ultimate purifier in that regard. For the purposes of kriyā yoga, the mantras are only Call Prayers.

Śrī Krishna wants us to regard Him as being represented in the Sāma Veda, the Gayatri Mantra, the November—December period of the year when the stars shine their brightest, and the Spring season when the vegetation springs to life each year.

By studying these representations, we get an idea of how to be Krishna conscious even in respect to mundane objects like the sun and the moon and in respect to the passing year and the seasonal changes.

द्यूतं छलयतामस्मि
तेजस्तेजस्विनामहम् ।
जयोऽस्मि व्यवसायोऽस्मि
सत्त्वं सत्त्ववतामहम् ॥ १०.३६॥

dyūtam — gambling skill; chalayatām — of the swindlers; asmi — I am; tejaḥ — splendor; tejasvinām — of the splendid things; aham — I; jayo = jayaḥ — victory;

dyūtaṁ chalayatāmasmi
tejastejasvināmaham
jayo'smi vyavasāyo'smi
sattvaṁ sattvavatāmaham (10.36)

'smi = asmi — I am; vyavasāyo = vyavasāyaḥ — endeavor; 'smi = asmi — I am; sattvam — reality; sattvavatām — of the real things; aham — I

I am represented as the gambling skill of the swindlers. I am compared to the splendor of the splendid things. I am compared to victory and endeavor. I am the reality of the realistic things. (10.36)

Commentary:

Śrī Krishna even posits Himself in reference to the gambling skill of swindlers, a ruinous thing indeed. He shows clearly how we may be Krishna conscious in every regard. In the course of kriyā yoga, a person moves away from the mundane situation. Eventually the mundane objects pale in their significance. The yogi's progress accelerates. He begins to observe how the mind and buddhi organ function. He pays less and less attention to what they interact with. Instead he studies their methods of operation. So long as the yogi continues to struggle with the interacting mind and remains baffled by its contents, he gains considerably by putting into practice this elementary Krishna consciousness. He remains linked to this associative thinking about Śrī Krishna, by using the analogies given here to assign everything a representation of Śrī Krishna.

Śrī Krishna gave value to the splendor of splendid things, to victory and endeavor, and to realism.

वृष्णीनां वासुदेवोऽस्मि
पाण्डवानां धनंजयः ।
मुनीनामप्यहं व्यासः
कवीनामुशना कविः ॥१०.३७॥
vṛṣṇīnāṁ vāsudevo'smi
pāṇḍavānāṁ dhanaṁjayaḥ
munīnāmapyahaṁ vyāsaḥ
kavīnāmuśanā kaviḥ (10.37)

vṛṣṇīnām — of the Vrishnis; vāsudevo = vāsudevaḥ — the son of Vasudeva; 'smi = asmi — I am; pāṇḍavānām — of the Pandavas; dhanaṁjayaḥ — Arjuna; munīnām — of the yogi philosophers; apy = api — also; aham — I; vyāsaḥ — Vyasa; kavīnām — of poets; uśanā — Ushana; kaviḥ — respected poet

Of the Vṛṣṇis, I am the son of Vasudeva. Of the Pāṇḍavas, I am represented by Arjuna. Of the yogi philosophers, I am compared to Vyāsa. Of the poets, I am represented by the respected poet Uśanā. (10.37)

Commentary:

It is interesting that Śrī Krishna posited Himself as the son of Vasudeva among the Vrishnis, because Śrī Krishna was in fact, just that, the son of Vasudeva of the Vrishni clan. The significance is that in so far as taking a body from a human male and female, Śrī Krishna was the best of the children of Vasudeva.

Of the sons of Pāndu, Śrī Krishna was represented by Arjuna, the very person whom He first tutored in this Krishna consciousness. Śrī Krishna directly used Arjuna to play out the karma yoga functions which Krishna Himself organized and designed as divine actions on earth. Of the yogi philosophers, Śrī Krishna was represented by Śrīla Vyāsadeva, the person who is accredited with the authorship of the *Mahābhārata* of which this *Bhagavad Gītā* is a part. Of the poets, it is Ushana or Pandit Shukracharya, a poetic genius of the past.

दण्डो दमयतामस्मि
नीतिरस्मि जिगीषताम् ।
मौनं चैवास्मि गुह्यानां
ज्ञानं ज्ञानवतामहम् ॥ १०.३८॥
daṇḍo damayatāmasmi
nītirasmi jigīṣatām
maunaṁ caivāsmi guhyānāṁ
jñānaṁ jñānavatāmaham (10.38)

daṇdo = daṇḍaḥ — authority to punish; damayatām — of the rulers; asmi — I am; nītir = nītiḥ — morality; asmi — I am; jigīṣatām — of those seeking victory; maunam — silence; caivāsmi = ca — and + eva — indeed + asmi — I am; guhyānām — of secrets; jñānam — knowledge; jñānavatām — of those who know; aham — I

Of rulers, I am the authority to punish. For those seeking victory, I may be compared to the means of morality; of secrets, I am represented by silence. In wise men, I am represented as knowledge. (10.38)

Commentary:

Śrī Krishna's authority to punish is not just an analogy as the history of the *Mahābhārata* shows and as the *Gītā* illustrates in the dramatic and brash display of the Universal Form, which is revealed in the next chapter. There Śrī Krishna told Arjuna why He came to scare any and everyone who opposed His will.

For methods of attaining victory, none is so certain and so enduring as morality. It is through morality that one eventually rules over in any given situation. Thus Śrī Krishna posits Himself as being represented by that. In the *Gītā*, which is a textbook about karma yoga, Krishna's style of morality stands out as the method of victory used by King Yudhiṣṭhira. It is because of Yudhiṣṭhira's persistent moral stance, that Śrī Krishna was so attached to that prince and supported him in the Kuru Civil War.

Of secrets, it is silence, and of the wise men, it is their knowledge.

यच्चापि सर्वभूतानां
बीजं तदहमर्जुन ।
न तदस्ति विना यत्स्यान्
मया भूतं चराचरम् ॥ १०.३९॥
yaccāpi sarvabhūtānāṁ
bījaṁ tadahamarjuna
na tadasti vinā yatsyān
mayā bhūtaṁ carācaram (10.39)

yac = yad — which; cāpi = ca — and + api — also; sarvabhūtānām — of all created beings; bījam — origin point; tad — that; aham — I; arjuna — Arjuna; na — not; tad — that; asti — is; vinā — without; yat = yad — which; syān = syāt — should be; mayā — through My influence; bhūtam — existing; carācaram — active or stationary

And O Arjuna, I am the origin of all created beings. There is nothing active or stationary which could exist without My influence. (10.39)

Commentary:

Here again as before in the *Gītā*, and as will be expressed further on, Śrī Krishna established Himself as the be-all and end-all of this gross and subtle existence with which we are somewhat familiar. He cites Himself as the origin of all created beings and as the causal influence in whatever is active or stationary. Again there is no proof, other than Śrī Krishna's credibility.

In kriyā yoga, at a certain stage, it becomes important to know if Someone in particular is the Cause of all causes. The yogi acknowledges that Person and gets His permission to advance to even higher stages. Such a person, the Supreme Personality of Godhead, as Śrīla Bhaktivedanta Swami so aptly addressed Him, would be the right person as the ultimate focus of a kriyā yogi, for the yogi's understanding of his relationship with that God.

नान्तोऽस्ति मम दिव्यानां
विभूतीनां परंतप ।
एष तूद्देशतः प्रोक्तो
विभूतेर्विस्तरो मया ॥ १०.४० ॥
nānto'sti mama divyānāṁ
vibhūtīnāṁ paraṁtapa
eṣa tūddeśataḥ prokto
vibhūtervistaro mayā (10.40)

nānto (nāntaḥ) = na — no + antaḥ — end; 'sti = asti — is; mama — of My; divyānām — of the supernatural; vibhūtīnām — manifestations; paraṁtapa — burner of enemy forces; eṣa — this; tūddeśataḥ = tu — but + uddeśataḥ — for a sample; prokto = proktaḥ — explained; vibhūter = vibhūteḥ — of the opulences; vistaro = vistaraḥ — of the spreading, extensive; mayā — by Me

There is no end to My supernatural manifestations, O burner of the enemy forces. This was explained by Me as a sampling of My extensive opulence. (10.40)

Commentary:

Śrī Krishna spoke of the supernatural manifestations which give rise to these subtle and gross worlds which we experience outside and inside our psychology. Whatever Śrī Krishna described previously in giving the elementary lessons on Krishna consciousness, was only a sampling of his extensive opulence. From that sampling, a devotee can expand the Krishna consciousness idea to everything encountered in the material world.

यद्यद्विभूतिमत्सत्त्वं
श्रीमदूर्जितमेव वा ।
तत्तदेवावगच्छ त्वं
मम तेजोंशसंभवम् ॥ १०.४१ ॥
yadyadvibhūtimatsattvaṁ
śrīmadūrjitameva vā
tattadevāvagaccha tvaṁ
mama tejoṁśasaṁbhavam (10.41)

yad yad — what, whatever; vibhūtimat — fantastic; sattvam — real object; śrīmad = śrīmat — prosperous; ūrjitam — powerful; eva — indeed; vā — or; tat tad = tat tat — this, that, any case; evāvagaccha = eva — indeed + avagaccha — realize; tvam — you; mama — of Me; tejo = tejaḥ — splendor; 'ṁśasaṁbhavam (aṁśasaṁbhavam) = aṁśa — fraction + saṁbhavam — origin

You should realize that whatever fantastic existence, whatever prosperous or powerful object there is, in any case, it originates from a fraction of My splendor. (10.41)

Commentary:

Elsewhere in the Śrīmad Bhagavata Purāṇa and the Vishnu Purāṇa, the factor which Śrī Krishna listed as a fraction of His splendor, is named as divine persons, namely Lord Mahavishnu or Lord Karanadakashayi Vishnu. Thus Śrī Krishna awards that Supergod as only a trifling portion of His glory. This is a person.

How great, therefore, is Śrī Krishna? Or rather, how great does Śrī Krishna consider Himself to be? Again we have no proof yet besides Śrī Krishna's word.

अथ वा बहुनैतेन
किं ज्ञातेन तवार्जुन ।
विष्टभ्याहमिदं कृत्स्नम्
एकांशेन स्थितो जगत् ॥ १०.४२ ॥
atha vā bahunaitena
kiṁ jñātena tavārjuna
viṣṭabhyāhamidaṁ kṛtsnam
ekāṁśena sthito jagat (10.42)

atha vā — but; bahunaitena = bahunā — with extensive + etena — with this; kim — what is the value?; jñātena — with information; tavārjuna = tava — of you + arjuna — Arjuna; viṣṭabhyāham = viṣṭabhya — supporting + aham — I; idam — this; kṛtsnam — entire; ekāṁśena = eka — one + aṁśena — by a fraction; sthito = sthitaḥ — based, standing; jagat — world

But Arjuna, what is the value of this extensive information? As the foundation, I support this entire universe with a fraction of Myself. (10.42)

__Commentary:__

This is a very good question that Śrī Krishna asked Arjuna because this information, which to Śrī Krishna was elementary, is important to us as kriyā yogis. The value of the extensive information, which Arjuna requested and which Śrī Krishna graciously and willingly gave, is this: We must understand how these subtle and gross material objects are produced by the Supreme Being. How have they entered into our purview?

CHAPTER 11

The Universal Form*

अर्जुन उवाच
मदनुग्रहाय परमं
गुह्यमध्यात्मसंज्ञितम् ।
यत्त्वयोक्तं वचस्तेन
मोहोऽयं विगतो मम ॥११.१॥
arjuna uvāca
madanugrahāya paramaṁ
guhyamadhyātmasaṁjñitam
yattvayoktaṁ vacastena
moho'yaṁ vigato mama (11.1)

arjuna — Arjuna: uvāca — said; madanugrahāya — kindness to me, as a matter of mercy to me; paramaṁ — highest; guhyam — private; adhyātmasaṁjñitam = adhyātma — Supersoul + samjnitam — known as; yad — which; tvayoktaṁ = tvaya — by you + uktam — explained; vacaḥ — lecture; tena — by this; moho = mohaḥ — delusion; 'yam = ayam — this; vigato = vigataḥ — departed; mama — of me (11.1)

Arjuna said: As a matter of mercy to me, the highest, most private information of the Supreme Soul was explained by You in this lecture. Subsequently, the delusion departed from me. (11.1)

Commentary:

What Arjuna acclaims as the highest, most private information of the Supreme Soul, is considered to be merely external information about Śrī Krishna. Why then did Arjuna give the previous chapter so much value? Some modern Vaishnava teachers, following the lead of Lord Śrī Chaitanya Mahaprabhu, say that the highest most private information deals with the relationship with Śrī Krishna, a relationship based on devotional service, either as His servant, friend, relative or lover, all based on eternal spiritual connections, something that the modern teachers say will help the devotee to reawaken his dormant love for Śrī Krishna.

This view is based on a question and answer session between Śrī Caitanya Mahāprabhu and Śrī Rāmananda Raya who is said to be the incarnation of Arjuna. Interestingly, in that conversation, Lord Chaitanya, whose Personality is a delicate combination of Radha and Krishna, inquired from Rāmananda Raya, an expert on bhaktisiddhānta, the theology of Vaishnavism. When hearing about the value of certain things, Lord Chaitanya rebuffs every answer given by Śrī Rāmananda Raya indicating that such things were external, pertaining to the subtle or gross material worlds. Śrī Caitanya only accepted the answers when Rāmananda Raya cited the loving relationships with Lord Krishna. Being relieved to hear something which He considered to be truly transcendental, Lord Chaitanya told Rāmananda to speak on, until Rāmananda cited the sexual love the gopis had for Śrī Krishna.

However here, in the *Bhagavad Gītā*, we do not hear a word about the gopis or about their sexuality towards Krishna. What exactly is the connection? Is Arjuna not really understanding the discourse? Has Arjuna overrated the elementary information?

**The Mahābhārata contains no chapter headings. This title was assigned by the translator on the basis of verse 16 of this chapter.*

The answer is that Arjuna is right on the mark. As a practicing kriyā yogi, he lived in the time of the gopis and was aware of their romance with Krishna. Still he cited Chapter Ten as being the highest, most private information. If we look closely at verses 10 and 11, we will have no doubt as to Arjuna's assessment of this chapter. Those two verses hint at a kriyā technique which would give us the break to discover and utilize the affectionate relationship each of us might have with Śrī Krishna, either directly or through an agent. Here are those two verses:

teṣāṁ satatayuktānāṁ bhajatāṁ prītipūrvakam
dadāmi buddhiyogaṁ taṁ yena māmupayānti te (10.10)
teṣāmevānukampārtham ahamajñānajaṁ tamaḥ
nāśayāmyātmabhāvastho jñānadīpena bhāsvatā (10.11)

Of those who are constantly disciplined, who worship with affection, I give the technique by which they draw near to Me. (10.10)

In the interest of assisting them, I who am situated within their beings, cause the ignorance, produced by the stupefying influence of material nature to be banished by their clear realized insight. (10.11)

As kriyā yogis, we follow in the footsteps of Arjuna, wanting to know of our relationship to Śrī Krishna, and not so much to focus on the relationship of the gopis. Their relationship was already attained. For us we try to activate a relationship by getting from Śrī Krishna or from his agent, the technique by which we can draw near to Him.

In assisting us one by one, individually, Śrī Krishna is supposed to banish the ignorance produced by the stupefying influence of material nature, so we could have clear insight. This happens when we master the last three stages, namely dhāraṇa, dhyāna and samādhi, when our buddhi organ is freed up from its absorption with the sensual energies, so it can perceive directly the supernatural and spiritual realities.

Śrī Krishna's lecture of elementary Krishna consciousness forms the bulk of Chapter Ten but verses 7 through 11, five verses in all, give us the highest most private information that Arjuna acclaimed.

Arjuna accepted that information from Śrī Krishna as a matter of mercy, because even though Arjuna had to a degree, mastered the advanced practices, he did not apply them to Śrī Krishna as described in those verses. He was thankful for the techniques. He said that his delusion departed, not just the delusion about his role at Kurukṣetra, but his delusion in terms of how to use his yoga skill to develop the divine loving relationship with God. That was solved for Arjuna. Essentially Arjuna said, "I did not know before that I could apply yoga skills to the mystery of Your own and my own existence and the connection between us as well. Before, I applied yoga to get weapons from Lord Shiva and Lord Indra for the sake of becoming the foremost warrior and for assisting my eldest brother. Now I hear of another, most relevant use of yoga skills."

Śrī Krishna, up to this Chapter Eleven, instructed Arjuna not only in karma yoga but in psyche yoga.

भवाप्ययौ हि भूतानां
श्रुतौ विस्तरशो मया ।
त्वत्तः कमलपत्राक्ष
माहात्म्यमपि चाव्ययम् ॥ ११.२॥

bhavāpyayau = bhava — origin + apy (api) – also + ayau — ruination; hi — indeed; bhūtānām — of the beings; śrutau — both were heard; vistaraśo = vistaraśaḥ — in detail; mayā — by me; tvattaḥ — from you; kamalapatrākṣa = kamala – lotus + patra –

bhavāpyayau hi bhūtānāṁ
śrutau vistaraśo mayā
tvattaḥ kamalapatrākṣa
māhātmyamapi cāvyayam (11.2)

petal + akṣa — eyed; māhātmyam — majestic glory; api — also; cāvyayam = ca — and + avyayam — eternally

The description of the origin and ruination of the beings was heard in detail by me, O Person Whose eyes are shaped like lotus petals. You also described Your eternal majestic glory. (11.2)

Commentary:

Śrī Krishna, a very handsome and pretty man, the Supreme Being as He depicted Himself, was being both admired and feared by Arjuna, because Krishna described Himself as the origin and ruination of the living beings. Śrī Krishna was pretty handsome as Arjuna viewed Him but Arjuna understood that He was quite dangerous as well.

एवमेतद्यथात्थ त्वम्
आत्मानं परमेश्वर ।
द्रष्टुमिच्छामि ते रूपम्
ऐश्वरं पुरुषोत्तम ॥ ११.३ ॥
evametadyathāttha tvam
ātmānaṁ parameśvara
draṣṭumicchāmi te rūpam
ěśvaraṁ puruṣottama (11.3)

evam — thus; etad — this; yathāttha = yathā — as + attha — you explain; tvam — you; ātmānam — yourself; parameśvara — O Supreme Lord; draṣṭum — to see; icchāmi — I wish; te — your; rūpam — form; aiśvaram — majesty; puruṣottama — O Supreme Person

This is as You explained about Yourself, O Supreme Lord. I wish to see Your Majestic Form, O Supreme Person. (11.3)

Commentary:

Arjuna therefore asked to see the Majestic Form of Śrī Krishna, the Form which carries out the origination and ruination of all beings. It is clear now that Śrī Krishna used a physical body which was not the form used by Him to execute the creative-destructive functions described. Śrī Krishna's physical form was both handsome and dangerous but not as awe—inspiring as the form that Arjuna requested to see.

In a very frank talk, plain and simple, Arjuna said that Śrī Krishna gave sufficient information but information is only just that. It is not the experience. Arjuna said, "You said everything about your supernatural power over these beings. You described your extensive control over everything, O glorious personality with the beautiful lotus eyes. If it is as you say, O God, let me experience this with certainty."

मन्यसे यदि तच्छक्यं
मया द्रष्टुमिति प्रभो ।
योगेश्वर ततो मे त्वं
दर्शयात्मानमव्ययम् ॥ ११.४ ॥
manyase yadi tacchakyaṁ
mayā draṣṭumiti prabho
yogeśvara tato me tvaṁ
darśayātmānamavyayam (11.4)

manyase — you think; yadi — if; tac = tad — that; chakyam = sakyam — possible; mayā — by me; draṣṭum — to see; iti — thus; prabho — O Lord; yogeśvara — Master of yoga technique; tato = tataḥ — then; me — to me; tvam — you; darśayātmānam = darśayā — make it be seen + ātmānam — self; avyayam — eternal

If You think that it is possible for me to see this, O Lord, Master of the yoga technique, then make me see You in that Eternal Form. (11.4)

Commentary:

Śrī Krishna was a master of the yoga technique because He mastered the techniques of His time. In just five or six months, an incredibly short time, He was given the techniques by Mahāyogī Rishi Upamanyu. A skill that takes us many lives to master, Śrī Krishna completed in just five months. Thus it is not simply a name that Arjuna gave Śrī Krishna as Yogeshwara. Śrī Krishna by physical and mystic actions in performance of the yoga kriyās, did in fact, master the art of it in the nick of time.

This particular request of Arjuna is craved by many neophyte kriyā yogis who hunt down famous kriyā masters to give shaktipat initiation. Recently in the subtle world I spoke to Siddha Swami Muktananda, a famous modern siddha, who departed his physical body. I discussed this shaktipat with him because he was one of the teachers who popularized it. In a list he explained that it was reliant on both the spiritual master who is a mahāyogī and the disciple who is a serious practicing yogi. Swami Muktananda feels that unless the spiritual master has a sealed celibate physical form, he cannot impart shaktipat. He claims that it can hardly be given to a student who also does not possess a sealed physical form.

If that is true, it means that most of us cannot get shaktipat in this life because we do not have such forms. Now the question is this: What is a sealed celibate physical form? The Swami told me this: "If you are born from parents who follow the Vedic regulative principles regarding sexual intercourse and if you yourself never had any such intercourse in the new body assumed, and if again you practiced yoga from childhood, then you would have such a form, otherwise no."

On the other hand, opposed to these siddhas are persons like our Vaishnava spiritual master, Śrīla Bhaktivedanta Swami. They bear the view that shaktipat initiation is mostly hocus pocus. They feel that the idea of being touched by a guru and then becoming enlightened is nonsense.

What Swami Muktananda told me makes sense. I myself do not have such a sealed celibate physical form. I am not empowered in this physical form to give shaktipat initiation. Many people who approached me over the years have hinted that I should give them that sort of initiation but I am unable to do it. However that does not mean that I am not a yogi of worth. It simply means that my physical body has those limitations.

I specialize in helping students who do not have a sealed physical form as described. They are not likely to absorb shaktipat initiations. Therefore they can use the kriyās which I successfully practiced.

Śrī Krishna will give Arjuna that shaktipat initiation but after all, they were born in the Vedic setting from parents who followed the regulations according to that lifestyle, and they were both yogis of repute. To boot, Śrī Krishna portrayed Himself as the Supreme Being.

Strikingly, Śrī Krishna was requested to make Arjuna see that supernatural form which causes the creation and destruction of these living beings. For those of us who do not have the sealed celibate physical form, Swami Muktananda feels that we have to purify our subtle and physical bodies to a greater degree before our vision opens up into the supernatural world.

There is a misunderstanding that shaktipat initiation is given by a kriyā master for the purpose of proving that the spiritual master is God. Generally when shaktipat is given it is designed to accelerate the samādhi experience of the disciple, to allow him to use his buddhi organ as a supernatural eye for seeing supernatural objects. At present we cannot see into that world. We rely on information from scripture and testimony of realized yogis but when the buddhi organ is restricted in kriyā yoga practices, we can view the supernatural objects.

That Śrī Krishna awarded Arjuna the supernatural vision to see the beings who comprise Śrī Krishna's Universal Form, does not imply that every yogin awards that or desires to award something like that. A yogi is not God. If he is a true yogi, his purpose in awarding shaktipat would not be to prove that he is God but rather to accelerate the purification of a student yogi.

श्रीभगवानुवाच
पश्य मे पार्थ रूपाणि
शतशोऽथ सहस्रशः ।
नानाविधानि दिव्यानि
नानावर्णाकृतीनि च ॥ ११.५॥
śrībhagavānuvāca
paśya me pārtha rūpāṇi
śataśo'tha sahasraśaḥ
nānāvidhāni divyāni
nānāvarṇākṛtīni ca (11.5)

śrībhagavān — the Blessed Lord; uvāca — said; paśya — see; me — My; pārtha — son of Pṛthā; rūpāṇi — forms; śataśo = śataśaḥ — hundred; 'tha = atha — or; sahasraśaḥ — thousand; nānāvidhāni — variously manifested; divyāni — supernatural; nānāvarṇākṛtīni = nānā — various + varṇa — color + ākṛtīni — shapes + ca — and

The Blessed Lord said: O son of Pṛthā, see My forms in the hundreds or rather in the thousands, variously manifested, supernatural and of the various colors and shapes. (11.5)

Commentary:

At first Śrī Krishna mentioned the hundreds of supernatural beings. Then He said there were thousands. This is because there are different categories of these beings all beginning with the Central Figure of the Universal Form, Who is Śrī Krishna Himself. There are those who are close to Him, whose power level is closer to His. For others, the power trails off.

Recently in this life, using this body, I saw that Universal Form once but before in former lives I have seen it in entirety. I can make a few statements based on seeing it in the past life, according to the recall coming up from my subtle body. When Śrī Krishna called each of these forms His own form, we have to understand that the empowerment of these forms are His own to a degree, otherwise each of the Beings except the Central Figure have their own power which is boosted authentically by Śrī Krishna's empowerment. Practically speaking, in the whole vision of it, every living creature everywhere is a part of that Universal Form, even ants and bacteria. It is a very awesome vision. The vision should not be desired by persons of fickle heart. It is very frightening to see such a form in a contrasting way. Everyone is located somewhere in that Form, even though most of us are not aware of our position in it. Still, if one happens to view it in a contrasting way, one will become afraid of the apparition.

What is wonderful about revelation, what we must agree with modern Vaishnava teachers on, is Śrī Krishna's nonchalant cool display of the Form. There was no preparation by Śrī Krishna. Arjuna asked on the spur of the moment and without hesitation, Śrī Krishna displayed the Form. This proves that Śrī Krishna was not limited by the physical body He used. Śrī Balarāma, Śrī Krishna's elder brother, used to do supernatural things just like that, spontaneously. However such displays cannot be exhibited by most other persons, even though others are part of the Form.

Śrī Krishna alerted Arjuna that some of the figures would not be recognizable. There would also be wonderful aspects of the natural and supernatural worlds, which Arjuna would see that might terrify him. Thus Śrī Krishna warned Arjuna to look out for the unusual.

पश्यादित्यान्वसून्रुद्रान्
अश्विनौ मरुतस्तथा ।
बहून्यदृष्टपूर्वाणि
पश्याश्चर्याणि भारत ॥ ११.६ ॥
paśyādityānvasūnrudrān
aśvinau marutastathā
bahūnyadṛṣṭapūrvāṇi
paśyāścaryāṇi bhārata (11.6)

paśyādityān = paśya — look at + ādityān — supernatural rulers; vasūn — Vasus; rudrān — supernatural destroyers; aśvinau — two supernatural doctors; marutaḥ — supernatural stormers; tathā — also; bahūny = bahūni — many; adṛṣṭapūrvāṇi = adṛṣṭa — unseen + pūrvāṇi — before; paśyāścaryāṇi = paśya — view + āścaryāṇi — wonders; bhārata — O relation of the Bharata family

Look at the supernatural rulers, the supernatural destroyers, the two supernatural doctors and the supernatural stormers. View many wonders which were unseen before, O relation of the Bharata family. (11.6)

Commentary:

Śrī Krishna wanted Arjuna to take a good look at the personalities who were under Śrī Krishna's control. As the Central Personality, the Ultimate Controller, Śrī Krishna regulated all that was enacted in the material world. Thus Arjuna was to draw the conclusion that Śrī Krishna's will was absolute. It is not that Śrī Krishna alone has autonomy but rather, other supernatural rulers and even the supernatural destroyers were all circumspect in relation to Śrī Krishna. After seeing this, Arjuna would understand that it was in his best interest to cooperate with Śrī Krishna.

इहैकस्थं जगत्कृत्स्नं
पश्याद्य सचराचरम् ।
मम देहे गुडाकेश
यच्चान्यद्द्रष्टुमिच्छसि ॥ ११.७ ॥
ihaikasthaṁ jagatkṛtsnaṁ
paśyādya sacarācaram
mama dehe guḍākeśa
yaccānyaddraṣṭumicchasi (11.7)

ihaikastham = iha — here + ekastham — situated in one reality; jagat — universe; kṛtsnam — entire; paśyādya = pasya — see + adya — now; sacarācaram – with active and inactive; mama — of Me; dehe — in the body; guḍākeśa — O conqueror of sleep; yac = yad — what; cānyad = cānyat = ca — and + anyat — other; draṣṭum — to see; icchasi — you desire

Here, O conqueror of sleep, you see the entire universe with all active and inactive manifestations, situated as one reality, in My body. And observe any other manifestations which you desire to see. (11.7)

Commentary:

By stringent practice, Arjuna conquered sleep but still those austerities did not give him the ability to see the Universal Form of Śrī Krishna, except if he was allowed to view it by Krishna. Thus by addressing Arjuna as the conqueror of sleep, Śrī Krishna hints at the limitations of Arjuna's former yoga practice which did not reveal Krishna's Universal Form.

Over the years of teaching and having the opportunity to introduce and encourage people to take up yoga, I found that many people have an idea of what they want to derive from the practice. Here, we see that yoga practice does not give one everything. Sometimes one has to get help from a mahāyogīn, just as Śrī Krishna assisted Arjuna to see that Form. Yoga is relevant but it will not give one everything. Some association with great souls is required. Yoga is there for self or psyche purification mostly and for little else.

What Śrī Krishna displayed was situated as one reality in His body. The interesting thing is that "body" in the verse means the physical body Śrī Krishna used, because the Sanskrit term is dehe. Thus we must understand that Śrī Krishna, as He walked around in that physical form, carried with Him all powers and glories in full. He was that Person even though He used a physical form. Everything, even what was situated in distant places, was located supernaturally in that Universal Form.

न तु मां शक्यसे द्रष्टुम्
अनेनैव स्वचक्षुषा ।
दिव्यं ददामि ते चक्षुः
पश्य मे योगमैश्वरम् ॥ ११.८ ॥ ॥
na tu māṁ śakyase draṣṭum
anenaiva svacakṣuṣā
divyaṁ dadāmi te cakṣuḥ
paśya me yogamaiśvaram (11.8)

na — not; tu — but; mām — Me; śakyase — you can; draṣṭum — to see; anenaiva = anena — by this + iva (eva) — indeed; svacakṣuṣā — with your vision; divyam — supernatural; dadāmi — I give; te — to you; cakṣuḥ — sight; paśya — look at; me — Me; yogam - mystic power; aiśvaram — majesty

But you cannot see with your vision. I give you supernatural sight to look at My mystic majesty. (11.8)

Commentary:

With physical vision, Arjuna could not see the Universal Form, even though Śrī Krishna displayed it. This means that the Form was not to be seen physically. Arjuna was staring at Śrī Krishna but he could not see anything besides Krishna's physical body. Noticing this, Śrī Krishna decided to award Arjuna supernatural vision and to blank out for the time being Arjuna's physical sight. Sometimes an artist depicts the scene of the Universal Form and conveys the idea that Arjuna, as well as others on the warfield, were seeing the Form with physical eyes. Such illustrations are misleading because the Form cannot be seen with physical vision. Physical eyes have nothing to do with supernatural vision. When one gets the vision, he sees it even with his eyelids closed.

Śrīla Bhaktivedanta Swami did write in his commentary that those who were spiritually awakened saw the Universal Form. What exactly does he mean by spiritually—awake? Was the Swami seeing the Form? Were his disciples whom he accredited as being pure devotees seeing the Form? One sees such a Form when supernatural vision becomes available. It does not happen ordinarily even to devotees of Krishna, even to pure devotees. After all, who can be a purer devotee than Arjuna?

By using the terms svacakṣuṣā, Śrī Krishna made a demarcation between Arjuna and Himself. Śrī Krishna did that when He spoke of Arjuna's perpetual lack of recall of past lives. Thus it is obvious that even a pure devotee may not have the supernatural eyes. The term sva means something that is one's own, something natural.

संजय उवाच
एवमुक्त्वा ततो राजन्
महायोगेश्वरो हरिः ।
दर्शयामास पार्थाय
परमं रूपमैश्वरम् ॥ ११.९॥
saṁjaya uvāca
evamuktvā tato rājan
mahāyogeśvaro hariḥ
darśayāmāsa pārthāya
paramaṁ rūpamaiśvaram (11.9)

saṁjaya – Sanjaya; uvāca — said; evam — thus; uktvā — having said; tato = tataḥ — then; rājan — O King; mahāyogeśvaro = mahāyogeśvaraḥ — the great master of yoga; hariḥ — Hari, the God Vishnu; darśayāmāsa — reveals; pārthāya — to the son of Pritha; paramam — supreme; rūpam – form; aiśvaram — supernatural glory

Sanjaya said: O King, having said that, the great Master of yoga, Hari, the God Vishnu, revealed to the son of Pṛthā, the Supreme Form, the supernatural glory. (11.9)

Commentary:

Sanjaya took a pause to stress to King Dhṛtarāṣṭra that Arjuna was shown the Form. Śrī Krishna was everything He claimed. He gave the supernatural vision in order to convince Arjuna of the supremacy extolled. Sanjaya wanted to impress upon King Dhṛtarāṣṭra, that Śrī Krishna was for real. Here was no mock God. This was the Supreme Person present physically at Kurukṣetra. In this way, Sanjaya tried to shock King Dhṛtarāṣṭra. However Dhṛtarāṣṭra did not budge from his position of supporting his sons against Yudhiṣṭhira whom Śrī Krishna backed. Dhṛtarāṣṭra was unable to put to use the facts which were presented to him respectfully by Sanjaya. Sanjaya reminded Dhṛtarāṣṭra that Śrī Krishna was both a practical great yogin as well as the God Vishnu who according to Vedic scriptures is supposed to be the creator of these material worlds.

अनेकवक्त्रनयनम्
अनेकाद्भुतदर्शनम् ।
अनेकदिव्याभरणं
दिव्यानेकोद्यतायुधम् ॥ ११.१०॥
anekavaktranayanam
anekādbhutadarśanam
anekadivyābharaṇaṁ
divyānekodyatāyudham (11.10)

anekavaktranayanam = aneka — countless + vaktra — mouth + nayanam — eye; anekādbhutadarśanam = aneka — countless + adbhuta — wonders + darśanam — vision; anekadivyābharaṇaṁ = aneka — countless + divya — supernatural + ābharaṇam — ornament; divyānekodyatāyudham = divya — supernatural + aneka — countless + udyata — uplifted + āyudham — weapon

Countless mouths, eyes, wondrous visions, countless supernatural ornaments, supernatural uplifted weapons, (11.10)

Commentary:

Sanjaya did see the Universal Form. Therefore we have to assume that he had the supernatural vision. He was awarded it just as Arjuna was. In either case, Sanjaya was a practicing yogi. His teacher was the great yogin named Krishna Dvaipāyana Vyāsadeva, the writer of the *Mahābhārata* history.

Dhṛtarāṣṭra could not see the Form. He relied on what Sanjaya described to him. This had nothing to do with Dhṛtarāṣṭra's blind physical condition. The supernatural vision has nothing to do with physical sight. A person who is blind physically can be a kriyā yogi. Or he can be graced by Śrī Krishna, supernaturally.

The supernatural vision is based on using the imagination orb in the buddhi organ of the subtle body. Even a blind man has such an orb. It is a technique of using that orb to see into the chit shakti or the sky of consciousness which usually appears to be just darkness. In fact most human beings are blind supernaturally.

दिव्यमाल्याम्बरधरं
दिव्यगन्धानुलेपनम् ।
सर्वाश्चर्यमयं देवम्
अनन्तं विश्वतोमुखम् ॥ ११.११ ॥
divyamālyāmbaradharaṁ
divyagandhānulepanam
sarvāścaryamayaṁ devam
anantaṁ viśvatomukham (11.11)

divyamālyāmbaradharam = divya — supernatural + mālya — garland + ambara — garment + dharam — wearing; divyagandhānulepanam = divya — supernatural + gandha — perfume + anulepanam — ointment; sarvāścaryamayam = sarvaścarya – all wonder + mayam — made of; devam — God; anantam — infinite; viśvatomukham — facing all directions

...wearing supernatural garlands and garments, with supernatural perfumes and ointments, appearing all wonderful, the God appeared infinite as He faced all directions. (11.11)

Commentary:

Interestingly, the Universal Form with expansions of personalities as well with its varied powers, was adorned fittingly. The central figure of it appeared to be infinite, as He faced all directions simultaneously.

This is why artists have depicted the Universal form showing faces in all directions, peering spherically.

दिवि सूर्यसहस्रस्य
भवेद्युगपदुत्थिता ।
यदि भाः सदृशी सा स्याद्
भासस्तस्य महात्मनः ॥ ११.१२ ॥
divi sūryasahasrasya
bhavedyugapadutthitā
yadi bhāḥ sadṛśī sā syād
bhāsastasya mahātmanaḥ (11.12)

divi — in the sky; sūryasahasrasya = sūrya — sun + sahasrasya — of one thousand; bhaved = bhavet — should be; yugapad — at once; utthitā — risen; yadi — if; bhāḥ — brilliance; sadṛśi — such; sā — it; syād — it might be; bhāsaḥ — of brightness; tasya — of it; mahātmanaḥ — of the great personality

Imagine in the sky, a thousand suns, being at once risen together. If such a brilliance were to be, it might be compared to that Great Personality. (11.12)

Commentary:

This is a very apt comparison, except that the light seen by Sanjaya was a supernatural illumination which is different from the physical luminescence that we know. However, it gave Dhṛtarāṣṭra some idea of Who he opposed in the person of Śrī Krishna. Sanjaya told him, "Just you try to imagine what sort of light it would be if a thousand suns were risen at once. That is the brilliance of the Universal Personality."

Of course the irony of this is that Sanjaya forgot that Dhṛtarāṣṭra was born blind, so the King's concept of the sun was reduced only to the heat radiating from it. We can understand however that Sanjaya was trying his best to convey to Dhṛtarāṣṭra what brilliance there was in the supernatural world as a result of the presence of Krishna.

तत्रैकस्थं जगत्कृत्स्नं
प्रविभक्तमनेकधा ।
अपश्यद्देवदेवस्य
शरीरे पाण्डवस्तदा ॥ ११.१३ ॥
tatraikasthaṁ jagatkṛtsnaṁ
pravibhaktamanekadhā
apaśyaddevadevasya
śarīre pāṇḍavastadā (11.13)

tatraikastham = tatra – there + ekastham — one position; jagat — universe; kṛtsnam — entire; pravibhaktam — divided; anekadhā — in many ways; apaśyad = apaśyat — he saw; devadevasya — of the God of gods; śarīre — in the body; pāṇḍavas — Arjuna Pandava; tadā — then

There the entire universe existed as one reality divided in many ways. Arjuna Pandava then saw the God of gods in that body. (11.13)

Commentary:

Again Sanjaya brings it to our attention that the Universal Form was present there in the physical body which Śrī Krishna manifested. It was not something apart. It was not another person. It was Śrī Krishna Himself, there, as the one reality divided into many, many parts, exhibited variously.

Arjuna was convinced by direct experience that He saw the God of gods, and it was Śrī Krishna and no one else, even the same Śrī Krishna who manifested a physical form as the son of Devakī and Vasudeva.

ततः स विस्मयाविष्टो
हृष्टरोमा धनंजयः ।
प्रणम्य शिरसा देवं
कृताञ्जलिरभाषत ॥ ११.१४॥
tataḥ sa vismayāviṣṭo
hṛṣṭaromā dhanaṁjayaḥ
praṇamya śirasā devaṁ
kṛtāñjalirabhāṣata (11.14)

tataḥ — then; sa = saḥ — he; vismayāviṣṭo = vismayāviṣṭaḥ — one who is amazed; hṛṣṭaromā — one whose hair is bristled; dhanamjayaḥ — Arjuna, conqueror of rich countries; praṇamya — bowing; śirasā — with the head; devam — God; kṛtāñjalir = kṛtāñjaliḥ — making reverence with palms pressed for prayers; abhāsata — he spoke

Then he, who was amazed, whose hair bristled, Arjuna, the conqueror of rich countries, bowing his head to the God, with palm pressed for prayers, spoke. (11.14)

Commentary:

Arjuna's hair stood on end because that is the nature of such an experience. Thus Vaishnava authorities downplayed the importance of the vision of the Universal Form and took steps to discourage their disciples from wanting to view it. Such an apparition is frightening to anyone who is not prepared to view it and who might experience themselves as being threatened by it.

Sanjaya, with intention to jolt King Dhṛtarāṣṭra to sanity, mentioned that Arjuna, the conqueror of rich countries, bowed his head to the God, with palms pressed for offering prayers. Arjuna was a conqueror of rich countries. He did such things for the Kuru ruling family, but still in the face of the Universal Form, this conqueror trembled.

अर्जुन उवाच
पश्यामि देवांस्तव देव देहे
सर्वांस्तथा भूतविशेषसंघान् ।
ब्रह्माणमीशं कमलासनस्थम्
ऋषींश्च सर्वानुरगांश्च दिव्यान् ॥ ११.१५॥
arjuna uvāca
paśyāmi devāṁstava deva dehe
sarvāṁstathā bhūtaviśeṣasaṁghān
brahmāṇamīśaṁ kamalāsanastham
ṛṣīṁśca sarvānuragāṁśca divyān
(11.15)

arjuna – Arjuna; uvāca — said; paśyāmi — I see; devāṁs — spiritual rulers; tava — your; deva — O God; dehe — in the body; sarvāṁs — all; tathā — as well as; bhūtaviśeṣasaṁghān = bhūta — being + viśeṣa – variety + saṁghān — assembled; brahmāṇam — Lord Brahmā; īśam — Lord; kamalāsanastham = kamala – lotus + āsana – seat + stham — situated; ṛṣīṁśca = ṛṣīn — yogi sages + ca — and; sarvān — all; uragāṁśca = uragān — serpents + ca — and; divyān — supernatural

Arjuna said: I see the supernatural rulers in Your body, O God, as well as all varieties of beings assembled there, Lord Brahmā, who is lotus—seated, all the yogi sages and the supernatural serpents. (11.15)

Commentary:

According to the *Mahābhārata* history, Arjuna knew the supernatural rulers personally. Arjuna by advanced yoga practice, had left his physical body on the earth for some months and had journeyed on and lived in the Swārga heavenly places, visiting with the supernatural rulers in those locales. Arjuna even fought and displaced many of their opponents from that subtle world. Thus he knew some of the celestial people personally. He could recognize the ones he met before.

The significance is that such persons form the first-level array of individuals who serve under the Universal Form and who function as prominent parts of it. These people are not Śrī Krishna Himself, but they are empowered by Him, and apart from that empowerment they have an unusual power of their own.

अनेकबाहूदरवक्त्रनेत्रं
पश्यामि त्वां सर्वतोऽनन्तरूपम् ।
नान्तं न मध्यं न पुनस्तवादिं
पश्यामि विश्वेश्वर विश्वरूप ॥ ११.१६ ॥
anekabāhūdaravaktranetraṁ
paśyāmi tvām sarvato'nantarūpam
nāntaṁ na madhyaṁ na
punastavādiṁ
paśyāmi viśveśvara viśvarūpa
(11.16)

anekabāhūdaravaktranetram = aneka — countless + bāhu — arm + udara — belly + vaktra — face + netram — eye; paśyāmi — I see; tvām — you; sarvato = sarvataḥ — all directions; 'nantarūpam = anantarūpam = ananta – infinite + rūpam — form; nāntam = na – not + antam — end; na – not; madhyam — middle; na – no; punas = punar — again even; tavādim = tava — of you + ādim — beginning; paśyāmi — I observe; viśveśvara — O Lord of all; viśvarūpa — form of everything

There are countless arms, bellies, faces, and eyes. I see You in all directions, O person of infinite form. There is no end, middle, or even a beginning of You. I observe You, O Lord of all, O Form of everything. (11.16)

Commentary:

This particular vision of the Central Person in the Universal Form, as far as I can recall from the memory vision in my subtle body, is a vision of seeing the Central Figure as each of the other persons in the Form. In other words from a certain supernatural perspective, one sees the empowerment as Śrī Krishna Himself. It is said that Śrī Aurobindo of Pondicherry, a successful yogin in India, did have a similar vision when he was tried in a court. At that time the judge, the lawyers, himself and everyone else appeared to be Śrī Krishna.

The point is that the Central Person in the Universal Form, Śrī Krishna Himself, is prefaced in every other person who comprises the Form. That means that the face, the very Form of Śrī Krishna is pushed to the limit or the edge of all other personalities, such that from a certain supernatural perspective, everyone is an expression of Śrī Krishna Himself.

All the same Śrī Krishna, and Arjuna as well, will deny Śrī Krishna as being liable for the actions of everyone. Lord Caitanya Mahāprabhu, in helping us to understand this, calls it the inconceivable oneness and difference with the Supreme Being, acintabhedabheda tattva.

किरीटिनं गदिनं चक्रिणं च
तेजोराशिं सर्वतो दीप्तिमन्तम् ।
पश्यामि त्वां दुर्निरीक्ष्यं समन्ताद्
दीप्तानलार्कद्युतिमप्रमेयम् ॥११.१७॥

kirīṭinaṁ gadinaṁ cakriṇaṁ ca
tejorāśiṁ sarvato dīptimantam
paśyāmi tvāṁ durnirīkṣyaṁ samantād
dīptānalārkadyutim aprameyam
(11.17)

kirīṭinam — crowned; gadinam — armed with a club; cakriṇam — bearing a discus; ca — and; tejo – splendor; rāśim — a mass; sarvato = sarvataḥ — on all sides; dīptimantam — shining wondrously; paśyāmi — I see; tvām — you; durnirīkṣyam — difficult to behold; samantāt — in entirety; dīptānalārkadyutim = dīpta – blazing + anala — fire + arka — sun + dyutim — effulgence; aprameyam — immeasurable

This Form is crowned, armed with a club, bearing a discus, a mass of splendor on all sides, shining wondrously with immeasurable radiance of the sun and blazing fire. I see You in entirety, You Who are difficult to behold. (11.17)

Commentary:

As Arjuna is bowing down to Śrī Krishna, we must also be bowing down to Arjuna for having borne the ability to see the form in its entirety. That is not an ordinary capacity to bear. It is not that every limited entity can bear the wide angle of supernatural vision required to see the Form in its entirety. That is something special. Thus Arjuna is special and deserves honor.

Arjuna admired his friend Śrī Krishna with the crowned head, with armaments, being a mass of supernatural splendor on all sides, shining with immeasurable radiance spherically. The supernatural bodies which Arjuna saw had their own light emitted from them, such that there was no need for illumination from a sun, moon or electricity. Light poured out of those forms naturally.

त्वमक्षरं परमं वेदितव्यं
त्वमस्य विश्वस्य परं निधानम् ।
त्वमव्ययः शाश्वतधर्मगोप्ता
सनातनस्त्वं पुरुषो मतो मे ॥११.१८॥

tvamakṣaraṁ paramaṁ veditavyaṁ
tvamasya viśvasya paraṁ nidhānam
tvamavyayaḥ śāśvatadharmagoptā
sanātanastvaṁ puruṣo mato me
(11.18)

tvam — you; akṣaram — imperishable; paramam — supreme; veditavyam — to be revealed; tvam — you; asya — of it; viśvasya — of all; param — ultimate; nidhānam — shelter; tvam — you; avyayaḥ — imperishable; śāśvatadharmagoptā = śāśvata – eternal + dharma – law + goptā — guardian; sanātanaḥ — most ancient; tvam — you; puruṣo = puruṣaḥ — person; mato = mataḥ — thought; me — of me

You are the indestructible Supreme Reality, to be revealed. You are the ultimate shelter of all. You are the imperishable, eternal guardian of law. It seems to me that You are the most ancient person. (11.18)

Commentary:

Arjuna hailed Śrī Krishna's Universal Form as the indestructible background upon which this destructible reality is based, and as the most ancient of the persons who form the core of this existence in its gross, subtle and causal compartments. Śrī Krishna, Arjuna said, is the ultimate shelter and the imperishable eternal guardian of law. Krishna is the ultimate reference, the final say and the existential backdrop of everyone.

अनादिमध्यान्तमनन्तवीर्यम्
अनन्तबाहुं शशिसूर्यनेत्रम्
पश्यामि त्वां दीप्तहुताशवक्त्रं
स्वतेजसा विश्वमिदं तपन्तम् ॥ ११.१९ ॥

anādimadhyāntam anantavīryam
anantabāhuṁ śaśisūryanetram
paśyāmi tvāṁ dīptahutāśavaktraṁ
svatejasā viśvamidaṁ tapantam
(11.19)

anādimadhyāntam = an – without + ādi — beginning + madhya — middle + antam — end; anantavīryam = ananta — unlimited + vīryam — manly power; anantabāhuṁ = ananta — unlimited + bāhum — arm; śaśisūryanetram = śaśi — moon + sūrya — sun + netram — eye; paśyāmi — I see; tvām — you; dīptahutāśavaktraṁ = dīpta — blazing + hutāśa – oblation—eating + vaktram — mouth; svatejasā — with Your splendor; viśvam — universe; idam — this; tapantam — heating

You who are without beginning, middle, or ending, Who has infinite manly power, Who has unlimited arms, Who has the sun and moon as Your eyes, I see You, with the blazing oblation—eating mouth, heating this universe with Your Own splendor. (11.19)

Commentary:

This is a supernatural heat which mobilizes pranic energy or very subtle emotional force. When we do yoga austerities in prāṇāyāma, we energize the tiny amount of the energy that is in our subtle bodies. Arjuna saw that energy on a cosmic scale. He could see that the energy was not being heated supernaturally by itself. It was charged by Śrī Krishna.

It appeared to Arjuna that the sun and moon were eyes of Śrī Krishna. To Arjuna, Śrī Krishna's manly power (virya) was infinite. He was the ultimate man.

This has value in kriyā yoga when one begins to research both what is driving this universe as well as who is driving one through the various incarnations in numerous bodies and cultural situations. One tries to come to terms with those forces and persons in order to get a release from the endless social involvements which continually consume one's energy.

The sociality exists even in the subtle world. As kriyā yogis we do not think that it will end merely at the death of our present bodies. The rigors of relationship which we endure here exists elsewhere, even in the hereafter. Ultimately each yogi appeals to the Supreme God for a waiver from the complications of these existences.

द्यावापृथिव्योरिदमन्तरं हि
व्याप्तं त्वयैकेन दिशश्च सर्वाः ।
दृष्ट्वाद्भुतं रूपम् उग्रं तवेदं
लोकत्रयं प्रव्यथितं महात्मन् ॥ ११.२० ॥

dyāvāpṛthivyor = dyāvāpṛthivyoḥ — of heaven and earth; idam — this; antaram — space between; hi — indeed; vyāptam — pervaded; tvayaikena = tvaya — by you + ekena — alone; diśaḥ — directions; ca — and; sarvāḥ — all;

dyāvāpṛthivyoridam antaraṁ hi
vyāptaṁ tvayaikena diśaścasarvāḥ
dṛṣṭvādbhutaṁ rūpam ugraṁ
tavedaṁ
lokatrayaṁ pravyathitaṁ
mahātman (11.20)

dṛṣtvā — having seen + adbhutam — marvelous; rūpam — form; ugram — terrible; tavedam = tava — your + idam — this; lokatrayam = loka — world + trayam — three; pravyathitam — trembling; mahātman — O great personality

In all directions, the space between heaven and earth is pervaded by You alone. Seeing Your marvelous Form, of a terrible feature, the three worlds tremble, O great Personality. (11.20)

Commentary:

The trembling of the worlds, though perceived as a fact by Arjuna was not felt by every living being everywhere. Arjuna perceived on the supernatural level which translates differently in the gross perception of other creatures who are not in tune with the mystic side. The terrible feature perceived by Arjuna was the ultimatum of power that Śrī Krishna wielded as the Central Figure in that Universal Form. It was the ghastly realisation that the one person, Śrī Krishna, could withdraw His energy and cause the collapse of numerous world systems. For everything to rely on one individual is, from a certain perspective, a terrible thing indeed.

अमी हि त्वा सुरसंघा विशन्ति
केचिद्भीताः प्राञ्जलयो गृणन्ति ।
स्वस्तीत्युक्त्वा महर्षिसिद्धसंघाः
स्तुवन्ति त्वां स्तुतिभिः पुष्कलाभिः ॥
११.२१॥

amī hi tvā surasaṁghā viśanti
kecidbhītāḥ prāñjalayo gṛṇanti
svastītyuktvā
maharṣisiddhasaṁghāḥ
stuvanti tvāṁ stutibhiḥ
puṣkalābhiḥ (11.21)

amī — those; hi — truly; tvā — you; surasaṁghā = sura – supernatural ruler + saṁghā — groups; viśanti — they enter; kecid — some; bhītāḥ — terrified; prāñjalayo = prāñjalayaḥ — bowing with palms pressed together; gṛṇanti — they offer praise; svastīty = svastīti = sv (su) — suitable + asti — there be + iti — thus; uktvā — saying; maharṣisiddhasaṁghāḥ = mahārṣi — great yogi sages + siddha — perfected yogis + saṁghāḥ — groups; stuvanti — they praise; tvām — you; stutibhiḥ — with glorification; puṣkalābhiḥ — with lavish

Those groups of supernatural rulers enter You. Some being terrified, bowing with palms pressed together, offer praise. "May everything be suitable," they say. The groups of great yogi sages and perfected yogis praise You with lavish glorification. (11.21)

Commentary:

These were the people who perceived that aspect of the Universal Form which was revealed to Arjuna. It was the groups of supernatural rulers in the astral dimensions. It was the perfected sages, the great rishis, and siddhas. They, and they alone, had the vision to see what was being shown to Arjuna. It appears that even though they were conscious of the Universal Form, still they did not perceive that controlling feature of it, before this. The exposure of the finalizing power of Śrī Krishna was something they were unaware of at the time. They were not thinking that Śrī Krishna, as the Central Figure, could close down everything or bring everything in line with His desire. They were taking everything for granted, feeling that the world situations and the social formations would continue going on forever. Now they realized that there might be an abrupt adjustment by the Central Figure.

Thus we hear that in the supernatural world, the spiritually—realized beings offered prayers to Śrī Krishna. The rulers promised everything would conform to Krishna.

रुद्रादित्या वसवो ये च साध्या
विश्वेऽश्विनौ मरुतश्चोष्मपाश्च ।
गन्धर्वयक्षासुरसिद्धसंघा
वीक्षन्ते त्वां विस्मिताश्चैव सर्वे ॥
११.२२॥

rudrādityā vasavo
ye ca sādhyā
viśve'śvinau
marutaścoṣmapāśca
gandharvayakṣā
surasiddhasaṁghā
vīkṣante tvām vismitāś
caiva sarve (11.22)

rudrādityā = rudra — supernatural destroyers + ādityāḥ — supernatural rulers; vasavo = vasavaḥ — Vasus, assistants to supernatural rulers; ye — who; ca — and; sādhyā — Sādhya, guardian angels; viśve — Vishvadeva supernatural priests; 'śvinau = aśvinau — two primal supernatural doctors; marutaścoṣmapāś = marutaḥ — supernatural stormers + ca — and + uṣmapāḥ — spirits who take vapor bodies; ca — and; gandharvayakṣāsurasiddhasaṁghā = gandharva — celestial musicians + yakṣa — spirits guarding natural resources + asura — supernatural rebels + siddha — perfected souls + saṁghā — groups; vīkṣante — they behold; tvām — you; vismitāścaiva = vismitāḥ — amazed + ca — and + iva (eva) — indeed; sarve — all

The supernatural destroyers, the supernatural rulers, the assistants to those rulers, these and the Sādhya guardian angels, the Vishvadeva supernatural priests, the two primal supernatural doctors, the supernatural stormers, the spirits who take vapor bodies, the groups of celestial musicians, the spirits guarding natural resources, the supernatural rebels and the perfected souls, behold You. And they are all amazed. (11.22)

Commentary:

These, except for the supernatural rebels, are mostly pious beings who use subtle bodies and live in subtle dimensions where they are permanent residents. Usually these persons do not take gross forms but they affect this gross world. We must deal with them when we depart from a gross body and have to assume a subtle form for some time.

The supernatural rebels are also permanent residents of the astral world. They are not in agreement with the Central Figure, with Śrī Krishna. They live in opposition to the deva people who cooperate with the lifestyle which is recommended by Śrī Krishna. In all cases, however, of those who were compatible with Śrī Krishna and those who were opposed, Arjuna perceived that after the exhibition of Krishna's controlling power, they looked on in wonder and were all amazed at Krishna's glory and power.

रूपं महत्ते बहुवक्त्रनेत्रं
महाबाहो बहुबाहूरुपादम् ।
बहूदरं बहुदंष्ट्राकरालं
दृष्ट्वा लोकाः प्रव्यथितास्तथाहम्॥ ११.२३॥

rūpaṁ mahatte bahuvaktranetraṁ
mahābāho bahubāhūrupādam
bahūdaraṁ bahudaṁṣṭrākarālaṁ
dṛṣṭvā lokāḥ pravyathitās tathāham
(11.23)

rūpam — form; mahat — great; te — your; bahuvaktranetram = bahu — many + vaktra — mouth + netram — eye; mahābāho — O mighty—armed Person; bahubāhūrupādam = bahu — many + bāhu — arm + ūru — thigh + pādam — foot; bahūdaram = bahu – many + udaram — belly; bahudaṁṣṭrākarālam = bahu – many + daṁṣṭrā — teeth + karālam — terrible; dṛṣṭvā — having seen; lokāḥ — the world; pravyathitāḥ — trembling; tathā — as well as; 'ham = aham — I

O mighty—armed Person, having seen Your great Form with many mouths and eyes, and many arms, thighs, and feet, many bellies and many terrible teeth, the worlds tremble as well as I. (11.23)

Commentary:

This statement of Arjuna is a generality. We must remember that Arjuna is looking through supernatural vision which is different to physical eyesight. Even though he perceived that all the worlds were trembling, seeing the many mouths, eyes, arms, thighs, feet, bellies and terrible teeth, still on the gross level it was not a fact that everyone was aware of the display of that awesome power. What Arjuna saw was not a hallucination, but what is seen and what transpires on the supernatural plane, does not necessarily translate into the physical world in the same way that it occurred supernaturally.

नभःस्पृशं दीप्तमनेकवर्णं
व्यात्ताननं दीप्तविशालनेत्रम् ।
दृष्ट्वा हि त्वां प्रव्यथितान्तरात्मा
धृतिं न विन्दामि शमं च विष्णो ॥ ११.२४ ॥
nabhaḥspṛśaṁ dīptamanekavarṇaṁ
vyāttānanaṁ dīptaviśālanetram
dṛṣṭvā hi tvāṁ pravyathitāntarātmā
dhṛtiṁ na vindāmi śamaṁ ca viṣṇo
(11.24)

nabhaḥspṛśaṁ = nabhaḥ — sky + spṛśaṁ — touching, extending; dīptam — glowing; aneka — many; varṇam — colors; vyātta — open; ānanam — mouths; dīpta — glowing; viśāla — very great; netram — eyes; dṛṣṭvā — seeing; hi — certainly; tvām — You; pravyathita — perturbed; antaḥ — within; ātmā — soul; dhṛtim — steadiness; na — not; vindāmi — I have; śamam — mental tranquility; ca — also; viṣṇo — O Lord Viṣṇu.

Having seen You, sky extending, blazing, multi—colored, with gaping mouths and blazing vast eyes, there is a shivering in my soul. I find no courage, or stability, O God Vishnu. (11.24)

Commentary:

Arjuna made an adjustment because he addressed Śrī Krishna as the God Vishnu. At first when Arjuna broke down in tears, he was not perceiving Śrī Krishna as the God Vishnu but rather as a friend who was driving his chariot. Arjuna had heard that Śrī Krishna was the God Vishnu. He believed it. Still he never did realize it to this extent. Now when he says God Vishnu he actually means it because he experienced the power of God Vishnu as Krishna's power on the supernatural level.

The lesson is that even though many people accept Śrī Krishna as God or as the Supreme Personality of Godhead, still they do not really accept Him, because they believe only and have no experience of Him as such.

Arjuna suddenly began to experience a supernatural shivering, which caused him to reconsider his position in relationship to Śrī Krishna. Was Śrī Krishna really his friend, Who could be requested to drive the chariot? Or was Śrī Krishna someone who was so vast and infinite that Arjuna was not really His friend? How was Arjuna to reconcile the role of Śrī Krishna as a friend and cousin and as the Central Person in the awesome Universal Form?

दंष्ट्राकरालानि च ते मुखानि
दृष्ट्वैव कालानलसंनिभानि ।
दिशो न जाने न लभे च शर्म
प्रसीद देवेश जगन्निवास ॥ ११.२५ ॥

damṣṭrā — teeth; karālāni — terrible; ca — also; te — Your; mukhāni — faces; dṛṣṭvā — seeing; eva — thus; kāla—anala — the fire of death; sannibhāni — as if; diśaḥ — the directions; na — not; jāne — I know; na — not;

daṁṣṭrākarālāni ca te mukhāni
dṛṣṭvaiva kālānalasaṁnibhāni
diśo na jāne na labhe ca śarma
prasīda deveśa jagannivāsa (11.25)

labhe — I obtain; ca — and; śarma — grace; prasīda — be pleased; deva—īśa — O Lord of all lords; jagat—nivāsa — O refuge of the worlds

And seeing Your Form with many mouths, having terrible teeth, glowing like the fire of universal destruction, I cannot determine the cardinal points. I do not find any peace of mind. Have mercy, O Lord of the gods, Abode of the universe. (11.25)

Commentary:

To Arjuna, it appeared that the universe would shut down at any moment. But nowadays we understand from the astronomers that parts of the galaxies are on continual review, either being created, sustained for the time being or moved into non-existence, at least in so far as our gross perception and electronic instruments can detect. From Arjuna's experience we can safely deduce that the gross cosmic operations, which the astronomers view, are being triggered by the minds of the supernatural persons, either by Śrī Krishna or by one of His expansions or parallel divinities. We should understand that behind the material display of power, there is supernatural force coming from specific persons who operate through the Universal Forms which govern those particular parts of the cosmos.

For the time being, this must be our belief. As kriyā yogis, we cannot afford to feel that everything is merely subtle or gross mundane energy in turmoil. There has to be some personal force in the operation. We experience this on a small scale in our meditations. From that we deduce that the personality factor must be considered in all circumstances. The facts established by the astronomers with their accurate instruments, do not deny the personal factor. In fact for us, it asserts it. In deeper meditations and in samadhis where supernatural vision becomes operative, we begin to perceive the gods and the God behind what the astronomers perceive. Arjuna lost his sense of balance after seeing the ghastly aspects of the Universal Form. The important realization is that this turmoil of energies transpires at every moment. We are simply unaware of it.

So long as we are not aware of it, it will not disturb us. Arjuna was troubled because he perceived it. Sometimes when we enter deep meditation or when our supernatural vision becomes operative, we see the ghastly aspect of it and we become afraid. But we learn to see it and not be fearful by shifting our viewing position from an objective to a subjective stance. After all, each of us, no matter how minute, no matter how insignificant, is a part of the Universal Form.

A limited being might not be a speck in that Form but even if he is a speck of a speck of a speck, still his spiritual existence is assured. The destruction and turmoil enacted by that Form do not affect the bare spirituality of any individual soul.

Kriyā yoga, unlike the faith-belief systems, is the definite way to realize one's spirituality and to face such specters as the ghastly aspect of the Universal Form.

अमी च त्वां धृतराष्ट्रस्य पुत्राः
सर्वे सहैवावनिपालसंघैः ।
भीष्मो द्रोणः सूतपुत्रस्तथासौ
सहास्मदीयैरपि योधमुख्यैः ॥११.२६॥

amī — those; ca — and; tvāṁ — you; dhṛtarāṣṭrasya — of Dhṛtarāṣṭra; putrāḥ — sons; sarve — all; sahaivāvanipālasaṁghaiḥ = saha — with + eva — indeed+avāvanipāla — rulers of the earth + saṁghaiḥ — with groups; bhīṣmo =

amī ca tvāṁ dhṛtarāṣṭrasya putrāḥ
sarve sahaivāvanipālasaṁghaiḥ
bhīṣmo droṇaḥ sūtaputrastathāsau
sahāsmadīyairapi yodhamukhyaiḥ
(11.26)

bhīṣmaḥ — Bhishma; droṇaḥ — Droṇa; sūtaputraḥ — Karna, son of the charioteer; tathāsau = tathā — as well as + asau — that; saha — along with; asmadīyaiḥ — with ours; api — also; yodhamukhyaiḥ — with chief warriors

And those, all the sons of Dhṛtarāṣṭra, along with the groups of rulers, Bhishma, Droṇa, as well as that son of the charioteer, along with our men and also our chief warriors, are in contrast to You. (11.26)

<u>Commentary:</u>

The contrasting relationship between Śrī Krishna and the Kauravas and their supporters like Karṇa, the son of the charioteer, was obvious on the physical level. Arjuna began to see it on the supernatural plane as well. There Arjuna saw that many of his men and even his chief warriors were in contrast to Śrī Krishna, even though physically they were supportive of Arjuna's team. This meant that some of his allies had reservations about Śrī Krishna and did not want to fight at Kurukṣetra.

Krishna may or may not be God, but still each and every person did not agree with His opinions and decisions. They simply did not like the idea of the civil war. They sensed that Krishna came there to enforce His will for the war in order to settle the rulership in favor of His choice who was Prince Yudhiṣṭhira, the eldest brother of Arjuna. Arjuna could see in the Universal Form that Śrī Krishna was in contrast to nearly every man on that battlefield and that Śrī Krishna exerted a power to force on the battle. Arjuna was amazed.

वक्त्राणि ते त्वरमाणा विशन्ति
दंष्ट्राकरालानि भयानकानि ।
केचिद्विलग्ना दशनान्तरेषु
संदृश्यन्ते चूर्णितैरुत्तमाङ्गैः ॥११.२७॥
vaktrāṇi te tvaramāṇā viśanti
daṁṣṭrākarālāni bhayānakāni
kecidvilagnā daśanāntareṣu
saṁdṛśyante cūrṇitair uttamāṅgaiḥ
(11.27)

vaktrāṇi — mouths; te — your; tvaramāṇā — speedily; viśanti — they enter; daṁṣṭrākarālāni = daṁṣṭrā — teeth + karālāni — dreadful; bhayānakāni – fearful; kecid (kecit) — some; vilagnā — clinging: daśanāntareṣu = daśana — tooth + antareṣu — in between; saṁdṛśyante — they are seen; cūrṇitaiḥ — with crushed; uttamāṅgaiḥ — with heads

They speedily enter Your fearful mouths, which have dreadful teeth. Some cling between the teeth. They are seen with crushed heads. (11.27)

<u>Commentary:</u>

This describes the contrasting desires of ourselves and Śrī Krishna. Normally this manifests in our lives as numerous obstacles and problems that arise and cause stress when we try to fulfill desires. There is a contrast between us and God, between us and one another, and between us and other persons with more power, who supersede us physically by political, social and emotional force or supernaturally by bringing on natural disasters and by contorting our minds with depression and fatigue. No matter where we turn, we run into obstacles in this existence. Our personalities contrast with those of others who are on par, less than or greater in power. Arjuna saw this on the supernatural plane. He saw that in the hassle between God and man, God, a ghastly superbeing, was prepared to eat up the psychologies of those who opposed His will. That God bit some and crunched some between His teeth. This is because Śrī Krishna told many human beings what He required of them.

They became disappointed and considered Him to be inconsiderate. Thus they aimed resentment at His mouth which had told them much of what He disapproved in their behavior. That resentment manifested on the supernatural plane as an attack on His mouth. He responded by biting and crunching down on their subtle bodies.

Arjuna considered that the battle was inevitable. No limited being had the power to stop it. Śrī Krishna wanted it. The resentments caused them to attack Krishna's body on the supernatural plane. As they approached His mouths, He torched them.

यथा नदीनां बहवोऽम्बुवेगाः
समुद्रमेवाभिमुखा द्रवन्ति ।
तथा तवामी नरलोकवीरा
विशन्ति वक्त्राण्यभिविज्वलन्ति ॥११.२८॥
yathā nadīnāṁ bahavo'mbuvegāḥ
samudramevābhimukhā dravanti
tathā tavāmī naralokavīrā
viśanti vaktrāṇyabhivijvalanti (11.28)

yathā — as; nadīnāṁ — of the rivers; bahavo – bahavaḥ — many; 'mbuvegāḥ = ambuvegāḥ — water currents; samudram — sea; evābhimukhā = eva — indeed + abhimukhā — facing towards; dravanti — they flow; tathā —so; tavāmī — tava — of you + amī — those; naralokavīrā = nara — man + loka — world +vīrā—heroes; viśanti — they enter; vaktràni — mouths; abhivijvalanti — they are flaming

As the water currents of many rivers flow to the sea, so the earthly heroes enter Your mouths, which are flaming. (11.28)

Commentary:

The movement of Śrī Krishna's opponents was irreversible. A great magnetic force drew those warriors into Śrī Krishna's mouth on the supernatural plane. But Arjuna saw more than the warriors he knew. He saw worlds moving to their destruction being inevitably drawn into Śrī Krishna's supernatural body. This is similar to what our astronomers see via telescopes and describe as galaxies moving into black holes and disappearing, except that Arjuna was viewing the apparition on the supernatural plane.

यथा प्रदीप्तं ज्वलनं पतंगा
विशन्ति नाशाय समृद्धवेगाः ।
तथैव नाशाय विशन्ति लोकास्
तवापि वक्त्राणि समृद्धवेगाः ॥११.२९॥
yathā pradīptaṁ jvalanaṁ pataṁgā
viśanti nāśāya samṛddhavegāḥ
tathaiva nāśāya viśanti lokās
tavāpi vaktrāṇi samṛddhavegāḥ (11.29)

yathā — as; pradīptaṁ — blazing; jvalanaṁ —fire; pataṁgā — moths; viśanti — enter; nāśāya — to destruction; samṛddhavegāḥ — with great speed; tathaiva = tathā —so + iva (eva) — indeed; nāśāya — to ruination; viśanti —enter; lokāh — worlds; tavāpi = tava — you + api — also; vaktrāṇi — mouths; samṛddhavegāḥ — with great speed

As moths speedily enter a blazing fire to destruction, so to ruination, the worlds enter Your mouths with great speed. (11.29)

Commentary:

Arjuna then saw that in addition to the local situation in the area of India where he lived, other social systems also contrasted the desire of Śrī Krishna. Those not having His approval were torched by supernatural fire which emanated from Śrī Krishna's mouths.

लेलिह्यसे ग्रसमानः समन्ताल्
लोकान्समग्रान्वदनैर्ज्वलद्भिः ।
तेजोभिरापूर्य जगत्समग्रं
भासस्तवोग्राः प्रतपन्ति विष्णो ॥ ११.३० ॥
lelihyase grasamānaḥ samantāl
lokānsamagrānvadanair jvaladbhiḥ
tejobhirāpūrya jagatsamagraṁ
bhāsastavogrāḥ pratapanti viṣṇo (11.30)

lelihyase — you lick; grasamānaḥ — swallow; samantāt — from all sides; lokān — the worlds; samagrān — all: vadanaiḥ — with mouths; jvaladbhiḥ — with flaming; tejobhiḥ — with splendor; āpūrya — filling; jagat — universe; samagraṁ — all; bhāsaḥ — rays; tavogrāḥ = tava — your + ugrāh — horrible; pratapanti — burns; viṣṇo — O Lord Vishnu

You lick, swallowing from all sides, all the worlds with Your flaming mouths, filling the universe with splendor. Your horrible blazing rays burn it, O Lord Vishnu . (11.30)

Commentary:

Arjuna lost track of his friend Śrī Krishna. He saw only the God Vishnu. He did not see Śrī Krishna as his friend any longer. At that point, Arjuna lost the footing as a human being. He was totally integrated on the supernatural plane. He experienced himself as a supernatural being with a supernatural body, as if he were a permanent resident in that other world.

आख्याहि मे को भवानुग्ररूपो
नमोऽस्तु ते देववर प्रसीद ।
विज्ञातुमिच्छामि भवन्तमाद्यं
न हि प्रजानामि तव प्रवृत्तिम् ॥ ११.३१ ॥
ākhyāhi me ko bhavānugrarūpo
namo'stu te devavara prasīda
vijñātumicchāmi bhavantamādyaṁ
na hi prajānāmi tava pravṛttim
(11.31)

ākhyāhi — explain; me — to me; ko = kaḥ— who; bhavān — respected person; ugrarūpo – ugrarūpaḥ — of terrible form; namo = namaḥ — homage; 'stu — astu— may it be; te — to you; devavara — best of the gods; prasīda — have mercy; vijñātum — to understand; icchāmi — I want; bhavantam — Your lordship; ādyaṁ — primal person; na — not; hi — indeed; prajānāmi — I know; tava — your; pravṛttim — intention

Explain to me who You are, O respected Person of terrible form. I gave my homage to You, O best of gods. Have mercy! I want to understand You, O Primal Person. I do not know Your intention. (11.31)

Commentary:

Having lost footing as a human being, Arjuna tried to gain a grip in the world to which he was transferred after requesting that Śrī Krishna should display the origin and ruination of the living beings. Arjuna now tries to fulfill his essential being as someone who requires relationships with others. In that supernatural dimension he found no one to relate to besides the Central Figure in the Universal Form. All the other persons in that Form ignored him and went about their business of smashing resistances and enforcing their views. No one had time for Arjuna. Since he caught the eye of the Central Figure, he began to request a relationship with that God.

Arjuna wanted some kind of rapport, so that the Person could speak of Himself and His intentions. Arjuna wanted to find a place to fit in, with something to do just as the other persons in the form. He did not want to be in contrast to the Central Person.

श्रीभगवानुवाच
कालोऽस्मि लोकक्षयकृत्प्रवृद्धो
लोकान्समाहर्तुमिह प्रवृत्तः ।
ऋतेऽपि त्वा न भविष्यन्ति सर्वे
येऽवस्थिताः प्रत्यनीकेषु योधाः ॥११.३२॥
śrībhagavānuvāca
kālo'smi lokakṣayakṛt pravṛddho
lokānsamāhartumiha pravṛttaḥ
ṛte'pi tvāṁ na bhaviṣyanti sarve
ye'vasthitāḥ pratyanīkeṣu yodhāḥ
(11.32)

śrī bhagavān — the Blessed Lord; uvāca — said; kālo = kālah — time—limit; 'smi = asmi — I am; lokaksayakrt = loka — world + ksaya — destruction + kṛt— causing; pravṛddho — pravṛddhaḥ — mighty; lokān — worlds; samāhartum — to annihilate; iha — here; pravṛttaḥ — appeared; ṛte — without; 'pi = api — also; tvāṁ — you na — not, cease; bhaviṣyanti — they will live; sarve — all; ye — who; 'vasthitāḥ = avasthitāḥ — armored; pratyanīkeṣu — on both armies; yodhāḥ — warriors

The Blessed Lord said: I am the time limit, the mighty world—destroying Cause, appearing here to annihilate the worlds. Even without you, all the armored warriors, in both armies will cease to live. (11.32)

Commentary:

His appearing there at Kurukṣetra to annihilate the world could not be taken literally because we know for a fact that these worlds were not annihilated since their continuation is factual by virtue of our existence in these bodies. However we may understand that wherever Śrī Krishna is, the potential for such annihilation exists, since He is in fact, according to the experience of Arjuna, the walking potential for the world's ruination.

In fact, the majority of the soldiers at Kurukṣetra did lose their bodies in the battle. That is factual. As the time limit, Śrī Krishna is a moving factor, both annihilating and creating. When someone loses a body, he does not lose his individuality but rather he is displaced from a locale. From there he moves on or is forcefully shifted into another dimension.

तस्मात्त्वमुत्तिष्ठ यशो लभस्व
जित्वा शत्रून्भुङ्क्ष्व राज्यं समृद्धम् ।
मयैवैते निहताः पूर्वमेव
निमित्तमात्रं भव सव्यसाचिन् ॥११.३३॥
tasmāttvamuttiṣṭha yaśo labhasva
jitvā śatrūnbhuṅkṣva rājyaṁ samṛddham
mayaivaite nihatāḥ pūrvameva
nimittamātraṁ bhava savyasācin
(11.33)

tasmāt — therefore; tvam — you; uttiṣṭha — stand; yaśo = yaśaḥ — glory; labhasva — get; jitvā — having conquered; śatrūn — enemies; bhuṅkṣva — enjoy; rājyaṁ — country; samṛddham — prosperous; mayaivaite = mayā — by me + eva — indeed + ete — these; nihatāḥ — supernaturally destroyed; pūrvam — already; eva — indeed; nimittamātraṁ = nimitta—agent + mātraṁ — only; bhava — be; savyasācin — O ambidextrous archer

Therefore you should stand up! Get the glory! Having conquered the enemies, enjoy a prosperous country. These fellows are supernaturally disposed by Me already. Be only the agent, O ambidextrous archer. (11.33)

Commentary:

The God Vishnu as exhibited by Śrī Krishna, gave Arjuna the order to stand up and conquer the enemies, since the God said that they were supernaturally killed by Him already. This meant that in His supernatural mind, their material bodies had already reached their respective time limits and would be destroyed very soon on the physical level.

द्रोणं च भीष्मं च जयद्रथं च
कर्णं तथान्यानपि योधवीरान् ।
मया हतांस्त्वं जहि मा व्यथिष्ठा
युध्यस्व जेतासि रणे सपत्नान् ॥ ११.३४॥
droṇaṁ ca bhīṣmaṁ ca jayadrathaṁ ca
karṇaṁ tathānyānapi yodhavīrān
mayā hatāṁstvaṁ jahi mā vyathiṣṭhā
yudhyasva jetāsi raṇe sapatnān
(11.34)

droṇaḥ — Droṇa; ca — and; bhīṣmaṁ — Bhishma; ca — and; jayadrathaṁ — Jayadratha; ca — and; karṇaṁ — Karṇa; tathānyān = tathā — as well as; anyān— others; api — also; yodhavīrān — battle heroes; mayā — by me; hatāṁ — supernaturally hurt; tvaṁ — you; jahi — physically kill; mā — not; vyathiṣṭhā — hesitate; yudhyasva — fight; jetāsi — you will conquer; raṇe — in battle; sapatnān — enemies

Droṇa, Bhishma, Jayadratha, and Karṇa, as well as other battle heroes, were supernaturally hurt by Me. You may physically kill them. Do not hesitate. Fight! You will conquer the enemies in battle. (11.34)

Commentary:

Droṇa, Bhīṣma, Jayadratha, Karṇa and other powerful warriors were supernaturally hurt by the God Vishnu, by Krishna as the Central Figure of the Universal Form. For all practical purposes their physical bodies were dead. Arjuna was told to be a superficial instrument in the affair of settling the difference of opinion between Śrī Krishna and those heroes.

It was an argument regarding their lifestyles and the lifestyles they promoted and encouraged in human society. Since Śrī Krishna failed to convince them to change their ideas to His preferences, He decided to remove them from the physical scene so that their influence would be reduced and His views would prevail.

संजय उवाच
एतच्छ्रुत्वा वचनं केशवस्य
कृताञ्जलिर्वेपमानः किरीटी ।
नमस्कृत्वा भूय एवाह कृष्णं
सगद्गदं भीतभीतः प्रणम्य ॥ ११.३५॥
saṁjaya uvāca
etacchrutvā vacanaṁ keśavasya
kṛtāñjalirvepamānaḥ kirīṭī
namaskṛtvā bhūya evāha kṛṣṇaṁ
sagadgadaṁ bhītabhītaḥ praṇamya
(11.35)

saṁjaya — Sanjaya; uvāca — said; etat — this; śrutvā — having heard; vacanaṁ — speech; keśavasya — of the handsome—haired Krsna; kṛtāñjalil— offering respects with joined palms; vepamānah — trembling; kirīṭī — Arjuna, the crowned one; namaskṛtvā = namaḥ — obeisances + krtvā — having made; bhūya — again; evāha = eva— indeed + aha — said; kṛṣṇaṁ — Kṛṣṇaṁ; sagadgadaṁ — stutteringly; bhītabhītaḥ — very frightened; praṇamya — prostrations

Sanjaya said: Having heard the speech of the handsome—haired Krishna, Arjuna, the crowned one, who was trembling, offered respect with joined palms. Bowing again, he stutteringly, with much fright and prostrations, spoke to Krishna. (11.35)

Commentary:

Sanjaya informed King Dhṛtarāṣṭra that the speech relayed, which was given by the God Vishnu in the apparition seen by Arjuna, also came from the mouth of the handsome—haired Śrī Krishna who stood in a physical body on the battlefield. This is because the God Vishnu was in fact Śrī Krishna Himself and no other person. Sanjaya noted that in spite of the beauty of Śrī Krishna, who is called Keshava for the same reason, still the supreme power was present along with that indescribable beauty.

Arjuna was crowned because he was a prince and a military officer. Still he was terribly frightened. In the Universal Form he met Someone who scared him. Spontaneously, Arjuna began to offer prayers. The fear he had of fighting the Kurus was nothing in comparison to the fear he felt while viewing the Universal Form of Śrī Krishna.

अर्जुन उवाच
स्थाने हृषीकेश तव प्रकीर्त्या
जगत्प्रहृष्यत्यनुरज्यते च ।
रक्षांसि भीतानि दिशो द्रवन्ति
सर्वे नमस्यन्ति च सिद्धसंघाः ॥११.३६॥

arjuna uvāca
sthāne hṛṣīkeśa tava prakīrtyā
jagatprahṛṣyatyanurajyate ca
rakṣāṁsi bhītāni diśo dravanti
sarve namasyanti ca siddhasaṁghāḥ
(11.36)

arjuna—Arjuna; uvāca — said; sthāne — in position; hṛṣīkeśa — masterful controller of the senses; tava — your; prakīrtyā — by fame; jagat — universe; prahṛṣyati — rejoices; anurajyate — is delighted; ca — and; rakṣāṁsi — demons; bhītāni — terrified; diśo = diśaḥ — directions; dravanti — they flee; sarve—all; namasyanti — they will reverentially bow; ca — and; siddhasaṁghāḥ — groups of perfected souls

Arjuna said: Everything is in position, O Hṛṣīkeśa, masterful controller of the senses. The universe rejoices and is delighted by Your fame. The demons being terrified, flee in all directions. All the groups of perfected souls will reverentially bow to You. (11.36)

Commentary:

As he looked around, Arjuna saw others on the supernatural plane. They too viewed the Universal Form. Some of them were not fearful. These admired the Form and offered prayers in admiration of the Personalities who composed that Divine Hierarchy.

Arjuna then saw that everything was in its proper position as arranged out of the personality—spread that divested from the Central Figure. Nothing was disorderly. Everyone was positioned in some relationship to the Central Personality, Śrī Krishna. No one could be in any other position but the one to which he was initially emitted from the Form. There was no disorder whatsoever.

Whosoever opposed the Form was regarded as deviant. They ran here and there, scattering to avoid clashes with the Form. The perfected souls (the siddhas) were reverentially bowing to the Form. Due to compliance with the divine will, they were in the good graces of the Form.

कस्माच्च ते न नमेरन्महात्मन्
गरीयसे ब्रह्मणोऽप्यादिकर्त्रे ।
अनन्त देवेश जगन्निवास
त्वमक्षरं सदसत्तत्परं यत् ॥११.३७॥

kasmācca te na nameran
mahātman
garīyase brahmaṇo'pyādikartre
ananta deveśa jagannivāsa
tvamakṣaraṁ sadasattat paraṁ
yat (11.37)

kasmāt — why; ca — and; te — to you; na—not; nameran — they should bow; mahātmān — O great soul; garīyase — greater; brahmaṇaḥ — than Brahma; 'pi = api — also; ādikartre — ādi — original + kartre — to the creator; ananta — infinite; deveśa — lord of the gods; jagan (jagat) —universe + nivāsa — resort; tvam — you; akṣaraṁ— imperishable basis of energies; sat — sum total permanent life; asat — sum total temporary existence; tatparaṁ— that which is beyond; yat = yad — whatever

And why should they not bow to You, O great soul, original creator, Who is also greater than Brahmā, Who is the infinite Lord of the gods, the resort of the world? You are the imperishable basis of energies, the sum total permanent life, the sum total temporary existence, and whatever is beyond all that. (11.37)

Commentary:

In consideration of what he saw, Arjuna felt that there was sufficient justification for the siddhas to bow down. As the imperishable basis of the energies, as the sum total permanent life, as the functioning sustainer of the sum total temporary manifestation, Arjuna felt that the God Vishnu was deserving of the respect offered to Him by the perfected beings.

त्वमादिदेवः पुरुषः पुराणस्
त्वमस्य विश्वस्य परं निधानम् ।
वेत्तासि वेद्यं च परं च धाम
त्वया ततं विश्वमनन्तरूप ॥ ११.३८॥
tvamādidevaḥ puruṣaḥ purāṇas
tvamasya viśvasya paraṁ nidhānam
vettāsi vedyaṁ ca paraṁ ca dhāma
tvayā tataṁ viśvamanantarūpa
(11.38)

tvam — you; ādidevaḥ— first God; puruṣaḥ— spirit; purāṇaḥ— most ancient; tvam—you; asya — of it; viśvasya— of the universe; paraṁ — supreme; nidhānam — refuge; vettāsi = vettā— knower + asi — you are; vedyaṁ — that which is to be known; ca — and; paraṁ — ultimate; ca —and; dhāma— sanctuary; tvayā— by you; tataṁ— pervaded; viśvam — universe; anantarūpa — Person of Infinite Form

You are the first God, the most ancient spirit. You are the knower, You are the supreme refuge of all the worlds. You are that which is to be known. You are the ultimate sanctuary. By You, the universe is pervaded, O Person of Infinite Form. (11.38)

Commentary

We must keep in mind that Arjuna viewed the gigantic Universal Form and not the human body of Śrī Krishna. He saw something cosmic as he looked with supernatural eyes. At a certain point, Arjuna was switched out from the supernatural vision and resumed the normal physical view with which we are familiar. This is important so that as kriyā yogis we do not confuse the two perceptions or feel, as some do, that Arjuna is now seeing the physical body of Śrī Krishna which is a temporary form standing on the warfield of Kurukṣetra. Arjuna viewed what he considered to be the God Vishnu, the ādideva, the First God and the most ancient of the spirits. The anantarūpa is the Person of Infinite Form. Arjuna here addressed that Cosmic Person with His expansions, that are spread out everywhere.

वायुर्यमोऽग्निर्वरुणः शशाङ्कः
प्रजापतिस्त्वं प्रपितामहश्च ।
नमो नमस्तेऽस्तु सहस्रकृत्वः
पुनश्च भूयोऽपि नमो नमस्ते ॥ ११.३९॥
vāyuryamo'gnirvaruṇaḥ
śaśāṅkaḥ
prajāpatistvaṁ prapitāmahaśca
namo namaste'stu
sahasrakṛtvaḥ
punaśca bhūyo'pi namo
namaste (11.39)

vāyuḥ — Vāyu wind regulator; yamo = yamaḥ — Yama, Death Supervisor; 'gniḥ = agniḥ — Agni, fire controller; varuṇaḥ —Varuṇa, Master of the waters; śaśāṅkaḥ — Śaśāṅka moon lord; prajāpatiḥ — procreator Brahmā; tvaṁ — you; prapitāmahaḥ — father of Brahmā; ca — and; namo = namaḥ — obeisances; namaḥ — obeisances repeated; te — to you; 'stu = astu — let it be; sahasrakṛtvaḥ — a thousand times made; punasca = punaḥ (punar) — again + ca — and; bhūyo = bhuyaḥ — again; 'pi = api — also; namo = namaḥ — obeisances repeated; te — to you

You are represented by Vāyu, the wind regulator; Yama, the death supervisor; Agni, the fire controller; Varuṇa, the master of the waters; Śāśaṅka, the moon Lord; Procreator Brahmā; and you are the father of Brahmā. Obeisances unto You a thousand times repeatedly. Again and again, honor to You! (11.39)

Commentary:

The Śrīmad Bhagavata Purāṇa and the Vishnu Purāṇa gave Lord Garbhodakaśāyī Viṣṇu as the father of Brahmā. Brahmā is said to have emerged from the lotus shaped navel of this God. Arjuna addressed the Central Figure of the Universal Form as this Vishnu. Repeatedly, over and over, a thousand times and more, Arjuna offers obeisances to that Super—Person.

नमः पुरस्तादथ पृष्ठतस्ते
नमोऽस्तु ते सर्वत एव सर्व ।
अनन्तवीर्यामितविक्रमस्त्वं
सर्वं समाप्नोषि ततोऽसि सर्वः ॥ ११.४० ॥
namaḥ purastādatha pṛṣṭhataste
namo'stu te sarvata eva sarva
anantavīryāmitavikramastvaṁ
sarvaṁ samāpnoṣi tato'si sarvaḥ
(11.40)

namaḥ— reverence; purastāt — from in front; atha — and then; pṛṣṭhataḥ — from behind; te — to you; namo = namaḥ — obeisances; 'stu = astu — let there be; te — to you; sarvata — on all sides; eva — also; sarva — sum total reality; anantavīryāmitavikramaḥ = ananta — infinite + vīrya — power + amita — immeasurable + vikramaḥ — might; tvaṁ — you; sarvaṁ — everything; samāpnoṣi — you penetrate; tato = tataḥ — thus, in that sense; 'si = asi — you are; sarvaḥ — everything

Reverence to You from the front, from behind. Let there be obeisances to You on all sides, O sum total Reality. You are infinite power, immeasurable might. You penetrate everything. In that sense, You are Everything. (11.40)

Commentary:

Arjuna is stunned. He finds that he can do nothing else but to join the siddhas in the glorification of that Cosmic Person. From the front, from behind, from all sides, Arjuna is going through the motions of offering sincere and deep respects to that God. He regards the God as everything, as sarva, the Sum—total Reality. In this vision when one has it, it feels as if everything else does not exist by itself and that only the God Himself is everything. Nothing feels as being objective or contrasted to that God. In such a vision, one's individual existence is for the time being suspended because one loses track of desires while the vision is seen.

सखेति मत्वा प्रसभं यदुक्तं
हे कृष्ण हे यादव हे सखेति.।
अजानता महिमानं तवेदं
मया प्रमादात्प्रणयेन वापि ॥ ११.४१ ॥
sakheti matvā prasabhaṁ
yaduktaṁ
he kṛṣṇa he yādava he sakheti
ajānatā mahimānaṁ tavedaṁ
mayā pramādāt praṇayena vāpi
(11.41)

sakheti = sakhā — friend + iti — such as; matvā — considering; prasabhaṁ — impulsively; yat — whatever; uktaṁ — was said; he — hey; kṛṣṇa — Kṛṣṇa; he — hey; yādava — family man of the Yadus; he — hey; sakheti = sakhā — buddy + iti — thus; ajānatā — through ignorance; mahimānaṁ — majestic supernatural glory; tavedaṁ = tava — your + idam — this; mayā — by me; pramādāt — from familiarity; pranayena — with affection; vāpi = va — or + api — even

Whatever was said impulsively, considering You as a friend, such as, "Hey, Krishna! Hey, family man of the Yadus! Hey, buddy!" was done by me through ignorance of Your majestic supernatural glory or even by affectionate familiarity. (11.41)

Commentary:

Even though he viewed the Universal Form, he realized the Central Personality as the God Vishnu, the father of the creator—god Brahmā. Arjuna also realized that this was the same Śrī Krishna, his friend and cousin. To that Central Figure, Arjuna offered an apology. The significance of this is that Arjuna did not lose total touch with his earthly reference point. Frequently, when a yogi gets such a vision or is transferred out of this existence for a time, he loses touch with his earthly rationale. Forgetting the person he functioned as on earth, he tunes into the new locale and plays out whatever role he is circumstantially positioned for there. He loses the earthly perspective and acts in a way that may not be consistent with his earthly values and culture. Arjuna retained the earthly awareness.

Arjuna apologized to the Central Figure. He spoke to the gigantic Form just as if he were speaking to Śrī Krishna, the human being. This is because Arjuna integrated into his understanding that the Central Figure was in fact Śrī Krishna, the human being. Arjuna asked to be pardoned for being casual with Krishna in the social relationship they enjoyed on earth. Arjuna regarded Śrī Krishna as his cousin and dear friend only and not as the God Vishnu to whom the people prayed, not as the Almighty Supreme Personality from Whom all originated. Because of ignorance and familiarity, Arjuna did not take Śrī Krishna seriously when He suggested that Arjuna should fight. Arjuna simply refused. There were other occasions when Arjuna had either slighted Śrī Krishna, denied Him or just outright rejected whatever Śrī Krishna had to say. Arjuna apologized for that too.

This is significant to a kriyā yogi since it means that someone whom we might consider to be ordinary might be God or might be a god or a supernatural ruler. So long as we are not perceiving supernaturally, we cannot understand the status of each individual. We might reject a divine instruction merely because of perceptual ignorance or because of social familiarity. If Arjuna could do this to Śrī Krishna, certainly we are capable of it too.

यच्चावहासार्थमसत्कृतोऽसि
विहारशय्यासनभोजनेषु ।
एकोऽथ वाप्यच्युत तत्समक्षं
तत्क्षामये त्वामहमप्रमेयम् ॥ ११.४२ ॥
yaccāvahāsārthamasatkṛto'si
vihāraśayyāsanabhojaneṣu
eko'tha vāpyacyut tatsamakṣaṁ
tatkṣāmaye tvām aham
aprameyam (11.42)

yat— that; cāvahāsārtham = ca — and + avahāsa — joking + artham — intention; asatkṛto = asatkṛtaḥ — disrespectfully; 'si = asi — you are; vihāraśayyāsanabhojaneṣu = vihāra — play + śayyā — couch + āsana — sitting + bhojaneṣu — in dining; eko = ekaḥ — alone, privately; 'thavāpi = athavāpi = athava — nor + api — also; acyuta — O infallible Kṛṣṇa; tatsamakṣaṁ — before the public; tat — that; kṣāmaye — I ask forgiveness; tvām — of you; aham — I; aprameyam — one who is boundless

And with intent to joke, You were disrespectfully treated, while playing, while on a couch, while sitting, while dining privately or even in public, O infallible Krishna. For that I ask forgiveness of You Who are boundless. (11.42)

Commentary:

Arjuna still spoke to the Central Figure in the Universal Form but with the understanding of that Cosmic Person as Śrī Krishna. Arjuna remembered incidences when he slighted Śrī

Krishna or regarded the God as just some other human being who was his friend and relative. Recognizing that Śrī Krishna knew Himself all along and that Śrī Krishna realized all along that Arjuna was slighting Him but still never complained about it, Arjuna felt that apologies were due.

पितासि लोकस्य चराचरस्य
त्वमस्य पूज्यश्च गुरुर्गरीयान् ।
न त्वत्समोऽस्त्यभ्यधिकः कुतोऽन्यो
लोकत्रयेऽप्यप्रतिमप्रभाव ॥ ११.४३ ॥
pitāsi lokasya carācarasya
tvamasya pūjyaśca gururgarīyān
na tvatsamo
'styabhyadhikaḥ kuto'nyo
lokatraye'pyapratim aprabhāva
(11.43)

pitāsi = pitā — father + asi — you are; lokasya — of the world; carācarasya — of the moving and non — moving; tvam — you; asya — of this; pūjyaśca — pūjyaḥ — worshipable + ca — and; guruḥ — spiritual master; garīyān — gravest; na — not; tvatsamo = tvatsamaḥ = tyat (tvam) — you + samaḥ — similar, like; 'sti = asti — there is; abhyadhikaḥ — greater; kuto = kutaḥ — how; 'nyo = anyaḥ — other; lokatraye — in the three partitions of the universe; 'pi = api — also; apratimaprabhāva — person of uncomparable splendor

You are the father of the world, of the moving and non—moving objects. You are the worshipable and gravest spiritual master. There is none like You in the three partitions of the universe. How could anyone be greater, O person of uncomparable splendor? (11.43)

Commentary:

Arjuna continues to glorify Śrī Krishna, the Central Figure of the Universal Form. He addressed Śrī Krishna as the father of the moving and non—moving objects, as the worshipable and gravest of the spiritual masters, as being incomparable in splendor and as being the greatest Personality in the three partitions of the universe, the upper, median and lower planetary systems according to the description in the Vedic literatures and the experience of the yogin mystics.

तस्मात्प्रणम्य प्रणिधाय कायं
प्रसादये त्वामहमीशमीड्यम् ।
पितेव पुत्रस्य सखेव सख्युः
प्रियः प्रियायार्हसि देव सोढुम् ॥ ११.४४ ॥
tasmātpraṇamya praṇidhāya kāyaṁ
prasādaye tvāmahamīśamīḍyam
piteva putrasya sakheva sakhyuḥ
priyaḥ priyāyārhasi deva soḍhum
(11.44)

tasmāt — therefore; praṇamya — bowing with reverence; praṇidhāya — lying down; kāyaṁ — body; prasādaye — I ask mercy; tvām — you; aham — of you; īśam — Lord; īḍyam — to be praised; piteva = pitā— father + eva — as; putrasya — of a son; sakheva = sakhā — friend + eva — as; sakhyuḥ — of a chum; priyaḥ — beloved; priyāyārhasi = priyāya — to a lover + arhasi — you should; deva — O God; soḍhum — to be merciful

Therefore, bowing with reverence, lying my body down, I ask for mercy of You, O Lord Who is to be praised. As a father to a son, as a friend to his chum, as a beloved to a lover, You should be merciful, O God. (11.44)

Commentary:

Bowing with reverence and lying his body down before Śrī Krishna were more supernatural acts than physical ones. His physical body went through the motions because it mimicked his supernatural form. This is an important notation for kriyā practice, since we should learn to differentiate between the various bodies.

A kriyā yogi may bow with his subtle form and not bow with the gross one. Or he may bow with the gross form and not move the subtle one. Arjuna's consciousness, that was now shifted over to his energized supernatural form, bowed in reverence.

Arjuna asked for mercy since he felt uneasy about his familiar and sometimes callous regard for Śrī Krishna. Appealing in an emotional way, he wanted to be forgiven as father would forgive a son, or a friend his chum or a beloved the lover. Arjuna did not want to be in contrast to Śrī Krishna or to be chewed up by any of the supernatural mouths. He wanted to be on the good side of Śrī Krishna.

अदृष्टपूर्वं हृषितोऽस्मि दृष्ट्वा
भयेन च प्रव्यथितं मनो मे ।
तदेव मे दर्शय देव रूपं
प्रसीद देवेश जगन्निवास ॥ ११.४५॥
adṛṣṭapūrvaṁ hṛṣito'smi dṛṣṭvā
bhayena ca pravyathitaṁ mano me
tadeva me darśaya deva rūpaṁ
prasīda deveśa jagannivāsa (11.45)

adṛṣṭapūrvaṁ = adṛṣṭa — never seen + pūrvaṁ — previously; hṛṣito = hṛṣitaḥ — delighted; 'smi = asmi — I am; dṛṣṭvā— having seen; bhayena — with fear; ca — and, but; pravyathitaṁ — trembling; mano = manaḥ — mind; me — my; tat — that; eva — indeed; me — to me; darśaya — to see; deva — O God; rūpaṁ — God-form; prasīda — have mercy; deveśa — Lord of gods; jagannivāsa — shelter of the world

Seeing what was never seen before, I am delighted but my mind trembles with fear. Now, O God, cause me to see the God—form. Have mercy, O Lord of the gods, shelter of the world. (11.45)

Commentary:

Arjuna was both delighted and frightened. In the kriyā yoga perspective this must be considered since we must prepare ourselves for the revelation of the same Form if perchance we are graced to see it. Then we too would be delighted and frightened. The fright is a natural reaction of our limited psyche. We should not be embarrassed about it. We should be willing to endure it, knowing fully well that we are not really in danger.

As kriyā yogis we would also be delighted in so far as we have cooperated with and fulfilled the will of Śrī Krishna. According to what we learned so far in the *Gītā*, we are on the right track in taking up the purificatory disciplines. Śrī Krishna approves this. As Arjuna said, from seeing what was never seen before, one part of him, the higher part of his psyche, was delighted but his lower mind trembled with fear.

Originally Arjuna only wanted to see how Krishna controlled the material world and the circumstances that occur within it. After getting that vision, Arjuna took the opportunity to ask to see something that He had always desired to view, which was the form of the God without reference to controlling this material world. That was Arjuna's foremost desire.

Arjuna asked to see the devarūpa, the form of God. This means that Arjuna was conscious of a difference between the varying features of the Godhead. He knew that beyond the Universal Form, the God existed free from those disciplinary tasks.

किरीटिनं गदिनं चक्रहस्तम्
इच्छामि त्वां द्रष्टुमहं तथैव ।
तेनैव रूपेण चतुर्भुजेन
सहस्रबाहो भव विश्वमूर्ते ॥ ११.४६॥

kirīṭinaṁ — form which wears a crown, gadinaṁ — form which is armed with a club; cakrahastaṁ — form with a disc in hand; icchāmi — I wish; tvāṁ — you; draṣṭum — to see; aham — I; tathaiva = tathā — as requested + eva — indeed;

kirīṭinaṁ gadinaṁ cakrahastam
icchāmi tvāṁ draṣṭumahaṁ tathaiva
tenaiva rūpeṇa caturbhujena
sahasrabāho bhava viśvamūrte
(11.46)

tenaiva = tena — with this + eva — indeed; rūpeṇa — with the form; caturbhujena — with four arms; sahasrabāho — O thousand-armed person; bhava — become; viśvamūrte — person of universal dimensions

I wish to see You wearing a crown, armed with a club, and with a disc in hand, as requested. Please become that four—armed form, O thousand—armed Person, O Person of universal dimensions. (11.46)

Commentary:

By yoga austerities, Arjuna saw many of the supernatural rulers like Lord Shiva, Indra and Varuṇa. He did not see Lord Vishnu. Thus this desire to see Lord Vishnu persisted in his mind. He took the opportunity to get this boon from Śrī Krishna for a vision of Lord Vishnu. It was an easy thing to ask for, now that he had supernatural eyes. Now he knew for sure that his friend and cousin, Śrī Krishna, was, in fact, Lord Vishnu posing on earth as a human being, hiding His divine glories by coming down to the human plane as an Avatar or divine person who appears to be reduced by physical limitations.

Arjuna heard of that Vishnu Person from others. He knew the descriptions of the God's divine attire and form. He had information from scriptures and from the eyewitness accounts of great yogins like Nārada and Markandeya. He requested to see that God Vishnu with four arms, wearing a crown. He no longer wanted to see thousands of arms of the Universal Form with its multidimensional significance and its inclusion of everything in the material world.

श्रीभगवानुवाच
मया प्रसन्नेन तवार्जुनेदं
रूपं परं दर्शितमात्मयोगात् ।
तेजोमयं विश्वमनन्तमाद्यं
यन्मे त्वदन्येन न दृष्टपूर्वम् ॥ ११.४७॥
śrībhagavānuvāca
mayā prasannena tavārjunedaṁ
rūpaṁ paraṁ darśitam ātmayogāt
tejomayaṁ viśvamanantam ādyaṁ
yanme tvadanyena na dṛṣṭapūrvam
(11.47)

śrī bhagavān — the Blessed Lord; uvāca — said; mayā — by me; prasannena — by grace; tavārjunedaṁ = tava — to you + arjuna — Arjuna+ idam — this; rūpaṁ — form; param — supreme; darśitaṁ — manifested; ātmayogāt — from my yoga power; tejomayaṁ — made of supernatural energy; viśvam — universal; anantam — infinite; ādyaṁ — primal; yat — which; me — my; tvadanyena = tvad — besides you + anyena — by any other; na — not; dṛṣṭapūrvam = dṛṣṭa — seen + pūrvam — before

The Blessed Lord said: By My grace to you Arjuna, this Supreme Form was manifested from My yoga power. This Form of Mine which is made of supernatural energy, being universal, infinite and primal, was never seen by any other person besides you. (11.47)

Commentary:

The supernatural energy of the Form is called tejomaya in Sanskrit. This means a form which was made of light only and nothing gross. It is a supernatural form. Presently we cannot understand such a form because our psyche leans downward into gross matter. If by kriyā yoga, we perform sufficient austerities, the forms of light will be manifested and we would then be suited to such forms ourselves and can lay aside the gross existence we presently endure.

The supernatural form which Śrī Krishna showed Arjuna was seen by others before and would be seen by others afterwards, but the particular phase of it was never seen at any other time. Arjuna saw a phase that related directly to the situation at Kurukṣetra. That was unique. As the Blessed Lord said, it was a special grace to Arjuna, that the Form was manifested by Krishna's yoga power, by His psychological control.

न वेदयज्ञाध्ययनैर्न दानैर्
न च क्रियाभिर्न तपोभिरुग्रैः ।
एवंरूपः शक्य अहं नृलोके
द्रष्टुं त्वदन्येन कुरुप्रवीर ॥११.४८॥

na vedayajñādhyayanairna dānair
na ca kriyābhirna tapobhirugraiḥ
evaṁrūpaḥ śakya ahaṁ nṛloke
draṣṭuṁ tvadanyena kurupravīra (11.48)

na — not; vedayajñādhyayanaiḥ = veda — Veda + yajñā — by sacrificial ceremonies + adyayanaiḥ — by education; na — nor; danaiḥ — by charity as recommended in the Vedic literature; na — not; ca — and; kriyābhiḥ — by special ritual acts; na — not; tapobhiḥ — by austerities; ugraiḥ — by strenuous; evam — as such; rūpaḥ — form; śakya = śakye — can; ahaṁ — I; nṛloke — in the world of human beings; draṣṭuṁ — to see; tvadanyena = tvad — except you + anyena — by another; kurupravīra — great hero of the Kurus

Not by Vedic sacrificial ceremonies, nor by Vedic education, not by offering charity as recommended in the Vedic literatures and not by special ritual acts, nor by strenuous austerities, can I be seen in such a form in this world of human beings except through the method used by you, O great hero of the Kurus. (11.48)

Commentary:

This statement must be taken seriously. This means that by austerities we will not be able to see what Arjuna saw. Such an apparition is manifested only by special grace to the devotee of Śrī Krishna. It is a fact.

For that matter when a great yogin gives shaktipat initiation it concerns the experience of the subtle body or causal form, all depending on the level of practice of the student. It usually does not concern the facet of our individual or joint resistance to the Supreme will. What Arjuna saw had to do with conjointed resistance to the divinity, as well as a show of the majesty of God as it relates to this material world. In kriyā yoga practice, this is not the primary concern of the neophyte yogi. His main interest is self purification, the removal of psychological impurities which cause him to remain on lower planes.

We must also note that a vision of the Universal Form would not be given to a devotee or a yogi—devotee unless he had a mission to serve that Form in a big way, as Arjuna was destined to perform. As such if we are not warriors, or if we are not political leaders, then it is hardly likely that we would get the vision of that Form. Arjuna saw the phase of the Form that related to what he was involved in, which was the Kuru civil war.

One cannot see such a Form merely by becoming an expert at Vedic sacrificial ceremonies. This means that an expert priest cannot see such a Form. He cannot make himself see it directly. God would not allow him to see it either, because his duties do not require its perception. It cannot be seen whimsically or merely based on one's desire.

A pandit who is very educated in Sanskrit and in the *Vedas* and Vedic literatures would not see the Form, nor would a devotee who offers Vedic style charity, nor would a tantric expert who can perform special ritual acts which are complicated and which if done improperly ruins the performers and causes twists in their destinies.

Even a yogi who performed the most strenuous austerities would not see such a Form. In fact he might be the least qualified to see it. His reductions in the performance of karma yoga disqualifies him.

Even though Śrī Krishna said that the Form can only be seen by the method conducted by Arjuna, still the Form is rarely revealed to anyone besides Arjuna. After all, who is as close as Arjuna? Who is as useful politically? Who is willing to fight relatives, to even displace them for the sake of Śrī Krishna? Śrī Krishna undoubtedly has millions of devotees in this world, but that does not mean that the vast majority would kill relatives just to satisfy the chastening moods of the Universal Form.

मा ते व्यथा मा च विमूढभावो
दृष्ट्वा रूपं घोरमीदृङ्ममेदम् ।
व्यपेतभीः प्रीतमनाः पुनस्त्वं
तदेव मे रूपमिदं प्रपश्य ॥ ११.४९॥

mā te vyathā mā ca vimūḍhabhāvo
dṛṣṭvā rūpaṁ ghoramīdṛṅmamedam
vyapetabhīḥ prītamanāḥ punastvaṁ
tadeva me rūpamidaṁ prapaśya
(11.49)

mā— not; te— of you; vyathā— should tremble; mā— not; ca — and; vimūḍhabhāvo = vimūḍhabhāvaḥ — confused state; dṛṣṭvā— having seen; rūpam — form; ghoram —ghastly; īdṛn = īdṛḥ— such; mamedam = mama—of my + idam — this; vyapetabhīḥ= vyapeta — freed from + bhīḥ— fear; prītamanāḥ— cheerful in mind; punaḥ — again; tvam — you; tat — you; eva — indeed; me — of me; rūpam —form; idam— this; prapaśya — look at

You should not tremble or be confused after seeing this, My ghastly form. Be free from fear and be cheerful of mind. Again look at this form of Mine. (11.49)

Commentary:

Śrī Krishna phased out the supernatural vision which Arjuna was awarded and gave Arjuna a different vision, divine eyesight to see the Divine Form of Lord Vishnu with four arms. Krishna asked Arjuna to look again and see that Divine Form which was most dear to Arjuna and which Arjuna always wanted to view.

संजय उवाच
इत्यर्जुनं वासुदेवस्तथोक्त्वा
स्वकं रूपं दर्शयामास भूयः ।
आश्वासयामास च भीतमेनं
भूत्वा पुनः सौम्यवपुर्महात्मा ॥ ११.५०॥

saṁjaya uvāca
ityarjunaṁ vāsudevas tathoktvā
svakaṁ rūpaṁ darśayāmāsa bhūyaḥ
āśvāsayāmāsa ca bhītamenaṁ
bhūtvā punaḥ saumyavapur
mahātmā (11.50)

Saṁjaya — Sanjaya; uvāca — said; iti — thus; arjunam = Arjuna; vāsudevaḥ — Kṛṣṇa, the son of Vasudeva; tathoktvā= tathā — thus + uktvā — having said; svakaṁ — his own; rūpaṁ — divine form; darśayāmāsa — he revealed; bhūyaḥ — again; āsvāsayāmāsa — he caused to be calm; ca — and; bhītam — frightened person; enam — this; bhūtvā — having assumed; punaḥ = punar — again; saumyavapuḥ = saumya — pleasing + vapuḥ — attractive appearance; mahātmā — great person

Sanjaya said: Krishna, the son of Vasudeva, having said this to Arjuna, revealed His own Divine Form. And once again that great person assumed the pleasing, attractive form and caused the frightened Arjuna to be calm. (11.50)

Commentary:

This verse 50 is the highlight of the kriyā yoga practice in the sense that ultimately the kriyā yogi wants to develop or be transferred into a spiritual body, a divine form, made of his own spirit only and nothing else, no causal, subtle or gross material elements or even pranic gases and energies. Ultimately the aim of kriyā yoga is for the yogi to assume a spiritual form with limbs and senses. We have to deduce that Arjuna used such a form for viewing that Divine Form of Śrī Krishna, the four handed Vishnu Form.

Some contend that this verse indicates that Arjuna just saw the same Krishna, the human historic body but that is not true since this form is not the same as the body produced from Devakī and Vasudeva. This is a Divine Form which has nothing to do with affairs in this world. It is even different to the supernatural Universal Form which Arjuna viewed.

Arjuna assumed spiritual eyes with a spiritual body as himself. He stared through spiritual eyes due to an energization put on him by Śrī Krishna. For us it may be that we must achieve this by yoga practice. It is not that we are working to see Krishna's form even though that might be attained in the process. We are working to integrate into our own spiritual forms without being hooked up to causal, subtle or gross material forms. Arjuna did not request his spiritual form but rather to see Krishna's. To achieve that, Arjuna was transferred into his spiritual body. In our case, the objective is to realize our individual spiritual form. We do not know as yet which Personality of Godhead, which Divinity we are connected to, and where in this spiritual domain we will be transferred to, once this occurs. It is not important that we know this beforehand.

Some say that we should be Krishna's devotees; others say, "No, it is better to be a Rāma bhakta." And yet others say that it is better to be nobody's worshipper. These arguments have no value because the important thing is to develop or assume or be transferred into the spiritual form. Once that is attained our relationship with God and our position in the spiritual domains will be automatically revealed. Arjuna was very satisfied to see that Lord of his life, his cherished deity (ishtadeva), Who had four hands. This also means that Arjuna was not like the cowherd boys of Vṛndāvana whose Lord was Krishna, the divine cowherd boy with two hands. Śrī Bhīṣmadeva too, was very satisfied at the end of his life, when this same historic Śrī Krishna revealed this same four-handed form of Lord Vishnu. Thus for them that form of the Divine is the person for whom they have the most divine affection, the One to Whom their devotional service is best suited. Each devotee, each yogi, must individually reach the stage of meeting that Lord of his life, thereby escaping the theoretical presentations and impositions about spiritual development and relationship.

Even though his devotional relationship was best suited to the four-handed form of Lord Vishnu which Śrī Krishna revealed, still Arjuna had to work in this world to please the Universal Form, the Vishvarupa. Take note of this. We should be practical. We do not want to reject the Universal Form's demands just because we are related to another feature of the Godhead. Like Arjuna we may have to serve in the social, cultural and political fields under the supervision of the Universal Form so that ultimately we can reach the Divine Person Who is most dear to us.

अर्जुन उवाच
दृष्ट्वेदं मानुषं रूपं
तव सौम्यं जनार्दन ।
इदानीमस्मि संवृत्तः
सचेताः प्रकृतिं गतः ॥ ११.५१ ॥
arjuna uvāca
dṛṣṭvedaṁ mānuṣaṁ rūpaṁ
tava saumyaṁ janārdana
idānīmasmi saṁvṛttaḥ
sacetāḥ prakṛtiṁ gataḥ (11.51)

arjuna — Arjuna; uvāca — said; dṛṣṭvedaṁ = dṛṣṭvā — having seen + idam —— this; mānuṣaṁ — human; rūpaṁ — form; tava — of you; saumyam — gentle; janārdana — O motivator of human beings; idānīm — now; asmi — I am; saṁvṛttaḥ — satisfied; sacetāḥ — with mind; prakṛtiṁ — to human nature, to normal condition; gataḥ — gone back, returned

Arjuna said: Seeing this gentle, human-like Form of Yours, O Janardana, motivator of human beings, I am satisfied with my mind returned to the normal condition. (11.51)

Commentary:

The Divine Vishnu Form which Arjuna saw, the one with four hands, had a human appearance. He was not gigantic and multi-personed like the Universal Form. He did not threaten anyone or engage in disciplinary responses. This is because that particular Vishnu Form is detached from the material world and does not respond to it with disapproval. That Form does not try to counteract our defiance. Thus Arjuna's mind had no reason to be repulsed from or frightened of Him.

श्रीभगवानुवाच
सुदुर्दर्शमिदं रूपं
दृष्टवानसि यन्मम ।
देवा अप्यस्य रूपस्य
नित्यं दर्शनकाङ्क्षिणः ॥ ११.५२ ॥
śrībhagavānuvāca
sudurdarśamidaṁ rūpaṁ
dṛṣṭavānasi yanmama
devā apyasya rūpasya
nityaṁ darśanakāṅkṣiṇaḥ (11.52)

śrī bhagavān — The Blessed Lord; uvāca — said; sudurdarśam — difficult to perceive; idam — this; rūpaṁ — form; dṛṣṭvān — having seen; asi — you are; yat — which; mamā — of mine; devā — supernatural rulers; api — also; asya — of this; rūpasya — of the form; nityam — always; darśanakāṅkṣiṇaḥ = darśana — sight + kāṅkṣiṇaḥ — wishing

The Blessed Lord said: This Form of Mine which you saw, is difficult to perceive. Even the supernatural rulers always wish for the sight of this Form. (11.52)

Commentary:

Indeed that is because most of the supernatural rulers are related devotionally to that four-handed Vishnu Form. The body Arjuna used to view that Form was not only different from his material body, but different from the supernatural one he used to see the Universal Form. The supernatural rulers are agents for that Vishnu Form but since they are engaged in mundane affairs, they lose touch with Him. They long to get out of the material world and to relocate to the spiritual provinces where that Form is available for loving devotional service.

We may see such a form momentarily just as Arjuna did but not otherwise. Presently, if perchance we are permitted to see that Form, then it will be in a flash and that is all. It will hardly be maintained for more than seconds. I say this from experience.

Once the Lord Padmanabha, a particular version of the four—handed Vishnu appeared to me. He came very close. His spiritual body had a pleasing appearance. I used spiritual eyes which focused on Him but they were only available for about 35 seconds. After that I was transferred back into astral vision and then into physical vision to which I remained time-bound.

At another time, the two—handed cowherd divine Krishna was seen by me. During the vision, I was in my spiritual body with spiritual vision, but that lasted for about three minutes while Śrī Krishna, the divine cowherd boy, kept himself at a distance from me. He moved further and further away as if He did not desire that I should embrace Him. None of these visions were controlled by me nor did I specifically desire to see Them at the time when they occurred. Up to the publication of this commentary, I have not found a definite method through which I could transfer myself into the spiritual body. However recently Lord Krishna of my Śrī Śrī Krishna and Balarāma Deities said that certainly, He feels that I will soon get a method. In addition Swami Muktananda, a siddha who left a physical body recently, told me that he has a method through which he sees Śrī Hari, the divine boy Krishna.

As Śrī Krishna told Arjuna, the supernatural rulers wish to see that Form. They are barred from the perception because they are too preoccupied with subtle mundane affairs in the supernatural world which is directly adjacent to the physical dimensions we live in. Their condition is to be regretted. A kriyā yogi should not aspire to become a deva supernatural ruler, because then he would be just as they are.

नाहं वेदैर्न तपसा
न दानेन न चेज्यया ।
शक्य एवंविधो द्रष्टुं
दृष्टवानसि मां यथा ॥११.५३॥
nāhaṁ vedairna tapasā
na dānena na cejyayā
śakya evaṁvidho draṣṭuṁ
dṛṣṭavānasi māṁ yathā (11.53)

nāhaṁ = na — neither + aham — I; vedaiḥ — by Vedic study; na — nor; tapasā — by austerity; na — nor; dānena — by charity; na — not; cejyayā = ca — and + ijyayā — by sacrificial ceremony; śakya = śakye — I can; evaṁvidho = evaṁvidhaḥ — in that way; draṣṭuṁ — to see; dṛṣṭavān — having seen; asi — you are; mām — me; yathā — as

Neither by Vedic study, nor by austerity, nor by charity, and not by sacrificial ceremony, can I be seen in the way you saw Me. (11.53)

<u>Commentary:</u>

Here, the restrictions are given, but this does not mean that we should abandon Vedic study, austerity, charity and sacrificial ceremony, because elsewhere in the *Gītā*, the same Śrī Krishna advised their adoption. It means however that we must know for certain that these will not yield such a vision. We should do this but not with the motivation to get such a vision or to be transferred into a spiritual body in the way Arjuna was when Śrī Krishna transferred him into it.

Austerity in particular, which is basically the territory of yoga, when done correctly, causes purification of the psyche. From that purification other benefits come into play.

भक्त्या त्वनन्यया शक्य
अहमेवंविधोऽर्जुन ।
ज्ञातुं द्रष्टुं च तत्त्वेन
प्रवेष्टुं च परंतप ॥११.५४॥

bhaktyā — by devotion; tu — only; ananyayā — not in another way, undistracted; śakya = śakye — I can; aham — I; evaṁvidho = evaṁvidhaḥ — in that way; 'rjuna = arjuna — Arjuna; jñātuṁ — to be known; draṣṭuṁ — to see; ca — and; tattvena — by reality;

bhaktyā tvananyayā śakya
ahamevaṁvidho'rjuna
jñātuṁ draṣṭuṁ ca tattvena
praveṣṭuṁ ca paraṁtapa (11.54)

praveṣṭuṁ — to communicate with; ca — and; paraṁtapa — scorcher of the enemies

By undistracted devotion only, O Arjuna, can I be known, seen in reality, and communicated with, O scorcher of enemies. (11.54)

Commentary:

The method for seeing that Divine Form is undistracted devotion. Thus we may ask how it is that Arjuna saw the Form merely upon request. Some Vaishnava preachers sell unfulfilled promises to devotees. Their chief slogan is this undistracted devotion to Śrī Krishna, bhaktyā ananyayā. However, many teachers do not have the undistracted devotion. Since many ordinary devotees do not know what it is, they are fooled by the teachers and tricked into serving their missionary intentions.

Let us note that Arjuna merely asked Śrī Krishna for the vision. Arjuna was not selling *Bhagavad Gītā* books to thousands of people. Arjuna was not building temples, or carving deities or doing Deity ceremonies. Arjuna was not chanting his teacher's glory—prayers. He was not attending lectures by self-proclaimed pure devotees. He was not chanting the Hare Krishna Mantra or any Mahamantra of a Vaishnava sect. How then was Arjuna qualified with undistracted devotion? Arjuna was the very person who refused to fight, who in effect, told Śrī Krishna that he was nervous about the battle. Arjuna was not convinced that Śrī Krishna was right. He regarded war as a cruelty to family members and friends.

In the case of the writer, he too saw divine forms in this body on two occasions. At both times, he was not doing anything especially devotional. In the first case when I saw the Lord Padmanabha, one of the four-handed Vishnu Forms, I was not even in a Vaishnava Sampradāya. I was practicing yoga and mysticism, but I had not formally accepted a spiritual master in disciplic succession from Śrī Krishna. Later, when I saw the Divine cowherd boy with the divine iridescent glowing deep blue body, I worked as a janitor in a Christian Church and had laid my physical body in a small dining room of that worship facility. It had nothing to do with the devotional service of the Vaishnava sects. In fact, I had recently left one such sect.

Without comparing myself to Arjuna, these incidences, his and mine, show that undistracted devotion has to mean something other than what some Vaishnava leaders are telling us. The majority of their followers do not get such experiences, despite the fact that the leaders keep saying that they are engaging them in undistracted devotion.

Now after presenting this information and going in a round about way, I will clearly define for the readers that undistracted devotion. It is simply one's relationship with the Divine Person, Who is revealed. In other words, it has nothing to do with one's present designation as a human being or as a disciple in a disciplic succession. If one's spirit has the relationship with the four-handed Form, it has it, regardless of a current affiliation with a lineage. This is not to say that the succession and the leaders of it have no value. I am saying that the actual meaning hinges on a spiritual relation that was emitted long, long ago even before this gross creation came about. It is not something that might be or could be created now.

मत्कर्मकृन्मत्परमो
मद्भक्तः सङ्गवर्जितः ।
निर्वैरः सर्वभूतेषु
यः स मामेति पाण्डव ॥११.५५॥
matkarmakṛnmatparamo
madbhaktaḥ saṅgavarjitaḥ
nirvairaḥ sarvabhūteṣu
yaḥ sa māmeti pāṇḍava (11.55)

matkarmakṛt — doing my work; matparamo = matparamaḥ — depending on me; madbhaktaḥ — being devoted to me; saṅgavarjitaḥ = saṅga — attachment + varjitaḥ — abandoned; nirvairaḥ — free from hostility; sarvabhūteṣu — to all beings; yah — who; sa = saḥ — he; mām — to me; eti — comes; pāṇḍava — son of Pandu

Whosoever does My work, depending on Me, being devoted to Me, abandoning attachment, being freed from hostility towards all beings, comes to Me, O son of Pandu. (11.55)

Commentary:

Some commentators and lecturers on the *Gītā* assure audiences that if they tow the line of the particular missions and adhere to its advices regarding how to attain Śrī Krishna, then certainly at least at the time of death, they will go to Śrī Krishna. However, most of these promises are so much hype that will get us nowhere, not a step closer to Śrī Krishna. Here is why:

Śrī Krishna speaks here of His work which is described already in Chapter Four, the work of karma yoga, the kind of work He cited Janaka as having done, the kind of work He instigated that Arjuna should perform. In Chapter Four, Śrī Krishna called this His personal way of yoga, or rather His personal course for teaching persons like Manu and Ikṣvāku, on how to apply yoga disciplines to rulership duties. From this Chapter Eleven, we gained more insight on this to see that this is actually traceable to the Universal Form which Arjuna saw and which bore resentments towards the pee-wee spirits who flout His authority by doing whatever they want whenever they are manifested in this world by Him. He then takes steps to discipline them. He expects persons like Arjuna to assist Him in this disciplinary approach.

To do this means to depend on Him. Otherwise one would not have the strength to do His work since it sometimes involves callous actions in respect to one's relatives and friends. We would all break down emotionally if we did not have that dependence on the Universal Form, through which the required chivalry and psychological strength would be imparted into us, as it was into the soft—hearted Arjuna.

Sir Paul Castagna, whose sparse remarks appear in this book, has called this "the path of no return". According to him, to adapt the karma yoga that Śrī Krishna introduced, a person must see himself as taking a path through this world, once and for all, without ever having to return to face the people he has hurt on behalf of God. We know, however, that it is on behalf of the ghastly Universal Form which Arjuna saw, the one which bit, crunched, burned and scalded the opponents of the divine will.

To go on such a path one would have to abandon attachment to all social norms and to one's peers and relatives, but one would also have to be freed from hostility. If one maintains personal likes and dislikes, one would be distracted and would not become absorbed with the likes and dislikes of the Central Figure in the Universal Form. In other words if He disliked something, one would have to turn away from it. If he liked something, one would have to select it, even if personally one disliked it. Such a person who could do all these things would go to that Lord Vishnu eventually, just as Arjuna was destined to, after his life as a member of the Kuru family.

CHAPTER 12

The Most Disciplined Yogi*

अर्जुन उवाच
एवं सततयुक्ता ये
भक्तास्त्वां पर्युपासते ।
ये चाप्यक्षरमव्यक्तं
तेषां के योगवित्तमाः ॥ १२.१ ॥
arjuna uvāca
evaṁ satatayuktā ye
bhaktāstvāṁ paryupāsate
ye cāpyakṣaramavyaktaṁ
teṣāṁ ke yogavittamāḥ (12.1)

arjuna — Arjuna; uvāca — said; evaṁ — thus; satatayuktā = satata — constantly + yuktā — disciplined in yoga; ye — who; bhaktāh — devoted; tvam —you; paryupāsate — they cherish; ye — who; cāpi = ca — and + api — also; akṣaram — imperishable; avyaktaṁ — invisible existence; teṣāṁ — of them; ke — which; yogavittamāḥ — those who have the highest knowledge of yoga

Arjuna said: Of those who are constantly disciplined in yoga, being also devoted to You, and those who cherish the imperishable invisible existence, which of these two have the highest knowledge of the yoga techniques? (12.1)

Commentary:

Here Arjuna spoke of devotion. He spoke of being disciplined in yoga and being devoted to Śrī Krishna. He does not mix one with the other. They are both different practices which are accommodated in the path to full Krishna consciousness.

Arjuna formed a contrast between yogi devotees and yogis who focus on the imperishable invisible existence. In both cases these persons are yogis but their aspirations are different. Some commentators, however, would have us believe that the first group is devotees not yogis and the second group is yogis with impersonalist bias. Both groups are yogis because in the time of Arjuna both groups specialized in yoga practice, while nowadays most of the devotees either avoid yoga or detest it altogether.

The interesting thing is this: The Divine Four—handed Form which Arjuna saw, exists in and is comprised of the same imperishable invisible existence, the akṣaram avyaktam. If a person does not have spiritual eyes, he will not perceive divine forms but will regard all as being abstract and inconceivable. Thus many who are impersonal in their aspirations are so because they do not have access to spiritual perception. The purpose of kriyā yoga is to cause a psychological purification through which we can be energized into a perception—capable spiritual body.

The most interesting thing is that Arjuna wanted to know which of the two groups of transcendentalists have the highest knowledge of the yoga techniques. The Sanskrit is yogavittamah. Directly speaking, this is a question about who has the highest yoga kriyās. That is basically what Arjuna asked.

**The Mahābhārata contains no chapter headings. This title was assigned by the translator on the basis of verse 2 of this chapter.*

श्रीभगवानुवाच
मय्यावेश्य मनो ये मां
नित्ययुक्ता उपासते ।
श्रद्धया परयोपेतास्
ते.मे युक्ततमा मताः ॥१२.२॥
śrībhagavānuvāca
mayyāveśya mano ye māṁ
nityayuktā upāsate
śraddhayā parayopetās
te me yuktatamā matāḥ (12.2)

śrībhagavān — the Blessed Lord; uvāca — said; mayyāveśya = mayi — on me + āveśya — focusing on; mano = manaḥ — mind; ye — who; māṁ — me; nityayuktā — those who are always disciplined in yoga; upāsate — they worship; śraddhayā — with faith; parayopetās = parayā — with the highest degree; upetāḥ — endowed; te — they; me — to me; yuktatamā — most disciplined; matāḥ — considered

The Blessed Lord said: Those whose minds are focused on Me, who are always disciplined in yoga, who are always involved in worship of Me, who are endowed with the highest degree of faith, they are considered to be the most disciplined. (12.2)

Commentary:

A personal reliance on someone else, on others who progressed before and who mastered the craft, can inspire, guide and accelerate the progression of an aspiring yogi. Without such assistance, one would have to be a genius to make rapid advancement. There are a few such geniuses. The example of Śrī Gautama Buddha stands out. Recently Guruji Rāmana Maharshi stood out.

Because we are persons, it is easy and natural for us to rely on persons. We find this on the mundane level as well as on the spiritual side. Thus undoubtedly those who are focused on Śrī Krishna, always disciplined in yoga and involved in worship of Krishna, having the highest degree of faith, will certainly make the most progress and acquire the most advanced techniques.

From this twelfth chapter onward, Śrī Krishna having shed his disguise as a human being, as just a cousin and friend of Arjuna, spoke as Lord Vishnu, the Four—handed Divine Person, and as the Central Figure of the Universal Form. From this point onward, Śrī Krishna spoke even more authoritatively than before, because He revealed divinity on the battlefield and cleared Arjuna's doubts. Arjuna also, with that clarity, speaks from the perspective of knowing for sure that the person whom he approached in the form of Śrī Krishna, the human son of Vasudeva and Devakī, is the Supreme God Vishnu.

When Śrī Krishna says "Me" from here on, it has more potency because of the revelation of the Universal Form and the Four—handed Divine Lord Vishnu. Śrī Krishna will no longer be accommodating to Arjuna's ignorance and familiarity. With this is mind, we can seriously study the remaining portions of the *Bhagavad Gītā*.

ये त्वक्षरमनिर्देश्यम्
अव्यक्तं पर्युपासते ।
सर्वत्रगमचिन्त्यं च
कूटस्थमचलं ध्रुवम् ॥१२.३॥
ye tvakṣaramanirdeśyam
avyaktaṁ paryupāsate
sarvatragamacintyaṁ ca
kūṭasthamacalaṁ dhruvam (12.3)

ye — who; tu — but; akṣaram — imperishable; anirdeśyam — undefinable; avyaktaṁ— invisible; paryupāsate — they cherish; sarvatragam — all—pervading; acintyam — inconceivable; ca — and; kūṭastham — unchanging; acalaṁ —— immovable; dhruvam— constant

But those who cherish the imperishable, undefinable, invisible, all—pervading, inconceivable, unchanging, immovable, constant reality, (12.3)

Commentary:

We must understand that in the imperishable, indefinable, invisible, all—pervading, inconceivable, unchanging, immovable constant reality, there might be, in fact there is, form, but it is not seen easily. One has to be equipped with a certain vision to see there.

Thus, generally, that appears to be abstract. For instance, even in this world, if we look into thin air, we do not see anything. And yet air, dust, light and even radio waves with information, are there. Spirits hover there whom we cannot perceive. Thus something might be termed as undefinable merely because we are not equipped to perceive it.

संनियम्येन्द्रियग्रामं
सर्वत्र समबुद्धयः ।
ते प्राप्नुवन्ति मामेव
सर्वभूतहिते रताः ॥१२.४॥
saṁniyamyendriyagrāmaṁ
sarvatra samabuddhayaḥ
te prāpnuvanti māmeva
sarvabhūtahite ratāḥ (12.4)

saṁniyamyendriyagrāmaṁ = saṁniyamya— controlling + indriyagrāmaṁ — all sensual energies; sarvatra — in all respects; samabuddhayaḥ — even—minded; te — them; prāpnuvanti — they attain; mām — me; eva — also; sarvabhūtahite = sarvabhūta — all creatures + hite — in the welfare; ratāḥ — rejoicing

...by controlling all sensual energies, being even—minded in all respects, rejoicing in the welfare of all creatures, they also attain Me. (12.4)

Commentary:

Even though at this point, Śrī Krishna did not state how they attain Him, He admits the achievement. Such persons must be expert in higher yoga, being detached and disinterested in potential disturbances. They must feel satisfied in the welfare of all creatures, bearing malice to none. In other words, such a person must feel a kinship with all creatures.

क्लेशोऽधिकतरस्तेषाम्
अव्यक्तासक्तचेतसाम् ।
अव्यक्ता हि गतिर्दुःखं
देहवद्भिरवाप्यते ॥१२.५॥
kleśo'dhikatarasteṣām
avyaktāsaktacetasām
avyaktā hi gatirduḥkhaṁ
dehavadbhiravāpyate (12.5)

kleśo = kleśaḥ — exertion; 'dhikataraḥ = adhikataraḥ — greater; tesam — of them; avyaktāsaktacetasām = avyakta — invisible existence + āsakta — attached + cetasām — of minds; avyaktā — invisible reality; hi — truly; gatiḥ — goal; duḥkhaṁ — difficult; dehavadbhiḥ — by the human beings; avāpyate — is attained

The mental exertion of those whose minds are attached to the invisible existence is greater. The goal of reaching that invisible reality is attained with difficulty by the human beings. (12.5)

Commentary:

Those who strive for the invisible existence without taking association from great devotees and from the Deity Forms of the Lord, must strain a lot more for the attainments. This is because those who strive for the invisible existence, do, by their attitude, debar themselves from getting assistance which would accelerate spiritual progress. It is not because they are impersonalists. It is because their mood makes them averse to taking help from mahāyogīns who could give them techniques which they might otherwise spend years discovering.

After all if one takes advice from someone who is expert in a certain field, one will be accelerated in that area and will progress faster than a person who tries to do so only through self—study and self—discovery. There are exceptions such as Gautama Buddha. Generally, those who do not take help because they feel no one is God and that no one is good enough to be trusted, take on more strain in their austerities, make more mistakes, waste more time and take longer to perfect the disciplines. By the same token, if a person is a devotee and does not do yoga, seeking only an easy way, he will not make substantial progress.

ये तु सर्वाणि कर्माणि
मयि संन्यस्य मत्पराः ।
अनन्येनैव योगेन
मां ध्यायन्त उपासते ॥ १२.६ ॥
ye tu sarvāṇi karmāṇi
mayi saṁnyasya matparāḥ
ananyenaiva yogena
māṁ dhyāyanta upāsate (12.6)

ye — who; tu — but; sarvāṇi — all; karmāṇi — actions; mayi — in me; saṁnyasya — deferring: matparāḥ — regarding me as the most important factor; ananyenaiva = ananyena — without another, undistracted + eva — indeed; yogena — with yoga discipline; māṁ — me; dhyayānta — meditating on; upāsate — they worship

But those who defer all actions to Me, regarding Me as the most important factor, who meditate on Me with undistracted yoga discipline, do worship Me. (12.6)

Commentary:

Here Śrī Krishna described the path of the neophyte kriyā yogis who do not have an exemption from cultural activities. They must do both karma yoga and kriyā yoga side by side with stress on karma yoga to please the Central Person in the Universal Form. They should do kriyā yoga in spare time to accelerate purification. This was discussed before when Arjuna declared a contradiction in Krishna's instruction that he should fight and do yoga simultaneously.

Both paths are reconciled in this verse. One has to worship Śrī Krishna. This means Deity Worship, Vaishnava style. One must also do kriyā yoga. One must also perform in the social and cultural fields to please the Central Figure in the Universal Form. Deity worship is not sufficient by itself. Yoga austerities are not sufficient. Karma yoga as described in Chapter Four is not sufficient either. These three must be done in a balanced way if we want success. That is the whole story.

तेषामहं समुद्धर्ता
मृत्युसंसारसागरात् ।
भवामि नचिरात्पार्थ
मय्यावेशितचेतसाम् ॥ १२.७ ॥
teṣāmahaṁ samuddhartā
mṛtyusaṁsārasāgarāt
bhavāmi nacirātpārtha
mayyāveśitacetasām (12.7)

teṣām — of those; aham — I; samuddhartā — delivered; mṛtyusaṁsārasāgarāt = mṛtyu — death + saṁsāra — reincarnations + sāgarāt — from the vast existence; bhavāmi — I am; nacirāt — soon; pārtha — son of Pṛthā; mayyāveśitacetasām = mayi — in me + āveśita — intently, invested in + cetasām — of thoughts

I am the deliverer of those devotees, rescuing them from the vast existence of death and reincarnation. O son of Pṛthā, I soon deliver those devotees whose thoughts are intently invested in Me. (12.7)

Commentary:

The devotees mentioned here and covered by the guarantee of this verse, are those who do karma yoga, do Deity Worship of the Vishnu or Krishna Mūrti and who do kriyā yoga also. We should not subtract anything from the qualifications nor try to contort the Sanskrit.

The investment of thoughts on Śrī Krishna occurs when we perform all those activities, not just one or the other. The three form the proper balance to attract Śrī Krishna for an early deliverance from the vast existence of death of gross bodies and reincarnation of the subtle ones into newly—formed gross ones.

मय्येव मन आधत्स्व
मयि बुद्धिं निवेशय ।
निवसिष्यसि मय्येव
अत ऊर्ध्वं न संशयः ॥१२.८॥
mayyeva mana ādhatsva
mayi buddhiṁ niveśaya
nivasiṣyasi mayyeva
ata ūrdhvaṁ na saṁśayaḥ (12.8)

mayyeva = mayi — on me + eva — alone; mana — mind; ādhatsva — place; mayi — on me; buddhiṁ — intellect; niveśaya — cause to be absorbed; nivasiṣyasi — you will be focused; mayyeva = mayi — in me + eva — indeed; ata ūrdhvaṁ — from now onwards; na — not; saṁśayaḥ— doubt

Placing your mind on Me alone, causing your intellect to be absorbed in Me alone, you will be focused on Me from now onward. There is no doubt about this. (12.8)

Commentary:

This is a kriyā yoga process and not a bhakti process. Śrī Krishna spoke here of a yoga meditation process which is practiced in the four higher states of yoga, namely pratyāhār, dhāraṇa, dhyāna, and samādhi.

The mind and the intellect are separated here as they are in mystic kriyā practice. Both are placed on Śrī Krishna, on His Mūrti and most of all on His Vishnu Form. This can only be done in the highest practice of yoga, namely samādhi. When it is a consistent practice, then later it becomes part of the lifestyle. It is not an easy process. It is not the same as the practice done with devotion to Krishna without yoga expertise.

अथ चित्तं समाधातुं
न शक्नोषि मयि स्थिरम् ।
अभ्यासयोगेन ततो
मामिच्छाप्तुं धनंजय ॥१२.९॥
atha cittaṁ samādhātuṁ
na śaknoṣi mayi sthiram
abhyāsayogena tato
māmicchāptuṁ dhanaṁjaya (12.9)

atha — if however; cittam — thought; samādhātum — to anchor; na — not; śaknoṣi — you can; mayi — on me; sthiram — steadily; abhyāsayogena = abhyāsa — practice + yogena — by yoga; tato = tataḥ — then; mām — me; icchāptum = iccha — with + āptuṁ — to attain; dhanaṁjaya — conqueror of wealthy countries

If, however, you cannot steadily anchor your thoughts on Me, then by yoga practice, try to attain Me, O conqueror of wealthy countries. (12.9)

Commentary:

We must remember that in the first verse, Arjuna inquired of the contrast between yogi devotees and non-devotee yogis.

Śrī Krishna said that the yogi devotees have higher techniques in comparison to the non-devotee yogis. I cited that there are exceptions like Gautama Buddha, even though generally a non-devotee yogi cannot make as rapid an advancement because he does not get assistance to accelerate his progress. He relies on self discovery which usually takes a tremendous amount of time.

Śrī Krishna gave some insight into the process used by the yogi devotees. In this verse, He gave advice for devotees who do no yoga. If such a devotee cannot steadily anchor his thoughts on Śrī Krishna, then he should begin yoga practice (yogena).

अभ्यासेऽप्यसमर्थोऽसि
मत्कर्मपरमो भव ।
मदर्थमपि कर्माणि
कुर्वन्सिद्धिमवाप्स्यसि ॥१२.१०॥
abhyāse'pyasamartho'si
matkarmaparamo bhava
madarthamapi karmāṇi
kurvansiddhimavāpsyasi (12.10)

abhyāse — in practice; 'pi = api — perchance; asamartho = asamarthaḥ— incapable; 'si = asi — you are; matkarmaparamo = matkarmaparamaḥ = matkarma—my work + paramaḥ — be absorbed; bhava — be; madartham — for my sake; api —— even; karmāṇi — activities; kurvan — doing; siddhim — perfection; avāpsyasi —you will attain

But if perchance, you are incapable of such practice, then by being absorbed in My work, or even by doing activities for My sake, you will attain perfection. (12.10)

Commentary:

Now if a devotee feels that he cannot practice yoga or if his practice is haphazard, then Śrī Krishna advised that he take to karma yoga. That means he should shift over more to doing social, cultural or political work for the pleasure of the Central Figure in the Universal Form. He should not do anything to irritate that Personality but should always do whatever is approved by that Lord, just as Arjuna had to fight because that was the divine will.

This tallies with what Śrī Krishna said before in Chapter Six:

ārurukṣormuneryogaṁ karma kāraṇamucyate
yogārūḍhasya tasyaiva śamaḥ kāraṇamucyate (6.3)

For a philosophical man who strives for yoga expertise, cultural activity is recommended. For one who has mastered yoga already, the tranquil reserved method is the means. (6.3)

Those who are neophyte must take up cultural activity and do the yoga in their spare time, while those who are proficient, can practice the higher stages which culminate in samādhi trances.

In this Chapter Twelve, in the verse above, Lord Krishna stated that by doing His work, one will attain perfection but it does not mean that one will not have to do yoga. It means that one will eventually attain yoga perfection by the practice of yoga. The techniques will be given by Śrī Krishna Himself and by other advanced yogi devotees.

अथैतदप्यशक्तोऽसि
कर्तुं मद्योगमाश्रितः ।
सर्वकर्मफलत्यागं
ततः कुरु यतात्मवान् ॥ १२.११ ॥
athaitadapyaśakto'si
kartuṁ madyogamāśritaḥ
sarvakarmaphalatyāgaṁ
tataḥ kuru yatātmavān (12.11)

athaitat = atha — if + etat — this; api — even; aśakto = aśaktaḥ — unable; 'si = asi — — you are; kartum — to do; madyogam — my yoga; aśritaḥ — resorting to; sarvakarmaphalatyāgaṁ = sarvakarmaphala — all results of action + tyāgam — abandoning; tataḥ — then; kuru — act; yatātmavān — with restraint

If you are unable to even do this, then resorting to My yoga process, abandoning all results of action, act with self restraint. (12.11)

Commentary:

Here again Śrī Krishna digresses consider the person who cannot do the recommended yoga austerities, and cannot help Krishna in the social, cultural and political way. That person can resort to working in the world with self restraint and by abandoning the benefits of his actions.

This person cannot fight directly for the Universal Form. He cannot do yoga either, but he can work in the social, cultural and political field. Whatever benefits he receives, he is supposed to contribute to good causes according to the regulations in the Vedic literature. Generally he should act with self restraint in observation of moral principles, being humble and modest in behavior.

श्रेयो हि ज्ञानमभ्यासाज्
ज्ञानाद्ध्यानं विशिष्यते ।
ध्यानात्कर्मफलत्यागस्
त्यागाच्छान्तिरनन्तरम् ॥ १२.१२ ॥
śreyo hi jñānamabhyāsāj
jñānāddhyānaṁ viśiṣyate
dhyānātkarmaphalatyāgas
tyāgācchāntiranantaram (12.12)

śreyo = śreyaḥ — better; hi—indeed; jñānam— derived knowledge, experience; abhyāsāt — from the practice; jñānāt — than derived knowledge; dhyānaṁ — meditation; viśiṣyate — is superior; dhyānāt — than meditation; karmaphalatyāgaḥ = karmaphala — results of action + tyāgaḥ — renunciation; tyāgāt — from renunciation; śāntiḥ— spiritual peace; anantaram — instantly

Indeed, derived knowledge is better than practice. Meditation is superior to derived knowledge. Renunciation of results is better than meditation. From such renunciation, spiritual peace is instantly gained. (12.12)

Commentary:

In this statement, Śrī Krishna explained why He charted out the course above, giving one compromise after the other, but in such a way whereby the person can gradually progress upwards.

By working in the world, one will eventually, if one has any sense or consideration, derive a certain philosophy (jñānam). Those conclusions being the result of experience are better than the actions from which they were derived, just as a fruit may be regarded as being better than the tree which produced it.

From that philosophical knowledge, one should develop a habit of mental reflection. This leads to meditation which is better than mere philosophy. From meditation one develops detachment. From that one exhibits practical renunciation which is even better. From practical renunciation, one simplifies the life style. That brings on spiritual peace.

Śrī Krishna recommended a process of getting to Him gradually, by working dutifully according to one's station in life, and then by working on God's behalf in terms of law and order for the sake of morality and all that God prefers. Later, one should practice yoga to learn how to focus the psyche on God so that one can get a clear idea of what God wants one to do for perfection.

अद्वेष्टा सर्वभूतानां
मैत्रः करुण एव च ।
निर्ममो निरहंकारः
समदुःखसुखः क्षमी ॥१२.१३॥
adveṣṭā sarvabhūtānāṁ
maitraḥ karuṇa eva ca
nirmamo nirahaṁkāraḥ
samaduḥkhasukhaḥ kṣamī (12.13)

adveṣṭā — one who does not dislike; sarvabhūtānāṁ — all creatures; maitraḥ — friendly; karuṇa — compassionate; eva — indeed; ca — and; nirmamo = nirmamaḥ — free from attachment to possessions; nirahaṁkāraḥ — free from the propensity of, "I am the creator of my actions"; samaduḥkhasukhaḥ = sama — equally disposed + duḥkha — pain + sukhaḥ — pleasure; kṣamī — be patient

One who does not dislike any of the creatures, who is friendly and compassionate, free from attachment to possessions, free from the propensity of "I am the creator of my actions," being equally disposed towards pain and pleasure, being patient, (12.13)

Commentary:

One should certainly aspire for being friendly and compassionate to all creatures and to be free from attachment to possessions, free from the propensity of thinking that one is actually the total creator of one's actions, but that does not mean that one can do this as thoroughly as an advanced yogi. His adoption of a pacifist stance is derived from the psychological purification which he gains by virtue of advanced yoga practice.

To accept these instructions as if Śrī Krishna meant it for non—yogis, is inconsistent with the *Gītā*, because Śrī Krishna meant that it is done in the process of yoga expertise. Let us look at the next verse to understand this.

संतुष्टः सततं योगी
यतात्मा दृढनिश्चयः ।
मय्यर्पितमनोबुद्धिर्
यो मद्भक्तः स मे प्रियः ॥१२.१४॥
saṁtuṣṭaḥ satataṁ yogī
yatātmā dṛḍhaniścayaḥ
mayyarpitamanobuddhir
yo madbhaktaḥ sa me priyaḥ (12.14)

saṁtuṣṭaḥ — contented; satataṁ — always; yogī — yogi; yatātmā — one with a controlled self; dṛḍhaniścayaḥ — determined; mayi — on me; arpitamanobuddhiḥ = arpita — focused + mano = manas — mind + buddhiḥ — intellect; yo = yaḥ — who; madbhaktaḥ — devoted to me; sa = saḥ — he; me — of me; priyaḥ — dear

...the yogi who is always content, who has a controlled self, who is determined, whose mind and intellect are focused on Me, who is devoted to Me, is dear to Me. (12.14)

Commentary:

Take notice of the Sanskrit word yogi. These verses apply to the yogi devotee. Other devotees may cull beneficial practices from these verses and try to use this advice without doing yoga but the public should not be fooled into thinking that Śrī Krishna meant for this to be practiced without yoga.

These qualities mentioned, even the devotion to Krishna is the type given by a yogi devotee who is consistent in the practice of yoga as it is defined in Chapter Six of the *Gītā*.

Other devotees can practice as much of this as they can comprehend and implement but that does not mean that Śrī Krishna discussed their practice.

यस्मान्नोद्विजते लोको
लोकान्नोद्विजते च यः ।
हर्षामर्षभयोद्वेगैर्
मुक्तो यः स च मे प्रियः ॥१२.१५॥
yasmānnodvijate loko
lokānnodvijate ca yaḥ
harṣāmarṣabhayodvegair
mukto yaḥ sa ca me priyaḥ (12.15)

yasmāt — from whom; nodvijate = na — not + udvijate — is repulsed; loko = lokaḥ — world; lokat — from the world; nodvijate = na — not + udvijate — is repulsed; ca — and; yaḥ — who; harṣāmarṣabhayodvegaiḥ = harṣa — excitement + amarṣa — impatience + bhaya — fear + udvegaiḥ — with distress; mukto = muktaḥ — freed; yaḥ — who; sa = saḥ — he; ca — and; me — of me; priyaḥ — dear

He from whom the world is not repulsed, and who is not repulsed from the world, who is free from excitement, impatience, fear and distress, is dear to Me. (12.15)

Commentary:

This is a high stage of yoga practice, in which the yogi devotee passes the stage of running away from the world. He can be in the world and not be antagonistic towards it. This comes about after one attained the samādhis.

अनपेक्षः शुचिर्दक्ष
उदासीनो गतव्यथः ।
सर्वारम्भपरित्यागी
यो मद्भक्तः स मे प्रियः ॥१२.१६॥
anapekṣaḥ śucirdakṣa
udāsīno gatavyathaḥ
sarvārambhaparityāgī
yo madbhaktaḥ sa me priyaḥ (12.16)

anapekṣaḥ — impartial; śuciḥ — hygienic; dakṣa — competent; udāsīno = udasīnāḥ — indifferent; gatavyathaḥ — one whose anxieties are gone; sarvārambhaparityāgī = sarva — all + ārambha — undertaking + parityāgī — abandoning; yo = yaḥ — who; madbhaktaḥ — devoted to me; sa = saḥ — he; me — of me; priyaḥ — dear

He who is impartial, hygienic, competent, indifferent, whose anxieties are gone, who abandoned all personal undertakings, and who is devoted to Me, is dear to Me. (12.16)

Commentary:

This again pertains to yogi devotees who mastered the samadhis. It is improper to apply this verse to others, even though it is good to encourage others to adopt these dispositions.

यो न हृष्यति न द्वेष्टि
न शोचति न काङ्क्षति ।
शुभाशुभपरित्यागी
भक्तिमान्यः स मे प्रियः ॥१२.१७॥
yo na hṛṣyati na dveṣṭi
na śocati na kāṅkṣati
śubhāśubhaparityāgī
bhaktimānyaḥ sa me priyaḥ (12.17)

yo = yaḥ — who; na — not; hṛṣyāti — rejoice; na — not; dveṣṭi — hates; na — not; śocati — laments; na — not; kāṅkṣati — craves; śubhāśubhaparityāgī = subhasubha — agreeable and disagreeable + parityāgī — leaving aside; bhaktimān — full of devotion; yaḥ — who; sa = saḥ — he; me — of me; priyaḥ — dear

One who does not rejoice, or hate, or lament, or crave, who left aside what is agreeable and disagreeable, who is full of devotion, is dear to Me. (12.17)

Commentary:

In these verses, the devotion to Śrī Krishna is included. Thus these individuals must be both yogis and devotees. For those who are only yogis and who are not devotees, these verses do not apply. And the same goes for those who are devotees and not yogis. They will not consistently feel like this because their basis is not yoga but rather mood adoption and attitude adjustment.

समः शत्रौ च मित्रे च
तथा मानावमानयोः ।
शीतोष्णसुखदुःखेषु
समः सङ्गविवर्जितः ॥१२.१८॥
samaḥ śatrau ca mitre ca
tathā mānāvamānayoḥ
śītoṣṇasukhaduḥkheṣu
samaḥ saṅgavivarjitaḥ (12.18)

samaḥ — equally disposed; śatrau — and to an enemy; ca — and; mitre — to friend; ca — and; tathā — similar; mānāvamānayoḥ — in honor and dishonor; śītoṣṇasukhaduḥkheṣu = śīta — cold + uṣṇa — heat + sukha — happiness + duḥkheṣu — in distress; samaḥ — same; saṅgavivarjitaḥ = saṅga — attachment + vivarjitaḥ — freedom from

Being equally disposed to an enemy and a friend, with a similar attitude in honor and dishonor, in cold and heat, happiness and distress, being free from attachment, (12.18)

Commentary:

This comes from slowing down the psyche in its rush for sense fulfillment. This only happens after mastering the pratyāhār stage of yoga practice.

तुल्यनिन्दास्तुतिर्मौनी
संतुष्टो येन केनचित् ।
अनिकेतः स्थिरमतिर्
भक्तिमान्मे प्रियो नरः ॥१२.१९॥
tulyanindāstutirmaunī
saṁtuṣṭo yena kenacit
aniketaḥ sthiramatir
bhaktimānme priyo naraḥ (12.19)

tulyanindāstutiḥ = tulya — relates to + nindā — condemnation + stutiḥ — glorification; maunī — silent; saṁtuṣṭo = saṁtuṣṭaḥ — content; yena — with what; kenacit = kenacid — with anything; aniketaḥ — without a house; sthiramatiḥ = sthira — steady + matiḥ — mind; bhaktimān — full of devotion; me — of me; priyo = priyaḥ — dear; naraḥ — person

...one who relates equally to condemnation and glorification, who is silent, content with anything, who is unattached to home, who has a steady mind, and who is full of devotion, that person is dear to Me. (12.19)

Commentary:

Conveniently, some Vaishnava teachers say that maunī (silence) means being silent about everything except Śrī Krishna, but that is not what Śrī Krishna meant here. He discussed the silence adopted at a certain stage of practice, when the yogi silences his mind in order to concentrate it away from the disturbing sensuality which is aggravated by mundane sense perception. In regards to "being content", those Vaishnava teachers say that we should be content with whatever facilitates Krishna consciousness and that we should not reject anything that furthers the preaching activities. However, in reality this verse is referring to an absolute contentment. This type of yogi devotee is not eager to preach because he has no commission to do so. He focuses on psyche purification and spiritual self development in isolation as yoga practice requires.

He is unattached to home but that does not mean he becomes attached to a room in the temple compound or thinks that since the temple and ashram are for Krishna, the attachment is legitimate. No, this type of yogi devotee becomes detached from everything in the material world, even the temple and ashram, because his preparation is not to stay here to preach but to move on to the spiritual locales. Just as Arjuna was shifted from this place for a short time when he used a supernatural and then a spiritual body to view what was shown to him by Śrī Krishna, so the yogi devotee gets ready to shift entirely from this world along with its temples and ashrams. The kriyā yogi, unlike so many non—yogi devotees, is not satisfied merely with the temple in this world or with the properly—installed Krishna Icon form of marble or other materials of this world. Thus his perspective is different.

It may be hard to believe that Śrī Krishna accredits these yogis as being dear to him, very, very dear, but that is what the Sanskrit states. Thus, we kriyā yogis must take heart and not abandon our practice on the basis of the ridicule and discouragement for which we are targeted.

ये तु धर्म्यामृतमिदं
यथोक्तं पर्युपासते ।
श्रद्दधाना मत्परमा
भक्तास्तेऽतीव मे प्रियाः ॥१२.२०॥
ye tu dharmyāmṛtamidaṁ
yathoktaṁ paryupāsate
śraddadhānā matparamā
bhaktāste'tīva me priyāḥ (12.20)

ye — who; tu — but; dharmyāmṛtam — dharmya — codes of behavior + amṛtam — life — giving; idam — this; yathoktaṁ = yathā — as + uktaṁ — declared; paryupāsate — they honor; śraddadhānā — having confidence; matparamā — absorbed in me as top priority; bhaktāḥ — be devoted; te — they; 'tīva = atīva — very very; me — to me; priyaḥ — dear

Those who honor these life—giving codes of behavior, who have confidence, being intent on Me as top—priority, being devoted, are very dear. (12.20)

<u>Commentary:</u>

If Śrī Krishna issued such a statement about the yogi devotee, why should any other person state otherwise or take steps to delete yoga as a valid and essential portion of Krishna consciousness?

CHAPTER 13

Material Nature

The Person

The Living Space*

अर्जुन उवाच
प्रकृतिं पुरुषं चैव
क्षेत्रं क्षेत्रज्ञमेव च ।
एतद्वेदितुमिच्छामि
ज्ञानं ज्ञेयं च केशव ॥१३.१॥
arjuna uvāca
prakṛtiṁ puruṣaṁ caiva
kṣetraṁ kṣetrajñameva ca
etadveditumicchāmi
jñānaṁ jñeyaṁ ca keśava (13.1)

arjuna — Arjuna; uvāca — said; prakṛtiṁ — material nature; puruṣaṁ — person; caiva — and indeed; kṣetraṁ — the living space; kṣetrajñam — the experiencer of the living space; eva — indeed; ca — and; etad — this; veditum — to know; icchāmi — I wish; jñānaṁ — conclusion; jñeyaṁ — what is to be experienced; ca — and; keśava — pretty — haired one

Arjuna said: What is material nature? What is the person? What is the living space? Who is the experiencer of the living space? I wish to know this. What is a conclusion? And what is experienced, O Keshava, pretty—haired One? (13.1)

Commentary:

There is no difference between the authority Śrī Krishna exhibited before the revelation of the Universal Form and thereafter. Still we must feel a difference in order to understand what is explained after the Form was displayed. Śrī Krishna spoke with more penetration thereafter because He established His position as the God Vishnu during the revelation, as well as the Central Figure in the supernatural political control of the mundane existence. It means therefore, that Arjuna developed a change of attitude. While before, Arjuna spoke to a friend of his in whom he had great confidence, afterwards, he knowingly spoke to the Supreme Person, to God, as far as he experienced in the revelation. From Chapter Eleven onwards everything takes on a greater significance.

Whatever Śrī Krishna said thereafter is graver. It should be taken more seriously, assuming that we gained some conviction from hearing Arjuna's revelation. It is not our revelation but on the basis of faith in the kriyā process, as well as on the basis of Arjuna's success with it and Lord Krishna's studentship under Mahāyogī Rishi Upamanyu, we should develop deeper faith in Krishna and in Arjuna as well.

**The Mahābhārata contains no chapter headings. This title was assigned by the translator on the basis of verse 1. of this chapter.*

The questions of Arjuna in this first verse of Chapter Thirteen are about the topics of Samkhya yoga. These are ancient questions. They will remain inquiries so long as there are human beings anywhere in the material world. Of course, other philosophers might have entirely different answers to these questions. Regardless, as aspiring yogis, we wish to hear what Śrī Krishna said since He defined these in respect to yoga practice.

Arjuna asked about material nature. This is not only gross material nature but subtle and causal material nature as well. Arjuna asked of the person, the puruṣa. This is important because according to common usage, the person is regarded as his material body. Furthermore, people feel that the person is also his emotions and mentality. In kriyā yoga we find out that the mentality is just an organ in the subtle body and that emotions are more or less types of subtle energy. The question remains: What exactly is the person?

Arjuna asked of the living space. Right now the living space seems to be this earthly environment. In kriyā yoga we discover that the earthly environment is a remote living space. The immediate one is our psyche. The spirit lives in that psyche which consists of a subtle and causal body. In the Śrīmad Bhāgavatam, Śrī Nārada Muni, a yogi devotee of repute, explained this to King Prachinabarhi in the analogy of Puranjana.

Arjuna asked about the experiencer of the living space. Who is he? Is he the spirit? Or is it the buddhi (analyzing organ)? Is it a combination of those two principles? Who experiences the living space? Are the spirits observers that supply energy and enthusiasm, like spectators cheering at a sports event?

Arjuna asked about a conclusion. What conclusion should we formulate? What experiences should we gain?

श्रीभगवानुवाच
इदं शरीरं कौन्तेय
क्षेत्रमित्यभिधीयते ।
एतद्यो वेत्ति तं प्राहुः
क्षेत्रज्ञ इति तद्विदः. ॥ १३.२ ॥
śrībhagavānuvāca
idaṁ śarīraṁ kaunteya
kṣetramityabhidhīyate
etadyo vetti taṁ prāhuḥ
kṣetrajña iti tadvidaḥ(13.2)

śrī bhagavān — The Blessed Lord; uvāca — said; idaṁ — this; śarīraṁ — earthly body; kaunteya — O son of Kuntī; kṣetraṁ — the living space; iti — thus; abhidhīyate — it is called; etat — this; yo = yaḥ — who; vetti — knows; taṁ — him; prāhuḥ — they declare; kṣetrajña — experiencer of the living space; iti — thus; tadvidaḥ — of those knowledgeable of that

The Blessed Lord said: This, the earthly body, O son of Kuntī, is called the living space. Those who are knowledgeable of this, declare the person who understands this to be the experiencer of the living space. (13.2)

Commentary:

It depends on where you are living at the time of inquiry. For instance, for the supernatural people Arjuna saw, the living space was just a subtle body and not a gross one. For them that subtle body was the place. For the Lord Vishnu whom Arjuna saw, His spiritual body was the place.

Many people take this word shariram to mean the earthly body but they are mistaken if they do not understand that a living body is different to a dead one. In other words, the gross material comprises the dead body but the gross, subtle and causal forms comprise the living body. Thus the living space or environment of an earthly creature means the earthly form plus the subtle and causal bodies. That is the immediate environment. In kriyā yoga we are not interested in the external environment or the outdoors. Such interest will not help us in kriyā yoga practice. Our primary concern is the subtle and causal forms. It is the subtle form that causes us to transmigrate regardless of whether we desire to or not. And it is the causal form that causes the development of the subtle one.

We have to understand one thing. We usually transmigrate helplessly without having any say in the matter. Many speakers about reincarnation indulge their audiences in the belief that transmigration is done selectively. Moving from a dying material body to a newly—formed one is such a natural and impulsive instinct, that a spirit can go through it involuntarily. It is not something that we usually control. Just as a body cries automatically if it hears a harsh voice or if it is struck, so transmigration takes place effortlessly by the grace of the subtle material nature, with or without our preference. For the most part, we are helplessly dragged into these transmigrations.

In kriyā yoga, we have to understand these things and know for sure that we reside in the wrong living space. It is not simply a matter of wishing to get out or imagining that we will get out. We have to take up hardcore austerities to achieve that feat. We have to follow in the footsteps of the mahāyogīs; otherwise we will remain time bound, being flung here or there by the whims of the subtle body on the basis of the need for fulfillment in the causal form.

When Śrī Krishna says "those who are in knowledge of this", some commentators explain that He meant those who have heard of this in disciplic succession and are faithfully repeating it. That explanation is inadequate. To be in knowledge of this, one has to realize it by the mystic process of kriyā yoga or by getting a revelation just as Arjuna experienced. This has to be an experience, not a hearing of evidence based on faith in a guru, an institution or a succession of teachers.

Nowadays, "imparting" has come to mean that the teacher speaks convincingly and the student believes and then serves the teacher but that is not meant here. Imparting means what Arjuna received which is revelation. If the teacher cannot give that, then he must be capable of giving the next best thing, the disciplines through which the students will get the revelation or will get the purity to open or develop subtle and supernatural vision.

The person who understands what the living space is, in terms of mystic experience in clarity, after his chakras are cleansed and after his buddhi organ converts into a supernatural eye, is the experiencer of the living space.

क्षेत्रज्ञं चापि मां विद्धि
सर्वक्षेत्रेषु भारत ।
क्षेत्रक्षेत्रज्ञयोर्ज्ञानं
यत्तज्ज्ञानं मतं मम ॥ १३.३

kṣetrajñaṁ cāpi māṁ viddhi
sarvakṣetreṣu bhārata
kṣetrakṣetrajñayorjñānaṁ
yattajjñānaṁ mataṁ mama (13.3)

kṣetrajñam — the experiencer of the living space; cāpi = ca — and + api — also; māṁ — me; viddhi — know; sarvakṣetreṣu — in all living spaces; bhārata — O man of the Bhārata family; kṣetrakṣetrajñayoḥ — of the living space and the experiencer of it; jñānaṁ — information; yat — which; tat — that; jñānaṁ — knowledge; mataṁ — considered; mama — by me

Know also, that I am the experiencer of all living spaces, O man of the Bharata family. Information of the living space and the experiencer of it, is considered by Me to be knowledge. (13.3)

Commentary:

The fact that Śrī Krishna is the mystic knower of all the living spaces is evident from what Arjuna saw when viewing the Universal Form. Arjuna declared in verse 40 Chapter Eleven that Śrī Krishna had infinite power and immeasurable might. Śrī Krishna penetrated everything. In that sense, Śrī Krishna was in touch with everything.

तत्क्षेत्रं यच्च यादृक् च
यद्विकारि यतश्च यत् ।
स च यो यत्प्रभावश्च
तत्समासेन मे शृणु ॥१३.४॥
tatkṣetraṁ yacca yādṛk ca
yadvikāri yataśca yat
sa ca yo yatprabhāvaśca
tatsamāsena me śṛṇu (13.4)

tat — tad — this; kṣetraṁ — living space; yat — what; ca — and; yadṛk — what kind?; ca — and; yadvikāri = yad — what + vikāri — changes; yataśca = yataḥ — what causes?; ca — and; yat — what; sa = saḥ — he; ca — and; yo = yaḥ — who; yatprabhāvaḥ = yat (yad) — what + prabhāvaḥ — potential + ca — and; tat = tad — that; samāsena — with brevity, in brief; me — of me; śṛṇu — hear

As for this living space, as for what is, as for what kind of environment it is, as for the changes it endures, as to what causes it to change, as for he who is involved, as for his potential, hear from Me of that in brief. (13.4)

Commentary:

Śrī Krishna, an ultimate authority on this material world, will give us an explanation in brief. Persons like Śrī Balarāmaji, Lord Shiva, Śrī Agastya Muni and others, are the ones who are the ultimate authorities on such matters. These also include Lord Kapila, Śrī Nārada Muni and Śrīla Vyasaji.

ऋषिभिर्बहुधा गीतं
छन्दोभिर्विविधैः पृथक् ।
ब्रह्मसूत्रपदैश्चैव
हेतुमद्भिर्विनिश्चितैः ॥१३.५॥
ṛṣibhirbahudhā gītaṁ
chandobhirvividhaiḥ pṛthak
brahmasūtrapadaiścaiva
hetumadbhirviniścitaiḥ (13.5)

ṛṣibhiḥ — by the yogī sages; bahudhā — many times; gītaṁ — recited; chandobhiḥ — with Vedic hymns; vividhaiḥ — with various; pṛthak — distinctly; brahmasūtrapadaiścaiva = brahmasūtrapadaiḥ — with Brahma — sūtra verses + ca — and, eva — indeed; hetumadbhiḥ — with sound logic; viniścitaiḥ — with definite, conclusive

This was distinctly recited many times with the various Vedic hymns and with the Brahma Sūtras, conclusively with sound logic, by the great yogi sages. (13.5)

Commentary:

Śrī Krishna informed Arjuna that these matters were discussed at length by great sages before their time and were recorded in Vedic scriptures conclusively with sound logic. The sages from the Upanishadic period did the mystic research into this. They were pioneers just before the time of Śrī Krishna. The sages mentioned in the Valmiki Rāmāyaṇa, persons like Agastya Muni and Śrī Matanga Rishi, mystically perceived this even before the time of the *Upanishads*.

महाभूतान्यहंकारो
बुद्धिरव्यक्तमेव च ।
इन्द्रियाणि दशैकं च
पञ्च चेन्द्रियगोचराः ॥ १३.६ ॥
mahābhūtānyahaṁkāro
buddhiravyaktameva ca
indriyāṇi daśaikaṁ ca
pañca cendriyagocarāḥ (13.6)

mahābhūtāni — major elements; ahaṁkāro = ahaṁkāraḥ— ahaṁ— I, person + kāraḥ— doing, initiative to act; buddhiḥ— intellect; avyaktam — unmanifested energy; eva—indeed; ca — and; indriyāṇi — senses; daśaikaṁ= dasa — ten + ekam—one; ca — and; pañca — five; cendriyagocarāḥ = ca — and + indriyagocarāḥ— attractive objects

The major categories of the elements, the personal initiative, the intellect, the unmanifested energy, the ten and one senses, the five attractive objects, (13.6)

Commentary:

This comprises the psyche of the spirit, his living space, his psychological environment. This is what we call a person but which in fact is a conglomeration of causal, subtle and gross energies which use some energy of the spirit in a cohesive way.

Each of the subtle and gross bodies have within them a minute portion of the major elements which are solid substances, liquids, fiery materials, gases and rarified spaces. These exist in the subtle world as prāṇas or subtle elements.

The personal initiative is the will to act which we experience as a need for doing things. The intellect is an analyzing light in the brain of the subtle form. The unmanifested energy resides in the causal body but it seeps into the subtle form and motivates it. Known as chitta in Sanskrit, Western psychologists regard this as the unconscious and subconscious.

The ten and one senses are the five perceiving senses, the five utilizing organs and the mind which is an overall sensing device that houses the intellect with the sensing mechanisms. The five senses are the five sensing organs, namely the nose, tongue, eye, skin and ear. These have subtle source forms as light-emitting orbs in the mind of the subtle body. These orbs can be seen by prāṇa vision or by subtle piercing vision in the advanced stages of yoga practice.

The five utilising sense organs are the hand, foot, vocal cord, anus and genital. These too have their orbs in the mind of the subtle body. These can be seen by prāṇa vision and chakra vision. One can do this in the advanced stages of mystic yoga practice.

The five attractive objects are odor, flavor, color, surface and sound. These abound everywhere in the material world on every level in every gross and subtle dimension. One needs the appropriate sense which may detect particular frequencies. These are also part of the psyche of the individual being.

इच्छा द्वेषः सुखं दुःखं
संघातश्चेतना धृतिः ।
एतत्क्षेत्रं समासेन
सविकारमुदाहृतम् ॥ १३.७ ॥
icchā dveṣaḥ sukhaṁ duḥkhaṁ
saṁghātaścetanā dhṛtiḥ
etatkṣetraṁ samāsena
savikāramudāhṛtam (13.7)

icchā — desire; dveṣaḥ — hatred; sukhaṁ — pleasure; duḥkhaṁ — pain; saṁghātaścetanā = saṁghātaḥ — the whole body + cetana — consciousness; dhṛtiḥ — conviction: etat = etad — this; kṣetraṁ — living space; samāsena — with brevity, briefly; savikāram — with changes; udāhṛtam — described

...desire, hatred, pleasure, pain, the whole body, consciousness and conviction; this is described with brevity, as the living space with its changes. (13.7)

Commentary:

Desire is part of the essential subtle being because the cosmic causal body is comprised of desire energy only. From this cosmic pool of desire energy, our individual causal forms are derived. From those individual forms, the subtle bodies are derived. We are thus driven to fulfill the desires stockpiled in our causal forms. It so happens that the seedlings of desire are endless. Thus if we remain under the influence of that desire energy our transmigrations would never end. In kriyā yoga, we seek to slide away from the desire force which seeps into our subtle bodies and drives those forms into various pleasant and unpleasant transmigrations. This can be achieved by mastery of higher yoga.

Śrīla Yogeshwarananda, a great yogin, informed me that it is nearly impossible for any of us, the limited beings, to completely escape the pressures of the desire force. He says that even if a yogin becomes liberated, he will likely become conditioned again, as soon as he relaxes or is forced to relax. The limited being never has an absolute control over the course of destiny. In the meantime, however, he extols all yogis to make the effort to free themselves from being stooges of the causal desire force.

Śrīla Yogeshwarananda did not advise that a yogin aspire to go live with the supernatural rulers in their paradise. He said that in such a situation, the subtle body is just concerned with fulfillments. One's discrimination becomes inactive. But if one gets a human body, he said, the rough life may develop discrimination which could lead to paravairāgya, acute dispassion, through which one can do the austerities for liberation.

Even though the subtle bodies of the devas last for millions of years, still those bodies engage in bhogas or experiences for fulfillments to satisfy the seed desires which ooze from the causal body and impregnate the subtle forms.

Hatred for persons, things or circumstances exists in the nature of every living being. We heard about the Universal Form's reaction to limited beings whose actions He did not approve. Hatred is natural but in kriyā yoga, we try to squelch our hating or disliking tendencies. Gradually we are able to relinquish the lower bodies and reach a plane where we no longer react to favorable or unfavorable factors.

Pleasure and pain are permanent parts of the mundane psyche. These cannot be removed or washed out. A yogin learns how to use the pains of this life and how to reduce his responses to pleasurable things. The causal body enjoys the impressions received from the subtle form regardless of whether such impulses come from pleasurable or painful experiences. Since that causal form eats or takes in the impressions from such experiences, it does in fact, endorse these. It is not possible to elicit its assistance in avoiding pains and minimizing pleasures. Once a kriyā yogi observes how this operates, he begins to curb himself from all experiences which are to be gained in the mundane world. Śrī Patañjali Maharsi wrote this:

prakāśa kriyā sthiti śīlaṁ bhūtendriyātmakaṁ bhogāpavargārthaṁ dṛśyam

What is perceived is of the nature of the mundane elements and the sense organs and is formed in clear perception, action or stability. Its purpose is to give experience or to allow liberation.(Yoga Sūtra 2.18)

The whole body comprises three bodies in operation together. This is commonly called the healthy person in common usage. Actually, by kriyā yoga practice, we realized that it is not the person. We begin to see by mystic perception that many of the energies are being replaced daily, like items that are vended or sold at a shop. The shop's contents appear the same every day, but really many items were replaced by new ones which will soon be purchased by customers.

Daily the body eats, and daily the body evacuates parts of what is eaten. Daily, the body assimilates energy from what is eaten and daily much of the energy is converted into calories for mental, emotional and physical work. When we master Kuṇḍalinī yoga we see the energy entering and leaving the body. We see the gyrating charkas which act as valves to regulate energy flow, sort the various types of energies and regulate passage through the subtle body. In celibacy yoga we see how cells act as inhabitants in various parts of the body similar to a country with villages, towns and cities. In higher yoga we substitute the energies in the subtle body for higher energies. These energies fall under the general term of prāṇa in Sanskrit. After one learns how to do this, he can terminate his material existence by shedding the desires which enter his subtle form from the causal body.

Advanced yogins like Śrīla Yogeshwarananda put a stop to the transfer of energies from the causal body to the subtle one. In this way, they terminate the urges for transmigration on these levels. Generally the causal energy oozes out and enters the subtle form and motivate it but the causal energy is very concentrated and powerful. Even a tiny amount less than what would hold on the tip of a pin, can send the subtle body into millions of transmigrations all over the universe in varying species of life for millions and millions of years, thus forcing the spirit to ride along through pleasant and unpleasant experiences. This is like a person who enters an amusement park and boards a wild roller coaster. Though scared out of his wits, he has no power to escape from the experience.

Consciousness as we know it, is not pure spiritual energy. Spiritual energy is involved but conventional consciousness is mostly subtle material energy. It is only in the high end of yoga practice, in samādhi, that a person can experience pure spiritual consciousness. Many teachers err in saying that our consciousness is the spiritual part of the psyche. This is said mostly by persons who have not mastered yoga and who have no experience of samādhi trance states. Formerly the acharyas and gurus had to master samādhi trance before they could become popular teachers, but now anybody with a convincing and charismatic presentation can become a guru. Thus the situation is risky. Consciousness, as we know it, is only a reflection of spiritual energy and is not spiritual energy itself because the spiritual energy flashes and reflects into the subtle emotional and mental force. That force is what we experience as consciousness. In the *Upanishads,* it is shown that spiritual consciousness is never directly experienced through the subtle energy. What we experience now happens through the facility of subtle mundane energy.

Conviction is the sureness about existence in the subtle or gross material world. Conviction shifts, all according to where and how we are situated in particular bodies. All of this, as Śrī Krishna informs us, is the living space or the psychological environment that we currently use.

अमानित्वमदम्भित्वम्
अहिंसा क्षान्तिरार्जवम् ।
आचार्योपासनं शौचं
स्थैर्यमात्मविनिग्रहः ॥१३.८॥

amānitvaṁ — a lack of pride; adambhitvam — freedom from deceit; ahiṁsā — non — violence; kṣāntiḥ — patience; ārjavam — straightforwardness; ācāryopāsanaṁ — sitting near a teacher, attendance to a teacher; śaucaṁ

amānitvamadambhitvam
ahiṁsā kṣāntirārjavam
ācāryopāsanaṁ śaucaṁ
sthairyamātmavinigrahaḥ (13.8)

— *purity; sthairyam — stability; ātmavinigrahaḥ = ātma— self + vinigrahaḥ — restraint*

Lack of pride, freedom from deceit, non—violence, patience, straightforwardness, attendance to a teacher, purity, stability and self—restraint, (13.8)

Commentary:

This begins the definition of what Śrī Krishna defines as knowledge. This definition is quite different from the use of the word knowledge in common life. This is not a definition that suits the world. For the world, knowledge means whatever a man knows that can help him to earn a livelihood.

Lack of pride may be cultivated by being humble and realizing that one always needs assistance from nature, God and other limited beings. No one can act in this world without such assistance. Even if the help is not obvious, it is there on the subtle and supersubtle levels. In consideration, therefore, a lack of pride is appropriate. The practice of this, however, is not consistent because from time to time, one will be overpowered with the energy of pride which is in one's psychology.

In kriyā yoga, we work to change our psychology to remove the pride energies and to make the emotions resistant to the penetration of pride. In meditation, one works on this and rids the psyche of the pride energies. Sometimes in meditation, one sees small supernatural figures who use subtle forms and reside within the psyche. These persons emit certain constructive or destructive energies. One can learn how to dismiss them from one's form by asking them to leave.

Many such supernatural persons live in the psyche. Normally we are unaware of them. We feel that we are the only ones possessing these forms. However these persons influence our attitude and behavior. In yoga, in meditation, when one masters Kuṇḍalinī practice, one begins to see and hear them moving around in the psyche. One begins to dismiss them when one sees that they cause destructive behaviors. This sort of practice is totally different to the practice of trying to be moral and good as people usually do in popular religions.

Unless one develops subtle vision, either as prāṇa vision or as vision of the buddhi organ in the head of the subtle form, he will not be able to successfully purify his psyche. It will be impossible and no God or guru can effectively bless him and purify him. The individual has to endeavor for clarity. God and the religious teacher can help us to develop prāṇa vision but we must do the subtle work to gain purification. It is an individual achievement.

Freedom from deceit is practiced in the general religions, but such practice is, of necessity, a haphazard affair. It often depends on the peer pressure of one devotee or member of a religion watching the other. The leaders get a better opportunity from the inherent pressure of always having to do better than their congregations. They are isolated from the masses of devotees by the system of having to be honored as leaders. Usually the religious heads do not have to engage in business directly. They get money easily and do not have to cheat outright. It is seen, however, that when they desire big projects, they are invariably forced into dishonesty in one way or the other.

Peer pressure works well within popular systems of salvation but these methods do not penetrate deep within the psyche. Thus we see that an upright person in one life becomes evil and conniving in another, when the opportunities for money and fame are barred to him.

In kriyā yoga, the freedom from deceit is first tackled by simple living and high thinking, by stepping aside from civilization and greatly reducing one's needs. Sometimes those who follow a general religion, try to do this and they call it simple living, but lacking internalization, they again build up their desires with the belief that they are doing this for God and the salvation of humanity. They again end up in the process of using deceit to attract funds for temple buildings, book printing and numerous other expenses. They rationalize that it is alright to deceive since they preach about salvation and God.

In yoga practice, one escapes from deceit by following the rule of isolation. If one ignores this rule, then one falls back into the deceit pattern. Another facet of deceit that wipes out a yogi, is the teaching of yoga as a livelihood. In the Western countries we see many yogis who come from India. Some of these take up teaching for a livelihood. This happens under the pressure of Western economies. Once a yogi does this, he has to engage in a certain degree of deceit. He falls back in the practice. If he was very advanced before leaving India, he remembers his former accomplishment. With a pretence of not having fallen back, he teaches Westerners.

One should not mix his livelihood with his yoga practice. Stated differently, one should not charge fees for yoga lessons. One may accept voluntary donations and use these for the purpose of publishing books or building residences or temples, but one should not charge for yoga lessons. If one charges, it is a definite indication that one has fallen under the influence of deceit.

Apart from all this, Śrī Bābāji Mahasaya instructed that I receive donations on his behalf. I am to use the money as he instructs. For instance, sometimes someone reads one of these books and sends a donation. Śrī Bābāji Mahasaya told me to use such funds only to publish more books. This means that I cannot use the money to buy food for my belly, or a pair of shoes for my wife.

As a trick of chance, a yogi might be tempted to make money teaching. He runs here and there to give lectures for high fees and to hold sessions for training. This is sponsored by the power of deceit.

If one takes seriously to the 5th stage of yoga, that of pratyāhār sense withdrawal, one will not be tempted like this. Even so, one who masters pratyāhār can fall back from it and the deceit energy will again invade his psyche and pull him into worldly affairs.

Fascination with disciples and acceptance of praise cause a yogi to fall back to the plane where deceit overtakes him. One should not hanker for disciples. One should protect oneself by always profiling as a disciple of the mahāyogīns. It is a mistake to seek only one spiritual master but one must identify the main teacher. If one feels that he has only one spiritual master, he will debar other competent teachers from wishing him well. That will cause the invasion of the energy of deceit. I have written all this, not to lengthen these purports, but to give hints to neophyte yogis on how they might be successful.

Non-violence became popular in the Western countries through Mahatma Gandhi's passive resistance to British domination of India and due to the attitude of Lord Buddha. Buddha, the lordly person, was a mahāyogīn. He practiced kriyā yoga and discovered all that was required for liberation. Even though there were no detailed descriptions of his austerities in advanced yoga, a careful study of his realizations and visions tells us that he did perfect higher yoga. His pacifism, his nonviolence, was truly based on purification and was not a fanciful opinion or an adopted attitude towards life.

Since Buddha, many persons have hailed as pacifists. Most are farces, even if their endeavor can be admired. Becoming a pacifist after succeeding in yoga practice and doing so merely by hearing of nonviolence and feeling it is the best course, is not the same.

Mahatma Gandhi's story is different because he was not practicing kriyā yoga like Buddha. Gandhi, the great strategist who shattered British dominance in India, fasted but his fasting was not coordinated with prāṇāyāma practices. It was not kriyā yoga. It worked in a way but it is not the same type of nonviolence advocated by Buddha which, if practiced after mastering yoga, produces a different effect.

In Buddhism, there are two types of pacifism; one is practiced as a moral principle to decrease the amount of suffering in the world and the other is practiced as part of the yoga kriyās. Our interest here is in its practice in reference to the yoga kriyās.

Due to deep realization and visions related to the chain-like connections between all living beings, great, small, infinite and limited, a yogi develops a nature which is incapable of initiating violence on other creatures but that does not mean such a yogi may not exhibit violent acts. Śrī Krishna, the Mahāyogīn of all time, incited Arjuna to judicial violence. Even Lord Shiva from time to time leaves aside his samādhi and, for a corrective purpose, commits disciplinary violence.

In kriyā yoga, when one is advanced, violence decreases. When one degresses, it increases. This is due to the nature of the varying realities as one advances or descends. In isolation there are virtually no violent acts to be performed, even for survival of one's body. As soon as one begins to socialize, the potential for violence increases.

When I first took this body, I entered a lower way of life, because the parents from whom it was derived were involved in the violence of eating animal bodies. We lived in what was then part of the British Empire. Later on I decreased the violence by cultivating yoga and excelling in its elementary practices.

At this point in the life of this body, I hope to practice the advanced stages of yoga. If providence allows, the violence performed by this body will be considerably reduced. For spiritual non-violence one must excel at yoga practice and become expert in the kriyās. Other types of nonviolence are merely exhibitions of adopted attitudes which will be disrupted by rash movements of providence. Everything is in the hands of providence. As such, human determination accounts for very little.

Patience develops only in the last stages of pratyāhār sense withdrawal practice. Only then does one becomes patient with destiny by virtue of having quelled the senses and limited the seepage of desires which ooze out of the causal body into the subtle form. These desires cause an impatience which is interpreted as a scramble for existence.

The modern civilization with its geographic, ecological and technological conquest is a typical example of impatience. Since the expansion of the European influence, the whole planet was overrun with gadgets like cars, airplanes, televisions, and washing machines. This is because of impatience. It is due to the pressure of the oozing energy which comes out of the causal body and which oozes into the subtle form through an orifice. Under that pressure, all the living entities who get the chance scramble here and there for commodities.

In kriyā yoga, after one has quelled his sensual energies, he feels a relief. His subtle body becomes unfit for absorbing desires from the causal plane. He steps aside from the advancement of civilization, simplifies his life style and forgets all those desires which formerly motivated him and drove him to be ambitious about new commodities.

Purity is both internal and external. External purity is important when one follows the general paths of religion but its importance is supplanted by internal purity when one practices kriyā yoga. In kriyā yoga one becomes obsessed with internal purity. This begins with āsanas (postures). By āsana practice, one learns how to purify the blood stream and causes the cells and muscles to release toxins which are usually held in reserve.

By prāṇāyāma one learns how to clean out the toxic air in the gross and subtle bodies. By Kuṇḍalinī yoga, one learns how to clean out chakras which are energy-regulating valves on the spine of the subtle body. Halfway through the course in Kuṇḍalinī yoga, one learns celibacy yoga, an art introduced to me by Swami Shivananda who established the Divine Life Society. In celibacy yoga one learns how to clean out the subtle body, while in Kuṇḍalinī yoga one learns how to clean out the chakras.

Once a yogi becomes absorbed with this psychic cleaning, he loses the fanaticism about external bodily cleanliness. Thus, people may think he has become careless about external cleanliness which they feel is essential to religion and basic hygiene.

In my case, for example I really do not care at all about bathing, but I do, I am more concerned with psychological purification by virtue of practice. People do not always understand kriyā practice because it may not show external improvements. A kriyā yogi should act as people do when he is with them. There is no point in causing others to become disturbed. For peace sake, a kriyā yogi should either stay completely away from people or act in their style when he is with them.

Hare Krishna devotees who are following the line brought by His Divine Grace Śrīla Bhaktivedanta Swami, the Vaishnava spiritual master, claim to know about purity. When I see them, I let them talk for peace sake. Actually they hardly know anything about internal purity because the Swami never practiced nor recommended yoga. He made no positive appraisal of the purity derived from āsana and prāṇāyāma, what to speak of Kuṇḍalinī yoga, celibacy yoga and purity yoga. However if one reads verse 12 of Chapter Six, one will get Lord Krishna's view.

Stability in yoga practice deals not with being stable in the society of human beings, but with stable focus. This comes in the 6th stage of yoga, that of dhāraṇa, focus of the buddhi organ and parts of the mind within itself. If one lacks this focus, he cannot use his brow chakra, a subtle eye in the forehead, and he cannot direct his imagination faculty for use as a supernatural eye.

Self restraint comes initially in the 5th stage of practice when there is sense withdrawal from pleasures and attractive objects. This means restraint of the senses which continually seek to imbibe different sounds, surfaces, colors, flavors and odors. Advanced self restraint is attained in dhyāna, the 7th stage of yoga practice but hardly a yogi reaches this stage which precedes samādhi. This is why in India, the home of yoga practice, a yogi who enters samādhi is treated as a god. It is not easy to attain the 7th and 8th stages. One must practice but he also requires the grace of providence.

इन्द्रियार्थेषु वैराग्यम्
अनहंकार एव च ।
जन्ममृत्युजराव्याधि—
दुःखदोषानुदर्शनम् ॥१३.९॥

indriyārtheṣu — towards the attractive objects; vairāgyam — indifference; anahaṁkāra = an — absence of + ahaṁkāra — motivated initiative; eva — indeed; ca — and; janmamṛtyujarāvyādhi = janma — birth + mṛtyu — death + jarā — old age

indriyārtheṣu vairāgyam
anahaṁkāra eva ca
janmamṛtyujarāvyādhi—
duḥkhadoṣānudarśanam (13.9)

+ vyādhi — disease; duḥkhadoṣānudarśanam = duḥkha — suffering + doṣa — danger + anudarśanam — perception

..indifference towards the attractive objects, absence of motivated initiative, the perception of the danger of birth, death, old age, disease, and suffering, (13.9)

Commentary:

The indifference towards attractive objects is practiced in general religions. This mostly shows that one is more advanced than ordinary followers who attend the temple or church. However, that is not the real practice. For indifference towards attractive objects one has to develop paravairāgya, which is an acute dispassion or disinterest towards the attractive objects. This occurs when one transforms his energy intake in the subtle body through mastership of Kuṇḍalinī yoga and by using advanced mystic acts which are taught by mahāyogīs only.

When one has mastered it, he needs no effort to restrain his senses because they naturally lose interest in attractive objects. Such senses are no longer fueled or driven by matching prāṇas, energies which match the attractive objects or which are polarized negatively or positively towards them. At that point the whole world appears quite bland to the yogi, but he does not tell others how he feels since he does not want to disturb their ideas.

The absence of a motivated initiative fully manifests only after one mastered samādhi. Before that, it is displayed in part. However, in karma yoga one needs that initiative as one is pushed on by Śrī Krishna, the Central Person in the Universal Form. People everywhere like to talk about false ego but usually they babble some nonsense. When they are inspired to insult someone, they speak of a false ego.

So long as there is interest in this world, there will be ego in relation to this world, or assertion in this world. Lord Krishna asserted certain things which he required of Arjuna. Arjuna had to use an ego to fight at Kurukṣetra because that was the only way for him to gain the approval of the Central Person in the Universal Form.

In kriyā yoga we intend to reduce our participation in this world. We gradually and systematically reduce the assertions as we make an exit from this place.

The perception of the danger of birth, death, old age and disease was achieved by Gautama Buddha. Once he saw that danger, for him there was no turning back. Later after he gained enlightenment, he decided to take the role of a religious figurehead. He did this for the sake of teaching morality so that limited entities would, by moral acts, decrease their sufferings.

In reality, birth, death, old age and diseases are no threat to the eternal spirit. These factors become a distraction for the spirit if he thinks that he can solve or remove them. The danger of these factors is that we may become preoccupied trying to solve them when in reality they cannot be banished. One understands this by deep mystic penetration into the nature of subtle matter.

असक्तिरनभिष्वङ्गः
पुत्रदारगृहादिषु ।
नित्यं च समचित्तत्वम्
इष्टानिष्टोपपत्तिषु ॥१३.१०॥

asaktiḥ — non — attachment, social detachment; anabhiṣvaṅgaḥ — absence of emotional affection; putradāragṛhādiṣu = putra — child + dāra — wife + gṛha — home + ādiṣu — beginning with, whatever is related to; nityaṁ — always; ca —

asaktiranabhiṣvaṅgaḥ
putradāragṛhādiṣu
nityaṁ ca samacittatvam
iṣṭāniṣṭopapattiṣu (13.10)

and; samacittatvam — even — mindedness; iṣṭāniṣṭopapattiṣu — iṣṭa — desired + aniṣṭa — not wanted + upapattiṣu — in matters

...social and emotional detachment towards a child, a wife, a home and whatever is related to social life, being always even—minded towards what is desired and what is not wanted, (13.10)

Commentary:

Social and emotional detachment towards a child, a wife, a home and whatever is related to social life comes mainly from a long history of yoga practice in the past lives. This is something that cannot be achieved overnight. One is either born with this ability or not. One cannot develop this in the time it takes to beget children after getting a body. Usually a male begets the first child between 20 and 30 years of age but in 20 years in a body, one cannot develop that ability. If however one carries it in the subtle form from previous lives, it will automatically be exhibited.

Someone without that detachment may get hints of its cultivation from ascetics who are householders and who exhibit it effortlessly. Such teachers should act responsibly towards their family despite the detachment. It cannot be learned from those who are resentful towards householder life, or those who are irresponsible. Śrī Krishna does not like irresponsibility. He influenced Arjuna to act in a responsible way in the Kuru family. This is what the *Gītā* is all about. If we want the approval of Krishna, we have to be responsible. Detachment is not an excuse for being irresponsible.

Many gurus, even some of the Vaishnava acharyas who position themselves as pure devotees of Śrī Krishna, are found encouraging their householder disciples to be irresponsible towards their families. These acharyas do this because they are influenced by a desire for prominence. They encourage their householder disciples to work for the mission and to neglect their families. That is not really a part of Krishna consciousness, even though the errant acharyas are successful in defining it as such.

Being even—minded towards what is desired and what is not wanted, is attained only in the 7th stage of yoga practice, when by focusing the buddhi organ and stilling it, one is able to stop the psychological seepage from the causal form which drives the subtle body for fulfillment at all costs. This even—mindedness applies to both good and bad things, religious and irreligious accomplishments. These factors relate to results which come to an ascetic through yoga practice and not by trying to self-induce a particular saintly behavior. It is good that many devotees try to improve their moral stances and develop higher qualities but that is not what is discussed here.

मयि चानन्ययोगेन
भक्तिरव्यभिचारिणी ।
विविक्तदेशसेवित्वम्
अरतिर्जनसंसदि ॥१३.११॥

mayi — in me; cānanyayogena = ca — and + ananya — no other + yogena — with yoga practice; bhaktiḥ — devotion; avyabhicāriṇī — not wandering away, unwavering; viviktadeśasevitvam = vivikta — secluded +

mayi cānanyayogena
bhaktiravyabhicāriṇī
viviktadeśasevitvam
aratirjanasaṁsadi (13.11)

deśa — place + sevitvam — resorting; aratiḥ — having a dislike; janasaṁsadi — in crowds of human beings

...unswerving devotion to Me, with no other discipline but yoga practice, resorting to a secluded place, having a dislike for crowds of human beings, (13.11)

Commentary:

Unswerving devotion to Śrī Krishna, with no other discipline but yoga practice, is the sure way to perfection. This means bhakti and yoga practice. Both must be performed to qualify under these guarantees. One should not take the word yogena which means with yoga practice, and divert it to some other meaning or minimize it.

Resorting to a secluded place and having a dislike for crowds of human beings, is an absolute must if one is to attain the 7th and 8th stages of yoga practice which are dhyāna, mystic contemplation of what is perceived in the subtle, supernatural and spiritual world, as well as the samādhi trance to spend long periods of time in that dimension in either of the higher bodies. One cannot attain those stages if one remains as a preacher at public temples. One must take to seclusion, simply because that is the correct method.

अध्यात्मज्ञाननित्यत्वं
तत्त्वज्ञानार्थदर्शनम् ।
एतज्ज्ञानमिति प्रोक्तम्
अज्ञानं यदतोऽन्यथा ॥ १३.१२ ॥
adhyātmajñānanityatvaṁ
tattvajñānārthadarśanam
etajjñānamiti proktam
ajñānaṁ yadato'nyathā (13.12)

adhyātmajñānanityatvam = adhyātma — Supreme Spirit + jñana — information + nityatvam — constantly; tattvajñānārthadarśanam = tattva — reality + jñāna — science + artha — value+ darśanam — perceiving; etat— this; jñānam — knowledge; iti — thus; proktam — declared as; ajñānaṁ — ignorance; yat — whatever; ato = ataḥ — to this; 'nyathā = anyathā — otherwise, contrary

...constantly considering information about the Supreme Spirit, perceiving the value of the science of reality; this is declared as knowledge. Whatever is contrary to this, is ignorance. (13.12)

Commentary:

Constantly considering information about the Supreme Spirit is the stage after one attained samādhi (trance). Before that, whatever we hear is usually distorted by the mind, even if heard from someone who directly perceived the Supreme Lord. At first one has to psych out or peer into his own psychology, something which is a lot closer than the Supreme Being. After we master the lower realities, we may perceive what is higher.

It is very easy to feign knowledge about the Supreme Spirit and sell our intellectual grasp and sentimental attachment to Śrī Krishna, but it is entirely different to first realize by yoga practice and then teach properly without cheapening what Śrī Krishna offered in the *Bhagavad Gītā*.

The perception of the value in the science of reality comes to a yogin when he advances far into the practice of kriyā yoga, so far that the practice takes over his life and dictates what he should do to complete it. Otherwise one will have a tendency to play around with religion and mysticism and never get serious.

Śrī Krishna gave this listing from verse 8 to this verse 12 as being knowledge. So this is His definition.

ज्ञेयं यत्तत्प्रवक्ष्यामि
यज्ज्ञात्वामृतमश्नुते ।
अनादिमत्परं ब्रह्म
न सत्तन्नासदुच्यते ॥ १३.१३ ॥
jñeyaṁ yattatpravakṣyāmi
yajjñātvāmṛtamaśnute
anādimatparaṁ brahma
na sattannāsaducyate (13.13)

jṇeyaṁ — to be known, the desired subject; yat — which; tat — that; pravakṣyāmi — I will explain; yat — which; jñātvā — knowing; 'mṛtam = amṛtam — eternal life; aśnute — he gets in touch with; anādimat — beginningless; paraṁ — supreme; brahma — reality; na — not; sat — substantial; tat — this; nāsat = na — not + asat — non — substantial; ucyate — is said

I will explain that which is to be experienced; knowing this one gets in touch with eternal life. The beginningless Supreme Reality is said to be neither substantial nor unsubstantial. (13.13)

Commentary:

There are many experiences to be gained in the subtle and gross material energy. At the high end of yoga practice, one can gain experiences even in the chitta energy which is in the causal body. Most of these experiences do not lead to liberation. Their main inducement is for the limited being to become increasingly involved in some phase of mundane existence.

However, Śrī Krishna promised to explain the type of experience that puts one in touch with eternal life. The beginningless supreme reality, the parambrahma, is the main topic in the *Upanishads*. There, it is portrayed as a special reality beyond the material world. The *Upanishads* do not introduce a Supreme Personality as Śrī Krishna does in the next verse and elsewhere in the *Gītā*. According to the *Upanishads*, this reality is neither sat nor asat but it is advised that we regard it as sat. The word sat means reality. Śrī Krishna described the parambrahma in a very unique and novel way:

सर्वतःपाणिपादं तत्
सर्वतोक्षिशिरोमुखम् ।
सर्वतःश्रुतिमल्लोके
सर्वमावृत्य तिष्ठति ॥ १३.१४ ॥
sarvataḥpāṇipādaṁ tat
sarvatokṣiśiromukham
sarvataḥśrutimalloke
sarvamāvṛtya tiṣṭhati (13.14)

sarvataḥ — everywhere; pāṇi — hand; pādaṁ — foot; tat = tad — this; sarvato = sarvataḥ — everywhere; 'kṣiśiromukham = akṣiśiromukham = akṣi — eye + śiraḥ— head + mukham — face; sarvataḥśrutimat = sarvataḥ — everywhere + śrutimat — having hearing ability; loke — in the world; sarvam — all; āvṛtya — ranging over; tiṣṭhati — stands

Everywhere is Its hands and feet, everywhere Its eyes, head and face, everywhere is Its hearing ability in this world; It stands, ranging over all. (13.14)

Commentary:

This description is the practical definition of the parambrahma because that is what we must face in terms of this existence. Arjuna saw this firsthand when he viewed the Universal Form. We need to understand that everything we do is being checked and catalogued. There are supernatural persons overseeing everything. There is absolutely no privacy. Everything we do is open to scrutiny. The fact that we are not interrupted most of the time and that we feel that we can be private, is based on our insensitivity to the All—pervading Supreme Personality. That insensitivity affords us the ignorance of His presence.

सर्वेन्द्रियगुणाभासं
सर्वेन्द्रियविवर्जितम् ।
असक्तं सर्वभृच्चैव
निर्गुणं गुणभोक्तृ च ॥ १३.१५ ॥
sarvendriyaguṇābhāsaṁ
sarvendriyavivarjitam
asaktaṁ sarvabhṛccaiva
nirguṇaṁ guṇabhoktṛ ca (13.15)

sarvendriyaguṇābhāsaṁ = sarva — all + indriyaḥ — sensual + guṇa — mood + ābhāsaṁ — appearance; sarvendriyavivarjitam = sarva — all + indriya — sensuousness + vivarjitam — freedom from; asaktaṁ — unattached; sarvabhṛt — maintaining everything; caiva = ca — and + eva — indeed; nirguṇaṁ — free from the influence of material nature; guṇabhoktṛ — experiencer of the modes of material nature; ca — and

It has the appearance of having all sensual moods, and It is freed from sensuousness. Though unattached, It maintains everything. Though free from the influence of material nature, It is the experiencer of that influence nevertheless. (13.15)

Commentary:

The Supreme Person who supervises the material world seems to have a contrary psychology, since on one hand He can sense everything and on the other, He is not affected. In addition, He causes reactions, just as the Central Figure in the Universal Form acted supernaturally in response to whatever He disapproved.

As kriyā yogis we want to get on His better side. We certainly do not desire His disapproval. Whatever we should do to gain His favor, should be carried out.

बहिरन्तश्च भूतानाम्
अचरं चरमेव च ।
सूक्ष्मत्वात्तदविज्ञेयं
दूरस्थं चान्तिके च तत् ॥ १३.१६ ॥
bahirantaśca bhūtānām
acaraṁ carameva ca
sūkṣmatvāttadavijñeyaṁ
dūrasthaṁ cāntike ca tat (13.16)

bahiḥ — outside; antaḥ — inside; ca — and; bhūtānām — of the beings; acaraṁ — non — moving; caram — moving; eva — indeed; ca — and; sūkṣmatvāt — from subtlety; tat — this; avijñeyaṁ — not to be comprehended; dūrasthaṁ — situated far off; cāntike = ca — and + antike — in the location; ca — and; tat = tad — this

It is outside and inside the moving and non—moving beings. Because of Its subtlety, this beginningless Supreme Reality is not comprehended. This Reality is situated far away and it is in the location as well. (13.16)

Commentary:

The misunderstandings and the disagreements regarding the description of the beginningless Supreme Reality spring from Its subtlety (sūkṣma). Various philosophers argue over it, trying to establish their convictions and experiences as the truth. However, so long as it remains as something that is supersubtle, the disagreements will continue. Even among kriyā yogis, there are disputes about what is seen and detected in samādhi trance states. One yogi has a certain experience and then another opens his supernatural sense perception in a way that reveals the transcendence in an entirely different way. Thus sects are formed around various yogis of accomplishment. How then do we know who had the highest, most accurate experiences?

In kriyā yoga we are not concerned with the arguments or the contest between the teachers. We only want to learn from the teachers how we may open up our subtle perception. We should not become distracted by arguments or end up as argumentative followers of any particular teacher. Our concern with these teachers is the technique through which we can acquire psychic purity.

Every limited being has a certain potential. The potential will not increase merely by austerities. One's potential will expand within its own limits through practice, but one will not get infinite vision because even in the potential state, one is still a limited being. Arjuna or any other kriyā yogi will not become Lord Krishna or Lord Shiva merely by psychic purity gained in kriyā yoga practice. We have to be satisfied with a certain limitation even if we perfect the practice and acquire the subtle and spiritual vision.

What a yogi sees once his vision opens up, will be related to his category as a spirit, as well as how he becomes purified and the particular supernatural energy through which he perceives the other world. Thus the visions may be different for each yogi. Ideally one successful yogi should not argue with another but should instead exchange descriptions of their experiences, just like travelers who tour a foreign country and who meet thereafter to compare notes.

अविभक्तं च भूतेषु
विभक्तमिव च स्थितम् ।
भूतभर्तृ च तज्ज्ञेयं
ग्रसिष्णु प्रभविष्णु च ॥१३.१७॥
avibhaktaṁ ca bhūteṣu
vibhaktamiva ca sthitam
bhūtabhartṛ ca tajjñeyaṁ
grasiṣṇu prabhaviṣṇu ca (13.17)

avibhaktam — undivided; ca — and; bhūteṣu — among the beings; vibhaktam — divided; iva — as if; ca — and; sthitam — remaining; bhūtabhartṛ = bhūta — being + bhartṛ — sustainer; ca — and; tat — this; jñeyaṁ — to be known; grasiṣṇu — absorber; prabhaviṣṇu — producer; ca — and

It is undivided among the beings, but It appears as if It is divided in each. It is the sustainer of the beings and this should be known. It is the absorber and producer. (13.17)

Commentary:

The undividedness of this beginningless Supreme Reality is one feature agreed upon by all yogis. Each state that it is one reality, either as a Supreme Person or as sum total transcendental energy. They also agree that it is the sustainer of the beings as the ultimate absorber and producer by remote control and perpetual proximity.

ज्योतिषामपि तज्ज्योतिस्
तमसः परमुच्यते ।
ज्ञानं ज्ञेयं ज्ञानगम्यं
हृदि सर्वस्य विष्ठितम् ॥१३.१८॥
jyotiṣāmapi tajjyotis
tamasaḥ paramucyate
jñānaṁ jñeyaṁ jñānagamyaṁ
hṛdi sarvasya viṣṭhitam (13.18)

jyotiṣām — of luminaries; api — also; tat = tad — this; jyotiḥ — light; tamasaḥ — of gross or subtle darkness; param — beyond; ucyate — declared to be; jñānaṁ — information; jñeyaṁ — education; jñānagamyaṁ = jñāna — education + gamyam — goal; hṛdi — in the psychological core; sarvasya — of all; viṣṭhitam — situated

This is declared as the light of the luminaries, but It is beyond gross or subtle darkness. It is the information, the education and the goal of education. It is situated in the psychological core of all beings. (13.18)

Commentary:

All yogis agree that it is the actual light of the luminaries, because in their tracings, they find it to be the ultimate luminary support. Its light transcends the gross and the subtle darkness as well as the gross and the subtle luminaries. The first evidence of its existence beyond the subtle darkness comes to neophyte yogis when their brow chakras open unexpectedly, and suddenly, for a split second or longer, the darkness between their eyebrows parts and a clear space with perceptions appears for the viewing.

In the more advanced stages, the buddhi organ in the head of the subtle form is converted into a viewing instrument. This penetrates the psychic darkness and shows the yogi the worlds of subtle light where the devas and others are living.

Certainly we should also note the mention of Śrī Krishna that it is the information, the education and the ultimate objective of knowing. Śrī Krishna says this beginningless Supreme Reality exists in the psychological core (hṛdi) of all beings.

इति क्षेत्रं तथा ज्ञानं
ज्ञेयं चोक्तं समासतः ।
मद्भक्त एतद्विज्ञाय
मद्भावायोपपद्यते ॥ १३.१९ ॥
iti kṣetraṁ tathā jñānaṁ
jñeyaṁ coktaṁ samāsataḥ
madbhakta etadvijñāya
madbhāvāyopapadyate (13.19)

iti — thus; kṣetraṁ — the living space, the psychological environment; tathā — as well as; jñanaṁ — standard knowledge; jñeyaṁ — what is to be known; coktaṁ = ca — and + uktaṁ — described; samāsataḥ — in brief; madbhakta — my devotee; etad — this; vijñāya — experiencing; madbhāvāyopapadyate = madbhāvāya — to my state of being + upapadyate — draws near

Thus the psychological environment as well as the standard knowledge and what is to be known, was described in brief. Experiencing this, My devotee draws near to My state of being. (13.19)

Commentary:

Any yogi who experiences this by direct mystic perception, not merely by hearing of it, draws nearer and nearer to the Divinity, to Śrī Krishna, in so far as he accepts the information Śrī Krishna gave on Himself and the revelation that He awarded Arjuna.

प्रकृतिं पुरुषं चैव
विद्ध्यनादी उभावपि ।
विकारांश्च गुणांश्चैव
विद्धि प्रकृतिसंभवान्॥ १३.२० ॥
prakṛtiṁ puruṣaṁ caiva
viddhyanādī ubhāvapi
vikārāṁśca guṇāṁścaiva
viddhi prakṛtisaṁbhavān (13.20)

prakṛtiṁ — material nature; puruṣaṁ — spiritual personality; caiva = ca — and + eva — indeed; viddhi — know; anādī — beginningless; ubhau — both; api — also; vikārān — changes of the living space (see 13.4); ca — and; guṇāṁ — moods; caiva = ca — and + eva — indeed; viddhi — know; prakṛtisaṁbhavān = prakṛti — material nature + saṁbhavān — produced

Know that both material nature and the spiritual personality are beginningless, and know that the changes of the living space and the moods of material nature are produced from material nature. (13.20)

Commentary:

Material nature and the spiritual personality are perpetually contrasted by each generation of philosophers. When the cultural assets are stripped away, we get the puruṣa in pure form. This puruṣa is not the gross, subtle or causal body but the spirit in its isolated and raw state. To discover this person requires advanced yoga practice, because only in such practice can one effectively leave aside the gross and subtle cultural trappings.

Very few yogis were able to strip away the subtle cultural mores they picked up in thousands of transmigrations. Many only rid the ones picked up in the last one, two or three human births. Lord Buddha is the example of a yogi who stripped away all cultural prejudices in his subtle body. Normally, these subtle biases stick to a spirit for the duration of the universe. The subtle body lives for that long unless a yogi can destroy it, a feat that only a very few mahāyogīns are *allowed* to achieve. I use the word *'allowed'* because one has to get permission from the Central Figure in the Universal Form before one can fade out one's Kuṇḍalinī energy and then scrap the buddhi organ in the subtle body.

One cannot, even a yogi cannot, just give up his subtle body, because it is bothersome or because it causes one to enter undesirable life forms. This is due to the overriding authority of the Central Figure in the Universal Form, a person who Arjuna had cause to fear. The subtle body is a botheration. Its prejudices and culture cause our downfall. Thus we have to work in cooperation with the Central Figure in the Universal Form to get a waiver for its elimination. That is not easy to achieve. There are many yogis who speak of their impending liberation, but after they attain a samādhi state and master that practice, we see that they become like humble puppets of the Universal Form. They become teachers who create world missions in which they become preoccupied with reforming human society. This means that somehow they were unable to get a complete waiver. They even forgot their aspiration, which was to get away completely from this scene.

If by nature, an ascetic gravitates to fame, it is unlikely that he will become liberated. Fame is the sure way to magnify one's need to stay on in the material world in the name of being a world savior or universal teacher, a so—called jagat—guru. Such a person cannot and perhaps may never qualify for a complete waiver because his very nature is against it. He will become attracted to the reformatory energies emitted from the eyes of the Central Figure in the Universal Form or from one of the personalities who function as figure heads of the Form. This does not mean that the ascetic will consciously realize this.

Lord Kapila brought some of these truths to our attention when he alerted his mother and student, Queen Devahūti, that persons like Brahmā, Nārada, even Lord Shiva, though they were supernatural beings in their own right, would again revisit these subsequent creations, to stay on in the material worlds. They just cannot become liberated fully due to an innate interest in this place. They are linked to Lord Vishnu in such a way that they cannot be freed from duties in formulating, maintaining and destroying this type of creation.

It is not their defect, but rather their spiritual nature. They are regarded as being eternally-liberated. Lord Kapila wanted to give his mother the chance to bypass that group of divine people who return repeatedly. She was in a category of spirits who could sidestep the duties of the karma yoga which Śrī Krishna enforced for Arjuna.

Also under discussion in this verse, is what Śrī Krishna said about the changes of the living space and the moods of material nature. He says that they are produced from material nature. This becomes clear when one becomes an advanced practitioner. The changes we feel in our psyche, as well as the moods which we endure are being produced by material nature, not by any of us or by the Supreme Being. These changes and moods go on because of the fluctuations in subtle material nature. In kriyā yoga, we learn how to replace the subtle mundane energy in a way that improves the quality of the energy day by day, until we reach the causal body and become conscious of it. Undoubtedly, those who feel that the psychology is themselves, cannot in any way understand the higher aspects of yoga.

कार्यकारणकर्तृत्वे
हेतुः प्रकृतिरुच्यते ।
पुरुषः सुखदुःखानां
भोक्तृत्वे हेतुरुच्यते ॥१३.२१॥
kāryakāraṇakartṛtve
hetuḥ prakṛtirucyate
puruṣaḥ sukhaduḥkhānāṁ
bhoktṛtve heturucyate (13.21)

kāryakāraṇakartṛtve = kārya — created work + kāraṇa — sensual potency as a cause + kartṛtve — agency; hetuḥ — cause; prakṛtiḥ — material nature; ucyate — is said; puruṣaḥ — the spiritual personality; sukhaduḥkhānāṁ — of pleasure and pain; bhoktṛtve — in terms of experiencing; hetuḥ — cause; ucyate — is said

Material nature is said to be the cause in terms of created work, sensual potency and agency. The spiritual personality is said to be the cause in terms of experiencing pleasure and pain. (13.21)

Commentary:

When Śrī Krishna said that material nature is said to be the cause, He referred to the previous time when it was declared so by the mahāyogīs of the Upanishadic period, and before. Even in the time of Lord Śrī Rāma, the son of Dasharatha, this information was divested by great yogins who mystically researched the Absolute Truth.

Right now, in the conditioned state, without the superior experience gained in higher yoga, we feel that sensual potency is our power, something very near and dear to us. In fact the whole social and cultural setting is designed for the satisfaction and facilitation of the sensual potency. In reality, it is conducted by material nature in material nature. One realizes this when he changes out a lower type of subtle energy (prāṇa) for a higher type in his psyche.

Śrī Krishna said that the spiritual personality was stated to be the cause in terms of experiencing pleasure and pain. Experiences or bhogas are enjoyed or ingested by the causal body. It does not feel pains and pleasure. It only accepts the condensed impressions as fulfillments. These impressions, after entering the causal body, reach corresponding energies and cancel out as fulfillments. The pleasures and pains are detected by the puruṣa or the spiritual personality, through his subtle body which emits a range of enjoyable and painful frequencies.

पुरुषः प्रकृतिस्थो हि
भुङ्क्ते प्रकृतिजान्गुणान् ।
कारणं गुणसङ्गोऽस्य
सदसद्योनिजन्मसु ॥ १३.२२ ॥
puruṣaḥ prakṛtistho hi
bhuṅkte prakṛtijānguṇān
kāraṇaṁ guṇasaṅgo'sya
sadasadyonijanmasu (13.22)

puruṣaḥ — spirit; prakṛtistho = prakṛtisthaḥ — situated in material nature; hi — indeed: bhuṅkte — experiencing; prakṛtijān — produced on material nature; guṇān — the modes of material nature; kāraṇaṁ — the source; guṇasaṅgo = guṇasaṅgaḥ — attachment to the influence of material nature; 'sya = asya — of it; sadasadyonijanmasu = sad (sat) — reality + asad (asat) — unrealistic + yoni — birth situations + janmasu — birth

The spirit, being situated in material nature, experiences the modes which were produced by that nature. Attachment to the modes is the cause of the spirit's emergence from realistic and unrealistic birth situations. (13.22)

Commentary:

The spirit experiences the modes of material nature and more than often, identifies such modes as its own moods. Thus its focus of attention is placed here and there, causing it to enter and then emerge from realistic and unrealistic birth situations. When it feels disgusted with this process, it looks for methods of liberation.

उपद्रष्टानुमन्ता च
भर्ता भोक्ता महेश्वरः ।
परमात्मेति चाप्युक्तो
देहेऽस्मिन्पुरुषः परः ॥ १३.२३ ॥
upadraṣṭānumantā ca
bhartā bhoktā maheśvaraḥ
paramātmeti cāpyukto
dehe'sminpuruṣaḥ paraḥ (13.23)

upadraṣṭānumantā = upadraṣṭā — observer + anumantā — permitter; ca — and; bhartā — supporter; bhoktā — experiencer; maheśvaraḥ — Supreme Lord; paramātmeti = paramātmā — Supreme Soul + iti — thus; cāpi — and also; ukto = uktaḥ — is called; dehe — in the body; 'smin = asmin — in this; puruṣaḥ — spirit; paraḥ — highest

The observer, the permitter, the supporter, the experiencer, the Supreme Lord, and the Supreme Soul as He is called, is the highest spirit in the body. (13.23)

Commentary:

This statement should be accepted at face value until we can get some direct experience to verify it. That the Supreme Soul is in the limited body which we inhabit, is hard to believe, but this verse states that. He is described as the ultimate observer, the actual permitter, the supporter of life for the body, the ultimate experiencer of what it endures, the Supreme Lord (maheśvarah) and the Supreme Soul (paramātmā). He is said to be the highest spirit (puruṣah parah) in the body.

After mastering Kuṇḍalinī yoga, a yogi discovers that there are many supernatural persons in the body. Most of them use miniature forms no larger than the size of a thumb. One sees them in meditation from time to time. Sometimes they come into the body. Sometimes they are seen going out of it. Sometimes one leaves it permanently. Sometimes new ones enter and take special seats at the chakras. Sometimes one sees Lord Shiva or Lord Vishnu or Lord Brahmā in the Causal body which is in the chest region of the physical body form. Sometimes one sees yogis entering one's body in order to show one certain techniques or to hold a conversation or to use one's body to continue the practice of their austerities. Besides these persons, elemental spirits inhabit certain cells and organs of one's physical or subtle body.

य एवं वेत्ति पुरुषं
प्रकृतिं च गुणैः सह ।
सर्वथा वर्तमानोऽपि
न स भूयोऽभिजायते ॥ १३.२४॥
ya evaṁ vetti puruṣaṁ
prakṛtiṁ ca guṇaiḥ saha
sarvathā vartamāno'pi
na sa bhūyo'bhijāyate (13.24)

ya = yaḥ — who; evaṁ — thus; vetti — knows; puruṣaṁ — spiritual person; prakṛtiṁ — material nature; ca — and; guṇaiḥ — with the variations of material nature; saha — with; sarvathā — in whatever way; vartamāno = vartamānaḥ — existing presently, present condition; 'pi = api — also; na — not; sa = saḥ — he; bhūyo = bhūyaḥ — again; 'bhijāyate = abhijāyate — is born

He who knows the spiritual person and material nature, along with the variations of material nature, is not born again, regardless of his present condition. (13.24)

Commentary:

Vetti is knowing by accurate mystic perception which results from advanced austerities in yoga. It does not come from a spiritual teacher who heard in disciplic succession and repeated what he was told. Personal experience by mystic perception is the actual method. It develops privately from individual practice. The yoga teacher gives the technique and encouragement for practice, along with some empowerment to proceed with the austerities. There is always some resistance to the discipline in one's nature and human society emits a retarding force which can prevent one's success if one is not empowered by the great yogis.

ध्यानेनात्मनि पश्यन्ति
केचिदात्मानमात्मना ।
अन्ये सांख्येन योगेन
कर्मयोगेन चापरे ॥ १३.२५॥
dhyānenātmani paśyanti
kecidātmānamātmanā
anye sāṁkhyena yogena
karmayogena cāpare (13.25)

dhyānenātmani = dhyānena — through meditative perception + ātmani — in the spirit; paśyānti — they perceive; kecit — some; ātmānam — by the spirit; ātmanā — the spirit; anye — others; sāṁkhyena — by Sāṁkhya philosophical conclusions; yogena — by yoga practice; karmayogena — by yogically disciplined action; cāpare = ca — and + apare — others

Some perceive the spirit by the spirit through meditative perception of the spirit. Others do so with Sāṁkhya philosophical conclusions and others by yogically disciplined action. (13.25)

Commentary:

Let us pay close attention to four standard groups and the associated methods used for spiritual perception. Usually one spiritual group puts itself forward as having the only method, but here Śrī Krishna gave four ways, three in this verse and one in verse 26. These four are meditative perception (dhyānena), yoga and Samkhya (samkhyena yogena), yogicly—disciplined action (karma yogena), and hearing from authorities with confidence while doing worship (śrutvānyebhya upāsate śrutiparāyaṇāh).

The first is the highest groups of transcendentalists. This is not for the majority of people. The majority use the method which is described in the next verse. They are the least qualified and the least perceptive. They are attracted to the easiest process of religion.

The first group is in the minority, because most of the spirits in this world express a low grade of spiritual energy. Most of us are not Godhead Personalities. Most of us are not like Lord Vishnu or Lord Shiva or even Lord Brahmā. Most of us are below their status eternally.

This first group has no need for austerities, promises of salvation, or reliance on anyone to get them out of material existence. They do have to perform austerities, even though they usually pioneer and illustrate the ways of perfection.

They, Śrī Krishna said, perceive the spirit by the spirit through meditative perception of the spirit. They do not have to develop that perception by austerity. They have it naturally. This first group of entities are not limited beings. They are absolute or semi-absolute.

The second and third groups were mentioned in Chapter Three:

śrībhagavānuvāca
loke'smindvividhā niṣṭhāpurā proktā mayānagha
jñānayogena sāṁkhyānāṁ karmayogena yoginām (3.3)

The Blessed Lord said: In the physical world, a two—fold standard was previously taught by Me. O Arjuna, my good man. This was mind regulation by the yoga practice of the Sāṁkhya philosophical yogis and the action regulation by the yoga practice of the non-philosophical yogis. (3.3)

The second group is the most advanced of the limited beings. They perceive the spirit by yoga practice with Samkhya philosophical conclusions which are explained to them by their teachers and which they perceive directly by practicing mystic kriyās. Their yoga practice is greatly accelerated because they get much time to practice as contrasted to the third group which practices part time.

Some of the second group used to be in the third group but left the third group after getting approval from the Supervising Universal Lord who is the Central Figure in the Universal Form which Arjuna perceived.

The third group comprises those who perceived the spirit by their yogicly—disciplined actions in this world. They work as Arjuna did after he was schooled in the art of karma yoga by Śrī Krishna. By agreeing to help the Universal Form in its disciplinary tasks, they derive an upgrade in psychology. They practice yoga as much as they are allowed in spare time. Later when they are freed from cultural duties, they join the superior group of the Samkhya yogis and become firmly situated in full time spiritual perception by virtue of an intense yoga practice.

Many spiritual masters in the disciplic succession from Śrī Krishna pretend they are in the first group that can naturally perceive the spirit by the spirit without having to perform yoga austerities. Their claim is that they can do the 7th stage of yoga practice which is listed in this verse as dhyanena. Such claims are almost always a sheer farce.

Another obvious discrepancy is the claim of these teachers that their followers can have spiritual visions merely by serving the teacher. Usually the followers derive only a theoretical understanding but somehow the teachers convince the followers that this theoretical view is a spiritual experience.

The only group of persons who reach the state of perceiving the spirit by the spirit directly are those naturally in the divine category as superior spirits beyond the normal category, including those who take up and perfect yoga practice step by step. A haphazard course of yoga does not result in the yogi reaching the last two stages of dhyāna contemplation and samādhi trance states.

अन्ये त्वेवमजानन्तः
श्रुत्वान्येभ्य उपासते ।
तेऽपि चातितरन्त्येव
मृत्युं श्रुतिपरायणाः ॥ १३.२६ ॥
anye tvevamajānantaḥ
śrutvānyebhya upāsate
te'pi cātitarantyeva
mṛtyuṁ śrutiparāyaṇāḥ (13.26)

anye — others; tu — but; evam — thus; ajānantaḥ — not knowing; śrutvānyebhya = śrutvā — hearing + anyebhya — from others; upāsate — they worship; te — they; 'pi = api — also; cātitaranti = ca — and + atitaranti — transcend; eva — indeed; mṛtyuṁ — death: śrutiparāyaṇāḥ = śruti — hearing + parāyaṇāḥ — putting confidence in as the highest

But some, though they are ignorant, hear from others. They worship and by their confidence in what is heard, they also transcend death. (13.26)

Commentary:

This describes the broadest, most numbered group of transcendentalists. They do not practice yoga, and do not fall into the category of the absolute or semi—absolute spirits but they hear from others with great faith. They worship and by confidence in what is heard, they also transcend death. Readers must pay attention to their accomplishment which is to transcend the death experience. This does not mean that they will become liberated necessarily, or that they will go to the divine regions, but they will know at the time of death that only the body is being eliminated. They will not be fearful like other spirits who have no confidence in the Vedic scripture and its ideas.

Throughout the entire *Gītā*, only this verse substantiates the claim of those teachers who preach the easy path of simply hearing from the Vedic sources about transcendence. Śrī Krishna does not elaborate much on this path because it was not important for Him to do so. Arjuna was not attracted to such a path. Arjuna mastered yoga austerities. By soul category, he fell into the third group of spirits who usually work under the direction of the Supervising Universal Spirit for promotion of moral activities in righteous living, as Śrī Krishna described in Chapter Four:

yadā yadā hi dharmasya glānirbhavati bhārata
abhyutthānamadharmasya tadātmānaṁ sṛjāmyaham (4.7)
paritrāṇāya sādhūnāṁ vināśāya ca duṣkṛtām
dharmasaṁsthāpanārthāya saṁbhavāmi yuge yuge (4.8)

Whenever there is a decrease in righteousness, O son of the Bharata family, and when there is an increase of wickedness, then I show Myself. (4.7)

For protecting the saintly people, to destroy the wicked ones, and to establish righteousness, I come into the visible existence from era to era. (4.8)

Many preachers try to reduce the *Bhagavad Gītā* to a book that was originally meant for the last group mentioned, those who worship and have confidence in what is heard. In reality, the *Gītā* is meant for persons like Arjuna who accept Krishna's style of karma yoga, and for those even higher who can practice yoga full—time along the guidelines given in the Samkhya philosophy, guidelines which concern mysticism mostly. It is amazing in a way, that many *Gītā* translations take each verse of the *Gītā* or take selected verses and prove to readers that the *Gītā* was originally intended for the general mass of people.

यावत्संजायते किंचित्
सत्त्वं स्थावरजङ्गमम् ।
क्षेत्रक्षेत्रज्ञसंयोगात्
तद्विद्धि भरतर्षभ ॥ १३.२७
yāvatsaṁjāyate kiṁcit
sattvaṁ sthāvarajaṅgamam
kṣetrakṣetrajñasaṁyogāt
tadviddhi bharatarṣabha(13.27)

yāvat — as for; saṁjāyate — is born; kiṁcit = kiṁcid — anything, whatever; sattvaṁ — existence; sthāvarajaṅgamam = sthāvara — stationary + jaṅgamam — moving; kṣetrakṣetrajñasaṁyogāt = kṣetra — living space + kṣetrajña — experiencer + saṁyogāt — from the synthesis; tat — that; viddhi — know; bharatarṣabha — strong man of the Bharatas

As for anything that is produced in this existence, be it a stationary or moving object, know, O strong man of the Bharatas, that it is produced from a synthesis of the experiencer and the living space. (13.27)

Commentary:

This is a conclusion of the Samkhya philosophy, that anything produced in this existence, stationary or moving, is produced from a synthesis of the experiencer and the living space or psychology. This includes both gross and very dense objects. As soon as one opens the subtle vision by yoga austerities, one perceives this. Some perceived it by taking herbs but that method is temporary. It relies on the continual ingestion of the herbs or drugs and the body's ability to withstand the side effects.

It is interesting that when He listed the four methods for spiritual perception, Śrī Krishna did not list bhakti as one. Instead of listing devotion as a method of spiritual perception, Śrī Krishna listed the four standard procedures, namely meditative perception (dhyānena), yoga and Samkhya (samkhyena yogena), yogicly—disciplined action (karma yogena), and hearing from authorities with confidence while doing worship (śrutvāṇyebhya upāsate śrutiparāyaṇāh).

समं सर्वेषु भूतेषु
तिष्ठन्तं परमेश्वरम् ।
विनश्यत्स्वविनश्यन्तं
यः पश्यति स पश्यति ॥ १३.२८ ॥
samaṁ sarveṣu bhūteṣu
tiṣṭhantaṁ parameśvaram
vinaśyatsvavinaśyantaṁ
yaḥ paśyati sa paśyati (13.28)

samam — similar; sarveṣu — in all; bhūteṣu — in beings; tiṣṭhantaṁ — situated; parameśvaram — Supreme Lord; vinaśyatsu — in disintegration; avinaśyantaṁ — not perishing; yaḥ — who; paśyati — perceive; sa = saḥ — he; paśyati — really sees

The Supreme Lord is similarly situated in all beings without perishing when they disintegrate. He who perceives that, really sees. (13.28)

Commentary:

This is not an easy perception to achieve but one can conceive it in the mind and apply that conception by believing the Lord exists in every creature form. Usually people hear of this and are encouraged by teachers to believe and act as if they perceive it. The kriyā yogi hears of it in Samkhya descriptions. Then he works under close instructions from mahāyogīs so that he can develop the mystic view.

Not only the Supreme Lord but the spirit also, does not perish when the material body dies. In fact, the subtle body does not perish. It becomes displaced from a dead physical form. When the subtle body disintegrates after millions of years of existence the causal body remains and so does the spirit and the Supreme Spirit. If we cannot perceive the subtle form, the causal form or the spirit, we certainly cannot see the Supreme Spirit who is even subtler than the other factors which comprise those forms. There is no fault for those who believe this but there is a discrepancy for those who come to think that their belief is itself the mystic perception. They fool themselves and retard those to whom they preach.

समं पश्यन्हि सर्वत्र
समवस्थितमीश्वरम् ।
न हिनस्त्यात्मनात्मानं
ततो याति परां गतिम् ॥ १३.२९॥
samaṁ paśyanhi sarvatra
samavasthitamīśvaram
na hinastyātmanātmānaṁ
tato yāti parāṁ gatim (13.29)

samaṁ — same; paśyan — seeing; hi — indeed; sarvatra — everywhere; samavasthitam — same established; īśvaram — Lord; na — not; hinasti — degrade; ātmānātmānaṁ = ātmanā —by the soul + ātmānaṁ — the soul; tato = tataḥ — subsequently; yāti — goes; parām — supreme; gatim — destination

Seeing the same Lord being situated everywhere, he does not degrade the soul by his own soul. Subsequently, he goes to the supreme destination. (13.29)

Commentary:

Śrī Krishna said that a person who perceived this Supersoul Who resides in all beings, really sees the truth about how this existence takes place. Still, that does not mean a person who conceives of this on the basis of information only, actually sees the truth. That person does not. He does try to reform himself. He does try to consider that God is present in all psyches or psychological outfits which appear as individual creatures, but still he does not actually see the truth. He is better than someone who has not heard these truths but that does not mean he perceives it. This is why a person who merely heard but lacks the mystic perception must, degrade himself. He has no choice because he is not viewing it in fact. His subtle and supernatural vision were not energized even though his imagination organ and sense of confidence absorbed the information.

प्रकृत्यैव च कर्माणि
क्रियमाणानि सर्वशः ।
यः पश्यति तथात्मानम्
अकर्तारं स पश्यति ॥ १३.३०
prakṛtyaiva ca karmāṇi
kriyamāṇāni sarvaśaḥ
yaḥ paśyati tathātmānam
akartāraṁ sa paśyati (13.30)

prakṛtyaiva = prakṛtya — by material nature + eva — indeed; ca — and; karmāṇi — actions; kriyamāṇāni — performed; sarvaśaḥ — in all cases; yaḥ — who; paśyati — he sees; tathātmānam = tathā — as regarding + ātmānam — self; akartāraṁ — non — doer; sa = saḥ — he; paśyati — truly sees

He who sees, that in all cases, the actions are performed by material nature, and who regards himself as a non—doer, truly sees. (13.30)

Commentary:

This is from the Samkhya training given to advanced yogis where in their mystic research with prāṇa vision or with supernatural sight, they see that in all cases, the actions are performed by the subtle material nature and that the spirits are actually non—doers on the scene.

यदा भूतपृथग्भावम्
एकस्थमनुपश्यति ।
तत एव च विस्तारं
ब्रह्म संपद्यते तदा ॥ १३.३१ ॥
yadā bhūtapṛthagbhāvam
ekasthamanupaśyati
tata eva ca vistāraṁ
brahma saṁpadyate tadā (13.31)

yadā — when; bhūtapṛthagbhāvam = bhūta — being + pṛthak — various + bhāvam — existential state; ekastham — based in one foundation; anupaśyati — he sees; tata — from that conclusion; eva — only; ca — and; vistāraṁ — extending, emanating; brahma — spiritual plane; saṁpadyate — he reaches; tadā — then

When a person sees that all the various states of being are based on a single foundation, and only from that everything emanates, then he reaches the spiritual plane. (13.31)

Commentary:

These are not realizations, but rather supernatural visions. One may realize this by conclusion but that is not the same as the actual perception. Śrī Krishna spoke of the Samkhya system of training which means yoga austerities and the mystic capability to see by prāṇa vision and by direct sight using the buddhi organ in the subtle body.

अनादित्वान्निर्गुणत्वात्
परमात्मायमव्ययः ।
शरीरस्थोऽपि कौन्तेय
न करोति न लिप्यते ॥ १३.३२ ॥
anāditvānnirguṇatvāt
paramātmāyamavyayaḥ
śarīrastho'pi kaunteya
na karoti na lipyate (13.32)

anāditvāt = due to being without a beginning; nirguṇatvāt — due to being devoid of the influence of material nature; paramātmāyam = paramātmā — Supreme Soul + ayam — this; avyayaḥ — imperishable; śarīrastho = śarīrasthaḥ — situated in the material body; 'pi = api — even though; kaunteya — O son of Kuntī; na — not; karoti — he acts; na — not; lipyate — become contaminated

Since this imperishable Supreme Lord is beginningless and devoid of the influence of material nature, even though He is situated in the material body, O son of Kuntī, He does not act or become contaminated. (13.32)

Commentary:

The limited spirit does not act or become contaminated but ironically the limited spirit comes to believe that he is contaminated. He feels that he does act. He becomes hypnotized by proximity to and focus through the material nature. Thus, he must strive for liberation to free himself from this.

यथा सर्वगतं सौक्ष्म्याद्
आकाशं नोपलिप्यते ।
सर्वत्रावस्थितो देहे
तथात्मा नोपलिप्यते ॥ १३.३३ ॥
yathā sarvagataṁ saukṣmyād
ākāśaṁ nopalipyate
sarvatrāvasthito dehe
tathātmā nopalipyate (13.33)

yathā — as; sarvagataṁ — all—pervading; saukṣmyāt — as by subtlety; ākāśaṁ — sky; nopalipyate = na — not + upalipyate — is polluted; sarvatrāvasthito = sarvatra — all over + avasthitaḥ — situated; dehe — in the body; tathātmā = tathā — so + ātmā — soul; nopalipyate = na — not + upalipyate — affected

As by subtlety, the all—pervading space is not polluted, so the soul, though situated all over the body, is not affected actually. (13.33)

Commentary:

The soul is not really affected just as a crystal is not changed by its absorption and deflection of light. Still the soul feels affected. This is cleared up by the mystic practice of kriyā yoga or genuine revelation.

Even if a spirit thinks that it is affected, the affectation is removed when the Supreme Person causes material nature to be inactive.

यथा प्रकाशयत्येकः
कृत्स्नं लोकमिमं रविः ।
क्षेत्रं क्षेत्री तथा कृत्स्नं
प्रकाशयति भारत ॥ १३.३४॥
yathā prakāśayatyekaḥ
kṛtsnaṁ lokamimaṁ raviḥ
kṣetraṁ kṣetrī tathā kṛtsnaṁ
prakāśayati bhārata (13.34)

yathā — as; prakāśayati — illuminates; ekaḥ — one, alone; kṛtsnaṁ —— whole; lokam — world; imaṁ — this; raviḥ — sun; kṣetraṁ — living space; kṣetrī— the user of the living space; tathā— so; kṛtsnaṁ — entire; prakāśayati — gives feeling; bhārata — O man of the Bhārata family

As the sun alone illuminates the whole world, O man of the Bharata family, so the user of the living space gives feeling to the entire psyche. (13.34)

Commentary:

The user of the living space, the kṣetrī, is you or me. We are not the only ones who give feelings to the living space but we are the main contributors. The Supreme Being contributes in a supplementary way.

क्षेत्रक्षेत्रज्ञयोरेवम्
अन्तरं ज्ञानचक्षुषा ।
भूतप्रकृतिमोक्षं च
ये विदुर्यान्ति ते परम् ॥ १३.३५॥
kṣetrakṣetrajñayorevam
antaraṁ jñānacakṣuṣā
bhūtaprakṛtimokṣaṁ ca
ye viduryānti te param (13.35)

kṣetrakṣetrajñayoḥ — of the experiencer and the living space; evam — thus; antaraṁ — difference; jñānacakṣuṣā = jñāna — perceptive knowledge + cakṣuṣā — intuitive vision; bhūtaprakṛtimokṣaṁ = bhūta — being + prakṛti — material nature + mokṣaṁ — liberation; ca — and; ye — who; viduḥ — they know; yānti — they go; te — they; param — supreme

Those who by intuitive perception know the difference between the living space and the experiencer, as well as the liberation of the living being from material nature, go to the Supreme. (13.35)

Commentary:

Cakṣusā is the vision one gets when his imagination faculty turns into an eye. With this he sees directly through the darkness which we find in our heads when we close our eyes. This darkness may be dense. It may be speckled with light. When the imagination faculty subsides in meditation after attaining Kuṇḍalinī purity, one sees directly into the subtle, supernatural and spiritual realities.

One who has such a vision developed by sincere yoga practice does go to the Supreme. For him it is definite.

CHAPTER 14

The Extensive Mundane Reality*

श्रीभगवानुवाच
परं भूयः प्रवक्ष्यामि
ज्ञानानां ज्ञानमुत्तमम् ।
यज्ज्ञात्वा मुनयः सर्वे
परां सिद्धिमितो गताः ॥ १४.१ ॥
śrībhagavānuvāca
paraṁ bhūyaḥ pravakṣyāmi
jñānānāṁ jñānamuttamam
yajjñātvā munayaḥ sarve
parāṁ siddhimito gatāḥ (14.1)

śrī bhagavān — the Blessed Lord; uvāca — said; paraṁ — highest; bhūyaḥ— further; pravakṣyāmi — I will explain; jñānānāṁ— of the knowledges; jñānam — information; uttamam — the very best; yat — which; jñātvā— having experienced; munayaḥ— yogī philosophers; sarve — all; parāṁ — supreme; siddhim — perfection; ito = itaḥ — from here; gatāḥ — done

The Blessed Lord said: I will explain more, giving the highest information of all knowledges, the very best. Having experienced that, all the yogi philosophers went away from here to the Supreme Perfection. (14.1)

Commentary:

Śrī Krishna, the Blessed Lord that He is, promised more of the highest information (jñānam uttamam), the very best of the descriptions which are taught in the Samkhya philosophy. This, once experienced by the yogin philosophers (munayah), caused them to attain the supreme perfection (parām siddhim).

इदं ज्ञानमुपाश्रित्य
मम साधर्म्यमागताः ।
सर्गेऽपि नोपजायन्ते
प्रलये न व्यथन्ति च ॥ १४.२ ॥
idaṁ jñānamupāśritya
mama sādharmyamāgatāḥ
sarge'pi nopajāyante
pralaye na vyathanti ca (14.2)

idaṁ—this; jñānam — experience; upāśritya — resorting to; mama — my; sādharmyam — a nature that is similar; āgatāḥ — transformed into; sarge — at the time of the universal creation; 'pi = api — even; nopajāyante = na — not + upajāyante — they are born; pralaye — at the time of universal dissolution; na — not; vyathanti — disturbed; ca — and

Resorting to this experience, being transformed into a nature that is similar to My own, they are not born even at the time of the universal creation, nor are they disturbed at the time of dissolution. (14.2)

**The Mahābhārata contains no chapter headings. This title was assigned by the translator on the basis of verse 3 of this chapter.*

Commentary:

This refers to those great yogins who completed the kriyā yoga course and who went beyond the causal plane. Such persons, according to Śrīla Yogeshwarananda, stay away from the subtle and gross material universe for millions and millions of years. Sometimes they come back into the world as saviors. Most of them do not return.

As Śrī Krishna stated, they were transformed into a nature that is similar to His own. Thus they are not born even at the time when Lord Vishnu starts up a new creation in which he impregnates that world with the unliberated souls from the last creation. Neither are they disturbed by the dissolution of the creation they were in, because they have ridden themselves of the subtle bodies. So long as we have subtle bodies, we will be disturbed when Lord Vishnu shuts down the creation.

Many devotees of Lord Vishnu, believing their spiritual masters, think that when the universe is destroyed they will be spared the suffering felt through the subtle bodies which are then destroyed. Most of these devotees are merely fooling themselves. They assume a false sense of confidence and try to offset their insecurities. They will not be spared the suffering any more than they will be spared some type of suffering when passing from their present physical bodies. Being a devotee does not guarantee that there will be no casualty.

मम योनिर्महद्ब्रह्म
तस्मिन्गर्भं दधाम्यहम् ।
संभवः सर्वभूतानां
ततो भवति भारत ॥ १४.३ ॥
mama yonirmahadbrahma
tasmingarbhaṁ dadhāmyaham
saṁbhavaḥ sarvabhūtānāṁ
tato bhavati bhārata (14.3)

mama — my; yoniḥ — womb; mahat — extensive; brahma — reality; tasmin — into it; garbhaṁ — essence; dadhāmi — I impregnate; aham — I; saṁbhavaḥ — origin; sarvabhūtānāṁ — of all beings; tato = tataḥ — from that; bhavati — comes into being; bhārata — O man of the Bharata family

The extensive mundane reality is My womb. I impregnate the essence into it. The origin of all beings comes from that reality, O man of the Bharata family. (14.3)

Commentary:

Mahad brahma or mahat brahma is the responsive form of the cosmic material nature. It is comparable to a woman. Śrī Krishna named it as a womb or vagina. It has cosmic proportions. This same energy is personified in Goddess Durga.

In His lectures to Uddhava which are in the Eleventh Canto of the Śrīmad Bhāgavatam, Śrī Krishna gave many more details and graphic descriptions of how this impregnation takes place. The conjunction of the responsive material nature and the Supreme Lord is what functions as the origin (sambhavah) of all beings in the causal, subtle and gross material nature.

At a certain point in mystic research in kriyā yoga, one reaches a point at which one is unable to see any longer. This is not due to voidness but due to a lack of very subtle perception. Just as a child cannot see how he became an embryo in the belly of his mother, so we are unable to see how Lord Vishnu impregnated the sexually—responsive material nature.

According to the Śrīmad Bhāgavatam, Śrīla Dvaipāyana Vyāsadeva did see this in a personal way, when he saw the Mahavishnu glancing at Goddess Durga.

सर्वयोनिषु कौन्तेय
मूर्तयः संभवन्ति याः ।
तासां ब्रह्म महद्योनिर्
अहं बीजप्रदः पिता ॥ १४.४॥
sarvayoniṣu kaunteya
mūrtayaḥ saṁbhavanti yāḥ
tāsāṁ brahma mahadyonir
ahaṁ bījapradaḥ pitā (14.4)

sarvayoniṣu — in all wombs; kaunteya — O son of Kuntī; mūrtayaḥ — forms; saṁbhavanti — they are produced; yāḥ — which; tāsāṁ — of them; brahmā — mundane reality; mahat — great; yoniḥ — giving; aham — I; bījapradaḥ — seed — giving; pitā — father

Forms are produced in all types of wombs, O son of Kuntī, I am the seed-giving father. The extensive mundane reality is the great womb. (14.4)

Commentary:

The brahma mahad or brahma mahat is the sexually-responsive material nature. This is a living power. Normally we dismiss matter as a dead force. However this merely oversimplifies matter in relation to the spirit. Matter is also a living force. Matter always works in conjunction with the spirits and the Supreme Spirit. It is always electricized and sexualised by their proximity. At no time is matter merely a dead force.

सत्त्वं रजस्तम इति
गुणाः प्रकृतिसंभवाः ।
निबध्नन्ति महाबाहो
देहे देहिनमव्ययम् ॥ १४.५॥
sattvaṁ rajastama iti
guṇāḥ prakṛtisaṁbhavāḥ
nibadhnanti mahābāho
dehe dehinamavyayam (14.5)

sattvaṁ — clarity; rajaḥ — impulsion; tama — retardation; iti — thus; guṇāḥ — influences; prakṛtisaṁbhavāḥ = prakṛti — material nature + saṁbhavāḥ — produced of; nibadhnanti — they captivate; mahābāho — O great — armed hero; dehe — in the body; dehinaṁ — embodied soul; avyayam — imperishable

Clarity, impulsion and retardation are the influences produced of material nature. They captivate the imperishable embodied soul in the body, O strong—armed hero. (14.5)

Commentary:

At present, we depend on material nature for clarity of perception, for focusing on activity and for retardation to either sleep or be dull for one reason or another. All this hinges on the sexuality and sensuality of material nature, according to different combinations of her numerous types of energy. In kriyā yoga, we learn to make a preference and get hints from advanced yogis on how we may procure the clarifying energies and leave aside the impulsive and retarding ones.

तत्र सत्त्वं निर्मलत्वात्
प्रकाशकमनामयम् ।
सुखसङ्गेन बध्नाति
ज्ञानसङ्गेन चानघ ॥ १४.६ ॥

tatra — regarding these; sattvaṁ — clarifying influence; nirmalatvāt — relatively free from perceptive impurities; prakāśakam — illuminating; anāmayam — free from disease; sukhasaṅgena = sukha — happiness + saṅgena — by attachment;

tatra sattvaṁ nirmalatvāt
prakāśakamanāmayam
sukhasaṅgena badhnāti
jñānasaṅgena cānagha (14.6)

badhnāti — it binds; jñānasaṅgena = jñāna — knowledge of expertise + saṅgena — by attachment; cānagha = ca — and + anagha — sinless one

Regarding these influences, the clarifying one is relatively free from perceptive impurities. It is illuminating and free from disease, but by granting an attachment to happiness and to expertise, it captivates a person, O sinless one. (14.6)

Commentary:

The clarifying energies are the best but these energies carry a flaw, just as the lower ones certainly cause our degradation. This is why many preachers hawk us about giving up material nature and going over to the transcendence fully. Of course most of these preachers are just talking, because it is not simply a matter of wishful thinking or of joining their institutions. One cannot go to the transcendental side or consistently imbibe transcendental energy from this side without doing hard-core austerities. It is simply impossible.

The clarifying energies are relatively free of impurities when compared to the impulsive and retarding forces, but the clarifying ones have the flaw of making us feel secured and happy. It gives us expertise from which we derive prestige and pride. These factors cause us to become careless and to exploit other living entities in lower modes. This results in sure degradation. This is why in kriyā yoga, we never stop the disciplines. We continue them on and on to reach higher and higher states, so that we can make the leap once and for all from the clarifying powers. At first one must use these powers to advance beyond the impulsions and retarding forces, but later one must get beyond the clarifying assistance given by material nature. One must work for the exemption from cultural activities. Even though cultural activities are requested of us by Śrī Krishna, still these are mostly operative through and in the clarifying energies. Anytime we are not vigilant they victimize us, even though we may be working in karma yoga for Śrī Krishna. This happened many times to Arjuna when he fought at Kurukṣetra with Śrī Krishna at his side.

The attachment and expertise is based on our need for fulfillment and status. This is called self—esteem. The fulfillments we crave, are a need of the causal body, but until we accelerate the yoga practice, we cannot understand this. Until such time, we will be victimized by it. The expertise lies mainly in the power of the subtle form and its adaptability to the varying cultural situations. So long as the subtle body can maintain a high adaptability to varying cultural situations, it predominates any type of material form, it creates. This causes pride, which ultimately leads to degradation. We have to curb the subtle body by advanced mystic practice.

रजो रागात्मकंविद्धि
तृष्णासङ्गसमुद्भवम् ।
तन्निबध्नाति कौन्तेय
कर्मसङ्गेन देहिनम् ॥१४.७॥
rajo rāgātmakaṁviddhi
tṛṣṇāsaṅgasamudbhavam
tannibadhnāti kaunteya
karmasaṅgena dehinam (14.7)

rajo = rajaḥ — impulsive influence; rāgātmakaṁ — characterized by passion; viddhi — know; tṛṣṇāsaṅgasamudbhavam = tṛṣṇā — desire + saṅga — earnest + samudbhavam — produced from; tat — this; nibadhnāti — it captivates; kaunteya — O son of Kuntī; karmasaṅgena — by attachment to activity; dehinaṁ — the embodied soul

Know that the impulsive influence is characterized by passion. It is produced from earnest desire and attachment. O son of Kuntī, this mode captivates the embodied soul by an attachment to activity. (14.7)

Commentary:

The impulsive influence is characterized by a passionate force which clearly manifests as the sex urge in the body. It functions through other energies but the predominance of the sex urge is the sure way of perceiving that force. This is why in kriyā yoga there is an emphasis on celibacy. One must master the sex urge before he can reach the higher stages.

The impulsive influence cannot be stopped entirely because at any given time, there is always a rush for gross bodies. In other words, there are always disembodied spirits who want gross bodies. These persons side with and are empowered in and by the impulsive force. They force their way into any gross manifestation by entering the emotions of those who use physical bodies. This applies to all species of life.

The impulsive forces sponsor earnest desire and attachment, which possess a person regardless of whether he likes it or not. One becomes attached to activity, because by activity one achieves the fulfillments which satisfy the causal body. Only a yogin who passed the causal level can step aside from this fulfillment business in the material world.

तमस्त्वज्ञानजं विद्धि
मोहनं सर्वदेहिनाम् ।
प्रमादालस्यनिद्राभिस्
तन्निबध्नाति भारत ॥ १४.८॥
tamastvajñānajaṁ viddhi
mohanaṁ sarvadehinām
pramādālasyanidrābhis
tannibadhnāti bhārata (14.8)

tamaḥ — depressing mode; tu — but; ajñānajaṁ — produced of insensibility; viddhi — know; mohanam — confusion; sarvadehināṁ — of all embodied beings; pramādālasyanidrābhiḥ = pramāda — inattentiveness + ālasya — laziness + nidrābhiḥ — sleep; tat — this; nibadhnāti — captivates; bhārata — O man of the Bharata family

But know that the depressing mode is produced of insensibility which is the confusion of all embodied beings. This captivates by inattentiveness, laziness and sleep, O man of the Bharata family. (14.8)

Commentary:

The depressing mode cannot be avoided altogether unless we reach beyond the causal plane. This is because it serves a useful function to shift out exhausted subtle energy and replace it with new vitality. This is how we stay psychologically fit. It is the depressing or retarding force in its positive aspect that causes resting and renewal of energies in sleep.

However that force also has a negative feature in the form of inattentiveness, laziness and drowsiness. In kriyā yoga we learn how to decrease the negative application of this force and how to increase its contribution to our well being.

The average human being is captivated by the depressive forces which cause one to be inattentive and lazy. It causes one to oversleep or to stay awake even when he is fatigued.

सत्त्वं सुखे सञ्जयति
रजः कर्मणि भारत ।
ज्ञानमावृत्य तु तमः
प्रमादे सञ्जयत्युत ॥ १४.९॥

sattvaṁ — clarifying influence; sukhe — in happiness; sañjayati — causes attachment; rajaḥ — impulsive influence; karmaṇi — to action; bhārata — O Bharata family man; jñānam —

sattvaṁ sukhe sañjayati
rajaḥ karmaṇi bhārata
jñānamāvṛtya tu tamaḥ
pramāde sañjayatyuta (14.9)

experience; āvṛtya — obscuring; tu — but; tamaḥ — depressing mode; pramāde — to negligence; sañjayati — causes attachment; uta — even

The clarifying influence causes attachment to happiness. The impulsive one causes a need for action, O Bharata family man. But the depressing mode obscures experience and causes attachment to negligence. (14.9)

Commentary:

The need for action cannot be justly criticized except when the action is destructive of the spiritual interest of the living entities concerned. After all, as we heard, the Universal Form itself, pushes for actions. Thus even the Divine Being is a motivator. However, each person must guard against impulsions which are not inspired by the Universal Form. That Lord is not the only force that pushes.

Each of us must do kriyā yoga to understand what portion of the energies we are motivated by. By the recommendation from great yogins, we should perform purificatory actions upon the gross and subtle bodies.

रजस्तमश्चाभिभूय
सत्त्वं भवति भारत ।
रजः सत्त्वं तमश्चैव
तमः सत्त्वं रजस्तथा ॥ १४.१० ॥
rajastamaścābhibhūya
sattvaṁ bhavati bhārata
rajaḥ sattvaṁ tamaścaiva
tamaḥ sattvaṁ rajastathā (14.10)

rajaḥ — impulsiveness; tamaścābhibhūya = tamaḥ — depression + ca — and + abhibhūya — predominating over; sattvaṁ — clarity; bhavati — emerges; bhārata — O Bharata family man; rajaḥ — impulsiveness; sattvaṁ — clarity; tamaścaiva = tamaḥ — depression + caiva — and indeed; tamaḥ — depression; sattvaṁ — clarity; rajaḥ — impulsion; tathā — similarly

When predominating over impulsiveness and depression, clarity emerges, O Bharata family man. Depression rises, predominating over impulsiveness and clarity. Similarly, impulsion takes control over depression and clarity. (14.10)

Commentary:

We cannot continue relying on the automatic system through which one mode takes precedence and then another in turn, predominates, to be overtaken by yet another. We have to try to get a handle on the influences. This is what the practice of kriyā yoga yields in the advanced stages.

Material nature will continue willy nilly to run the world in its own way but we should develop a power through which we can side—step it and move on to transcendence. Surely, we will not change the whole world or banish material nature in the lives of other living beings, yet we can do something about our personal condition if we take up yoga practice in earnest.

सर्वद्वारेषु देहेऽस्मिन्
प्रकाश उपजायते ।
ज्ञानं यदा तदा विद्याद्
विवृद्धं सत्त्वमित्युत ॥ १४.११ ॥

sarvadvāreṣu — in all openings; dehe — in the body; 'smin = asmin — in this; prakāśa — clear perception: upajāyate — is felt; jñānaṁ— true knowledge; yadā — when; tadā — then; vidyāt — it should be

sarvadvāreṣu dehe'smin
prakāśa upajāyate
jñānaṁ yadā tadā vidyād
vivṛddhaṁ sattvamityuta (14.11)

concluded; vivṛddhaṁ — dominant; sattvam — clarifying mode; iti — thus; uta — indeed

When clear perception, true knowledge, is felt in all openings of the body, then it should be concluded that the clarifying mode is predominant. (14.11)

Commentary:

Śrī Krishna gave a guideline for understanding what He meant by the clarifying force. This is the soberness in clear perception in a healthy human form. This is just to give us some idea of the topic under discussion. There are various levels of clarity. The higher ones are not experienced by mere soberness in a healthy body. To experience higher levels, one must practice kriyā yoga and change the subtle body's intake of energy. This involves prāṇāyāma.

लोभः प्रवृत्तिरारम्भः
कर्मणामशमः स्पृहा ।
रजस्येतानि जायन्ते
विवृद्धे भरतर्षभ ॥१४.१२॥
lobhaḥ pravṛttirārambhaḥ
karmaṇāmaśamaḥ spṛhā
rajasyetāni jāyante
vivṛddhe bharatarṣabha (14.12)

lobhaḥ = greed; pravṛttiḥ — over — exertion; ārambhaḥ — rash undertaking; karmaṇām — of action; aśamaḥ — restlessness; spṛhā — craving; rājasī — in impulsiveness; etāni — those; jāyante — are produced; vivṛddhe — in the dominance; bharatarṣabha — strong man of the Bharatas

Greed, overexertion, rash undertakings, restlessness and craving, these are produced when impulsiveness is predominant, O strong man of the Bharatas. (14.12)

Commentary:

A beginner should learn to recognize the more obvious manifestations of the passionate force by studying the psychological conditions of greed, overexertion, rash undertaking, restlessness and craving. At first it is easy to recognize these moods in others, but as one advances, it becomes imperative to observe them in one's psyche. One simply tracks how such moods arise, and how the intellect and life force indulge in them.

अप्रकाशोऽप्रवृत्तिश्च
प्रमादो मोह एव च ।
तमस्येतानि जायन्ते
विवृद्धे कुरुनन्दन ॥१४.१३॥
aprakāśo'pravṛttiśca
pramādo moha eva ca
tamasyetāni jāyante
vivṛddhe kurunandana (14.13)

aprakāśo = aprakāśaḥ — lack of clarity; 'pravṛttiśca = apravṛttiśca = apravṛttiḥ — lack of energy + ca — and; pramādo = pramādaḥ — inattentiveness; mohā — confusion; eva — indeed; ca — and; tamasī — in depression; etāni — these; jāyante — they emerge; vivṛddhe — in the dominance; kurunandana — O dear son of the Kurus

Lack of clarity, lack of energy, inattentiveness and confusion emerge when depression is predominant, O dear son of the Kurus. (14.13)

Commentary:

Instead of relying on the normal course of material nature, a yogi does kuṇḍalinī yoga to surcharge the gross and subtle body with oxygen and energized subtle air (prāṇa) respectively. This takes those bodies away from the lack of positive energy which they are normally afflicted with. Even when the body is alive and well, it is to a degree starved for energy. One realizes this when he does bhastrik prāṇāyāma as a daily practice in the morning and afternoon. One finds that the body absorbs much more air and prāṇa than it would acquire by normal breathing.

यदा सत्त्वे प्रवृद्धे तु
प्रलयं याति देहभृत् ।
तदोत्तमविदां लोकान्
अमलान्प्रतिपद्यते ॥ १४.१४ ॥

yadā sattve pravṛddhe tu
pralayaṁ yāti dehabhṛt
tadottamavidāṁ lokān
amalānpratipadyate (14.14)

yadā — when; sattve — in clarity; pravṛddhe — under the dominance of; tu — but; pralayaṁ — death experience; yāti — he goes; dehabhṛt — the embodied soul; tadottamavidāṁ = tadā — then + uttamavidāṁ — of those who know the supreme; lokān — worlds; amalān — pure; pratipadyate — he is transferred

When the embodied soul goes through the death experience while under the dominance of the clarifying mode, he is transferred to the pure worlds of those who know the Supreme. (14.14)

Commentary:

Many devotees feel that since they are in the mode of clarity by virtue of eating sanctified dairy products and vegetarian foods, chanting holy names, doing worship ceremonies and submitting themselves for service to a spiritual master, they fall under the category described in this verse. However, they are mistaken. The clarity described here is not the mode of clarity we normally experience in a material body on earth. This pertains to the mode of clarity attained through hard core yoga austerities. Otherwise the devotee will again take another body on earth, because his consciousness is actually in the mode of passion. It is a higher version of the mode of passion, but still it is not actual clarity.

Some devotees are even more speculative since their teacher might assure them that they are beyond even clarity and that they are on the transcendental level. Most of this is imagination and belief only. One cannot enter higher modes that easily.

रजसि प्रलयं गत्वा
कर्मसङ्गिषु जायते ।
तथा प्रलीनस्तमसि
मूढयोनिषु जायते ॥ १४.१५ ॥

rajasi pralayaṁ gatvā
karmasaṅgiṣu jāyate
tathā pralīnastamasi
mūḍhayoniṣu jāyate (14.15)

rajasi — in the impulsive mode; pralayam — death experience; gatvā — having gone; karmasaṅgiṣu = karmā — work + saṅgiṣu — among people who are prone; jāyate — is born; tathā — likewise; pralīnaḥ — dying; tamasi — in the depressive mode; mūḍhayoniṣu = mūḍha — ignorant + yoniṣu — in the wombs of species; jāyate — is born

Having gone through the death experience in the impulsive mode, the soul is born among the work—prone people; likewise when dying in the depressive mode, the soul takes birth from the wombs of the ignorant species. (14.15)

Commentary:

Most devotees reside either in the impulsive or depressive mode. It is simply a matter of degree. Usually religious people on earth are at the high end of the impulsive mode, while the irreligious wickedly-inclined ones and the ones who are retarded, are in the depressive energy.

Taking birth among work—prone people means to take birth on an earthly planet. Taking birth in the ignorant species means an earthly body too, or it means taking birth in subterranean forms which are fearful of sunlight. I took birth in this life among work—prone people. Such folk may be religious or irreligious. The worlds which are in the mode of goodness are the celestial ones. It is not our habit to take such a birth, because we, like many devotees, are attached to a gross type of existence.

कर्मणः सुकृतस्याहुः
सात्त्विकं निर्मलं फलम् ।
रजसस्तु फलं दुःखम्
अज्ञानं तमसः फलम् ॥ १४.१६ ॥
karmaṇaḥ sukṛtasyāhuḥ
sāttvikaṁ nirmalaṁ phalam
rajasastu phalaṁ duḥkham
ajñānaṁ tamasaḥ phalam (14.16)

karmaṇaḥ — of action; sukṛtasyāhuḥ — sukṛtasya — of well—performed + āhuḥ— the authorities say; sāttvikaṁ — of the clarifying mode; nirmalaṁ — free of defects; phalam — result: rajasaḥ — of impulsion; tu — but; phalaṁ — result; duḥkham — distress; ajñānaṁ — ignorance; tamasaḥ — of the depressing mode; phalam — consequences

The authorities say that the result of a well—performed action is in the clarifying mode and is free of defects. But the result of an impulsive act is distress, while the consequence of a depressive act is ignorance. (14.16)

Commentary:

This clarifying mode governs the actions which are performed under the direct supervision of the Universal Form, for the satisfaction of the Central Figure of it. Someone may do something to please Him and may not be conscious of the righteousness of the act, but even that person will get benefits in the clarifying mode. One need not be aware of what he is doing or which mode he functions in, to derive benefits. A person gets the benefit according to how he is influenced.

Sometimes when fooled by a certain mode, a limited being gets the idea that he is in a higher energy. Then he assumes a very confident attitude, acts, and to his dismay finds out that the outcome is contrary. By the results achieved, he learns what mode he functioned in. In kriyā yoga, we use the guidelines given by Lord Krishna in this chapter and particularly in Chapter Eighteen to determine the influences. Gradually, by steady observation of how our tendencies are manifested, we get some idea of how we are influenced. Then by austerities, we fling ourselves into a higher mode and escape from the lower dominance.

Those who are male householder yogis have a good opportunity to study the nature of women. Females have a more energy—absorbing tendency. They usually function in the mode of passion but they do so without complaint. Generally, males by virtue of a strong sense of reason feel dissatisfied by the dominance of the lower modes. By observing women, a yogi gets more insight into the operations of the modes. In women, their influence is more obvious, more magnified.

Unmarried male yogis usually have less of an opportunity to observe this. They may take hints from advanced householders who advise them and who explain these matters in detail. In the advanced stages, a non—married yogi gets direct insight about females. This happens when he perfects the Kuṇḍalinī yoga portion of the practice. I myself, though functioning as a householder, took much help from many non—married yogis like Śrīla Yogeshwarananda Yogiraja. I took assistance from the siddha, Swami Muktananda, when he regularly entered my buddhi organ and showed me certain things.

Even though I am a householder, Swami Muktananda, who in his last body was not married, showed me certain ways of taking advantage of female exposure. Female exposure refers to the environment in Western countries or countries under Western dominance, where females wear skimpy clothing in public places. Swami Muktananda once showed me the Kuṇḍalinī Mātā deity who produces the female forms and who forces such forms to display sexuality. Once I saw her, I was able to take advantage of the exposure, because when seeing this deity, one is compelled to respect her, regardless of her sexually—aggressive behaviors.

If one sees one's mother taking bath, one does not disrespect her or consider her in a sexual way. She remains as one's mother with the full respect. Usually a child does not sexually disrespect his mother merely because her breasts are exposed. After all one is indebted to that organ for catering milk during infancy. When I see the female body parts, it does not disturb me because I see also the Kuṇḍalinī Mata deity who is my mother, who provided me with nourishment through Śrīmatī Pushti Ma, the goddess of nutrition. This maternal perception occured by the grace of Swami Muktananda, that accomplished siddha.

Kuṇḍalinī Shakti functions mostly from the mode of passion in terms of sexual polarity and from the mode of ignorance in terms of survival. This ignorance is removed in part by the buddhi organ which provides Kuṇḍalinī Ma with information from the senses. Hardly any of these faculties function from the clarifying mode. Therefore we have to make the effort of kriyā yoga to bring on the purity in which the clarifying energy becomes available.

सत्त्वात्संजायते ज्ञानं
रजसो लोभ एव च ।
प्रमाद्मोहौ तमसो
भवतोऽज्ञानमेव च ॥ १४.१७॥
sattvātsaṁjāyate jñānaṁ
rajaso lobha eva ca
pramādamohau tamaso
bhavato'jñānameva ca (14.17)

sattvāt —from clarity; saṁjāyate — is produced; jñānaṁ —factual knowledge; rajaso = rajasaḥ — from impulsion; lobha — greed; eva — indeed; ca — and; pramādamohau — inattentiveness and confusion; tamaso = tamasaḥ —from depression; bhavato = bhavataḥ — they come; 'jñānam = ajñānam — ignorance; eva — indeed; ca — and

Factual knowledge is produced from clarity. Greed comes from impulsion. Inattentiveness, confusion, and ignorance come from depression. (14.17)

Commentary:

This factual knowledge deals with the material world and with the spiritual realities as seen from the material perspective. One sees from the mode of goodness in its most purified form and then gets some idea of the spiritual realities. In kriyā yoga we first see through the brow chakra. This became famous as the third eye. It was made popular in the 1960s and 1970s by T. Lobsang Rampa who wrote a book about life in Tibetan monasteries. That book was titled *Third Eye*. After the popularity of that book, many yogis from India discussed the opening of the third eye through Kuṇḍalinī yoga and by meditative piercing of the darkness which one beholds when the eyelids are closed.

Śrīla Yogeshwarananda popularized prāṇa vision which is a more intricate and precise sight but which cannot be attained except by very advanced yoga practice in the samādhi stages. There is also buddhi vision. All these types of mystic perception utilize various purified types of pranic energy to give factual knowledge about the psyche, the world at large, and the other individuals who exist here. In taking help from the subtle material energy, we are still not seeing directly through spiritual eyes.

It should be noted that when Arjuna was awarded supernatural vision, it was not sufficient to perceive the spiritual body of the four—handed Lord Vishnu. Arjuna was given the ability to use his spiritual body to see that Lord. That type of sight is completely beyond the material energy, even the very subtle potencies.

Kriyā yogis cannot reject the material energy outright, because it has usefulness. We must use it to get out of the material world. We have no choice. One who ends up in a bad situation, must sometimes, use the same inconveniences to free himself. Thus we must learn how to use the material energy to get away from the very same power. In the case of the impulsive mode, it develops into greed. In all cases, if one is not frugal and exact in its usage, it leads to addiction which is furthered by the greedy attitude. However, impulsion is necessary even if we require a human form. It is by passion that our parents are motivated to beget infant bodies. As disembodied spirits requiring infant forms, we become *incarnations of passion*. Possessing our parents, we cause them to be lusty and to engage in the intercourse through which our bodies are formulated in the father's form as seminal fluid and then in the mother's form as an embryo.

The depressive mode has its usefulness also. It dulls the sense of activity, causing the gross body to rest and sleep. The retardative force causes negative attitudes like inattentiveness, confusion and ignorance. We should spare ourselves its negative applications.

ऊर्ध्वं गच्छन्ति सत्त्वस्था
मध्ये तिष्ठन्ति राजसाः ।
जघन्यगुणवृत्तस्था
अधो गच्छन्ति तामसाः ॥१४.१८॥
ūrdhvaṁ gacchanti sattvasthā
madhye tiṣṭhanti rājasāḥ
jaghanyaguṇavṛttasthā
adho gacchanti tāmasāḥ (14.18)

ūrdhvaṁ — upward; gacchanti — they go; sattvasthā — situated in clarity; madhye — in the middle; tiṣṭhanti — they are situated; rājasāḥ — those who are impulsive; jaghanyaguṇavṛttasthā = jaghanya — lowest + guṇavṛttasthā — situated in the influence of the material energy; adho = adhaḥ — downward; gacchanti — they go; tāmasāḥ — those who are retarded

Those who are anchored in clarity, go upward. Those who are impulsive are situated in the middle. Those who are habituated to the lowest influence of the material energy, the retarded people, go downward. (14.18)

Commentary:

This upward movement relates to people permanently situated in the higher celestial world and those aspiring for spiritual development by the numerous functional methods which apply to these gross situations and which, in fact, cause the spirits to go to the celestial regions. It is said that one can go directly to the kingdom of God by believing in a person like Jesus Christ or in Lord Krishna, for instance, but this is mostly belief.

One must pass through the celestial worlds on the way to the spiritual places. Thus if in passing through, one becomes attracted to any situation, one will go no higher but will immediately become involved there and will assume a form there for the time being. Since most human beings would not be able to resist the celestial pleasures, there is hardly any possibility of them going beyond to spiritual places.

This is why in kriyā yoga, one should attain a yoga—siddha body before passing from the gross human form. In a yoga—siddha body one can reach the celestial places, face the temptations they offer and work for the improved resistance required to rid the psyche of the attractions. As for the celestial people, they are unattracted to the spiritual places beyond their locales, because the subtle bodies they use celestial sense fulfillment. Thus some of these people aspire for human birth as a yogi, so that they can work for a yoga—siddha form and gain the resistance required to bypass those celestial zones. Overall the celestial people remain in their locales and do not evolve further.

The problem with the subtle body is its tendency for high—class sense fulfillment. That is its sole interest. Hence when one passes from his present gross body, if he assumes such a subtle form, his interest in liberation will be suspended for the time being, until his term of celestial residence is terminated and he must again come down to an earthly place to take up another body and become disgusted here.

Generally those who take birth on earthly planets, either in this dimension which we perceive or in others, are in the impulsive mode. Human beings like to portray themselves as being on the high end of the evolutionary cycle but this is in reference to trees and animals. In truth, the human situation is sponsored by and dominated by the impulsive mode. Most human beings perceive through the impulsive mode but they think that they view in clarity. A false pride endures which restricts self—correction and retards any effort that might be made for liberation.

The retarded people go downwards, because of the dragging influence of the depressive mode. The animals are in that mode. Many animals aspire and hope to get human incarnations. The power of the depressive mode pulls downwards in the mundane evolutionary cycle.

नान्यं गुणेभ्यः कर्तारं
यदा द्रष्टानुपश्यति ।
गुणेभ्यश्च परं वेत्ति
मद्भावं सोऽधिगच्छति ॥ १४.१९॥
nānyaṁ guṇebhyaḥ kartāraṁ
yadā draṣṭānupaśyati
guṇebhyaśca paraṁ vetti
madbhāvaṁ so'dhigacchati (14.19)

nānyaṁ = na — not + anyam — other; guṇebhyaḥ — than the influences of material nature; kartāraṁ — the performer; yadā — when; draṣṭānupaśyati = draṣṭā — observer + anupaśyati — he perceives; guṇebhyaḥ — than the influences of material nature + ca — and; paraṁ — higher; vetti — he knows; madbhāvaṁ — my level of existence; so = saḥ — he; 'dhigacchati = adhigacchati — he reaches

When the observer perceives no performer besides the influences of material nature and knows what is higher than those influences, he reaches My level of existence. (14.19)

Commentary:

This stage of observation is reached when one has mastered the samādhi trance states; otherwise one can understand this intellectually and also have visions of it periodically and so try to improve one's status. Ultimately if one does not achieve the samādhi stages, one cannot become anchored in this vision. To reach Śrī Krishna's level of perception, means to use spiritual senses in a spiritual body. We already heard that Arjuna was able to reach that status with the help of Śrī Krishna only. However, when Arjuna was performing yoga austerities in the Himalayas, he reached a stage where he developed sufficient spiritual perception to see Mahādeva. Arjuna saw Lord Shiva and his wife Umā in their locale where they live eternally. Thus Arjuna by yoga austerities attained that spiritual perception. It is only when one can see like this, that he has attained a state similar to Śrī Krishna or Lord Shiva.

गुणानेतानतीत्य त्रीन्
देही देहसमुद्भवान् ।
जन्ममृत्युजरादुःखैर्
विमुक्तोऽमृतमश्नुते ॥ १४.२० ॥
guṇānetānatītya trīn
dehī dehasamudbhavān
janmamṛtyujarāduḥkhair
vimukto'mṛtamaśnute (14.20)

guṇān — the influences of material nature; etān — these; atītya — transcends; trīn — three; dehī — embodied soul; dehasamudbhavān — deha — body + samudbhavān — formulated in; janmamṛtyujarāduḥkhaiḥ = janma — birth + mṛtyu — death + jarā — old age + duḥkhaiḥ — with distress; vimuktaḥ — released; 'mṛtam = amṛtam — immortality; aśnute — he attains

When the embodied soul transcends these three influences of material nature which are formulated in the body, he is released from birth, death, old age, and distress, and attains immortality. (14.20)

Commentary:

This is easy to discuss but few spirits attain immortality. In kriyā yoga, once the yogi becomes serious and has a consistent daily practice, he begins to understand that there are varying degrees of pollution. He has to work hard to remove these step by step. They are not removed by shortcuts or easy religions.

For success, a yogi has to agree to take the full course of yoga step by step. Then he will get success. Otherwise he will only achieve a partial purity. So long as one preaches to the public, one will be fooled because the tendency is to advance sufficiently, to be elevated above the public. This is not purity. It is merely a way of maintaining one's status as a religious leader.

अर्जुन उवाच
कैर्लिङ्गैस्त्रीन्गुणानेतान्
अतीतो भवति प्रभो ।
किमाचारः कथं चैतांस्
त्रीन्गुणानतिवर्तते ॥ १४.२१ ॥
arjuna uvāca
kairliṅgaistrīnguṇānetān
atīto bhavati prabho
kimācāraḥ kathaṁ caitāṁs
trīnguṇānativartate (14.21)

arjuna — Arjuna; uvāca — said; kaiḥ — by what; liṅgaiḥ— by features; trīn — three; guṇān — influences; etān— these; atīto = atītaḥ — transcending; bhavati —he is; prabho — respectful Lord; kimācāraḥ = kim — what + ācāraḥ — conduct; kathaṁ — how; caitān = ca — and + etān— these; trīn — three; guṇān — influences; ativartate — he transcends

Arjuna said: In regards to a person who transcended the three influences of material nature, by what features is he recognized, O respectful Lord? What is his conduct? And how does he transcend the three influences? (14.21)

Commentary:

These are an important questions for the novice yogi. The answers will give us some idea of who could be our teacher. Since so many people advertise themselves as competent spiritual leaders, we need to know how to find the true teacher, who can give us the disciplines that would cause us to transcend material nature. We cannot judge by external appearance. The qualifications of the teacher have to do with disciplines performed with the psyche. Thus we need some insight in how to recognize him or her.

श्रीभगवानुवाच
प्रकाशं च प्रवृत्तिं च
मोहमेव च पाण्डव ।
न द्वेष्टि संप्रवृत्तानि
न निवृत्तानि काङ्क्षति ॥ १४.२२ ॥
śrībhagavānuvāca
prakāśaṁ ca pravṛttiṁ ca
mohameva ca pāṇḍava
na dveṣṭi saṁpravṛttāni
na nivṛttāni kāṅkṣati (14.22)

śrī bhagavān — the Blessed Lord; uvāca — said; prakāśaṁ — enlightenment; ca — and; pravṛttiṁ — enthusiasm; ca — and; moham — depression; eva — indeed; ca — and; pāṇḍava — O son of Pāndu; na — not; dveṣṭi — scorns; saṁpravṛttāni — presence; na — nor; nivṛttāni — absence; kāṅkṣati — yearns for

The Blessed Lord said: O son of Pāndu, he does not scorn nor does he yearn for the presence or absence of enlightenment, enthusiasm or depression. (14.22)

Commentary:

Prakāśam means enlightenment, the very thing for which we hanker. Śrī Krishna said that the teacher should have passed the stage of hankering for enlightenment. The key issue in kriyā yoga is the practice, according to the stage of advancement. A teacher who is not absorbed into his practice is not a good example, but one can still learn from some one who has mastered yoga or who brings a message about the disciplines. As we learn from others, we should also recognize the exemplary teacher.

In my experience, while using this present body, Lord Shiva arranged many instances for me to learn from persons who were not competent teachers. Usually a novice shies away from such teachers, feeling that they are not competent enough to be masters and that they are cheaters, but that is a mistake. If Lord Shiva inspires the cheater to teach a particular technique, we should take the lesson from him. We should approach humbly, get the information of the practice and politely move on.

Sometimes a teacher, by bad motivation, masters a particular technique and then misuses it or becomes stagnant. Still he might take an inspiration to teach a novice. One should always be ready to learn one or two disciplines from such a person, while continuing to seek the ideal teacher.

दासीनवदासीनो
गुणैर्यो न विचाल्यते ।
गुणा वर्तन्त इत्येव
योऽवतिष्ठति नेङ्गते ॥ १४.२३ ॥
udāsīnavadāsīno
guṇairyo na vicālyate
guṇā vartanta ityeva
yo'vatiṣṭhati neṅgate (14.23)

udāsinavat — detached; āsīnaḥ — sitting, existing; guṇaiḥ — by the influences of material nature; yaḥ — who; na — not; vicālyate — he is affected; guṇā — the mundane influences; vartanta — they operate; iti — thus (thinking that); eva — indeed; yo = yaḥ — who; 'vatiṣṭhati = avatiṣṭhati — he is spiritually situated; neṅgate = na — not + iṅgate — he becomes excited

Being situated in the body, but being detached, not being affected by the influences of material nature, considering that the modes are operating naturally, he who is spiritually—situated, who does not become excited, (14.23)

Commentary:

In the advanced kriyā practice, the person sees that the modes are operating naturally. Therefore he does not become excited about anything rewarding or discouraging. He remains cool-headed. That is the mood of the really advanced person. Because he cut his relationship with material nature, she no longer excites him, but since he saw that her influences are extensive, he respects her in a very big way.

An example of a person who reached this stage of vision is Swami Muktananda, a siddha who recently left his gross body and who left his mission in the hands of a lady, Swami Chidvilasananda. Once, in 2002, when I spoke to the Swami, he showed me a technique for turning unfavorable female influences into favorable ones. As we discussed the matter, he suddenly said to me, "Look here, if the lady wants to undress in her own dressing room, then who are you to tell her to put on garments. It is her dressing room. You should try to leave that chamber, because you are an invader. In fact, she has every right to undress in there."

In that way he showed me how Ma Durga operates in the material world. He chastized me for criticizing the sexually-revealing clothing styles of ladies in the developed countries. The point is that such a siddha, as he, sees the modes of nature operating naturally. This is due to higher perception. He is not hung up on the idea that "This is illusion" or "That is illusion." He progressed beyond the neophyte stage.

समदुःखसुखः स्वस्थः
समलोष्टाश्मकाञ्चनः ।
तुल्यप्रियाप्रियो धीरस्
तुल्यनिन्दात्मसंस्तुतिः ॥१४.२४॥
samaduḥkhasukhaḥ svasthaḥ
samaloṣṭāśmakāñcanaḥ
tulyapriyāpriyo dhīras
tulyanindātmasaṁstutiḥ
(14.24)

samaduḥkhasukhaḥ = samā — equally regarded + duḥkha — pain + sukhaḥ — pleasure; svasthaḥ — self — situated; samaloṣṭāśmakāñcanaḥ = samā — regarded in the same way + loṣṭa — lump of clay + aśmā — stone + kāñcanaḥ — gold; tulyapriyāpriyo = tulyapriyāpriyaḥ = tulya — treated equally + priya — loved ones + apriyaḥ — despised person; dhīraḥ — one who is steady of mind; tulyanindātmasaṁstutiḥ = tulya — regarded equally + nindā — condemnation + ātmā — self + saṁstutiḥ — congratulation

...to whom pain and pleasure are equally regarded, who is self—situated, to whom a lump of clay, a stone or gold, are regarded in the same way, by whom a loved one and a despised person are treated equally, who is steady of mind, to whom condemnation and congratulation are regarded equally, (14.24)

Commentary:

Swami Vishnudevananda, my haţha yoga teacher, used to tell the story of how Swami Shivananda, his spiritual master, was spat upon in public by a man who verbally abused him. All the while, Swami Shivananda smiled and actually went so far as to bless and congratulate the man. Usually in India, the established gurus have disciples who defend them strongly. One dares not insult their guru. Even in the Vaishnava sampradayas one has to be careful saying anything against a guru. Even today this transpires. However in kriyā yoga, we are not interested in prestige. It has no significance. In fact, an interest in it is a sure sign of degression.

We have to study these descriptions given by Śrī Krishna carefully. Then we can begin the hunt for an advanced kriyā master. In the meantime, we should take an instruction from anyone if such an instruction would move us one step forward. We should not expect that we will have only one teacher. It might take years or lives to find the perfect teacher. In the meantime we should advance little by little.

मानावमानयोस्तुल्यस्
तुल्यो मित्रारिपक्षयोः ।
सर्वारम्भपरित्यागी
गुणातीतः स उच्यते ॥ १४.२५ ॥
mānāvamānayostulyas
tulyo mitrāripakṣayoḥ
sarvārambhaparityāgī
guṇātītaḥ sa ucyate (14.25)

mānāvamānayoḥ — in honor and dishonor; tulyaḥ — equally-disposed; tulyo = tulyaḥ — impartial; mitrāripakṣayoḥ — to friend or foe; sarvārambhaparityāgī = sarvā — all + ārambha — undertaking + parityāgī — renouncing; guṇatītaḥ = guṇa — mundane influence + atītaḥ — transcending; sa = saḥ — he; ucyate — is said to be

...who is equally disposed to honor and dishonor, who is impartial to friend or foe, who has renounced all undertakings, is said to have transcended the mundane influences. (14.25)

Commentary:

The quality of renouncing all undertakings is a key note for the advanced kriyā yogi. Such a person does not have a mission to perform except to teach those who are serious about yoga austerities. He does not start up a general preaching mission but he does not oppose those who establish that. He is not against the popular spiritual masters and he does not become their competitor.

Some commentators criticize the advanced yogi who does not take up any mundane undertakings. They feel that for Krishna, he should take on a huge preaching mission. These opinions come from the mouths of preachers who barely understand kriyā yoga.

In advanced kriyā yoga, one does not take on missionary work at all because such work is a grand delusion. It is not possible to liberate the entities in mass. It must be done through individual practice. The mass of people will not be inspired to do such austerities. Knowing this, a kriyā yogi does not begin an institution. However he is not against such missions. Sometimes, as forced by providence he openly supports such religious societies started by others. However, as soon as providence releases him, he eliminates such obligations. Once a kriyā yogi gets an exemption from cultural acts, he does not backtrack to the world of involvement. Instead he uses the exemption to institute a fulltime discipline.

मां च योऽव्यभिचारेण
भक्तियोगेन सेवते ।
स गुणान्समतीत्यैतान्
ब्रह्मभूयाय कल्पते ॥ १४.२६ ॥
māṁ ca yo'vyabhicāreṇa
bhaktiyogena sevate
sa guṇānsamatītyaitān
brahmabhūyāya kalpate (14.26)

māṁ — me; ca — and; yo = yaḥ — who; 'vyabhicāreṇa = avyabhicāreṇa — with unwavering; bhaktiyogena — by yogically-disciplined affection; sevate — serves; sa = saḥ — he; guṇān — the mundane influences; samatītyaitān = samatītya — transcending + etān — these; brahmabhūyāya — absorbing in spiritual existence; kalpate — is suited

And a person who serves Me with unwavering, yogically—disciplined affection and who transcends these mundane influences, is suited for absorption in spiritual existence, (14.26)

Commentary:

Bhakti yoga and bhakti are not one and the same thing. Yoga and bhakti are also different. Yoga is yoga, an eightfold process of progressively harder disciplines. Bhakti is affection for a divine personality. Bhakti has its stages of purity and impurity. When we coordinate bhakti and yoga we get bhakti yoga. One does not have to do yoga to be a devotee of Krishna or a bhakta, but to be a yogi devotee, one has to be a devotee and perform yoga. We have to be clear on these definitions. In this verse, the bhakti yoga process is not bhakti alone, but bhakti with yoga. Yogicly disciplined affection and affection which is disciplined by other methods is different. This verse accords the yogicly—disciplined affection. This was something that Arjuna was familiar with because he was a yogi. The gopis were not yogis and so their affection was not the yogicly—disciplined type.

A person who serves Śrī Krishna with unswerving, yogicly—disciplined affection, and who transcends these mundane influences discussed so far in the *Gītā*, is suited for absorption in spiritual existence. He is suited to the samadhis which will give him direct perception of the spiritual world.

Śrī Caitanya Mahāprabhu, a Yugavatar for this era, become absorbed in the spiritual existence to such an extent that He used to enter Śrī Krishna's eternal pastimes with the gopis. Amazingly, Lord Caitanya did not perform yoga. Still, this verse applies to those who will do the yoga practice. We do not have to make this verse match the example of Lord Caitanya. We should understand the *Gītā* in its own time and place without shifting its definitions into Śrī Caitanya līlā.

ब्रह्मणो हि प्रतिष्ठाहम्
अमृतस्याव्ययस्य च ।
शाश्वतस्य च धर्मस्य
सुखस्यैकान्तिकस्य च ॥१४.२७॥
brahmaṇo hi pratiṣṭhāham
amṛtasyāvyayasya ca
śāśvatasya ca dharmasya
sukhasyaikāntikasya ca (14.27)

brahmaṇo = brahmaṇaḥ — of spiritual existence; hi — indeed; pratiṣṭhāham = pratiṣṭhā — basis + aham — I; amṛtasyāvyayasya = amṛtasya — of the immortal + avyayasya — of the imperishable; ca — and; śāśvatasya — of the perpetual; ca — and; dharmasya — of the rules for social conduct; sukhasyaikāntikasya = sukhasya — of happiness + ekāntikasya — of the absolute; ca — and

...for I am the basis of the immortal, imperishable spiritual existence and of the perpetual rules of social conduct and of absolute happiness. (14.27)

Commentary:

As the pratiṣţha, the very basis of perfection, Śrī Krishna laid down the rules for elevation. Some realized souls do not accept Śrī Krishna as the basis for the immortal, imperishable spiritual existence. Their idea is that Śrī Krishna is a big aspect and nothing else. They feel that existence itself is the basis from which all individual spirits, even the Supreme Spirit, emanate. However it is not a cause for argument.

Each living entity, by its own experience, will testify to this or that according to its biases. That is natural. We have to get along with each other, respect each other and try to attain the highest possible state according to our category.

CHAPTER 15

Two Types of Spirits*

श्रीभगवानुवाच
ऊर्ध्वमूलमधःशाखम्
अश्वत्थं प्राहुरव्ययम् ।
छन्दांसि यस्य पर्णानि
यस्तं वेद स वेदवित् ॥ १५.१ ॥
śrībhagavānuvāca
ūrdhvamūlamadhaḥśākham
aśvatthaṁ prāhuravyayam
chandāṁsi yasya parṇāni
yastaṁ veda sa vedavit (15.1)

śrī bhagavān — The Blessed Lord; uvāca — said; ūrdhvamūlam = ūrdhva — upward + mūlam — root; adhaḥśākham = adhaḥ — below + śākham — branch; aśvatthaṁ — ashvattha tree; prāhuḥ — the yogī sages say; avyayam — imperishable; chandāṁsi — Vedic hymns; yasya — or what which; parṇāni — leaves; yaḥ — who; taṁ — this; veda — knows; sa = saḥ — he; vedavit — knower of the Vedas

The Blessed Lord said: The yogi sages say that there is an imperishable Ashvattha tree which has a root going upwards and a trunk downwards, the leaves of which are the Vedic hymns. He who knows this is a knower of the *Vedas*. (15.1)

Commentary:

This imperishable banyan tree represents the living material world. The yogi sages saw by mystic perception that the material situation is alive. It is not dead matter as we are usually told. It is alive, every part of it. It is only varying degrees of mobility and activity which fool us into thinking that it might be dead matter. There is not a scrap of anything anywhere which is dead in fact.

The root of the tree of the material existence goes upwards which is contrary to the way trees normally grow. From another aspect this is consistent with tree growth. Tree roots travel in whatever direction they sense nutrients. The material existence which is, in fact, an extensive vegetation, when seen from a certain mystic perspective, feeds on the proximity of the spiritual existence, which is upwards. Thus its roots do go up.

The trunk of the tree goes downwards, away from the immortal, imperishable spiritual existence because the trunk can develop in the material atmosphere. From that development comes many life forms, of which the human form is the best. The best production of the early human beings on this planet, was the *Vedas*, which are the manual for mundane existence, comprising of cultural life, religious life and the effort for liberation. These are described in the hymns of the *Vedas* by the first ritual mystics.

**The Mahābhārata contains no chapter headings. This title was assigned by the translator on the basis of verse 15 of this chapter.*

अधश्चोर्ध्वं प्रसृतास्तस्य शाखा
गुणप्रवृद्धा विषयप्रवालाः ।
अधश्च मूलान्यनुसंततानि
कर्मानुबन्धीनि मनुष्यलोके ॥ १५.२॥
adhaścordhvaṁ prasṛtāstasya śākhā
guṇapravṛddhā viṣayapravālāḥ
adhaśca mūlānyanusaṁtatāni
karmānubandhīni manuṣyaloke (15.2)

adhaścordhvaṁ = adhaḥ — downward + ca — and + urdhvam — upward; prasṛtāh — widely spreading; tasya — of it; śākhā — branches; guṇa — mundane influence; pravṛddhā — nourished; viṣayapravālāḥ = viṣaya — attractive objects + pravālāḥ — sprouts; adhaśca = adhaḥ — below + ca — and; mūlāni — roots; anusaṁtatāni — stretched out; karmānubandhīni = karmā — action + anubandhīni — promoting; manuṣyaloke = manuṣya — of human being + loke — in the world

Branches spread from it, upwards and downwards. It is nourished by the mundane influences and the attractive objects are its sprouts. The roots are spread below, promoting action in the world of human beings. (15.2)

Commentary:

The branches of the tree of mundane existence spread upward and downward, because the tree is intended to yield bondage or liberation. However the tree is also nourished by the mundane influences. These same influences absorb energy from the spiritual existence. This absorption of spiritual energy makes the material world capable of yielding self realization.

The main trunk of the tree produces sprouts on the basis of our attraction to its form. The more we are attracted, the more the tree expands and produces sprouts; the tree is impregnated for growth by its absorption of our energy. That is a sexual relationship between mundane existence and the spirits.

Even though the main root goes upward towards the spiritual existence, still there are subsidiary roots which go downward, and which promote action in the human world. These subsidiary roots feed on the causal bodies of the living beings, extracting subtle energy from which various desires are engendered, fostered and fulfilled.

न रूपमस्येह तथोपलभ्यते
नान्तो न चादिर्न च संप्रतिष्ठा ।
अश्वत्थमेनं सुविरूढमूलम्
असङ्गशस्त्रेण दृढेन छित्त्वा ॥ १५.३
na rūpamasyeha tathopalabhyate
nānto na cādirna ca saṁpratiṣṭhā
aśvatthamenaṁ suvirūḍhamūlam
asaṅgaśastreṇa dṛḍhena chittvā (15.3)

na — not; rūpam — form; asyeha = asya — of it + iha — in this dimension; tathopalabhyate = tathā — thus + upalabhyate — it is perceived; nānto = nāntah = na — not + antaḥ — end; na — nor; cādiḥ = ca — and + ādiḥ — end; na — nor; ca — and; saṁpratiṣṭhā — foundation; aśvatthaṁ — ashvattha tree; enam — this; suvirūḍhamūlam = suvirūḍha — well-developed + mūlam — root; asaṅgaśastreṇa = asaṅga — non-attachment + śastreṇa — with the axe; dṛḍhena — with the strong; chittvā — cutting down

Its form is not perceived in this dimension, nor its end, beginning or foundation. With the strong axe of non—attachment, cut down this Ashvattha tree with its well—developed roots. (15.3)

Commentary:

The tree of mundane existence cannot be seen from this dimension. We can be sure of this. It would take a special vision for the perception of it. In fact, one cannot see it unless allowed by Lord Krishna, Lord Balarāma, or Lord Shiva alternately. Even the great yogis cannot usually see the entire form of the colossal mundane existence. Just as the Universal Form could not be seen by Arjuna without supernatural vision from Śrī Krishna, so the Living Mundane Existence in its natural shape cannot be seen by anyone, even by a yogi, unless he takes assistance from a divinity.

However, even without seeing the tree in its entirety, a yogi can cut down his connection with it. He has to use the cutting tool of non—attachment. This non—attachment is the type attained by yoga practice rather than the type attained by adoption of indifferent mental attitudes.

A yogi does not have to see the entire mundane existence in its tree form to cut his connection with it, but he has to feel that connection. He must first admit it, trace it out properly and then use special purificatory actions to elevate himself on the mystic plane. Systematically, he may develop the subtle body which is capable of the necessary non—attachment.

Such a body is used by Swami Nityananda, the spiritual master of Siddha Muktananda. I was shown that body. In it there is no sexual potency, no sexual organ whatsoever, and its Kuṇḍalinī chakra was eliminated.

ततः पदं तत्परिमार्गितव्यं
यस्मिन्गता न निवर्तन्ति भूयः ।
तमेव चाद्यं पुरुषं प्रपद्ये
यतः प्रवृत्तिः प्रसृता पुराणी. ॥ १५.४॥
tataḥ padaṁ tatparimārgitavyaṁ
yasmingatā na nivartanti bhūyaḥ
tameva cādyaṁ puruṣaṁ prapadye
yataḥ pravṛttiḥ prasṛtā purāṇī(15.4)

tataḥ — then; padaṁ — place; tat — that; parimārgitavyaṁ — to be sought; yasmin — to which; gatā — some; na — not; nivartanti — they return; bhūyaḥ — again; tam — that; eva — indeed; cādyaṁ = ca — and + ādyaṁ — primal; puruṣaṁ — person; prapadye — I take shelter; yataḥ — from whom; pravṛttiḥ — creation; prasṛtā — emerged; purāṇī — in primeval times

Then that place is to be sought, to which having gone, the spirits do not return to this world again. One should think: I take shelter with that Primal Person, from Whom the creation emerged in primeval times. (15.4)

Commentary:

Once a spirit overcomes the attractions of the material existence, he can turn to the spiritual existence in earnest. Otherwise he will hang on here to further material existence and to work with the spiritual and the material realities side by side. For kriyā yoga, we should abandon the entire material existence. In other words, we should become qualified to go to that place from which the spirits do not return.

If we are attracted to Śrī Krishna, then we should aspire to be in close association with Him, regarding Him as the Primal Person, the ādyam puruṣam, from whom the creation emerged in primeval times. If we are not attracted to Him, then we would strive to find the root cause of the material existence, in order to pass beyond it, into the spiritual existence. In either case, this is nirvāṇa or the ending of our individual history in the material existence.

निर्मानमोहा जितसङ्गदोषा
अध्यात्मनित्या विनिवृत्तकामाः ।
द्वंद्वैर्विमुक्ताः सुखदुःखसंज्ञैर्
गच्छन्त्यमूढाः पदमव्ययं तत् ॥ १५.५

nirmāna — devoid of pride; mohā — confusion; jita — conquered; saṅga — attachment; doṣā — faults; adhyātmanityā = adhyātma — Supreme Spirit + nityā — constantly; vinivṛtta — ceased; kāmāḥ — cravings; dvandvaiḥ — by dualities;

nirmānamohā jitasaṅgadoṣā
adhyātmanityā vinivṛttakāmāḥ
dvaṁdvairvimuktāḥ
sukhaduḥkhasaṁjñair
gacchantyamūḍhāḥ
padamavyayaṁ tat (15.5)

vimuktāḥ — *freed; sukhaduḥkha* — *pleasure—pain; saṁjñaiḥ* — *known as; gacchanti* — *they go; amūḍhāḥ* — *the undeluded souls; padam* — *place; avyayam* — *imperishable; tat = tad* — *that*

Those who are devoid of pride and confusion, who have conquered the faults of attachment, who constantly stay with the Supreme Spirit, whose cravings have ceased, who are freed from the dualities known as pleasure and pain, these undeluded souls go to that imperishable place. (15.5)

Commentary:

Preachers who are absorbed in educating the population, building temples, creating institutions and making disciples, are not described in this verse. These verses pertain to those who are ending their material existence. That excludes limited spirits who take on savior roles in the cause of salvation as they defined it.

Going to the imperishable place, once and for all, means leaving behind disciples, institutions, temples and the like, including the interest in rescuing humanity. If a spiritual master's mind is bent into this world, then he will not be going to the spiritual place, due to the force of his interest in this world. A kriyā yoga student should be aware of this. We see that soon after some teachers attain samādhi, they turn away from kriyā practice, open institutions, begin teaching and then become fully preoccupied with their missions. They attempt continued practice but the truth is that they forsake the practice just to help beginners. In other words, they lose interest in going away from the tree of material existence and instead are sustained by the caring force of their disciples. That caring force effectively curtails progression.

A recent case illustrates this. In 2001, I visited Sacramento, California. Nearby on the edge of Nevada City, there a spiritual community established by Swami Kriyānanda, a disciple of Śrī Paramhansa Yogananda. Swami Kriyānanda faced some legal difficulties when some of his female disciples filed sexual complaints against him.

However, when I visited the place, the Swami was not in residence. On the subtle side of existence, Śrī Paramhansa Yogananda was there to greet me. We had some in-depth talks about kriyā yoga practice and about his contribution to its cultivation in the Western countries. Even though people believe that he merged into the Supreme, still the fact is that Śrī Paramhansaji uses a subtle body only. He lives on the subtle side at that community and at his other institutional places elsewhere in California.

I checked his subtle body carefully. It was not a yoga siddha form like the one Śrī Bābāji Mahasaya uses. It was a low energy subtle body. Because of disciples and the assumption of a savior role, Śrī Paramhansaji became slack in the practice. In fact, a lady who used a Jewish body who was an official at the spiritual community, spoke to me with authority and said that they do not focus on haţha yoga. She said some people do it there but that their process is simply meditation. However, meditation alone is not the complete kriyā practice. It is only part of the practice if the meditator mastered haţha yoga and prāṇāyāma beforehand.

Even though I went to California at the time, I had no plan to visit that spiritual community or to hold a discussion with the departed Yogananda. It was the desire Śrī Bābāji because he had advised me some months prior to the visit, to procure a copy of

Yogananda's *Bhagavad Gītā* translation and commentary. This was acquired for me by Sriman Bharat Patel, a disciple of Swami Rāma, another accomplished kriyā master.

Even though I had no plan to go to Nevada City, a daughter of my body, Bloom Beloved, insisted that I go to that community. Thus later I understood that she was in touch with Swami Yogananda and with Śrī Bābāji Mahasaya even though she was not fully conscious of such subtle associations.

Undoubtedly Swami Yogananda is a master of kriyā yoga, having practiced under Śrī Yuktesvara Giri; but that does not mean that Swami Yogananda completed the practice. He was diverted by the assumption of a Savior-of-Humanity role. That is to be regretted. It is however beneficial to us when we see these diversions. They forewarn of what would happen if we take the same course.

It is unfortunate that the lady using the Jewish body, did not recognize me, because I could have given her some important kriyās which would have accelerated her progress. Such is the kriyā path. One meets many proud people from day to day, people who latch onto an institution and who become stagnant as officials of it. In a sense, this means that I do not have to accept many disciples. They will remain in the material world with their favorite institutions life after life.

As Śrī Krishna said in this verse, those who are devoid of pride and confusion, who have conquered the faults of attachment, who consistently stay with the Supreme Spirit, whose cravings have ceased, who are freed from the dualities known as pleasure and pain, these undeluded souls go to that imperishable place. That is final. Others who are distracted by disciples must stay on here and gain reputations as Saviors of humanity.

In the process of getting an exemption from karma yoga as Śrī Krishna taught Arjuna, I do not have to take on disciples. In fact, some people reject me as a possible teacher. Others who acclaim me are unable to complete the disciplines through which they would qualify for more advanced kriyās. The Universal Form is pushing me out of the world. This is wonderful. For one reason or the other, He feels that I am not needed. He can do His disciplinary work by Himself and through others. So that is His blessing.

Having a family is one problem but a greater headache is disciples. By the grace of God, really, by the grace of God only, I am not having disciples. This is a most wonderful thing. For some reason, by an action of the Central Figure in the Universal Form, I am unable to make disciples. He definitely decided to give me the waiver from cultural and religious activity.

In kriyā yoga, this is regarded as the stage of throwing the tridents in a corner. Śrīla Gambhiranatha, a great Nath yogin in the lineage from Śrī Gorakshnath, used to stress this throwing of the tridents in a corner. It is the act of taking the tridents with which Lord Shiva pokes, and then throwing them away. Of course as soon as the novice throws away one of Shiva's tridents, that Lord produces another and pokes him again. So repeatedly one has to throw away these tridents. These are the miseries of this material world. They come disguised as legitimate responsibilities or as dharma. Once a yogi puts down his desire to participate in the world of dharma, the sphere of responsibility, he has it made as a yogi. Otherwise, he complete down his family responsibilities or he may do whatever he can to renounce the world, and then he will take up obligations for disciples and become stuck in some astral dimension, not doing his practices and pretending that he is the world's savior. Actually the Savior is already there. Arjuna saw Him, the Central Figure in the Universal Form, Śrī Krishna Himself, the Supreme Personality of Godhead, as Śrīla Bhaktivedanta Swami has so expertly addressed Him.

न तद्भासयते सूर्यो
न शशाङ्को न पावकः ।
यद्गत्वा न निवर्तन्ते
तद्धाम परमं मम ॥ १५.६ ॥
na tadbhāsayate sūryo
na śaśāṅko na pāvakaḥ
yadgatvā na nivartante
taddhāma paramaṁ mama (15.6)

na — not; tat —that; bhāsayate — illuminates; sūryo = sūryaḥ — the sun; na — nor; śaśāṅko = śaśāṅkaḥ — moon; na — nor; pāvakaḥ — fire; yat — which; gatvā — having gone; na — never; nivartante — they return; tat — that; dhāmā — residence; paramaṁ — supreme; mama — my

The sun does not illuminate that place, nor the moon, nor the fire. Having gone to that location, they never return. That is My supreme residence. (15.6)

Commentary:

The astral world where Swami Yogananda stays is not illuminated by the sun, moon or fire, but it is not the place from which souls never return. It is a place from which one can again take a human body. In fact, one must take a human body to be freed from that place, since it is nearly impossible to take up the advanced kriyās in that location. Śrīla Yogeshwarananda, a kriyā yoga master, did avoid such places. To complete the austerities, he went to the causal region, where one is not bothered by disciples.

Śrī Krishna described a place which He called His supreme residence, dhāma paramam mama. This is not the place in which I saw Śrīla Paramhansa Yogananda. That place Śrī Krishna described, is a spiritual locale not attainable except by exclusive focus on it by very advanced kriyā practice. One who is burdened by disciples and their problems, one who adjusts the kriyā path to make it easy for followers, cannot go to Krishna's spiritual place.

ममैवांशो जीवलोके
जीवभूतः सनातनः ।
मनःषष्ठानीन्द्रियाणि
प्रकृतिस्थानि कर्षति ॥ १५.७ ॥
mamaivāṁśo jīvaloke
jīvabhūtaḥ sanātanaḥ
manaḥṣaṣṭhānīndriyāṇi
prakṛtisthāni karṣati (15.7)

mamaivāṁśaḥ = mama — my + eva — indeed + aṁśaḥ — partner; jīvaloke = jīva — individualized conditioned being + loke — in the world; jīvabhūtaḥ — individual soul; sanātanaḥ — eternal; manaḥ — mind; ṣaṣṭhānindriyāṇi = saṣṭhāni — sixth + indriyāṇi — sense, detection device; prakṛtisthāni — mundane; karṣati — draws

My partner is in this world of individualized conditioned beings. He is an eternal individual soul but he draws to himself the mundane senses of which the mind is the sixth detection device. (15.7)

Commentary:

In terms of exploitation of the subtle and gross resources, that is done by material nature herself in conjunction with the individual spirits and the Supreme God. Since the Supreme Spirit is detached, the exploitive pursuits are enacted by the individual spirits in their conjunction with material nature. Śrī Krishna regards these spirits as His partners in this affair.

Even though both the Supreme Person and the individual limited spirits are eternal, the limited spirits have a way about them, that is distinctly different from the Supreme Spirit. This difference is no more clearer than described by Śrī Krishna in this verse. The kriyā yogis should make a thorough study of what Śrī Krishna explained here.

Our tendency to attract, the mundane senses is the very cause of our conditioning. Our ability to resist the senses and subsequently relinquish them, is the cause of our freedom from material existence.

So, how did we draw to ourselves the mundane senses, of which the mind is the sixth detection device? The answer is that we did not deliberately do this. This happened naturally by a primal instinct.

Even though the conditioning is non-deliberate, the freedom from it must be deliberate. Thus we have to study how we became conditioned in the first place. Then we may work to reverse the process. The 5th step of yoga, that of pratyāhār sense withdrawal is the preliminary work for removing ourselves from the mundane senses. These are subtle senses of the subtle body. The withdrawal is completed after one masters the full course of samādhi practice. It is not easy to attain this. Very few yogis do this, because the tendency to draw the subtle senses to ourselves is very innate.

Śrī Krishna graciously mentioned this to Arjuna to give the ultimate hint on how to become liberated from the emotional forces which affected Arjuna on the battlefield and to inform Arjuna of what he needed to complete kriyā practice.

शरीरं यदवाप्नोति
यच्चाप्युत्क्रामतीश्वरः ।
गृहीत्वैतानि संयाति
वायुर्गन्धानिवाशयात् ॥ १५.८॥
śarīraṁ yadavāpnoti
yaccāpyutkrāmatīśvaraḥ
gṛhītvaitāni saṁyāti
vāyurgandhānivāśayāt (15.8)

śarīraṁ — by body; yad — which; avāpnoti — he acquires; yat — which; cāpi — and also; utkrāmatīśvaraḥ = utkrāmati — departs from + īśvaraḥ — master; gṛhītvaitāni = gṛhītvā — taking + etāni — these; saṁyāti — he goes; vāyuḥ — wind; gandhān — perfumes; ivāśayāt — ivā — just as + āśayāt — from source

Regardless of whichever body that master acquires, or whichever one he departs from, he goes taking these senses along, just as the wind goes with the perfumes from their source. (15.8)

Commentary:

This is another very important piece of information. When the body dies, a spirit takes his psychology along with its imperfect sensing mechanisms. The psyche does not change merely because a spirit has left a gross body. The psyche will not improve or be divinized merely because a spirit shifted to the astral world. We will take our subtle senses as they are at the time of death of the body. It is an urgency for us to first improve that sensuality and then eventually get rid of it.

This does not mean no senses at all. It means assuming spiritual senses which can operate directly without taking help from the mundane sensuality which we know.

By a careful study of this verse, a kriyā yogi will understand that those teachers who tell us that our subtle psychology will suddenly become changed at death, merely because of faith and religious affiliation, are speaking falsely. According to Śrī Krishna, it does not work like that.

श्रोत्रं चक्षुः स्पर्शनं च
रसनं घ्राणमेव च ।
अधिष्ठाय मनश्चायं
विषयानुपसेवते ॥ १५.९ ॥
śrotraṁ cakṣuḥ sparśanaṁ ca
rasanaṁ ghrāṇameva ca
adhiṣṭhāya manaścāyaṁ
viṣayānupasevate (15.9)

śrotraṁ — hearing; cakṣuḥ — vision; sparśanaṁ — sense of touch; ca — and; rasanaṁ — taste; ghrāṇaṁ — smell; eva — indeed; ca — and; adhiṣṭhāya — governing; manaścāyaṁ = manaḥ — mind; ca — and + ayaṁ — this; viṣayān — attractive objects; upasevate — becomes addicted

While governing the sense of hearing, vision, touch, taste, smell and the mind, My partner becomes addicted to the attractive objects. (15.9)

Commentary:

Even though the spirit governs the senses and the mind, still he is usually conditioned by what he governs. That means that his governship is like that of an affectionate mother. Such a lady usually does exactly what her children desire. She is governed by her children.

Becoming addicted to the attractive objects, the soul merely sponsors the activities of the senses and so he becomes lost to himself and feels that he is the mind, the senses and their offshoot energies which form his psychology. Kriyā yoga is the sure way for eliminating this.

उत्क्रामन्तं स्थितं वापि
भुञ्जानं वा गुणान्वितम् ।
विमूढा नानुपश्यन्ति
पश्यन्ति ज्ञानचक्षुषः ॥ १५.१० ॥
utkrāmantaṁ sthitaṁ vāpi
bhuñjānaṁ vā guṇānvitam
vimūḍhā nānupaśyanti
paśyanti jñānacakṣuṣaḥ (15.10)

utkrāmantaṁ — departing; sthitaṁ — remaining; vāpi = vā — or + api — also; bhuñjānaṁ — exploiting; vā — or; guṇānvitam — under the influence of material nature; vimūḍhā — idiots; nānupaśyanti = na — not + anupaśyanti — they perceived; paśyanti — they perceive; jñānacakṣuṣaḥ — vision of reality

The idiots do not perceive how the spirit departs or remains or exploits under the influence of material nature. But those who have the vision of reality do perceive this. (15.10)

Commentary:

Jñānacakṣuh, the vision of reality, is not the conceptual knowledge from reading *Bhagavad Gītā* or from hearing lectures of self realized souls. It is rather a mystic perception attained by kriyā practice. If one has that, he will consistently perceive his connection with material nature and his addictive assumption of the mundane sensuality. In addition he will do something effective to alter this.

The idiots (vimūḍhā) are any of us who are not situated in the mystic perception. There are degrees of idiocy because some of us have the vision periodically, while others have it as a conception remembered after hearing from Śrī Krishna. There are others, the least of human beings, who have no perception or any type of conception of this.

यतन्तो योगिनश्चैनं
पश्यन्त्यात्मन्यवस्थितम् ।
यतन्तोऽप्यकृतात्मानो
नैनं पश्यन्त्यचेतसः ॥ १५.११ ॥
yatanto yoginaścainaṁ
paśyantyātmanyavasthitam
yatanto'pyakṛtātmāno
nainaṁ paśyantyacetasaḥ (15.11)

yatanto = yatantaḥ — endeavoring; yoginaścainaṁ = yoginaḥ — yogis + ca — and + enam — this (spirit); paśyānti — they see; ātmani — in the self; avasthitam — situated; yatanto = yatantaḥ — exertion; 'pi = api — even; akṛtātmāno = akṛtātmānaḥ = akṛta — not in order, imperfect + ātmānaḥ — self; nainaṁ = na — not + enam — this (spirit); paśyanti — they see; acetasaḥ — thoughtless ones

The endeavoring yogis see the spirit as being situated in itself; but even with exertion, the imperfected souls, the thoughtless ones, do not perceive it. (15.11)

Commentary:

There are the endeavoring yogis who are or are not devotees of Śrī Krishna. By striving hard in yoga practice, they begin to open the doors of mystic perception, through which they begin to perceive the operation of the subtle body. It is the subtle body which the ordinary man uses in dreams, thoughts, imaginations and plannings of all sorts. It sponsors the transmigrations from one form to another. By studying the operations of this form, the endeavoring yogi sees that the spirit is situated in itself mostly and is unreliant on any lower reality for its survival.

This is why some of these yogis do not see God as necessary. Perceiving that a spirit is eternal regardless of its relationship to anything or to anyone else, some yogis have a tendency not to believe in any God or gods. They form the conclusion that God is not necessary and that there is no singular Supreme Spirit. In actuality, however, the eternality of a spirit, as well as its eternal relationship to other personal and impersonal realities is a fact. The spirit is simultaneously eternal and is reliant on other realities all dependent on where it has objective or subjective display of consciousness. The limited spirit is not a reality unto itself but it is eternal nevertheless. Its survival is unquestioned by virtue of its key position in the existence. This position of it, however, does not guarantee for it, eternal objectiveness. It has eternity but it does not have autonomy or perpetual license for objectiveness.

The Supreme Being with His array of divine personages who are absolute and semi—absolute, are the ones with that license in varying degrees. Thus they are regarded as being the greatest of the personalities (puruṣottama) and as being the most ancient of the existences. They are the most objective. They are the most wise and knowledgeable. It is this array of divine personages who are called Krishna, Vishnu, Shiva and so on in the Vedic literature.

The layout of the personal existences is such that each person is yoked or joined to a specific personality in an Axis Supreme, with Śrī Krishna as the Center. This was shown by Arjuna when he saw the Universal Form. That Form showed the application of that Personality Axis to this material creation, particularly to Its concern with what took place in Arjuna's time. However the Axis of Personalities or the Universal Form applies to all situations in all time and at all places, in different functioning ways. It consists of all the personalities who exist everywhere, both embodied and disembodied.

The thoughtless souls are in the category of being either devotees of Krishna or persons who are not His admirers. For one reason or the other, they are not in the mystic perception of the spirit or its subtle body. They may or may not believe in the subtle body, but they do not understand its operations. As such they reduce this life into being a material effort only.

They are described as being imperfect in actions (akṛt), because their activities are regulated by their materialistic perception. Some of these souls believe in reincarnation and in Śrī Krishna too, but since they have no mystic perception, their materialistic demeanor overrules all that they do.

यदादित्यगतं तेजो
जगद्भासयतेऽखिलम् ।
यच्चन्द्रमसि यच्चाग्नौ
तत्तेजो विद्धि मामकम् ॥ १५.१२ ॥
yadādityagataṁ tejo
jagadbhāsayate'khilam
yaccandramasi yaccāgnau
tattejo viddhi māmakam (15.12)

yat — which; ādityagatam — sun-yielding; tejo = tejaḥ — splendor; jagat — universe; bhāsayate — illuminates; 'khilam = akhilam — completely; yat — which; candramasi — in the moon; yat — which; cāgnau = ca — and + āgnau — in fire; tat — that; tejo = tejaḥ — splendor; viddhi — knows; māmakam — mine

That sun—yielding splendor which illuminates the universe completely, which is in the moon and which is in fire; know that splendor to be Mine. (15.12)

Commentary:

We know today that the sun—yielding splendor emanates from atomic and nuclear energy, which is converted into gross heat through a series of changes in subtle matter. Śrī Krishna presents Himself as being the source of that energy. Such energy is researched by yogis using the intellect organ of the subtle body and by using prāṇa vision and other types of mystic perception. Prāṇa vision is sight through pranic energy without having to take recourse to an optic view.

These claims of Śrī Krishna have validity, except that each yogi should get evidence in the form of direct perception. That is the difference between being just a devotee and being a yogi devotee. The yogi devotee applies for a direct view. A yogi is not fanatical in the belief of Śrī Krishna. He is gentle with the information and open—minded. He waits for the time when he can see this directly.

गामाविश्य च भूतानि
धारयाम्यहमोजसा ।
पुष्णामि चौषधीः सर्वाः
सोमो भूत्वा रसात्मकः ॥ १५.१३ ॥
gāmāviśya ca bhūtāni
dhārayāmyahamojasā
puṣṇāmi cauṣadhīḥ sarvāḥ
somo bhūtvā rasātmakaḥ (15.13)

gām — the earth; āviśya — penetrating; ca — and; bhūtāni — beings; dhārayāmi — I support; aham — I; ojasā — with potency; puṣṇāmi — I cause to thrive; cauṣadhīḥ = ca — and + auṣadhīḥ — plants; sarvāḥ — all; somo = somaḥ — moon; bhūtvā — having influenced; rasātmakaḥ — sap-producing

And penetrating the earth, I support all beings with potency. And having influenced the sap—producing moon, I cause all plants to thrive. (15.13)

Commentary:

This potency of the earth is experienced commonly as the nourishment which comes into human bodies from food produce. When it enters the human form, it either kills, sustains or stuns it, all depending on the preferences of the body. If it nourishes the form, it forms hormones. These hormones are usually slanted in a sexual direction, and they cause a craving for sexual intercourse. By such intercourse infant forms are produced.

There is something supernatural in all this. Śrī Krishna claims the supernatural potency which penetrates the earth and influences the formation of living bodies. The sap—producing moon, as well as the radiant sun, influences all earthly life forms. When doing Kuṇḍalinī yoga, a yogi notices the influences of the sun and the moon by their effects on the right and left side of his subtle body. When the sun's energy is stronger, the right nostril remains open during prāṇāyāma exercise, but if the moon is predominant, the left side remains open. When in balance, both nostrils remain cleared.

By careful observation, the yogis understand how these influences bear upon every creature from day to day. Some of these influences are nullified by prāṇāyāma practices.

अहं वैश्वानरो भूत्वा
प्राणिनां देहमाश्रितः ।
प्राणापानसमायुक्तः
पचाम्यन्नं चतुर्विधम् ॥ १५.१४॥
ahaṁ vaiśvānaro bhūtvā
prāṇināṁ dehamāśritaḥ
prāṇāpānasamāyuktaḥ
pacāmyannaṁ caturvidham (15.14)

aham—I; vaiśvānaro = vaiśvānaraḥ — Vaiśvānara, a supernatural being, digestive heat; bhūtvā — becoming; prāṇināṁ — of the breathing beings; deham — body; āśritaḥ — entering; prāṇāpānasamāyuktaḥ = prāṇāpāna — inhaled and exhaled breath + samāyuktaḥ — combining; pacāmi — digest; annam — food; caturvidham — four kinds

Becoming the Vaiśvānara digestive heat, I, entering the body of all breathing beings and combining with the inhaled and exhaled breath, digest the four kinds of foodstuffs. (15.14)

Commentary:

In the Vedic literature, Vaishvanara is described as both a supernatural being and the digestive heat in mammalian bodies. When that heat combines with the inhaling and exhaling airs, it is known as the bhasvara heat. This is experienced in Kuṇḍalinī yoga. For that matter this energy is collectively known as the life force in a living body. In Kuṇḍalinī yoga, a yogi first tries to refine and purify this energy. Then at last, he seeks to eliminate it altogether. Kuṇḍalinī yoga is one of the elementary stages of kriyā yoga practice but for beginners it seems to be the full course. Haṭha yoga, which concerns the various postures for stretching and relaxing muscles and organs in the body, causes the refinement of the digestive organs in the body. Thus a yogi learns how he can eat less and less and still live in the body. In the advanced stages however, he foregoes the eating process and learns to live without physical foods. This happens when at first, he masters dhāraṇa focusing after he perfects Kuṇḍalinī yoga. At that time, the eating urges are controlled.

सर्वस्य चाहं हृदि संनिविष्टो
मत्तः स्मृतिर्ज्ञानमपोहनं च ।
वेदैश्च सर्वैरहमेव वेद्यो
वेदान्तकृद्वेदविदेव चाहम् ॥ १५.१५॥
sarvasya cāhaṁ hṛdi saṁniviṣṭo
mattaḥ smṛtirjñānam apohanaṁ ca
vedaiśca sarvairahameva vedyo
vedāntakṛdvedavideva cāham (15.15)

sarvasya — of all; cāhaṁ = ca — and + aham — I; hṛdi — in the central, psyche; saṁniviṣṭo = saṁniviṣṭaḥ — entered; mattaḥ — from me; smṛtiḥ — memory; jñānam — knowledge; apohanaṁ — reasoning; ca — and; vedaiśca = vedaiḥ — by the Vedas + ca — and; sarvaiḥ — by all; aham — I; eva — indeed; vedyo = vedyaḥ — to be known; vedāntakṛt = vedānta — Vedānta + kṛt — maker, author; vedavit — knower of the Vedas; eva — indeed; cāham = ca — and + aham — I

And I entered the central psyche of all beings. From Me comes memory, knowledge and reasoning. By all the *Vedas,* I am to be known. I am the author of *Vedānta* and the knower of the *Vedas.* (15.15)

Commentary:

The operation of memory, knowledge and reasoning are the functions of the buddhi organ and the causal body but modern psychologists related these functions to the conscious and subconscious mind. Because they lack mystic clarity and cannot perceive the intellect as a subtle organ, they rely on a vague feeling of viewing one mind with two compartments; one being conscious and the other subconscious. However this is insufficient knowledge for the purposes of kriyā yoga.

In the practice of kriyā, at the advanced stages one sees the organs of the subtle body just as a physician sees the physical organs during surgery. The mystic perception however, does not develop except through yoga practice. This is what yoga practice yields. This is its specialty.

Śrī Krishna's claim as the source of memory, knowledge and reasoning cannot be substantiated unless we can trace these psychological attributes. However in the meantime, we can know for sure that the limited spirit is not in charge of these. At any moment he may lose memory; he may lose knowledge; or he may lose his analytical ability. There are many cases of intelligent human beings who suddenly lose their minds altogether. Thus a limited spirit has no absolute control over these aspects, which are so vital to his status and well—being.

As Śrī Krishna claimed to be the original teacher of the karma yoga system, He also claimed to be the original author of *Vedānta* and the actual knower of Veda. He claimed that by the *Vedas* He is to be known.

द्वाविमौ पुरुषौ लोके
क्षरश्चाक्षर एव च ।
क्षरः सर्वाणि भूतानि
कूटस्थोऽक्षर उच्यते ॥ १५.१६ ॥
dvāvimau puruṣau loke
kṣaraścākṣara eva ca
kṣaraḥ sarvāṇi bhūtāni
kūṭastho'kṣara ucyate (15.16)

dvau — two; imau — these two; puruṣau — two spirits; loke — in the world; kṣaraścākṣara = kṣaraḥ — affected + ca — and + akṣara — unaffected; eva — indeed; ca — and; kṣaraḥ — affected; sarvāṇi — all; bhūtāni — mundane creatures; kūṭastho = kūṭasthaḥ — stable soul; 'kṣara = akṣara — unaffected; ucyate — is said to be

These two types of spirits are in this world, namely the affected ones and the unaffected ones. All mundane creatures are affected. The stable soul is said to be unaffected. (15.16)

Commentary:

Sanskrit terminology lists these two types of spirits as being those who are eternally—liberated and those who are eternally bound, all depending on the resistance of each group to material nature's influences. It is believed that those who emerged from Goddess Durga are mostly bound. Those who emerged from Shiva and from Lord Vishnu are mostly in the habit of exhibiting the qualities of liberation. However the demarcation between the two groups is not as distinct as it seems. Some of those who are supposed to be eternally liberated, appear to be bound. At other times those who are supposed to be eternally bound, appear to be liberated.

There is however a definite way of finding out whether a spirit is kṣara or akṣara, affected or unaffected, by knowing the category of the spirit. Those who are in a higher category, who are capable of displaying resistance to material nature, are the ones who are eternally liberated. No matter what they do, they cannot be held down for a very long time.

Conversely those who are prone to material nature's influence can only exhibit liberated qualities when they are buoyed up by the influence of a powerful divine personality and only for as long as he can boost them. Despite talk by spiritual masters about their respective Lords saving followers, generally the Divinities do not hold up the lowly entities. The reason is this: By their very nature, such entities cannot remain in the divine association alone. Their psyche cries out for fulfillments in lower psychological locales.

उत्तमः पुरुषस्त्वन्यः
परमात्मेत्युदाहृतः ।
यो लोकत्रयमाविश्य
बिभर्त्यव्यय ईश्वरः ॥१५.१७॥
uttamaḥ puruṣastvanyaḥ
paramātmetyudāhṛtaḥ
yo lokatrayamāviśya
bibhartyavyaya īśvaraḥ (15.17)

uttamaḥ — higher; puruṣaḥ — spirit; tu — but; anyaḥ — another; paramātmeti = paramātmā — Supreme Spirit + iti — thus; udāhṛtaḥ — is called; yo = yaḥ — who; lokatrayam — three worlds; āviśya — entering; bibharti — supports; avyaya — eternal; īśvaraḥ — Lord

But the highest spirit is in another category. He is called the Supreme Spirit, Who having entered the three worlds as the eternal Lord, supports it. (15.17)

Commentary:

Part of the kriyā yoga course involves knowing exactly what category one fits into, as well as what one's factual relationship is to the others. A person does not set out in kriyā yoga to find out that he is God or to find out that he might be this or might be that. Rather, he researches mystically for the truth.

Śrī Krishna has diagonally-opposed those philosophers, yogis and mystics who deny that there is a Supreme Being Who was the first to enter into these worlds. Krishna called that person the highest spirit who entered the material creation, supports it and functions here or there as the eternal Lord of this mundane place.

यस्मात्क्षरमतीतोऽहम्
अक्षरादपि चोत्तमः ।
अतोऽस्मि लोके वेदे च
प्रथितः पुरुषोत्तमः ॥१५.१८॥
yasmātkṣaramatīto'ham
akṣarādapi cottamaḥ
ato'smi loke vede ca
prathitaḥ puruṣottamaḥ (15.18)

yasmāt — since; kṣaram — effected; atīto — atītaḥ — beyond; 'ham — aham — I; akṣarāt — than the unaffected spirits; api — even; cottamaḥ = ca — and + uttamaḥ — higher; ato — ataḥ — hence; 'smi = asmi — I am; loke — in the world; vede — in the Veda; ca — and; prathitaḥ — known as; puruṣottamaḥ — Supreme Person

Since I am beyond the affected spirits and I am even higher than the unaffected ones, I am known in the world and in the *Vedas* as the Supreme Person. (15.18)

Commentary:

Actually in the *Vedas*, namely the Ṛg, Sāma, *Yajur* and Atharva *Vedas*, the declarations about the Supreme Person are written so that Śrī Krishna, the son of Devakī is not directly listed as the Supreme Lord. However the definition of that God as given in the *Gītā*, matches what was extolled in the *Vedas*.

Some teachers in disciplic succession say that this statement proves that the *Vedas* list Śrī Krishna as the Supreme Lord. They use this as support from antiquity, to prove Śrī Krishna's claims of divinity. Such a declaration is either due to ignorance of the *Vedas* or a deliberate effort to deny that the *Vedas* do not clearly explain the Supreme Being as Śrī Krishna. In fact the name of the Supreme Being in the *Vedas* as a whole is not at all clear, except as that person who is the Paramātma and Parambrahma.

What took place here in the *Gītā* is this: Śrī Krishna interjected Himself into these historic circumstances from the past, beginning with His declaration of having taught the Sun God which was mentioned in Chapter Four. We have to accept the *Gītā* in that way on a take—it or leave—it, believe it or reject it, wait—for—the—proof basis. It will do us no good to try to scrape through the *Vedas* to find Śrī Krishna there or to find some fact which substantiates what He said. Arjuna was aware of the histories, even more so than we, and he contested Krishna's claim about teaching Vivaswan, the Sun God.

Arjuna's misgivings were removed after he saw the Universal Form and saw what took place supernaturally. Understanding then that Śrī Krishna was really behind the scenes, even behind the most miniscule actions in the material world, Arjuna testified to Śrī Krishna's sovereignty. Our position is not exactly the same. We do not have the revelation. Until we acquire it, we have to either accept, reject or maintain an open mind about Śrī Krishna's declarations.

In kriyā yoga, the identity of that Supreme Being is irrelevant. What does it matter if it is Śrī Krishna or somebody else? The main concern of a kriyā yogi is to exist in harmony with that Supreme Being, Whoever He may be. The kriyā yogi is not a religious fanatic or an insecure person who must attribute his favorite deity as the Supreme. The kriyā yogi is dedicated to purifying his psychology no matter who that Supreme Person might be. It is irrelevant really whether that person is Śrī Krishna or some other. Ultimately we will have to get the waiver from that Person by following His stipulations. He will not allow us to avoid the obligations which He imposes, merely because we are fanatic about His sovereignty. Śrī Krishna, for example, was the good friend of Arjuna. He regarded Arjuna as His very dear devotee. Still, He did not give in to Arjuna's idea about avoiding unpalatable duty.

The avisya or entering into these mundane worlds is a subject of much controversy among yogis, mystics and religionists. The argument was there for some time. The religionists are usually arguing on the basis of what they read in scriptures. Some of these consider the *Vedas* to be infallible. Others regard the *Vedas* as being absolute but they use the *Vedas* as a reference and honor it as being the first authoritative scripture in the world. These religionists are usually offbeat because they have very little mystic perception. Being myopic in the mystic sense, they make up for their lack of perception by leaning heavily on the scriptures. Thus they argue about God's entry into the material world in a dogmatic way. Because these preachers stress dharma or responsible social life, they get the support of the females. By that contribution, they usually amass a large congregation, because after all, the females are the center of mundane social life, the focal point of the generation of infant bodies.

The mystics who do no yoga also formulate ideas about how God entered this world. Their ideas are vague, based on their haphazard and shifting perception. Sometimes they read the existence accurately. Sometimes they do not. They have no set way of curbing and improving their mystic perception. As a class of visionaries, they are unreliable. These people also hold a sizeable following because they have sufficient time to hold seminars and be available for consultation, especially to superstitious people who are interested in astrology, predictions and visions.

The yogis have a more accurate mystic perception. This is because of disciplines like Kuṇḍalinī and celibacy yoga, techniques through which their psychology becomes more and more clarified, leading to clear perception. Śrīla Yogeshwarananda used to stress the development of the ṛtambhāra buddhi, which is the truth (ṛta) — bearing (bhāra) intellect (buddhi). He said that this allows one who possesses clarity to see what is behind the mundane manifestation.

All the same the yogis do have their arguments about who entered, as to whether it is this or that person or influence. Śrī Krishna sounded certain in His declarations. It is up to each yogi to research those claims.

The Supreme Person is known, or rather is surmised, but not necessarily as Śrī Krishna. All through the centuries, human beings have surmised an ultimate person who is the source of all others but there is no unanimous agreement as to who that person is. Even today, there is disagreement among various philosophers, religious leaders and the like as to that identity.

The word Veda in this verse means more than the four *Vedas*. It means any scriptures and acclamations about that Supreme Person; but specifically in India in the time of Śrī Krishna, the *Vedas* were stressed. Today in India, preachers pay lip service to the *Vedas*. Most of them do not use the *Vedas* as their reference scriptures. This *Bhagavad Gītā*, the Rāmāyaṇa, the Bhagavata Purāṇa, the Shiva Purāṇa, Devi Purāṇa and other scriptures, even modern texts like the Śrī Caitanya Caritāmṛta, and the Vachnamrut are used as standard reference books, leaving aside the four *Vedas*. Śrī Krishna acknowledged Himself as the Supreme Person and showed Arjuna the Universal Form; but in other texts like the Devi Purāṇa, for instance, Ma Durga is acknowledged as such when she displayed her Universal Form. In the Shiva Purāṇa, Lord Shiva is presented as such.

The point remains that there is a Supreme Person, a Central Divinity from Whom all others derive existential security. To accept the *Gītā* means to accept Śrī Krishna as that Personality.

The Supreme Person whosoever He may be, must be beyond the affected spirits. He must also be higher than the unaffected ones.

यो मामेवमसंमूढो
जानाति पुरुषोत्तमम् ।
स सर्वविद्भजति मां
सर्वभावेन भारत ॥१५.१९॥
yo māmevamasaṁmūḍho
jānāti puruṣottamam
sa sarvavidbhajati māṁ
sarvabhāvena bhārata (15.19)

yo — yaḥ — who; mām — me; evam — in this way; asaṁmūḍho = asaṁmūḍhaḥ — undeluded; jānāti — knows; puruṣottamam — Supreme Person; sa — he; sarvavit — all — knowing, knowledgeable; bhajati — worships; mām — me; sarvabhāvena — with all being; bhārata — O man of the Bharata family

In this way, he who is undeluded, who knows Me as the Supreme Person, he being knowledgeable, worships Me with all his being, O man of the Bharata family. (15.19)

Commentary:

Some commentators who are not yogis but who have large followings, explain this verse as follows: They say that once a person enters the disciplic succession from Śrī Krishna, accepting a leader of the succession as a spiritual master and pure devotee of the Lord, then that disciple becomes undeluded, merely by that acceptance. They say that such disciples get the knowledge of Śrī Krishna by hearing from them, since they are the right source. Citing the analogy of the milk which spoiled after being licked by a serpent, they say that unless one hears from them, an audience with others is like taking milk licked by a snake. Fresh milk is wholesome but as soon as a reptile licks, the acidic saliva spoils it, such that anyone who drinks after the reptile is poisoned.

The idea is that one must hear from someone who is faithful to a certain spiritual master in the disciplic succession; otherwise if one hears from any other person even if he is in the succession, one will get misinformation and will not attain Śrī Krishna, due to the lack of proper connection in the parampara succession of teachers.

Such a proposal sounds good but it will not do in kriyā yoga. We are interested in techniques for psyche purification. Our interest in gurus is restricted to that only. We do not care what disciplic succession a person is in, or who he heard or did not hear from. If he has a valid technique, he is our teacher automatically. Furthermore a teacher who is not a yogi or a yogi devotee, cannot be of much assistance, because he does not practice the purificatory disciplines. He might be in the disciplic succession, he might have a good rhetoric, but nevertheless since he does not know the techniques, he cannot share them. At the same time, we do not begrudge him.

Even though many religious teachers hijack this verse and use it to give guarantees to their followings, still this verse pertains to yogi devotees only. A yogi devotee who is undeluded and who knows Śrī Krishna by direct mystic experience in advanced yoga practice, does worship Śrī Krishna with a purified psyche.

इति गुह्यतमं शास्त्रम्
इदमुक्तं मयानघ ।
एतद्बुद्ध्वा बुद्धिमान्स्यात्
कृतकृत्यश्च भारत ॥ १५.२० ॥
iti guhyatamaṁ śāstram
idamuktaṁ mayānagha
etadbuddhvā buddhimānsyāt
kṛtakṛtyaśca bhārata (15.20)

iti — thus; guhyatamaṁ — most secret; śāstram— teaching; idam — this; uktaṁ— is declared; mayā— by me; 'nagha= anagha — O blameless man; etat — this; buddhvā — having realized; buddhimān —wise; syāt — he should become; kṛtakṛtyaśca = kṛtakṛtyaḥ — with duties accomplished + ca — and; bhārata — O descendant of Bharata

Thus the most secret teaching is declared by Me, O blameless man. Having realized this, O descendant of the Bharatas, one becomes a wise person, whose duties are accomplished. (15.20)

Commentary:

At last Śrī Krishna told Arjuna how and when a yogi devotee would get the waiver from cultural activity. This was the thing that Arjuna wanted but could not get from Śrī Krishna just before the *Gītā* was spoken. At that time, Śrī Krishna was willing to give Arjuna two courses, either karma yoga practice or no association at all. That was the choice, as indicated by the vision of the Universal Form which scared Arjuna. It was as if Śrī Krishna had said, "Either you do what I suggest or you are on your own against Me."

When will our duties be accomplished to Śrī Krishna's satisfaction? That is the ultimate question.

CHAPTER 16

Two Types of Created Beings*

श्रीभगवानुवाच
अभयं सत्त्वसंशुद्धिर्
ज्ञानयोगव्यवस्थितिः ।
दानं दमश्च यज्ञश्च
स्वाध्यायस्तप आर्जवम् ॥१६.१॥
śrībhagavānuvāca
abhayaṁ sattvasaṁśuddhir
jñānayogavyavasthitiḥ
dānaṁ damaśca yajñaśca
svādhyāyastapa ārjavam (16.1)

śrī bhagavān — The Blessed Lord; uvāca — said; abhayaṁ — fearlessness; sattvasaṁśuddhiḥ = sattva — existence, being + saṁśuddhiḥ — purity; jñānayogavyavasthitiḥ = jñāna — mental concept + yoga — application of yoga + vyavasthitiḥ — consistence; dānaṁ — charity; damaśca — damaḥ — self-restraint + ca — and; yajñaśca — yajñaḥ — worship ceremony + ca — and; svādhyāyaḥ — recitation of scripture; tapa — austerity; ārjavam — straight-forwardness

The Blessed Lord said: Fearlessness, purity of being, consistency in application of yoga to mental concepts, charity, self-restraint, worship ceremony, recitation of scripture, austerity and straight-forwardness, (16.1)

Commentary:

These are some of the qualities which come from the godly nature. These comprise the psychology of godly people in a much greater proportion than in vindictive and criminally—minded humans. We should not make the mistake of thinking that since we are godly or good, we do not have wicked tendencies. The subtle body is such that in one life it might exhibit what is good and in the next, one might be evil. Such is the flexibility of that form. A person who is mostly good, misbehaves on occasion. One who is mostly evil, is good periodically. There is also the factor of good acts which appear to be evil, as well as bad ones which appear to be good. The *Bhagavad Gītā* shows that what Arjuna considered to be evil, was actually good; while his adoption of a pacifist stance was irresponsible.

Since one who is mostly good might do what is truly bad on occasion, some human beings ridicule good leaders as being capable of errors and not worthy of respect and honor. One who leads a family, village, a city or country, usually becomes the laughing stock of persons who are critical of human nature and who feel that everyone is in error, and that no one should be honored.

**The Mahābhārata contains no chapter headings. This title was assigned by the translator on the basis of verse 6 of this chapter.*

For example, Arjuna was imperfect initially and could not see what to do. He was childish and cowardly but still he was appointed by the Universal Form to represent divine objection to reckless human acts. This means that we should respect Arjuna as a leader, no matter what. To point at his frailties and to neglect him, would be a serious mistake. Despite his weakness, Arjuna was, for all practical purposes, the face of the Universal Form which confronted the warriors and dispensed what was due to them as divine approval or disapproval.

Śrī Krishna by listing off the godly qualities gave us something definite. We do not have to figure it out for ourselves or argue among ourselves as to what is godly and what is ungodly. God Himself, Śrī Krishna, gave the definitions directly.

Fearlessness: There are various types of fearlessness. Some of these border on stupidity. This fearlessness of the godly nature applies when doing what is stipulated by the Universal Form. Anyone, a good person or a predominantly bad one, who acts at any time as moved by the Universal Form, is fearless in the proper way. This is because whatever that Form dictates is the final say.

Purity of Being: Purity of being comes through advanced yoga practice. One gets this after mastering Kuṇḍalinī yoga. This is because in its primitive state, the Kuṇḍalinī force yearns for survival, which causes the psychology to be dirty. When that is cleansed, the survival anxieties leave a yogi. After the Kuṇḍalinī chakra is refined, one develops a mystic envelope body, a higher more purified energy. It is easy to recognize a yogi who attained that purity of being (sattvasamśuddhir). He gets the waiver from the Supreme Being so that he does not have to do karma yoga. He can and does dedicate himself to full time yoga practice. He does not crave or have many disciples. He does not become a big time missionary. He steps aside from the scope of material existence altogether.

A great yogi in India by the name of Neem Karoli Baba was one such being. One can also include Swami Nityananda, the spiritual master of the renowned siddha Swami Muktananda. These persons used such a purified subtle body.

After mastering Kuṇḍalinī yoga and celibacy yoga, one practices purity yoga. When that is mastered, one reaches the stage of purity of being.

Application of Yoga to Mental Concepts: Jñāna yoga or the application of yoga to mental concepts is not the same as mental or philosophical concepts all by themselves. With yoga, one can test the concepts to see whether they are right or wrong, realistic or unrealistic, applicable in this or that dimension or not applicable in any other. Without yoga, one cannot perform such tests.

Jñāna yoga is not speculation as some modem commentators suggest. Speculation is jñāna without yoga. When we add yoga to jñāna, we get something definite in the form of mystic perception. Jñāna is like having a map or blue-print and walking on the streets which are represented on the map or entering the building depicted on the blue-print. After that experience, then he knows for sure if the map or blue-print is accurately depicted.

For consistency in the application of yoga to mental concepts, the yogi should have an ongoing mystic development. This starts with Kuṇḍalinī yoga. It is fine-tuned when he masters celibacy and purity yoga. Gradually he develops keener and keener mystic perception until he reaches a stage where the speckled darkness, seen in the head behind closed eyelids, clears and the sky of consciousness opens up to supernatural vision.

Charity: Charity usually means a human action involving kindness to the needy. When we take the Universal Form into account, charity has another meaning to give to those in need, according to the command of the Universal Form. In that case, the human serves as an agent for the divine. Any charitable acts are merely echoes or after-shocks of a supernatural action of the Universal Form, just as Arjuna's battle performance mimicked events on the supernatural level.

In elementary religion, the human being thrives on charity, as a kindness to the needy, but in higher yoga, that method is abandoned. One acts as an agent of the Universal Form, doing charitable acts on His behalf. Such acts do not bear positive consequences for the yogi but carry a neutral charge. As such he is not required to take another body to reap compensations and rewards.

Self—restraint: Self—restraint is a godly quality because if we allow all natural tendencies to guide us indiscriminately, we will commit much evil in the course of time. The natural tendencies are not particularly discriminant of what is good and what is bad. Many tendencies are anti-social in application. Thus even in the elementary religions, there is stress on self-restraint, especially for the sake of morality and peaceful coexistence. In kriyā yoga, self-restraint involves more than moral values and related social behaviors. We are interested in self purification for a cleared-up psychology. Thus we apply much more restraint than the average religionist or believer.

Worship ceremony: According to the *Gītā in Chapter Three*, worship ceremony entails Brahmā's instructions to the first human beings whom he commanded to worship the supernatural rulers. In addition, Śrī Krishna suggested that He be worshiped. As we saw, most of these requests were made in respect to practicing yogi—devotees of Śrī Krishna.

We may use our own definition of worship according to preferences but still the actual meaning is tied to this:

sahayajñāḥ prajāḥ sṛṣṭvā purovāca prajāpatiḥ
anena prasaviṣyadhvam eṣa vo'stviṣṭakāmadhuk (3.10)
devānbhāvayatānena te devā bhāvayantu vaḥ
parasparaṁ bhāvayantaḥ śreyaḥ paramavāpsyatha (3.11)
iṣṭānbhogānhi vo devā dāsyante yajñabhāvitāḥ
tairdattānapradāyaibhyo yo bhuṅkte stena eva saḥ (3.12)

Long ago, having created the first human beings, along with religious fulfillment and ceremonies, the Procreator Brahmā said: By this worship procedure, you may be productive. May it cause the fulfillment of your desires. (3.10)

By this procedure, you may cause the supernatural rulers to flourish. They, in turn, may bless you. In favorably regarding each other, the highest well—being will be achieved. (3.11)

The supernatural rulers, being manifested through prescribed austerity and religious ceremony, will, indeed, give you the most desired people and things. Whosoever does not offer those given items to them, but who enjoys these, is certainly a thief. (3.12)

The act of worship implies the presence of higher personalities somewhere. The Deities may not be physical but they exist in the supernatural world. This recognition induces worship. Śrī Krishna prefers the type of worship which Brahmā introduced to his sons.

Recitation of scriptures: Recitation of scriptures was more relevant in the time of Śrī Krishna than it is now. Nowadays the academic education, the religious training, the disciplinary life for youths and the behavioral values are usually not taught together at one school or in one home. Nowadays the academic training is separated from religious orientation and indoctrination. In the time of Śrī Krishna, it was all put together.

Recently there were many attempts to reintroduce the old system. Such efforts have met with great opposition and sure failure in a losing battle against Western Civilization, with its liberal, commercial and technological ways. Swami Bhaktivedanta Prabhupāda, for example, tried to establish boarding schools which he called gurukulas but some students were victimized by homosexual and otherwise deviant acts of some disciples who were posted as teachers.

In some of his schools, the academic part of the training received lower priority than the religious part. Subsequently some students became resentful when they reached adult age and discovered that they were ill-equipped to fit into Western society, especially since the Swami and his senior men were all well educated in academic subjects in their youthful years.

Somehow or the other the Swami transmitted the idea that if the religious training was given top priority, the students would have everything by the grace of Śrī Krishna, but actually that grace manifested in an undesireable way. There were a few examples of success cited by the Swami and his core of leading disciples but generally it did not occur. The whole way of the world changed, even in India. Time did not bend to the will of the Swami.

Recitation of scripture closely relates to the language structure of Sanskrit, Hindi and their allied languages which has the conjunction of verbs and declension of nouns like that of Greek and other ancient languages. It includes a difficult grammar of an ancient language which cannot be learned unless one has a high aptitude or IQ.

Today with the profusion of books and the commonality of reading, it is more important to understand what a scripture states than it is to recite the words and commit them to memory. Still, is a superstition remains that formerly people learned verses from scripture for the purpose of quoting these, as many missionaries do today. The truth is that such learning was more for printing such information on the mind than for the sake of learning. Nowadays, we are freed from having to memorize scriptures. We can replace that habit with one of learning the meaning.

Regardless, many spiritual masters continue the oral system just as if the printed press was not invented, and just as if we were still dependent on keeping information printed in our minds. Many people are habituated to recitation of scripture cannot understand what I said above. This is caused by stubborn tendencies in their subtle bodies, traits which they have difficulty overcoming, because the subtle forms are stuck firmly to things of the past which are out of sequence with the flow of time.

For this recitation of scripture as Śrī Krishna states, we now have to learn the meanings of the words in the scripture. We have to become educated academically because now the academic part is separated. Priests and gurus no longer hold the monopoly over all types of education as they did before. Formerly even a priestly person like Paraśurāma was a military expert. So was Droṇāchārya, one of the instructors of the Kauravas. Nowadays a priest usually has no military expertise. Times changed. For the full recitation of scripture now, we should learn the meanings of the terms in the scripture. We should also acquire a proper education.

When Śrī Krishna's wife, Jāmbhavatī wanted a baby, she appealed to Śrī Krishna to petition Lord Shiva. Śrī Krishna, even though he was married, attended the school of the mahāyogī Upamanyu. Krishna became the yogin's student for the purpose of getting yoga techniques for entering the dimension where Lord Shiva lived with His wife, the goddess

Umā. Today if someone wants a baby, he can see a doctor if he wants advice for begetting children. Most of these procedures changed. It will do us no good to hang on to ancient methods which are irrelevant today, especially if we are simultaneously attracted to the advantages of modern society.

Austerity: Austerity is related to self restraint. In the yoga system one acquires more and more self restraint, as one applies more and more austerity on oneself. However, it is not haphazard. It must be done step by step in the various stages. Austerity gives one the ability to successfully restrain from lower habits. It causes the subtle body to change in such a way as to be freed from lower qualities.

If one does not perform the correct austerity for a sustained period of time, one's attempt at self restraint will fail. Self restraint without austerity causes one to return to old habits repeatedly. This is because by self restraint alone, bad habits only go into dormancy.

Straight-forwardness: Straightforwardness, though one of the godly qualities, is not a very practical quality in the social world. This is because various types of diplomacy, hypocritical courtesies and the like are required for success in that situation. Good people have this feeling that they should be straightforward and that one should not indulge in duplicity, but when such good people are involved in business or in anything that requires manipulation, they quickly excuse themselves from their self—made rule of absolute honesty. They engage in courteous or discourteous dishonesty. Much of this is indeliberate. It is inspired and urged on by inner energies of defense which overtake the conscious deliberate status—seeing mind of the human being.

In kriyā yoga we are subjected to the same type of force which causes a person to abandon straightforwardness. We gradually curb that force by psychological austerities and by adoption of a simple lifestyle. Ultimately a yogi is forced into isolation for the sake of adopting full—time straightforwardness. He can do this when he is freed from the need for the advantages of civilized living. Civilized living with its conveniences, which are supplied and maintained by entities who have engineering skill, is actually forwarded into human civilizations from the supernatural level. Still such life deters yoga practice. Hence a yogi should abandon it and go for a simple lifestyle just as the ancient ascetics did.

So long as we are involved in complexities of living, our bid for a simple lifestyle will be thwarted. So long as we associate with people who appreciate the conveniences of an advanced human civilization with all its accoutrements, we will be forced into diplomacy and methods of conniving just to compete and survive. These aspects discourage straightforwardness which is necessary for progression in advanced yoga practice. We should decide whether to pamper around with yoga or to complete it.

अहिंसा सत्यमक्रोधस्
त्यागः शान्तिरपैशुनम् ।
दया भूतेष्वलोलुप्त्वं
मार्दवं ह्रीरचापलम् ॥ १६.२ ॥
ahiṁsā satyamakrodhas
tyāgaḥ śāntirapaiśunam
dayā bhūteṣvaloluptvaṁ
mārdavaṁ hrīracāpalam (16.2)

ahiṁsā — non — violence; satyam — recognition of reality; akrodhaḥ — absence of anger; tyāgaḥ — abandonment of consequences; śāntiḥ — spiritual security; apaiśunam — absence of destructive criticism; dayā — compassion; bhūteṣu — in beings; aloluptvam — freedom from craving; mārdavaṁ — gentleness; hrīḥ — modesty; acāpalam —absence of fickleness

...non-violence, recognition of reality, absence of anger, abandonment of consequences, spiritual security, absence of destructive criticism, compassion for the beings, freedom from craving, gentleness, modesty, absence of fickleness, (16.2)

Commentary:

Nonviolence: Social nonviolence which deals with avoidance of all types of hurting actions is not the same as the nonviolence in the *Gītā*. In kriyā yoga, nonviolence is the same as it is in the *Gītā* within the context of Śrī Krishna's asking Arjuna to perform hurting acts for the sake of the dharma or righteous living. Good people, kind—hearted ones, feel that the ends should not justify the means. They criticize Śrī Krishna for inciting Arjuna into warfare. They feel that Śrī Krishna should have supported Arjuna's pacifist stance to avoid the warfare at all costs. However this life is not that simple of an equation. Unless we broaden the meaning of kindness, everything cannot be solved out by kind means.

Since the *Mahābhārata* reports that thousands of soldiers were killed in battle, and since in the end, Duryodhana held his views and did not compromise with Śrī Krishna or with Prince Yudhiṣṭhira, some peace—loving people form the view that the violence urged by Śrī Krishna served no useful purpose whatsoever. This type of logic holds good in limited considerations of life, when regarding people as their material bodies and their emotional psyches. It does not take into account reincarnation or the eternality of the spirit or the supervising role of a Supreme Personality.

When we figure that the subtle body lasts for millions of years, the death of one of its short-lived material forms, for the purpose of curbing the bad habits of that body, serves a useful purpose, especially if the subtle body will be curbed by no other means.

When we figure that the spirit is eternal, the significance of its adoption of temporary forms like the long—lived subtle bodies and the short—lived gross ones, changes completely. There arises the question of the value of the subtle body and its production, the gross form. What is their value in comparison to the spirit? Should a spirit be allowed to totally forget itself for the sake of its subtle body or its gross forms?

When we include a Supervising Supreme Person, then what is His role? What are His rights in the matter? Do His actions have to make sense to us? Should He be made to satisfy our opinion of what is right or wrong? What is the value of a short—lived human body? Is it so valuable that it should never be killed under any circumstance? Should the Supreme Person restrain Himself from disapproving certain human behaviors? Should He not express disapproval in a disciplinary way which might involve killing short—lived human bodies? These are the questions which challenge the stance of the pacifist.

There is a misunderstanding that, in India, all the people were once pacifists. It is only the brahmin caste who are pacifists, not the administrators and others. The administrators, as the histories in the *Puranas* show, were always involved in one type of violence or the other. Arjuna was in the administrative caste. He was the son of a king. His duty was to rule peaceably or by force of arms.

Kind-hearted people have to realize that a completely pacifist stance is not practical in a world where everyone is not very advanced in the evolutionary cycle. In so far as there is a Supreme Being, we have to realize that He will not adopt a pacifist stance, unless we adhere to the supreme will. He will, from time to time, discipline humanity. To Him a short—lifespan body is not worth the value, if it is misused. His definition of such misuse might, of necessity, be variant to ours. Still, He is the Supreme Being and has overall autonomy.

God can engage in such violence, as Śrī Krishna did, or as He urged Arjuna to do, because God does not regard the short—lived human body the way we do. The value we place on it and the endearing emotions we experience through the sensations in it, is not the way God regards it.

If we disconnect from our positions for just a second and if we could see God's, we would understand this, just as Arjuna comprehended it when he viewed the Universal Form's fussing and fuming about the deviant behavior of certain political leaders and their followers.

What about anger? Some feel that if someone is God He should never be angry, since anger is a bad quality. Such a feeling serves no practical purpose if the Supreme Being does get angry from time to time. To rate His anger as a bad quality is to latch on to an excuse for not understanding His perspective. Are we sure that His anger is not another form of His love and concern for human beings? Are we certain that His expression of dislike for certain human attitudes is not His way of saying that we are on the wrong track? These matters require a new view and some deep thinking.

Those ascetics who get the waiver from the Supreme Being, do not have to engage in violent acts as Arjuna was compelled to do. If an ascetic lacks the waiver he will have to be involved, because it is an integrated part of the social scene. We read of the vision of the Universal Form, how it was engaged in combat with opponents, how it burnt and chewed them up supernaturally.

If God is involved in violence on the supernatural level, as Śrī Krishna admitted and as He showed Arjuna, then how can we figure a total nonviolence in terms of not hurting anybody? The whole idea of nonviolence is merely a fantasy. Read this:

śrībhagavānuvāca
kālo'smi lokakṣayakṛt pravṛddho lokānsamāhartumiha pravṛttaḥ
ṛte'pi tvāṁ na bhaviṣyanti sarve ye'vasthitāḥ pratyanīkeṣu yodhāḥ (11.32)
tasmāttvamuttiṣṭha yaśo labhasva jitvā śatrūnbhuṅkṣva rājyaṁ samṛddham
mayaivaite nihatāḥ pūrvameva nimittamātraṁ bhava savyasācin (11.33)
droṇaṁ ca bhīṣmaṁ ca jayadrathaṁ ca karṇaṁ tathānyānapi yodhavīrān
mayā hatāṁstvaṁ jahi mā vyathiṣṭhā yudhyasva jetāsi raṇe sapatnān (11.34)

The Blessed Lord said: I am the time limit, the mighty world—destroying Cause, appearing here to annihilate the worlds. Even without you, all the armored warriors in both armies will cease to live. (11.32)

Therefore you should stand up! Get the glory! Having conquered the enemies, enjoy a prosperous country. These fellows are supernaturally disposed by Me already. Be only the agent, O ambidextrous archer. (11.33)

Droṇa, Bhishma, Jayadratha, and Karṇa, as well as other battle heroes, were supernaturally hurt by Me. You may physically kill them. Do not hesitate. Fight! You will conquer the enemies in battle. (11.34)

Śrī Krishna stated that the soul is eternal. He said that the soul could not be pierced by weapons, burnt by fire, wet by water, or dried by the wind. He also established indirectly that the soul could only be superficially affected by emotional attacks. His statement about supernaturally hurting the warriors pertains to their subtle psychology and not the spirits in fact. In all circumstances, it is not possible to be violent in the spiritual sense of killing the soul. Śrī Krishna stated this. But it is possible to hurt the supernatural compartment which the soul is housed in, even though that cannot be killed altogether so long as the subtle mundane world continues as it is.

For the purpose of kriyā yoga, we step aside from all types of judicial and non—judicial violent acts. If we have the waiver from the Supreme Being, then we step away from it all. If we do not have an exemption we should, upon His request, engage in judicial violence. Śrī Krishna told Arjuna that cultural activity is recommended for a philosophical person who strives for yoga expertise but the tranquil reserved method is for those who have mastery of yoga.

ārurukṣormuneryogaṁ karma kāraṇamucyate
yogārūḍhasya tasyaiva śamaḥ kāraṇamucyate (6.3)

For a philosophical man who strives for yoga expertise, cultural activity is recommended. For one who has mastered yoga already, the tranquil reserved method is the means. (6.3)

Nonviolence in kriyā yoga means to do nothing to deter someone's self realization. A person's self realization does not necessarily come about by kind acts alone. In fact, kindness may sometimes destroy self realization. It is very complicated.

Recognition of Reality: The recognition of reality, *satyam*, is sometimes mistaken for honesty and truthfulness. Many commentators make the mistake of saying that *satyam* is honesty. Honesty is covered in these verses under the quality of straightforwardness. This *satyam* concerns reality as a whole and not personal honesty.

On the social level, honesty is a component of action. For instance if a retarded person commits a crime he might admit honestly, saying, "I did it. Who cares? What does it matter? I did not hurt anyone." He might have killed 50 people by the action but he honestly feels that it was harmless. This is due to insanity. From a deeper view, however, a judge would determine that the retarded fellow was affected by a drug or possessed by a psychotic energy. The idiot's honesty was not factual. In that case he did it under an influence. Honesty is a good quality but it does not necessarily tally with reality. For instance: A man shoots the body of another person whom he does not like. When questioned, he replies, "I shot his body because he aggravated me by harsh words."

In that case such honesty would be shallow, if the real cause was a violent act perpetrated by the victim upon the assailant in a previous life. The reality of it would be that the man was shot because he shot the assailant in a previous life.

In kriyā yoga, we are more concerned with the deeper truths which are the reality of a matter and not so much with honesty which is rationalized on the basis of what occurs in this one life. As we practice, we develop deeper and deeper insight, more and more penetrating vision to see the reality. Arjuna saw the realism behind what was to transpire at Kurukṣetra, when he saw that the Universal Form was up—and—at—it with opponents, hurting them in any way possible. That is *satyam*.

Absence of Anger: The cultivation of absence of anger comes about in the advanced stages of *paravairāgya* extreme detachment from social circumstances. Right now, as directed by Śrīla Yogeshwarananda, I cultivate that disinterest. I mastered it before in many previous lives but in this life, due to taking a body in a non—yogi family, I again assumed the anger. To get rid of it, one has to eliminate the Kuṇḍalinī chakra. So long as the Kuṇḍalinī chakra is active, the potential of anger remains with us.

Generally good people regard anger as a bad force but judicial anger is good. The anger of the Universal Form is very good for human society. It shows God's concern for the world.

As Śrī Krishna stated, He is concerned to save the world from ruination. That is why He gets involved on the social scene, either directly or through an agent:

na me pārthāsti kartavyaṁ triṣu lokeṣu kiṁcana
nānavāptamavāptavyaṁ varta eva ca karmaṇi (3.22)
yadi hyahaṁ na varteyaṁ jātu karmaṇyatandritaḥ
mama vartmānuvartante manuṣyāḥ pārtha sarvaśaḥ (3.23)
utsīdeyurime lokā na kuryāṁ karma cedaham
saṁkarasya ca kartā syām upahanyāmimāḥ prajāḥ (3.24)

For Me, O son of Pṛthā, there is nothing specific that must be done in the three divisions of the universe. And there is nothing that I have not attained or should acquire, and yet I function in cultural activities. (3.22)

If perchance, I did not perform attentively, then all human beings, O son of Pṛthā, would follow Me in all respects. (3.23)

If I should not engage in cultural activity, these worlds would perish. And I would be a producer of social chaos. I would have destroyed these creatures. (3.24)

Generally anger which is derived from frustration is a bad force. In kriyā yoga, in personal practice, it is a good force. By this anger, an ascetic becomes serious about spiritual life, after he is frustrated again and again, trying to be successful in the social world. Sometimes a yogi in a former life takes a new body in ignorance. When he cannot function properly in the social world, he becomes dissatisfied. Somehow he begins to do yoga in an angry mood, feeling that his social life is a waste of time and that bad luck follows him. In that case, anger, which came from his frustrations, brought him back to the yoga practice which he partially mastered in a former life.

Abandonment of consequences: Abandonment of consequences is required. If one lacks an instinct for this, he cannot be a successful yogi. The ability for this indicates a potential for acute detachment. At first a neophyte is concerned with abandonment of bad consequences. When we get higher association we understand that there is a danger in good results also. Favorable responses are the ones we really need to cast aside. In the very advanced stages, when one gets the waiver from the Supreme Being, one is able to abandon all consequences, favorable or unfavorable.

An example from my life may explain this. Sometimes one of my body's children is successful in a particular venture. People inform me of this. They say, "You should be proud that your son has gone to the Academy. I can just imagine how happy you are about that. Your eldest daughter is now on her own in a Drafting Career. I think you are proud of her. Your last daughter is a leading Cadet in another institution and your second daughter followed her brother to the Academy. What a successful parent you are! Express some pride in your great children."

However I do not like anyone who speaks in this way. It is not realistic. These children are their own entities. What I did to assist them, was done with detachment. I do not care about it. I was simply a tool for social forces when I acted as parent. I do not take myself seriously in the matter. In fact I do not want to know what the children of my body are doing. I have no plan to keep track of their activities.

I abandoned the consequences of having raised them. These are both good and bad effects. I ran away from it all. One daughter of this body had many resentments for the disciplinary way in which she was raised. She has always wanted to settle the issue. Soliciting and courting her mother, they harangued me repeatedly about this. For me there is no issue to solve because I have abandoned the consequences, which in this case are negative ones. I am not interested in being the recipient of these. All the same I am also not interested in any good reactions either.

I cited this piece of personal history to show the practical layout of the quality of abandonment of consequences in the life of a yogi.

Spiritual security: Spiritual security is an obvious godly quality that comes when one advances beyond the 7th stage of yoga practice. In the lower stages, up the 6th stage of dhāraṇa, focus of the will through the curbed buddhi organ, one has to be insecure to a certain extent. It cannot be helped. On the lower levels one relies on unstable energies which nudge, pull and push the sensuality.

The disturbing sensuality is the keynote of a jittery psychology, but it cannot be solved out by wishful thinking or by mere faith in God. The methods of wishful thinking or religious confidence serve to make us forget the jittery condition but they do not remove the underlying nervousness.

In the 7th stage of yoga, that of dhyāna contemplation of supernatural and spiritual realities, one moves his buddhi organ from the disturbing lower planes. Then, the buddhi neither perceives nor desires interaction on the lower levels. It settles down viewing what is supernatural and spiritual. This is spiritual security. At such levels the advanced yogi is never tempted by sense objects from lower planes.

Absence of destructive criticism: Destructive criticism is a reflexive action which occurs in the lower modes of material nature. This is not controlled by the spirit. Such criticism is designed to retard the cultural progression of other entities. In the struggle for existence this makes sense, because unless one advances himself, his family and his race, they will be predominated by others. Material existence is more or less a territorial scene, a scramble for skills, pleasures and possessions. Thus we see that in spiritual societies, the territorial instinct continues in a very strong way with one guru outlawing others and with followers of gurus stating that their guru is the only authority.

In the political area everything is reduced to the adage that "might is right". Thus whosoever is the strongest prevails. This motivates even godly people to acquire weapons for defense lest they find themselves under the thumb of others. Many theories exists about living by peaceful co-existence but none can abolish the survival instinct of a human being. Thus in the *Gītā*, we see that Śrī Krishna did not touch any peace ideas, except those realized in the advanced stages of yoga practice by virtue of mystic perception of the spirits who are harnessed to similar types of psychic equipments, just like car drivers who are seat—belted behind steering wheels.

Destructive criticism cannot be stopped merely by joining a religion and following its methods for salvation. Within the nature, the urges of envy will continue even if one is religiously—inclined and follows an easy course of religion. One has to upgrade himself along the lines of yoga practice to gradually squeeze out the urges which cause a destructive concern for others.

In the neophyte stages, one observes how the psyche participates in destructive criticism. Then one decides how to curb himself from it, but he realizes that it is not an easy task because a neophyte does not have a waiver from cultural activity, and he does not understand how to do karma yoga in the technical way described in the *Gītā*.

When one first hears of these technicalities, one may become disheartened. It may seem that one's situation is hopeless. One may reason: "If Arjuna could not do it, then how can I? How would I determine what to do and what not to do? How would I know the opinion of the Central Figure in that Universal Form? I am unfortunate. I will transmigrate endlessly. Who will help me?"

The fact remains, however, that even in the neophyte stage one has a connection to the disciplines of kriyā yoga. It is not like other paths where one has a connection with this or that mediocre or advanced guru. The kriyā path puts the stress on practice. If one takes seriously to the practice, he is bound to make advancement. He will gradually move up day by day. He will get instructions from other yogis as he progresses.

I experienced this repeatedly, even though I did not have a physical spiritual master on hand to guide me. In the beginning, in this lifetime, I began yoga practice by unconscious subtle association of Swami Shivananda of Rishikesh. This happened because I used to be with him in the last body in India. Later on I took instruction from Rishi Singh Gherwal's American disciple, a martial arts master named Arthur Beverford. Rishi Singh was a master haţha and prāṇāyāma yogi. I did not reach his physical body. It had passed away by the time I found his American disciple. On the other hand, Teacher Beverford was more attentive to martial arts training than to yoga practice. However he explained what Rishi told him when they were in association physically. And he cultivated a meditation habit through the methods taught by his Guru.

I tried to track down Rishi Singh in the astral world but I could not find him. This is a regular occurrence where one cannot locate a great yogi, because he takes to isolation and does not take disciples. Later on, I used to practice at Yogi Bhajan's Kuṇḍalinī yoga ashram. There again it was mostly association with practice, because Yogi Bhajan was busy supervising and lecturing. I did not live in Los Angeles where he resided. I stayed there once for about three days. For about a year I lived at his Denver ashram in Colorado. I learned the bhastrika rapid breathing there and continued the practice on my own.

Generally, one must stick to the practice. If one does so, he will get help. Here is how that happens. Sometimes I used to be with Śrī Bābāji Mahasaya in the astral world. We would be there, several of us, listening to him or just being with him to get association and practice—sustaining vibrations. Then all of a sudden there would be a glow in the distance. Śrī Bābāji would then leave and go to the area where the glow was perceived or he would beckon one of his assistants to go to the glowing location.

So that is it. You practice. From your practice, there is a glow in the astral world. Śrī Bābāji or some other mahāyogīn sees it. He comes to assist you. I have seen this happen many times in the astral world. After Śrīla Paramhansa Yogananda popularized Śrī Bābāji Mahasaya's name in the Western countries, many youths went to India to find Bābāji in the Himalayas. Some of them thought they could find him as Haidakan Baba who was also known as Bābāji. Hardly any of them found him. This is because you cannot find him. He finds you. You practice. When you reach a certain stage you see him in his sunlight body.

From the very beginning of my practice in this life around 1970, I was able to find him but this is only because I am his perpetual dependent. It is not because I was looking for him. One does not find a great yogin by looking for him. If you want to find him then you practice whatever little you know about yoga sincerely. Eventually you will see him.

He is not a physical being. Your physical vision will not help you to find him. By the practice, your astral vision comes into play. Then you see him. You have relinquish your dependence and confidence in physical perception. Then you will find him.

This purport discusses destructive criticism. It is not that I diverted to the topic of finding Śrī Bābāji Mahasaya. Rather, he is the person who gives most of the assistance to eliminate the bad quality of always seeking to criticize a person in such a way as to stop his spiritual development. Śrī Bābāji gives out the self—critical energy. In the Samkhya system this is known as self-analysis. In the *rāja* yoga system this is now known as the neti neti process of "not this-not that."

In the Samkhya philosophy of non—yogis, it is merely analyzes oneself to find faults and to try to correct these by restraining oneself and adopting moral rules. However, far from kriyā yoga, this is merely a way of toying around with spiritual life by trying to cultivate a morality which will upgrade one on the social plane.

In some *rāja* yoga systems, one takes to meditation even without a purified psyche. Thus one fails at it. *Rāja* yoga without haţha yoga and prāṇāyāma is meditation without the blessings of the mahāyogīn Śrīla Gorakshnath. Without him one fails miserably. It is like neating up a dirty house. It simply does not make any sense to set everything neatly in an uncleaned place.

Yogi Gorakshnath, an intimate expansion of Lord Shiva, came into our world and boosted the haţha yoga and prāṇāyāma disciplines with new energy. Since many spiritual seekers do not like him, they do not practice. This is because of an ancient prejudice against Śrī Skanda Kumāra, a son of Lord Shiva. Mostly, people prefer Lord Ganesha because he is easy going. He has two attractive women for wives, Riddhi and Siddhi, who are respectively the embodiments of prosperity and secretarial skill. Since Skanda Kumāra has no wife, nobody likes him.

This preference is natural. After all, what is the use of a father who has no wife to assist with household tasks? Most of us prefer to be with affectionate young women rather than with disciplinary young men. Even yogis prefer such women. Such is our nature. Therefore the rejection of Śrī Gorakshnath is natural. Have you ever heard of Śrī Gorakshnath? What do you know about him? Hardly anybody, even in India, knows about him. But unless you take energy from him, you cannot succeed in yoga because he has the energy for our completion of haţha yoga and prāṇāyāma.

As Śrī Gorakshnath has that energy, so Bābāji has the self—critical energy. That energy curtails destructive criticism of others, so that we can focus on our own faults. In Sanskrit this is called gunadoshavicharakah. This is because you are going to take a good look at the faults (doshas) within your nature (guna). Fortunately for me, I got that energy from Śrī Bābāji Mahasaya not directly but through a bestowal from Śrīla Satyeshwarananda. I never met this yogi physically but Śrī Bābāji Mahasaya instructed him to give it to me in the astral world. Since then, I made some leaps and bounds in kriyā yoga practice.

When one reaches the advanced stages of kriyā yoga and gets the critical energy, he experiences the absence of destructive criticism because then the energy which sponsors that power leaves him. It goes away, departing from his psyche. Thus he is no longer driven by it. In my experience, one has to get the self—critical energy from someone else, someone like Śrī Bābāji.

Compassion for the beings: Compassion for the beings is a necessity. This has to be monitored by great yogis. To understand this, one should remember what happened to Arjuna. He had that compassion for the beings but his expression of it was in opposition to the mood of the Universal Form. The Form had that compassion also, but it was converted into corrective violent force. Arjuna remained unconvinced until Śrī Krishna subjected him to the shock—vision of the Universal Form.

One must, therefore, stay in tune with the Universal Form; otherwise one will run into problems being hurt supernaturally because of blind deviation from the plan of Śrī Krishna. If one's interest in others runs contrary to that of the Universal Form, one is placed in jeopardy.

For Arjuna the adjustment was easy because Śrī Krishna was present to assist him, to lift him up psychologically, to bring to his attention that he could upgrade himself by this knowledge of the psyche gained from yoga practice. For us, who would that lifting—personality be?

Freedom from craving: This has to do with covetousness, sexual lust and food greeds. Even though these habits are condemned, still they are natural tendencies. Apart from the living entities, there is the chitta (subtle emotional energy) which gets a fulfillment from these. This energy drives the subtle body to procure fulfillments in a variety of ways. Sometimes this driving force is interpreted incorrectly as a spiritual impetus. Some spiritual teachers feel that the driving force becomes positive when it is applied to missionary activities and temple services. They do not understand that whatever is driven by the chitta energy is in fact bad for a living entity and ultimately leads him downwards.

In kriyā yoga, one seeks to become purified so that one can correctly perceive the motivations and urges and trace their origins. It is not a matter of a good or bad motivation but rather the source of the motivation, because even a good motivation is bad if it originates in the wrong energy. A bad motivation is good if it comes from the right level of consciousness.

Covetousness, sexual lust and food greeds are constantly with us, because by these, the chitta energy in the causal body gets its fulfillment. So long as we are hooked up to such energy, we will be forced to serve as stooges who procure the fulfillments, even if these cause suffering or uncontrollable enjoyment. The sufferings are not desired. The uncontrollable enjoyments become obsessions. They cause addiction. Once an addiction is formed, we become crime-prone because when we cannot fulfill it, our buddhi organ induces us to commit criminal or perverted acts to procure it.

Covetousness means that I desire what someone else has. I desire it to the extent of resenting the person who has it. I take steps to acquire it by hook or crook. I will explain this in an example from my life. When this body was just about nine years old, it was living in Guyana. At the time it was not in a wealthy family. It did not have money. It was not given any more allowance than one cent each day. With that one cent, it could purchase one spoonful of fruit syrup.

The sister of this body used to get money in a much easier way. She got more of it. From time to time she bought chocolate bars. When she did not have money, she used to steal chocolate from shops. Once understood how she was procuring the bars, I thought that I should follow suit to acquire them. Once I stole a bar in a shop but before leaving the premises, I got an idea that I was being watched by the shopkeeper. I felt uncertain. I then put down the bar in another part of the shop. Soon after, the shopkeeper came from behind and held me. He said, "Where is the chocolate bar? I am going to hold you until the police officers arrive. Empty out your pockets." I then said to him, "I do not have a chocolate bar. I will empty my pockets."

After I emptied my pockets, the shopkeeper said, "I know you took the bar. You could not have eaten it that quickly. Where is it? If you do not show it, I will call the police and file a charge against you."

Realizing that he was serious, I said to him, "I took the bar but I placed it on another shelf."

The shopkeeper then said, "Show me where it is." I took him where it was placed. He smiled and released me. Now there are some lessons. First, the idea of eating the chocolate bar came because of association with my sister who used to either buy or steal such bars and eat them greedily. Seeing her enjoying the bars, I got a feeling for them. I acquired a craving to such a degree that I decided to risk stealing the bars. Once I decided to steal the bars, I entered a danger.

After the shopkeeper caught me, I technically lied because my intention was to steal the bar. I was overcome by food greed, but I did not have sufficient allowance for chocolate. My intellect helped me to get out of that tight situation by talking to the shopkeeper in such a way as to avoid any admittance. This is how the buddhi organ works its way out of an entanglement. The desire to steal the bar came from the life force's urge to procure the chocolate taste. Such a taste, if acquired, would give fulfillment to the chitta energy which takes the compressed impressions from the subtle form. In that way I was being victimized. In kriyā yoga, we study this carefully. By mystic perception we see how the psychological mechanism operates. Eventually we are able to curb its behavior.

After the incident with the shopkeeper, my intellect being strained to please the life force, which was pressured to satisfy the subtle body, came up with another plan for the chocolates. This is food greed. Instead of giving up the idea and accepting a poverty—stricken condition as something positive, my intellect simply considered a better plan for stealing the bars. I decided that since the storekeeper was vigilant it would be wise to go to another store. The intellect then perused and figured that it was better not to put any stolen chocolates in the pockets. It would be wiser, it considered, to push these under the waistband or stick them in socks.

With this plan in mind, I stole more chocolates from other stores. I was never caught. As I recalled, I must have stolen four or five more chocolates in that way. Somehow by the grace of Śrī Bābāji Mahasaya who was watching over my infant body, I gradually forgot about the chocolates. The question is: Who or what gets the fulfillments from these activities which are carefully and meticulously mapped out by the buddhi organ as urged by the life force?

Sexual lust works the same way except as a much stronger force. In infancy and early childhood, sexual lust does not occur except as a need for companionship. As soon as the body acquires the capacity for sexual expression, the lust pours in from the subtle body. It is important to understand that the subtle body carries the sexual lust with it at all times. As soon as a gross body can channel and contain such energy, it becomes manifested. The energy remains in the background at all times. It does not develop until the physical form reaches a certain age, but it is there nevertheless. It merely takes possession of the physical form when that form is capable of expressing it.

Let me cite a piece of my own life. In the immediate past life, my physical body was immune to sexuality due to yoga practice. When it was time to pass from that body, I realized I would have to take another physical form for teaching yoga to others. It was a trend in India at the time for able yogis to travel to the Western countries to teach yoga. I got caught in the flow of that energy to go West. In retrospect, I see that it was a mistake. Lord Shiva was not partial to the idea. As I recall, I saw Lord Shiva at the place called Kailash. That happened as soon as I passed from the last body. When I saw him, he showed no interest in me going to the Western countries. He felt that it was unnecessary. He had other plans but since I was determined, he did not object. When I said that I saw him at Kailash, you have to understand that I mean in the astral world. It was not a physical perception. Lord Shiva is not to be found nowadays at Kailash physically.

Because I had associated with some yogis who wanted to go West, I picked up the idea. This is a lesson: One must be careful in association with fellow seekers. In any case, because I expressed a desire to go West, the subtle energies began forming an opportunity to take birth somewhere either in a European country or in a country controlled by Europeans. I decided that I did not want to take birth in a European country. I was afraid of Western conditioning. Knowing that I would not be in control of my infant body and that the society of its birth would train it in its early years, I was deadly afraid of what would happen and what fix I would be in if I took birth in a European family. And to boot, Lord Shiva avoided me. I began to realize that I made a mistake but since the desire was there and since subtle forces were already conforming to it, I was stuck with it.

Somehow I met a lady in the astral world. Later on this lady turned out to be my eldest sister. She said to me, "I know how to do this. Do not worry. Follow me. We will get bodies." She was confident of herself. As it is in life, one follows a confident person who has the skill. It so happened that she took me to a family in which I had some slight karmic advantage. The family used black bodies but I had made a contribution to it. One of its members had studied yoga from me in India during World War II.

When that member studied yoga from me, it was not my intention to get a result by taking a body from his relatives, but this is exactly what happened. The point is that even if one does not intend to get a result from an action, one might be forced by providence to take a consequence. Everything is supervised by providence in such a way that even if one makes a selfless act, still one might be induced to take the benefit of it.

If for instance in one life I acquire some money by good or bad means and I donate that money freely to a charitable cause in a mood of selflessness, still my selfless intentions might be thwarted. In another life when I am poverty stricken or in need, providence might decide to award the result of my previous selfless act. In other words, providence pays a person from the pool of his pious activities. My sister was only the superficial cause of me being qualified to take this body. If I did not have some piety by training a family member in yoga practice, I could not take the opportunity. One cannot take birth in a family in which he has absolutely no piety.

My sister had lots of piety in the family into which my father was born. She went into my father's body and stayed there in his groin area. She did this by instinct. Somehow I did not know how to do that. It was because I was a practicing celibate. In celibacy yoga, one forgets about the groin area. To put it in the words of Śrīla Yogeshwarananda, the genitals are for urination only. That is how one sees it in celibacy yoga. Since I was a successful celibate, I lost the instinct for entering the subtle genital area of a man's body for taking a baby form. I saw my sister do this by instinct. Then I understood what I should do. I was however hesitant, because it seemed to me that she entered a dirty smelly area.

At that time I went away from her association as she stayed in the subtle groin of my father—to—be. I went to be with some Hindus in the astral world. They were doing various puja ceremonies. These were not yogis. They were just orthodox Hindus who attend temple services and invite priests to do home programs.

I inquired from many of the men if anyone could assist me because I needed a body but they all said that they could do nothing even though they wanted to help me. They realized that I was an ascetic; still they could not do anything, because for their ancestors, there was a shortage of bodies. They had no vacancy for me. A few of them said they knew for sure where I could easily get a body. When I asked them to show me those homes, they pointed to the area where the black—bodied human beings lived. That is how I was treated by the Hindus.

Even though I had many births in Indian bodies, still the Indians did not afford me a birth opportunity. The reason is this: I was a yogin by nature, a person who is a bad investment for householder life, a misfit who does not conform to the traditional ways of human society. Sensing my antisocial tendencies, no one compromised their ancestor's opportunities by permitting me to enter their family.

After trying and trying, asking and asking many Hindus, I resolved to find out if my sister had developed a body. By the time I returned she was in my would-be mother's womb. She was in the 4th month of formation of her embryo. I was amazed. Here I was, a proficient yogin, a successful spiritualist and here this lady already got a body. I tried to talk to her but she was so absorbed in her embryo that she could not relate to me. I watched from the astral world.

At that time, another lady came there and entered my father's groin area. She acted just like my sister as if she had instincts for this. Seeing me looking, she spoke as if she knew me or as if my sister had told her something to tell me. She said, "Do not worry. Hold this and come in after me. You will get through. We know how to do this."

And so it was that after the lady got through, I entered the groin of my would—be father and then was transferred into our mother's body through their sexual intercourse. I became forcibly involved in the formation of the embryo which turned out to be my present black body. When the other lady said hold this, she handed me an orange colored ribbon—like energy which she pulled out from my father's testes. This was an astral material through which I got connected to his sexual energy. None of this was physical. This was only on the subtle plane.

Needless to say I was not satisfied with the body after it was born. The environment was not a yogicly—inspiring one. Sensing that, I disliked it and did not trust it. However in such a situation what else can one do but to conform? I entered my father's body and due to the fact that his was a lusty form, the embryo which formed from it had strong sexual instincts which were activated when that body reached maturity. It altered my subtle form, making it lust-prone. Thus, after sexual maturity, I struggled with turbulent, demanding sexual energy. It was recently after this body reached forty years of age that I effectively curbed it.

Even though it only requires one fruitful intercourse to beget a child, and even though the parents do not have to prolong the act, still by the nature of sexual lust, one is induced to indulge it. This happens because in the causal body, a need exists for those varied or perverted fulfillments. In kriyā yoga one is trained in how to avoid having to fulfill perverted or excessive needs. Indeed, freedom from craving is a godly quality.

Gentleness: Gentleness is a big item in the advanced stages of yoga. This happens by receiving instruction of what to eat and what not to eat, and especially how to prepare food for offering to great yogins who use one's physical body to finish their austerities. Just as Śrī Krishna, as the Central Person in the Universal Form, wanted to use Arjuna's body and Arjuna's fighting skill and status as a member of a militant family, so a great yogin might want to use a neophyte's body for doing austerities on the physical plane. When this happens, the neophyte finds himself adopting certain superior techniques automatically.

An example of my own life would suffice. Once when I used to cut up vegetables for preparing offerings for my Śrī Śrī Radha—Krishna Deities, Śrī Bābāji Mahasaya got annoyed at me. He then said, "Do not use the knife in that way. This knife habit takes away whatever gentleness you are capable of. What do you think, you idiot? We are yogins. We are not supposed to be involved in cutting like warriors. Get rid of that knife. You can tear those green leafy vegetables with your fingers. There is no need for a blade."

Once again when I cut up squash on a cutting board, Śrī Bābāji stopped me. This happened about 3:30 *a.m.* one morning. He said, "Now of course a knife would be used in that case, but only as much as necessary. Cut a little and then break a piece of squash off by tilting the knife. Use that knife as little as possible. Remember that we are yogis. We want to get away from any type of violence. Eventually you want to go to a place where violence is absent."

There is however, another type of gentleness which is practiced from the sentimental level. This is mostly lived out by kind—hearted people. Their idea is that one should be gentle in dealings with others. However in kriyā yoga, we are not concerned with that because that would imply staying back in the material world to associate with those to whom we apply such gentle touches. Ultimately such gentleness is dictated by the feminine nature within us, a nature which requires soft touches for fulfillments.

It is not that in kriyā yoga there is no female association. In fact kriyā yoga is practiced by women as well as by men. Ma Durga and Ma Sarasvatī were the first ladies who mastered the art. Ma Sarasvatī became known as Arundhati. In higher yoga, one meets with the advanced ladies and one takes lessons from them.

These women are not interested in mundane gentleness at all. Sometimes early in the morning, when one does yoga practice, one of these ladies may come to teach how to stretch certain parts of one's physical and subtle bodies, so that one can make rapid advancement. This is the kind of female association that is good for a male yogin.

Modesty: Modesty is connected to the need for isolation. If one is not modest he will not be successful as a kriyā yogi and whatever success he gets by an ardent practice will be dissipated or traded off for fame. In yoga, fame is the way to destroy modesty. What happens is this: One learns yoga. As soon as one advances a little, one attracts disciples. People sense one's advancement. They come and ask for favors. They become fascinated with the results of yoga. If one ignores this, one will continue to advance; otherwise one will be diverted by an attraction to popularity. Fame is the highlight of many spiritual paths because in many, the main objective is to increase their following by proselytizing the mass of people. Kriyā yoga is different. If one falls for popularity, his modesty will be ruined. Modesty causes one to be loyal to the practice and to respect it as a thing in itself. Otherwise one acts like a prostitute and begins to petition people to make them disciples. Once this is done, one becomes immodest.

As soon as one begins to take many disciples, Śrī Bābāji Mahasaya goes away. It is interesting because Śrī Bābāji himself has thousands of disciples but yet, he retreats from many of his students who take disciples. He might say, "What are you doing? What happened to your practice? You ruined everything. You are no longer a student. Now that you are a master in your own right, you have no time for sitting at the feet of teachers. You posted yourself on a high seat! So many victims of your salvation plan are sitting at your lotus feet. How disgusting!"

Śrī Bābāji asked me to help many people but it is just as if a teacher asked a student to help another student. It was never in the mood of me becoming anyone's teacher forever, as their eternal guru or anything like that. We have to understand that there are certain Figure—head gurus. Śrī Bābāji is one of these. These persons are Over—lords of the creation. They are actually either the Supreme God or a god, either one. Śrī Lahiri Mahasaya regarded Śrī Bābāji Mahasaya as Śrī Krishna, as God.

The modern siddha Swami Muktananda regarded his guru, Swami Nityananda, as Śrī Krishna too. But I can say this. They regard them as such because these teachers were instrumental in giving them techniques for perfection. Neither Śrī Bābāji Mahasaya nor Swami Nityananda is Śrī Krishna. Śrī Krishna is another person. But the point is that if someone frees you from material existence, to you that person is a god, to you that person is as effective in your life as God would have been.

These Figure—head people are in the existence already. There is no need for any of us, the pee wee spirits, to pretend that we are in their position. If we do this, we will ruin advancement. One should be modest and not allow fame to carry one away from yoga practice into guruship.

Absence of fickleness: This absence of fickleness comes on by association with advanced yogins. The reason is this: On the lower levels of consciousness the mind is fickle. Its nature is jumpy like a squirrel. Even when its body remains in one position, a squirrel's form goes through numerous antics of muscular jerks. That is just the nature of it. Thus one has to get higher association. Through that one learns how to shift from the lower levels through mastery of prāṇāyāma. Many people have this idea of creating peace of mind but that is a misunderstanding. Peace of mind is already there on a higher energy level. What we have to do is relocate there. Remaining where we are and struggling with lower energies, trying always to adjust and change these, is like fighting a losing battle. We have to do austerities which shift us to a higher plane, to vacate ourselves from a lower psychology.

Patañjali, the mahāyogīn of repute, who wrote the *Yoga Sūtras*, points out clearly that yoga really means the stopping of the vrittis (mental fluctuations). But it is not that you are going to just stop the fickle, squirrel—like mind; rather you are going to move from the lower level and go where the fickleness does not manifest. This is done in deep meditation by shifting into higher planes.

Sometimes in meditation, all of a sudden, the darkness or speckled lights in the head, clear away. Then one sees through the sky of consciousness just like that and all fickleness goes away. This is actually a samādhi experience which might come by chance. In higher yoga, a yogi learns how to reach that clear sky of consciousness by certain mystic maneuvers and especially by situating himself in a particular place in the psyche.

तेजः क्षमा धृतिः शौचम्
अद्रोहो नातिमानिता ।
भवन्ति संपदं दैवीम्
अभिजातस्य भारत ॥ १६.३ ॥
tejaḥ kṣamā dhṛtiḥ śaucam
adroho nātimānitā
bhavanti saṁpadaṁ daivīm
abhijātasya bhārata (16.3)

tejaḥ — vigor; kṣamā — forbearance; dhṛtiḥ— strong — mindedness; śaucam — purity; adroho = adrohaḥ — freedom from hatred; nātimānitā = na — not + ātimānitā — conceit; bhavanti — they are; saṁpadaṁ — nature; daivīm — godly; abhijātasya — of those born; bhārata — O desendant of Bharata

...vigor, forbearance, strong—mindedness, purity, freedom from hatred, and the freedom from conceit; these are the talents of those born with the godly nature, O descendent of Bharata. (16.3)

Commentary:

Vigor: Vigor must be there for us to complete the austerities. To increase vigor one does prāṇāyāma and haṭha yoga. Meditation by itself does not increase vigor. Once in awhile, one gets a burst of energy from meditation but usually it calms the lower mental energy when it is practiced without yoga. Vigor is first understood through kuṇḍalinī yoga when the life force is energized by increased prāṇa. Then the kuṇḍalinī energy surges up the spine of the gross and subtle bodies.

This energy is known usually as sexual energy. It is felt during sexual intercourse as an uncontrollable, over—pleasurable, mind—dominating enjoyment. That is the vigor of the gross and subtle forms being used for sexuality. When this same energy moves upwards through the spine into the brain, it is said that Kuṇḍalinī passed through the central spine into the buddhi organ in the brain of the subtle body.

People with little vigor are usually not attracted to Kuṇḍalinī yoga but some of them either believe in Kuṇḍalinī or have experienced it by chance occurrence. Since one has to endeavor in haţha yoga and prāṇāyāma, some people do not practice these but instead meditate and try to raise Kuṇḍalinī by will power. There are many teachers who advocated this.

A yogi does, on occasion, experience a lack of vigor. This makes him oversleep, become lax with the exercises and relaxed with vigilance. A teacher might advise him to do prāṇāyāma to increase the vigor of the subtle body.

Forbearance: While for a kriyā yogin, forbearance must be practiced, for Arjuna who was a karma yogin, forbearance was discouraged. Arjuna was not to be forbearing towards the rival Kurus. He was to hurt and kill any of them who stood their ground in opposition to what the Universal Form desired. Forbearance is for yogis who have the waiver from cultural activities.

Strong—mindedness: A person can do kriyā yoga without being strong-minded, but only if he remains in the association of yogis who are strong—willed. Kriyā yoga goes against the natural way for accommodating desires which satisfy urges. Thus, unless one is strong—minded or unless one relies on someone who is, one cannot do kriyā yoga. The natural course of this existence is pravritti marga, which is the way of pushing on (pra) much desire for activity (vritti). Thus if one takes to the opposite course which is nirvritti marga or curtailing (nir) the desire energies (vrittis), then one has to be strong—willed. One must be tolerant of loneliness. Most of the living beings in this world are going for the fulfillment of desires. That is the natural way.

As aforementioned, everyone doing kriyā yoga does not have to be strong—minded; those who are weak-spirited by nature can succeed if they rely on the strong—minded yogis. It is not easy to fight the urges that come from the causal body. That cannot be successfully done by an ordinary entity unless he or she takes help from the Supreme Lord and other great persons. The causal body produced the subtle form which, in turn, produces numerous gross bodies. We can just imagine the potency of the causal form. It is something to contend with. Most living beings will have to act as motivated by the causal body. They have no choice in the matter.

Śrīla Yogeshwarananda, a divine being in his own right, outwitted the causal body, but that does not mean that we can challenge it in any way. It is too subtle and too remote of a thing for us to even tamper with the smallest part of it. However if we take help from him, there is a chance that we may transcend it.

Purity: Purity means purity of the psyche. It does not mean a basic thing like physical purity of the body by baths. That has nothing to do with it. Purity of the psyche is gained by a proper and aggressive haţha yoga and prāṇāyāma practice. I discussed this at length elsewhere in these commentaries.

Freedom from hatred: The freedom from hatred comes about by purity of the psyche. In common religions, one aspires for this by following certain moral rulings for behavior and by relying on the association of fellow religionists. However, in kriyā yoga we leave aside such awkward attempts at controlling the psychology. We opt for thorough control by cleaning the psyche by mystic means.

In kriyā yoga, we come to a stage of realization that all the negative qualities are ours when we are on the lower level. They are not someone else's. They are ours so long as we are in tune with the levels which foster these. Thus we work with the austerities and get to higher planes where more wholesome energies abound. We take assistance from haţha yoga and prāṇāyāma. That helps us to reach the higher stages.

Freedom from conceit: The freedom from conceit is also gained by internal purity which is attained by cleaning the psyche and moving the psyche a few notches up into higher energies. It is not just a moral and behavioral practice. In kriyā yoga, we focus on the internal energies to get rid of the ones which sponsor the lower stages of creature behavior. These are mystic processes.

Śrī Krishna listed these qualities as the talents of those born with a godly nature. This is interesting because in kriyā yoga we are not satisfied merely with prenatal or natal qualities. We check to see which natural qualities help us in the quest for spiritual vision and which do not; then we work to change the negative ones. The attitude of Śrī Krishna here is the attitude of His era, whereby if you were born with certain tendencies you were stigmatized or isolated as being in a certain caste.

For instance, in a popular story from the *Puranas*, Vishvamitra belonged to the warrior caste not only by birth as the son of a king, but by his mentality. He wanted to enter the brahmin caste because he felt that the warrior status was lower. Vishvamitra's idea was to abandon the warrior caste and adopt the brahmin way of life. He wanted supernatural power. He undertook austerities to attain this. It is said that after some 60,000 years he was successful in changing caste.

How long will it take to change tendencies and adopt something higher? Say for instance, that I was born with a wicked nature which will be described in the next verse. Then how long will it take for me to change? Will it take 60,000 years?

Śrī Krishna said in the *Gītā*, that Arjuna should not worry since he was born with the godly nature. But what about me? And what about you? My body was inclined to some ungodly habits. What is my status?

There is something funny. When I was in the society formed by my Vaishnava Spiritual Master, His Divine Grace A.C. Bhaktivedanta Swami Śrīla Prabhupāda, he assured us that we would have the godly nature just by joining his institution and following the path he chalked out. However with all due respect to him, for me that was just so much talk because my wicked nature did not go away that easily. It is by kriyā yoga in the methods given to me by Śrī Bābāji Mahasaya, Lord Shiva, Śrīla Yogeshwarananda and other mahāyogīns, that I could change out the wicked qualities and bring on the godly ones permanently with a shift in the mystic energies of consciousness. How long will a complete transformation take? This is a very good question.

दम्भो दर्पोऽतिमानश्च
क्रोधः पारुष्यमेव च ।
अज्ञानं चाभिजातस्य
पार्थ संपदमासुरीम् ॥ १६.४॥
dambho darpo'timānaśca
krodhaḥ pāruṣyameva ca
ajñānaṁ cābhijātasya
pārtha saṁpadamāsurīm (16.4)

dambho = dambhaḥ — deceit; darpo = darpaḥ — arrogance; 'bhimānaśca = abhimānaśca = abhimānaḥ — conceit + ca — and: krodhaḥ — anger; pāruṣyam — abusive language; eva — indeed; ca —and; ajñānaṁ — lack of knowledge; cābhijātasya = ca — and + abhijātasya — of those born; pārtha — son of Pṛthā; saṁpadam — tendency; āsurīm — those with a wicked nature

Deceit, arrogance, conceit, anger, abusive language, and lack of knowledge are the tendencies of those born with a wicked nature, O son of Pṛthā. (16.4)

Commentary:

Deceit: Deceit, though an ungodly quality, is absolutely necessary in the struggle for survival and for a decent placement in material life. It is part of the toolkit for living. One cannot function without it if one wants to be successful, even if one practices karma yoga, Krishna's style. Śrī Krishna employed deceitful tactics to outwit some opponents of the Pandavas during the battle. Once he engaged Bhīma in killing an elephant who was a namesake of the son of Droṇa. The purpose of this was to fool Droṇa into thinking that his son (by the same name of Ashvatthama) was killed in battle. It was calculated that once Droṇa heard of his son's death he would become discouraged. It was an effective ruse.

On another occasion, Śrī Krishna used mystic power to create a false sunset in order to give Arjuna a chance to kill Jayadratha, the person who caused Arjuna's son Abhimanyu to be killled. There were other occasions of deceit by Śrī Krishna. Thus in his course of karma yoga, of acting for the Universal Form, one may have to do some trickery.

This is not a fault of Śrī Krishna or the Universal Form. It is rather a result of the superior perception of Śrī Krishna and the application of His tit—for—tat attitude. Usually His deceits are reactions to particular entities who used deceit previously. Some good people feel that God would never employ deceit. They disavow Śrī Krishna as the Supreme Being.

For the purpose of kriyā yoga, deceit has to be admitted as part of the psyche. We are not concerned to point it out in others. We look to see the portion of it that functions in our nature and to gradually squeeze that out of ourselves and to remove ourselves from the levels where it is a portion of the natural energies.

Arrogance: Arrogance is another quality which is considered ungodly but which is in the toolkit of the psyche on lower levels. It is another necessary psychological tactic if one is to be successful in the material world. A person cannot be without it. As the common saying goes, one must have what it takes, to be successful.

Arjuna and his brother Bhīma had shown arrogance now and again. Bhīma, in particular, had the arrogance to say that he alone would kill off all the Kurus. Actually that was not possible for him. Some of the Kurus were protected by their log of piety in such a way that Bhīma's power, great as it was, could not counteract them. But Bhīma as he was possessed by the energy of the Universal Form, felt inflated in that empowerment.

In serving the Universal Form in karma yoga, one must be careful not to mistake the empowerment for personal power. If he does that, he will show certain arrogance which he will regret. The Universal Form empowers a man but when the mission is over, the boost of power is retracted from him. He then experiences a reduction in supernatural energy. As such, if he was arrogant when under its usage, he will feel undone or reduced when the energy is withdrawn. Such is the hard part of karma yoga.

In kriyā yoga, we see the necessity for arrogance, mostly by observing how it operates in others and how it causes them to predominate in the material world. We also see that the arrogance erases spiritual sensibility. Thus we desire to get rid of it. Understanding that we cannot be rid of it unless we get away from the mundane environment, we work hard to relocate our attention to higher planes.

Conceit: Usually religious people do not display blatant conceit. For them it is expressed very subtly. In kriyā yoga we introspect to find and then eliminate our own subtle bias. This occurs once we get separated from the intellect organ in the subtle body. So long as a person is glued to his intellect, whereby he cannot perceive it as an organ in the subtle body, as something distinctly separate, he will be victimized by conceit. This conceit is a conjoint energy from the buddhi organ and the life force. When this life force is unified with the buddhi organ in any venture to improve material existence, conceit comes into play.

Private conceit is actually worse than a public display of it. In a public display, the individual expressing it, has a chance of being corrected by others. In private in—the—mind conceit, hardly anyone helps the individual. He is left alone to be overtaken by the conceit—energy produced by his life force.

In kriyā yoga because of the clarity gained on the internal plane, one is able to observe this deceptive privacy. Gradually one learns how to eliminate it. In the field of karma yoga, it cannot be eliminated all together, but it can be reduced to a greater degree.

Anger: Anger stays in the nature at all times, even in the kriyā yogis at the advanced stages. One gets rid of it by abandonment of human society and by adoption of the association of the siddhas on the astral plane. Anger is there because it is a conversion of the lusty energy.

No matter where one goes on the subtle and gross planes, there will be pressure for bodies or appearances. This pressure from disembodied spirits is converted into lusty energy. When that energy is frustrated it converts into anger and resentment automatically. These are mostly indeliberate energies.

In the completion of celibacy yoga practice, one becomes exempt from the lust energy. This means that one gets out of the range of having to respond to the needs of the departed souls. Because of eliminating sexual polarity, one becomes neutral in sexual response. This is when anger comes to an end for a particular entity.

Moral ideas about the elimination of anger are mostly fantasy. Such methods are stop—gap only. They cannot get rid of it entirely. In morality, one tries to behave in a particular way and tries to curtail anti—social behavior. In kriyā yoga, one gets rid of the energies which cause or foster immoral behavior. These are psychological maneuvers.

Abusive language: Abusive language is also necessary in the material world. Despite the good people, and there are many of them, despite their ideas about politeness, even these people are stirred to express abusive language. It is not the language but the mood behind it. The human psyche has an abusive side for getting things done by force. When all else fails including politeness, pleasant requests and loving appeals, the energy converts into abusiveness. It happens indeliberately because it is an automatic emotional mechanism in the psyche.

For the purpose of kriyā yoga, abusive language which is motivated by a need for predominance, deters the advanced practice. Noticing this, the yogi watches his internal moods carefully. He takes hints from higher yogis on how to rid himself of the abusive capability. It takes two to tangle. A yogi seeks isolation and avoids confrontations. Both isolation and avoidance of confrontation are good but these by themselves do not eliminate the abusive capacity.

Lack of knowledge: Lack of knowledge is definitely a handicap in the social as well as the spiritual fields. However, many religious leaders gather masses of followers by stating that a lack of knowledge is not an impediment. They say that faith in their God is all that is required.

In kriyā yoga we have no use for ignorance nor do we have use for spiritual masters who say that it is alright. A yogi wants the information and the experience, both. He wants the experience most of all but he is practical and patient. First he takes the information by hearing of the experiences of great yogins who practiced before. Ignorance is confronted by close association with great yogis who experienced the reality. After that association, one takes up austerities and techniques through which one gains the experience.

At the end of Chapter Fifteen, Lord Krishna explained the affected and unaffected spirits. He stated that He was greater than either of these. Here he described the influences which prevail over the affected spirits. This is important for it tells us what conditions we are under.

When I got the instruction from Śrī Bābāji Mahasaya to write this commentary, I considered its relevance to the Gītā. However when Sir Paul Castagna heard of it he wondered what I was up to. In a conversation, he reminded me that in the purport to the last verse of my previous commentary on the *Gītā* (*Bhagavad Gītā Explained*), I stated the following:

> ***Let no one fool you. The Gītā is primarily a treatise on karma yoga, the type of yoga King Janak exemplified. Some modern teachers have said otherwise. In any case, yoga and its application are discussed in the Gītā as well. The central teaching was karma yoga and the objective of it was to get Arjuna to fight at Kurukṣetra. This is the truth of the matter.***

Sir Paul's objection was this: If indeed the *Gītā* is a treatise of karma yoga, then what is kriyā yoga? How does kriyā yoga fit it?

When we talk of karma yoga, we do not mean the modern idea of religious work without yoga. We discussed work with yoga or work which is done by a person who is somewhat expert at yoga, with the application of his emotional maturity in his work attitude and his dealing with others.

But what of yoga? Everyone has got some idea of what karma (work) is. What is yoga? This second commentary explains yoga. Sir Paul asked a tricky question as to whether kriyā yoga is mentioned in the *Gītā*. The joint term *kriyā yoga* is not mentioned in the *Gītā*. Only the term yoga is given. However in modem times, that type of yoga which Śrī Krishna explained in the *Gītā* has come to be known as kriyā yoga. This is why that term is used in this commentary. In addition kriyā yoga is mentioned in the *Mahābhārata* and in the instructions given to Śrī Uddhava in Canto 11 of the Śrīmad Bhagavata Purāṇa. When used in reference to religious ceremonies, the word kriyā means a ritual act which has a mystic effect to bring about a desired result.

दैवी संपद्विमोक्षाय
निबन्धायासुरी मता ।
मा शुचः संपदं दैवीम्
अभिजातोऽसि पाण्डव ॥१६.५॥
daivī sampadvimokṣāya
nibandhāyāsurī matā
mā śucaḥ sampadaṁ daivīm
abhijāto'si pāṇḍava (16.5)

daivī — godly; saṁpad — talent; vimokṣāya — to liberation; nibandhāyāsurī = nibandhāyā — to bondage + āsurī — wicked tendency; matā — considered to be; mā — not; śucaḥ — worry; saṁpadaṁ — nature; daivīm — godly; abhijāto = abhijātaḥ — born; 'si = asi — you are; pāṇḍava — son of Pāndu

The godly talent is conducive to liberation. It is considered that the wicked tendencies facilitate bondage. Do not worry. You are endowed with the godly nature, O son of Pāndu. (16.5)

Commentary:

Arjuna was endowed with the godly nature. What about us? Merely because we are yogins or because we are devotee yogins, does not mean that we exhibit the godly nature. In kriyā yoga it is not important that we start with a godly nature. The important thing is perseverance. We can move from being wicked to being godly if we persist. Arjuna had fortune. If any of us do not have it, then we need not despair. We should practice for purification.

द्वौ भूतसर्गौ लोकेऽस्मिन्
दैव आसुर एव च ।
दैवो विस्तरशः प्रोक्त
आसुरं पार्थ मे श्रृणु ॥ १६.६ ॥
dvau bhūtasargau loke'smin
daiva āsura eva ca
daivo vistaraśaḥ prokta
āsuraṁ pārtha me śṛṇu (16.6)

dvau — two; bhūtasargau = bhūta — being + sargau — two created types; loke — in the world; 'smin = asmin — in this; daiva — godly; āsura — wicked; eva — indeed; ca — and; daivo = daivah — godly type; viṣṭaraśaḥ — in detail; prokta — explained; āsuraṁ — wicked; pārtha — son of Pṛthā; me — from me; śṛṇu — hear

There are two types of created beings in this world, the godly type and the wicked. The godly type was explained in detail. Hear from me of the wicked, O son of Pṛthā. (16.6)

Commentary:

Śrī Krishna did explain much about the godly nature, about what is expected of it and how it expresses itself. He spoke of the great yogins who operate with it. Little detail was given about the wicked nature, which is now described.

प्रवृत्तिं च निवृत्तिं च
जना न विदुरासुराः ।
न शौचं नापि चाचारो
न सत्यं तेषु विद्यते ॥ १६.७ ॥
pravṛttiṁ ca nivṛttiṁ ca
janā na vidurāsurāḥ
na śaucaṁ nāpi cācāro
na satyaṁ teṣu vidyate (16.7)

pravṛttiṁ— what to do; ca — and; nivṛttiṁ— what not to do; ca — and; janā — people; na — not; viduḥ — they know; āsurāḥ— wicked; na — neither; śaucaṁ— cleanliness; nāpi = na — nor + api — also; cācāro = cācāraḥ = ca — and + ācāraḥ — good conduct; na — nor; satyam — realism; teṣu — in them; vidyate — is found

The wicked people do not know what to do and what not to do. Neither cleanliness or even good conduct, nor realism is found in them. (16.7)

Commentary:

Here Śrī Krishna spoke of those who are to a greater degree, asuric or demonic. The application of this to kriyā yoga is that even a godly person might, on occasion, behave badly. Even such a person might, on occasion, become confused. We heard that Arjuna did not know what to do. In fact he rejected the right action.

असत्यमप्रतिष्ठं ते
जगदाहुरनीश्वरम् ।
अपरस्परसंभूतं
किमन्यत्कामहैतुकम् ॥ १६.८ ॥

asatyam — unreal; apratiṣṭhaṁ — without a foundation; te — they; jagat — the world; āhuḥ — they say; anīśvaram — without a Supreme Lord; aparasparasaṁbhūtaṁ = aparaspara —

asatyamapratiṣṭhaṁ te
jagadāhuranīśvaram
aparasparasaṁbhūtaṁ
kimanyatkāmahaitukam (16.8)

without a series of causes + saṁbhūtaṁ — produced; kim — what?; anyat — other cause; kāmahaitukam = kāma — sensual urge + haitukam — caused

They say that the universe is unreal, without a foundation, without a Supreme Lord, without a series of causes. They explain, saying, "Sexual urge is the cause. What other basis could there be?" (16.8)

Commentary:

The perspective of seeing sexual nature as the cause comes from a certain level of consciousness. Anyone who takes energy from that level sees in that way. Even a kriyā yogin viewing from that plane will see in that way. The difference is that a kriyā yogi may take his memory of higher experiences with him to that lower level. He can analyze and understand that he descended to a place wherefrom, he is forced to perceive life as being caused by sexuality. He can then shift himself upwards or endeavor to relocate out of the lower level. Others who do not have the experience of something higher or who are not told about the higher realities, have no choice but to accept the lower views.

एतां दृष्टिमवष्टभ्य
नष्टात्मानोऽल्पबुद्धयः ।
प्रभवन्त्युग्रकर्माणः
क्षयाय जगतोऽहिताः ॥१६.९॥
etāṁ dṛṣṭimavaṣṭabhya
naṣṭātmāno'lpabuddhayaḥ
prabhavantyugrakarmāṇaḥ
kṣayāya jagato'hitāḥ (16.9)

etāṁ — this; dṛṣṭim — view; avaṣṭabhya — holding; naṣṭātmāno = naṣṭātmānaḥ = naṣṭa — lost + ātmānaḥ — to their spiritual selves; 'lpabuddhayaḥ= alpabuddhayaḥ = alpa — negligible + buddhayaḥ — intelligence; prabhavanti — they become; ugrakarmāṇaḥ = ugra — cruel + karmāṇaḥ — acts; kṣayāya — to destruction; jagato = jagataḥ — of the world; 'hitāḥ = ahitāḥ — enemies

Holding this view, men who lost track of their spirituality, who have negligible intelligence, who commit cruel acts, become enemies for the destruction of the world. (16.9)

Commentary:

Some of us do this on occasion, while others spend most of their lives striving for the physical or moral destruction of the world. In kriyā yoga we seek to see the system of degradation through which we may become ignorant of spirituality and hell bent upon a course for destruction of this created world. As one can go down, so he can climb out and achieve transcendental status. A human being can exert himself or herself for liberation.

I, for one, was degraded when I took this birth. By a careful study of my condition, and by seeing how I descended, I took certain steps to effect an elevation. It is not that you are demonic or he or they, but rather I am potentially evil. Therefore Śrī Krishna described my capacity. I can retrieve my spirituality and rekindle divine intelligence.

काममाश्रित्य दुष्पूरं
दम्भमानमदान्विताः ।
मोहाद्गृहीत्वासद्ग्राहान्
प्रवर्तन्तेऽशुचिव्रताः ॥१६.१०

kāmam — lusty urge; āśritya — relying; duṣpūraṁ — non-fulfilling; dambhamānamadānvitāḥ = dambba — hypocrisy + māna —pride + mada — intoxicated + anvitāḥ — possessed by; mohāt —from delusion; gṛhītvā — having accepted; 'sadgrāhān = asadgrāhān

kāmamāśritya duṣpūraṁ
dambhamānamadānvitāḥ
mohādgṛhītvāsadgrāhān
pravartante'śucivratāḥ (16.10)

= *asad (asat) — unrealistic + grāhān — views; pravartante — they proceed; 'śucivratāḥ = aśucivratāh = aśuci — impure + vratāḥ — objectives*

Being reliant on the non—fulfilling lusty urge, possessed of hypocrisy, pride, and intoxication, having accepted unrealistic views, through delusion, they proceed with impure objectives. (16.10)

Commentary:

In youth, because of its birth situation, this body was in association with persons who were primarily reliant on the nonfulfilling lusty urge. This is the sexual nature. However, by a careful study of how it operated, I gained ascendency over it by taking up relevant yoga practices in haṭha yoga, prāṇāyāma and mystic technique.

I remember when this body was in high school. It associated with persons of a lusty demeanor. Such persons were preoccupied with sexual desires, always wanting sexual intercourse. The urge is endless for those who are so afflicted. Through their association and by taking a body from parents who were affected, I myself came under its influence. It held me as its slave. It was by practicing haṭha yoga and prāṇāyāma and by fine—tuning the mystic perception, that I got away from it.

When one is spellbound by the lusty urge, it is to be understood that one is being directed by the ancestors who require baby forms. But even though one is directed like this, one does not realize it. This applies to religious and irreligious people. The sexual urge is not an isolated energy. It is powered by the departed souls who require new bodies. Any of us can become the driving force of the sexual urge of a man or woman if we lose our present body and crave a new one.

The sexual urge holds its own agenda upon a person, making him hypocritical in order to live by subterfuge so that he can beget children responsibly or irresponsibly. Those who have the financial or moral means to maintain a family, usually pretend that they are more elevated than their poor or vulgar counterparts who cannot adequately support the progeny their bodies generate.

The sexual urge produces a pride in one's sexuality, which amounts to nothing but pride over the animal urge of aroused sexual nature. When this takes over the mind, one loses the moral perspective or one exhibits morality in a superficial way. The sex urge is tallied to the taking of intoxicants, either liquor or herbs. Sex too, has its own natural intoxicant manifested by the romantic feelings it creates in the mind and emotions of the living beings.

By sexual power, one gets many unrealistic views and one does anything to get sexual intercourse, a thing which if done irresponsibly, brings on liabilities. One becomes reckless by the sexual urge so that he is unable to foresee the consequences of sexual connection.

Śrī Krishna alerted us that under the sexual influence we work for impure objectives. Kriyā yoga is for purifying the psyche so that there is clarity on the psychological plane. It begins with kuṇḍalinī yoga for cleaning out the energy gyrating centers in the subtle body. This advances to celibacy yoga to clean out the subtle groin area, thighs, buttocks, chest and breast of the subtle body. This moves the yogi into the practice of purity yoga to clean the entire psyche. That moves the yogi into brahma yoga which causes the subtle body to change so that the kuṇḍalinī chakra is eliminated. One then develops a subtle body with a brahmarandra hole at the top of it. It continues further.

चिन्तामपरिमेयां च
प्रलयान्तामुपाश्रिताः ।
कामोपभोगपरमा
एतावदिति निश्चिताः ॥ १६.११ ॥
cintāmaparimeyāṁ ca
pralayāntāmupāśritāḥ
kāmopabhogaparamā
etāvaditi niścitāḥ (16.11)

cintām — worry; aparimeyāṁ — endless; ca — and; pralayāntām — ending at death; upāśritāḥ — clinging; kāmopabhogaparamā = kāma — lust + upabhoga — enjoyment + paramā — highest aim; etāvat — so much; iti — thus; niścitāḥ — convinced

And clinging to endless worries which end at the time of death, with lusty enjoyment as the highest aim, being convinced that this is all there is, (16.11)

Commentary:

These worries begin in a particular body as soon as the sexual urge is manifested at the onset of puberty. We can recall an experience of this as we observed the effect of puberty on children. I recall specifically how the attitude of the children of my body changed towards me when their bodies reached puberty.

In my case, when my body reached puberty, I marveled at the transformation. One lady, a lusty woman who was addicted to sexual intercourse, made a remark when my body reached puberty. She said with glee, "His voice changed!" I remember clearly the joy on her face. At the time I did not know how to interpret that facial expression. In retrospect, I understand that her complete thought was this: "His voice changed which means he can now enjoy sexual expression. What a wonderful experience that will be for him. It is the greatest pleasure in life."

Behind the worries which come from sexual maturity is the worry for a family, for any children one's body produces. For those who have the advantage of birth control, there is the background worry because of circumventing Nature's reproductive functions. Even though modern civilization legitimatized the use of contraceptives, still that does not mean that material nature will let it pass unscathed. One should not fool the self by thinking that human opinion will forever hold sway. It is better to wise up, see material nature for what it is. Whatever material nature objects to, will find us sooner or later, in this life or the next. The human beings who excuse us now, will not be there to bar nature from inconveniencing us in the future. One should understand the views of material nature and work to suit. God may come and disapprove of what I am doing or He may come and punish as He did to the Kurus, but besides God there is nature which will act regardless. In a sense, material nature is a more exacting and consistent reactor to our activity. Nature is sure to act to balance out any tensions that she finds in her energy. That takes place automatically.

For the time being the worries over sex life will end at death, at least until a sex—prone person locates another environment where his sexual nature can express itself freely. Some find this soon after the body dies, when they end up in a subtle world where sexual indulgence transpires in excess without the moral restraints which restricted them in human society. Others must wait for another birth when they would acquire a human or animal form which is capable of sexual pleasure.

For a successful kriyā yogi who is a householder, his worries end when he becomes detached from the children produced from his body or when he becomes detached at the time of death. If he is successful his worries will end sooner than the time of death. Single men who practice kriyā yoga and who are preoccupied with sexual ideas, remain with the urge unfulfilled until they can gain proficiency in kuṇḍalinī yoga or until they become responsible householders who have facility for sexual contact.

Worries from the sexual urge are a concern about departed ancestors who need bodies. A kriyā yogi learns how to sidestep their influence. With all due respect to them and with appreciation for their pious services, he declines their influence and takes instead to the association of the mahāyogīns.

आशापाशशतैर्बद्धाः
कामक्रोधपरायणाः ।
ईहन्ते कामभोगार्थम्
अन्यायेनार्थसंचयान् ॥ १६.१२ ॥
āśāpāśaśatairbaddhāḥ
kāmakrodhaparāyaṇāḥ
īhante kāmabhogārtham
anyāyenārthasaṁcayān (16.12)

āśāpāśaśataiḥ = āśāpāśa — frustrating expectations + śataiḥ — by a hundred; baddhāḥ — bound; kāmakrodhaparāyaṇāḥ = kāma — craving + krodha — anger + parāyaṇāḥ — cherishing; īhante — they strive to acquire; kāmabhogārtham = kāma — craving + bhoga — pleasure + artham — fulfillment; anyāyenārthasañcayān = anyāyena — with any other + artha — money + sañcayān — huge sums

...bound by hundreds of frustrating expectations, cherishing craving and anger, using any means, they strive to acquire huge sums of money for the fulfillment of craving and pleasure. (16.12)

Commentary:

Most of the frustrating expectations which arise in a person's mind when he is under the lusty influence, come from the departed ancestors who are around us in the subtle atmosphere. Due to a lack of clarity in determining the sources of thoughts, one thinks that every thought which arises in one's mind should be identified with. This mistake is eliminated when one reaches the 6th stage of yoga, that of dhāraṇa, focus of the will through the buddhi organ.

Some teachers criticize the acquirement of siddhis, mystic powers, but accurate tracking is one of these. Unless one can track thoughts, he cannot free himself from the frustrating expectations. We must develop mystic perception if we are to become liberated. Without it, no one can get out of the material world.

Many of the cravings come from others and from such cravings arise frustrations and anger. This is because material nature is designed not to fulfill every urge.

Huge sums of money are required for the fulfillment of desires, such that even great religious leaders who should know better, crave money, and then induce followers to acquire it by hook or crook and legitimize it by saying that it is for God and for the salvation of human beings, as if the money fulfills a divine need.

इदमद्य मया लब्धम्
इदं प्राप्स्ये मनोरथम् ।
इदमस्तीदमपि मे
भविष्यति पुनर्धनम् ॥ १६.१३
idamadya mayā labdham
idaṁ prāpsye manoratham
idamastīdamapi me
bhaviṣyati punardhanam (16.13)

idam — this; adya — today; mayā — by me; labdham — obtained; idaṁ — this; prāpsye — I will fulfill; manoratham — fantasy; idam — this; astīdam = asti — it is + idam — this; api — also; me — mine; bhaviṣyati — willl be; punaḥ — again, also; dhanam — wealth

Thinking: "This was obtained by me today, I will fulfill this fantasy. This is it. This wealth will also be mine. (16.13)

Commentary:

The first attainment one gets is an education. But if one fails to get that, then one gets from material nature a sense of survival. Thus even an uneducated person prides in his ability to survive as a material body. After procuring an education one tries to get a job and form a family. These are status symbols. One feels a sense of completion when one acquires a good job and has a faithful spouse and some children.

Then one feels that this is it. Actually that is nothing. It is not an achievement because it comes about naturally even in the life of animals. A bird gets an education from its parents regarding how to fly, how to find food and how not to become the food of other creatures. This is also education. A bird builds a nest, takes a spouse and raises chicks. It is similar. It is the gift of nature. It is not something we human beings invented. When a bird finds a straw while building a nest, the creature also thinks, "This straw is mine. No one has the right to take it away from me."

असौ मया हतः शत्रुर्
हनिष्ये चापरानपि ।
ईश्वरोऽहमहं भोगी
सिद्धोऽहं बलवान्सुखी ॥१६.१४॥
asau mayā hataḥ śatrur
haniṣye cāparānapi
īśvaro'hamahaṁ bhogī
siddho'haṁ balavānsukhī (16.14)

asau — that; mayā — by me; hataḥ — was killed; śatruḥ — enemy; haniṣye — I will kill; cāparān = ca — and + aparān — others; api — as well as; īśvaro = īśvaraḥ — controller; 'ham = aham — I; aham — I; bhogī — enjoyer; siddho = siddhaḥ — successful; 'ham = aham — I; balavān — powerful; sukhī — happy

"That enemy was killed by me. I will kill others as well. I am the controller. I am the enjoyer. I am successful, powerful and happy. (16.14)

Commentary:

These feelings are there in the animal forms as well. We can realize this by developing deep meditations and going back to the time when we took animal bodies.

आढ्योऽभिजनवानस्मि
कोऽन्योऽस्ति सदृशो मया ।
यक्ष्ये दास्यामि मोदिष्य
इत्यज्ञानविमोहिताः ॥१६.१५॥
āḍhyo'bhijanavānasmi
ko'nyo'sti sadṛśo mayā
yakṣye dāsyāmi modiṣya
ityajñānavimohitāḥ (16.15)

āḍhyo = āḍhyaḥ — rich; 'bhijanavān = abhijanavān — upper class; asmi — I am; ko = kaḥ — who; 'nyo = anyaḥ — other; 'sti = asti — there is; sadṛśo = sadṛśaḥ — like; mayā — me; yakṣye — I will perform religious ceremony; dāsyāmi — I will give in, donate; modiṣya — I will make merry; iti — thus is said; ajñānavimohitāḥ = ajñāna — ignorance + vimohitāḥ — those who are deluded

"I am rich and upper class. Who is there besides me? I will perform religious ceremony. I will donate. I will make merry." This is what is said by those who are deluded by ignorance. (16.15)

Commentary:

Animals do not get involved in religious ceremonies but they do everything else that is listed in this verse. Lions and tigers, for instance, sometimes kill other animals when they are begged to do so by the animal cries of other predators like hyenas and carrion birds. Even the lions and tigers donate part of their kill to other animals who do not have the courage and prowess required to bring down huge elephants and swift deer.

When a big cat, lion, tiger or puma walks in the forest or on the plain, the creature walks with a certain confidence and with a sense of pride, feeling that it is lord of creation. I cited these examples to bring to fore that these are not human sentiments alone. These are urges felt by animals and human beings alike.

अनेकचित्तविभ्रान्ता
मोहजालसमावृताः ।
प्रसक्ताः कामभोगेषु
पतन्ति नरकेऽशुचौ ॥ १६.१६ ॥
anekacittavibhrāntā
mohajālasamāvṛtāḥ
prasaktāḥ kāmabhogeṣu
patanti narake'śucau (16.16)

anekacittavibhrāntā = aneka — many + citta — idea + vibhrāntā — carried away; mohajālasamāvṛtāh = moha — delusion + jāla — entanglement + samāvṛtāḥ — occupied by; prasaktāḥ — being attached; kāmabhogeṣu = kāma — craving + bhogeṣu — in enjoyments; patanti — they fall; narake — in hellish condition; 'śucau = aśucau – unclean

Being carried away by many ideas, being occupied by entangling delusions, being attached by cravings and enjoyments, they fall into an unclean, hellish condition. (16.16)

Commentary:

The quality of a person's consciousness and the motivational force behind his activities, determine his destination. A living being is never static. Whatever he does or does not do, has an impact. He becomes the focal point of that impact.

By unclean condition, Śrī Krishna meant the condition of the subtle body. It is that form which causes the transmigration of the soul. One falls into an unclean psychological condition and then enters a lower species of life or a lower type of human form.

I for one, took a lower human body in this life. It caused my subtle body to become unclean. By good luck, I got mystic techniques for cleaning the subtle form. Thus I repossessed my purity. One can also take an animal form. These are all possible futures for any living being who is careless in demeanor and actions.

आत्मसंभाविताः स्तब्धा
धनमानमदान्विताः ।
यजन्ते नामयज्ञैस्ते
दम्भेनाविधिपूर्वकम् ॥ १६.१७ ॥
ātmasaṁbhāvitāḥ stabdhā
dhanamānamadānvitāḥ
yajante nāmayajñaiste
dambhenāvidhipūrvakam (16.17)

ātmasaṁbhāvitāḥ — self-conceited; stabdhā — stubborn; dhanamānamadānvitāḥ = dhanamāna — arrogance of having money + mada — pride + anvitāḥ — possessed with; yajante — they worship in ceremony; nāmayajñaiḥ — with religious ceremony in name only; te — they; dambhenāvidhipūrvakam = dambhena — with hyprocrisy + avidhipurvakam — without reference to Vedic injunction

Self—conceited, stubborn, possessed of pride and the arrogance of having money, with hypocrisy and without reference to Vedic injunctions, they worship in ceremonies that are religious in name only. (16.17)

Commentary:

This condition is arrived at by the influence of the two lower modes of material nature, the passionate force and the retarding one. As human beings, we are under the passionate force. We are supposed to be guided in how to use that energy by the clarifying force which sponsors good acts or pious functions. However, the passionate energy has an affinity for both the clarifying and retarding functions. On its own, it will facilitate one or the other.

The unclean hellish condition may be taken to mean life in the animal world or life in a low class family which remains dirty and dingy externally. In kriyā yoga we take the higher meaning which refers to a dingy dirty psychology. This type of psyche is cleaned up by Kuṇḍalinī yoga, celibacy and purity yoga.

When a piously inclined person is overtaken by the passionate energies of material nature, he still sticks to religion but he does so with much self—conceit, being biased, feeling arrogant if he has a little money to donate to the church, temple or mosque, being hypocritical and cynical to anyone who has left aside passion and dull consciousness.

He worships and may even worship by Vedic stipulations but whatever he does in that way will be deviant.

अहंकारं बलं दर्पं
कामं क्रोधं च संश्रिताः ।
मामात्मपरदेहेषु
प्रद्विषन्तोऽभ्यसूयकाः ॥१६.१८॥
ahaṁkāraṁ balaṁ darpaṁ
kāmaṁ krodhaṁ ca saṁśritāḥ
māmātmaparadeheṣu
pradviṣanto'bhyasūyakāḥ (16.18)

ahaṁkāraṁ — misplaced self-identity; balam — brute force; darpaṁ — arrogance; kāmaṁ — craving; krodhaṁ — anger; ca — and; saṁśritāḥ — clinging to; mām — me; ātmaparadeheṣu = ātma — self + para — other + deheṣu — in bodies; pradviṣanto = pradviṣantaḥ — disliking; 'bhyasūyakāḥ = abhyasūyakāḥ — those who are envious

Clinging to a misplaced self—identity, brute force, arrogance, craving and anger, those who are envious dislike Me, in their own bodies and in those of others. (16.18)

Commentary:

When Śrī Krishna said that under the retarding influence, persons dislike Him in their own bodies as well as in the bodies of others, He must mean that their dislike is an unconscious but reflexive rejection of His presence. It cannot, in most cases, be a conscious one. In the case of persons like Duryodhana, Arjuna's cousin who was the rival of the Pandavas, the rejection was a conscious one. But for most others, it is a reflexive, albeit defensive mechanism designed to protect the person from having a guilty conscience, something that would drive them mad sooner or later, if not reformed.

The reason for the reflexive rejection is this: The psyche of the living being can sense when someone approves or disapproves of his or her views and behaviors. This conscience is guided by the life force. The intellect tries to protect it.

This is why the yogi steps aside from the social scene as soon as he gets a waiver from the Supreme Being. At the time the yogi is relieved from having to represent the Universal Form in cultural and political affairs. There is no point in being strung up like Jesus Christ. It is not required. The contention between the limited beings and the Supreme Person is on—going. Even if one is strung up, it will not stop the argument. It will not substantially decrease the resentments people feel towards the Supreme Being.

The example of Lord Jesus Christ is there. Since his crucifixion, people still continue in their resentments. Jesus' martyrdom did not stop it. Of course it eased the situation for a handful of people but still it did not end it. Thus for humanity one should not come into the view that if one is permitted to abandon the path of karma yoga, there will be something missing in the world. There are many living entities who are in the process of becoming qualified martyrs. There is no necessity for any of us to forestall the waiver from the Supreme Being.

If we can get it let us take it either conjointly or singly, because we are simply not needed. The business of the Central Figure in the Universal Form in terms of His disapproval of human acts, is just that; it is primarily God's concern, not ours.

The reflexive dislike that some human beings feel towards the Supreme Person, need not be directed to a saintly personality. A saint should act in order to get a waiver so that he can complete yoga practice and not have to be an agent of the disciplinary attitude of the Universal Form. Many great yogi-devotees of the past took that waiver, persons like Nārada, Śrīla Vyāsadeva, his son Shuka and others. Nārada, for example, knew Kansa who was instinctively hostile to Śrī Krishna. Nārada and Kansa were friends in a way. Kansa had no idea that Nārada was such a loyal and steadfast devotee of Krishna. In other words, Nārada did not vehemently reflect the disapproval of the Universal Form, when he was with Kansa.

When I began to write this book, I did not see that I would become a preacher as the book developed but now I am feeling as if I am a preacher. That is not the idea. This book is not for proselytizing. Readers should therefore accept my apologies. I just wanted to make some points clear about the kriyā path.

Even though Śrī Krishna said that one clings to a misplaced self—identity and to brute force, arrogance, craving and anger, in the experience we feel it as a mutual clinging. The lower energies cling to us just as much or even more than we embrace them. It is like electrical power. One gets the feeling that one cannot loosen one's grip from a live electric wire Sometimes we see that even though a person wants to get away from the lower influence, it holds him and does not permit his release.

तानहं द्विषतः क्रूरान्
संसारेषु नराधमान् ।
क्षिपाम्यजस्रमशुभान्
आसुरीष्वेव योनिषु ॥ १६.१९
tānahaṁ dviṣataḥ krūrān
saṁsāreṣu narādhamān
kṣipāmyajasramaśubhān
āsurīṣveva yoniṣu (16.19)

tān — them; aham — I; dviṣataḥ — those who are despising; krūrān — those who are cruel; saṁsāreṣu — in the cycles of rebirth; narādhamān — lowest of humans; kṣipāmi — I hurl; ajasram — constantly; aśubhān — the vicious; āsurīṣu — into the wicked people; eva — indeed; yoniṣu — in the wombs

I constantly hurl the despising, cruel, vicious, lowest of humans into the cycles of rebirth in the wombs of wicked people. (16.19)

Commentary:

This is some statement by Śrī Krishna! It demolishes any idea we might have entertained about a loving and kind God who is anxious to free us from the lower modes. It is also true that even if Śrī Krishna does not do this, then by the way of material nature, the person would be degraded. Śrī Krishna's hurling act would send the limited being down in the evolutionary cycle much quicker than the slow but sure process of nature.

While material nature may allow a wicked individual, who exerts himself and plays up to religion, to be promoted anyway as did Kansa and persons like Rāvaṇa, Śrī Krishna's preference is for such a person to be denied any higher births.

आसुरीं योनिमापन्ना
मूढा जन्मनि जन्मनि ।
मामप्राप्यैव कौन्तेय
ततो यान्त्यधमां गतिम् ॥ १६.२० ॥
āsurīṁ yonimāpannā
mūḍhā janmani janmani
māmaprāpyaiva kaunteya
tato yāntyadhamāṁ gatim (16.20)

āsurīṁ — the wicked people; yonim — womb; āpannā — entering; mūḍhā — the blockheads; janmani janmani — in birth, in birth again; mām — me; aprāpyaivā = aprāpya — associating + eva — indeed; kaunteya — O son of Kuntī; tato = tataḥ — thence; yānti — they traverse; adhamāṁ — lowest; gatim — route of transmigration

Thus, O son of Kuntī, entering the wombs of the wicked people, the blockheads, after not associating with Me in birth after birth, traverse the lowest route of transmigration. (16.20)

Commentary:

This association with Śrī Krishna is the Supersoul association which is manifested as a qualified sense of right and wrong in the average human being. We experience sometimes, that certain individuals do not have that conscience. Even some devotees seem to not have it. Anyone who has that sensitivity has great advantage. By instinct, he knows what is right or wrong, conducive or restrictive. Śrī Krishna stated that He bars the wicked people from having His association, which is the curative energy required for their reform. It is because their tendency is to misuse the divine association.

त्रिविधं नरकस्येदं
द्वारं नाशनमात्मनः ।
कामः क्रोधस्तथा लोभस्
तस्मादेतत्त्रयं त्यजेत् ॥ १६.२१ ॥
trividhaṁ narakasyedaṁ
dvāraṁ nāśanamātmanaḥ
kāmaḥ krodhastathā lobhas
tasmādetattrayaṁ tyajet (16.21)

trividhaṁ — threefold; narakasyedaṁ = narakasya — of hell + idam — this; dvāraṁ — avenues; nāśanam — destructive of, degrading towards; ātmanaḥ — of the self; kāmaḥ — craving; krodhaḥ — anger; tathā— as well; lobhaḥ — greed; tasmāt — therefore; etat — this; trayam — three — fold; tyajet — should abandon

Craving, anger and greed are the three avenues of hell which degrade the soul. Therefore one should abandon this threefold influence. (16.21)

Commentary:

This instruction is direct. How to do this is not spelled out in detail. Previously we were advised about this.

एतैर्विमुक्तः कौन्तेय
तमोद्वारैस्त्रिभिर्नरः ।
आचरत्यात्मनः श्रेयस्
ततो याति परां गतिम् ॥ १६.२२ ॥
etairvimuktaḥ kaunteya
tamodvāraistribhirnaraḥ
ācaratyātmanaḥ śreyas
tato yāti parāṁ gatim (16.22)

etair (etaiḥ) — by these; vimuktaḥ — released; kaunteya — son of Kuntī; tamodvārais = tamo (tamaḥ) — depression + dvāraiḥ — by avenues; tribhir (tribhiḥ) —by three; naraḥ — a person; ācaratyātmanaḥ = ācarati — he serves + ātmanaḥ — of the self; śreyaḥ — best interest; tato (tataḥ) — then; yāti — goes; parāṁ — supreme; gatim — destination

Being released from these three avenues of depression, O son of Kuntī, a person serves his best interest and then goes to the highest destination. (16.22)

Commentary:

This is a very down-to-earth statement. This is realized by one who shines the critical energy on himself or herself. Once we look inwards and take to criticising ourselves constructively, with a mood to do something about our condition, to reform, then we see that it is our own craving, anger and greed which degrade us.

These are deep-seated traits which do not leave us merely because we declare allegiance to a spiritual master. These traits leave us by hard core austerities in yoga practice, disciplines which bring on inner mystic perception and give us the psychic tools necessary to clean our psyche and move the focus of attention to the sky of consciousness, thus abandoning this sky of material air with its planets, suns and stars.

यः शास्त्रविधिमुत्सृज्य
वर्तते कामकारतः ।
न स सिद्धिमवाप्नोति
न सुखं न परां गतिम् ॥१६.२३॥
yaḥ śāstravidhimutsṛjya
vartate kāmakārataḥ
na sa siddhimavāpnoti
na sukhaṁ na parāṁ gatim (16.23)

yaḥ — who; śāstravidhim — scriptural injunction; utsṛjya — discarding; vartate — he follows; kāmakārataḥ — impulsion, inclination; na — not; sa = saḥ — he; siddhim — perfection; avāpnoti — attains; na — nor; sukhaṁ — happiness; na — nor; parāṁ — highest; gatim — destination

Whosoever discards the scriptural injunctions, and follows the impulsive inclinations, does not get perfection or happiness or the supreme destination. (16.23)

Commentary:

We should not discard the scriptural injunctions as being useless. They were put there for our benefit. A total reliance on one's insight, without checking what the great sages and Śrī Krishna said, is a serious mistake in judgment. We have to constantly check to be sure that our advancement was chalked out by the great sages and by Śrī Krishna. It is foolish to rely on sense perception and the intellect alone.

तस्माच्छास्त्रं प्रमाणं ते
कार्याकार्यव्यवस्थितौ ।
ज्ञात्वा शास्त्रविधानोक्तं
कर्म कर्तुमिहार्हसि ॥१६.२४॥
tasmācchāstraṁ pramāṇaṁ te
kāryākāryavyavasthitau
jñātvā śāstravidhānoktaṁ
karma kartumihārhasi (16.24)

tasmāt — therefore; śāstram — scripture; pramāṇaṁ — recommendation; te — your; karyākāryavyavasthitau = kārya — duty + akārya — non-duty + vyavasthitau— setting; jñātvā — knowing; śāstravidhānoktaṁ = śāstravidhāna — scriptural rules + uktaṁ — prescribed; karma — action; kartum — to perform; ihārhasi = ihā — here in this world + arhasi — you can

Therefore, setting your standard of duty and non—duty by scriptural recommendation, knowing the scriptural rules prescribed, you should perform actions in this world. (16.24)

Commentary:

This is an advice for Arjuna as a karma yogi. For those of us who have exemption from cultural and political acts, this advice applies as well. We too, must stick to duty, which is to consistently practice yoga disciplines and to advance as rapidly as possible. For Arjuna and any of us who do not have the waiver from karma yoga, we are advised to adhere to the scriptures to find out what should and should not be done.

CHAPTER 17

Three Types of Confidences*

अर्जुन उवाच
ये शास्त्रविधिमुत्सृज्य
यजन्ते श्रद्धयान्विताः ।
तेषां निष्ठा तु का कृष्ण
सत्त्वमाहो रजस्तमः ॥ १७.१ ॥
arjuna uvāca
ye śāstravidhimutsṛjya
yajante śraddhayānvitāḥ
teṣāṁ niṣṭhā tu kā kṛṣṇa
sattvamāho rajastamaḥ (17.1)

arjuna — Arjuna; uvāca — said; ye — who; śastravidhim — scriptural injunction; utsṛjya — disregarding; yajante — they perform religiously—motivated ceremony and austerity; śraddhayānvitāḥ — with full confidence; teṣāṁ— of them; niṣṭhā — position; tu—but; kā — what; kṛṣṇa — O Krishna; sattvaṁ — clarity; āho— is it?; rajaḥ — impulsion; tamaḥ—depression

Arjuna said: Concerning those who disregard scriptural injunction, but who with full confidence perform religiously—motivated ceremonies and austerities, what indeed, is their position, O Krishna? Is it clarity, impulsion or depression? (17.1)

Commentary:

This is an interesting question. Arjuna realized that human beings are psychotic. For them it is not simply a matter of being all religious or irreligious. They usually are not all compliant or non—compliant. Most human beings do a little of this and a little of that, not drawing a clear—cut line as Śrī Krishna did.

Someone may not be too particular about scriptural injunctions, but that does not mean that he does not have a sentiment for religion. He may attend the temple, church or mosque and do so with a declared and a seemingly—sincere faith. Such a person might even take up austerities at random and complete them fittingly.

श्रीभगवानुवाच
त्रिविधा भवति श्रद्धा
देहिनां सा स्वभावजा ।
सात्त्विकी राजसी चैव
तामसी चेति तां श्रृणु ॥ १७.२ ॥
śrībhagavānuvāca
trividhā bhavati śraddhā
dehināṁ sā svabhāvajā
sāttvikī rājasī caiva
tāmasī ceti tāṁ śṛṇu (17.2)

śrī bhagavān — The Blessed Lord; uvāca — said; trividhā — three types; bhavati — there is; śraddhā — confidence; dehināṁ — of the embodied souls; sā — anyone; svabhāvajā — produced from innate tendency; sāttvikī — clarifying; rājasī — motivating; caiva — and indeed; tāmasī — depression; ceti = ca — and + iti — thus; tāṁ — this; śṛṇu — hear

The Mahābhārata contains no chapter headings. This title was assigned by the translator on the basis of verse 2 of this chapter.

The Blessed Lord said: According to innate tendency, there are three types of confidences of the embodied souls. These are clarifying, motivating and depressing. Hear about this. (17.2)

Commentary:

The key Sanskrit term is svabhāvajā which means produced of one's inherent nature. Such a nature is the substance of the subtle body through which we transmigrate and get these gross forms. Such a nature changes from time to time. It is not, in all cases, a consistent or constant medium of the being.

A person's confidence hinges on how he feels within. Thus a person might whimsically reject something that is in his interest and take to something that ruins him. He may do that with confidence because confidence is always there lurking in the background of the psyche.

सत्त्वानुरूपा सर्वस्य
श्रद्धा भवति भारत ।
श्रद्धामयोऽयं पुरुषो
यो यच्छ्रद्धः स एव सः ॥१७.३॥
sattvānurūpā sarvasya
śraddhā bhavati bhārata
śraddhāmayo'yaṁ puruṣo
yo yacchraddhaḥ sa eva saḥ (17.3)

sattvānurūpā = sattva — essential nature + anurūpā — according to; sarvasya — of every person; śraddhā — confidence; bhavati — becomes manifest; bhārata — O man of the Bharata family; śraddhāmayaḥ — made of faith, trend of confidence; 'yaṁ = ayaṁ — this; puruṣo = puruṣaḥ — human being; yo = yaḥ — who; yacchraddhah = yac (yad) — which + chraddhah (śraddhaḥ) — faith; sa = saḥ — he; eva — only; saḥ — he

Confidence becomes manifest according to the essential nature of the person, O man of the Bharata family. A human being follows his trend of confidence. Whatever type of faith he has, that he expresses only. (17.3)

Commentary:

The essential nature, the fabric and texture of one's being may change from time to time, all depending on the influences that prevail. One's faith is expressed according to the particular energies which predominate at any given time and place.

As Śrī Krishna says, a human being follows a natural trend. Whatever type of faith a person has, that he expresses only. After all, what else can anyone do?

यजन्ते सात्त्विका देवान्
यक्षरक्षांसि राजसाः ।
प्रेतान्भूतगणांश्चान्ये
यजन्ते तामसा जनाः ॥१७.४॥
yajante sāttvikā devān
yakṣarakṣāṁsi rājasāḥ
pretānbhūtagaṇāṁścānye
yajante tāmasā janāḥ (17.4)

yajante — they worship; sāttvikā — clear-minded people; devān — supernatural rulers; yakṣarakṣāṁsi = yakṣa — passionate sorcerers + rakṣāṁsi — to cannibalistic powerful humans; rājasāḥ — impulsive people; pretān — the departed spirits; bhūtagaṇāṁścānye = bhūtagaṇān — hordes of ghosts + ca — and + anye — others; yajante — they petition; tāmasā = retarded; janāḥ — people

The clear—minded people worship the supernatural rulers. The impulsive ones worship the passionate sorcerers and the cannibalistic humans. The others, the retarded people, petition the departed spirits and the hordes of ghosts. (17.4)

Commentary:

This is a description of those human beings who are inclined to worship an authority. This does not cover the human beings who are averse to venerating a personality. Some human beings seek out an energy source or causal power which is not a personality. In some Vaishnava groups all persons who avoid personal authority are branded as impersonalists, in a "*we—are—devotees*" and "*they—are—impersonalists*" prejudice. In any case, the whole existence is still one reality. Whatever we find within it that is suitable to us and whatever we locate to which we form a bias, is still part of the whole reality.

The clear—minded people, due to higher perception, perceive the supernatural rulers. These gods are part of the Universal Form which Arjuna perceived. They regulate the existences. They are worthy of respect.

Persons who are dominated by the passionate energies take to worshipping powerful human beings who exhibit charismatic influence but who are not major components in the Universal Form. Such persons are throw—offs from the Form, separated aspects as they were. Since they are now disconnected but have great persuasive powers, they mistake themselves for being gods in their own right. Thus they form factions with those who are irresistably attracted to them. Creating their own religions or ideologies, these charismatic leaders act in opposition to the Universal Form. Usually they come to ruination.

Many retarded people have psychic sensitivity. They detect the departed spirits and the hordes of ghosts who hover in astral dimensions. Feeling akin to those, they worship for powers in the hope of gaining more intelligence so that they can better exploit human society, a community which sets them apart as being non—functional and idiotic.

Kriyā yogis come from every group of worshippers. The important thing is that a kriyā yogi works from where he is in his present life. He develops himself by constant practice. There are many yogis who started as simpletons and who by practice reclaimed their sensibilities and advanced to become masters. Some did yoga in order to gain cultural or political ascension. As soon as they attained that they gave up the kriyā practice, remained favorable to their teachers, but departed for fulfillments in the social and political arenas. Such persons will again return to kriyā practice in some future birth.

अशास्त्रविहितं घोरं
तप्यन्ते ये तपो जनाः ।
दम्भाहंकारसंयुक्ताः
कामरागबलान्विताः ॥ १७.५ ॥
aśāstravihitaṁ ghoraṁ
tapyante ye tapo janāḥ
dambhāhaṁkārasaṁyuktāḥ
kāmarāgabalānvitāḥ (17.5)

aśāstravihitaṁ = aśāstra — not of scripture + vihitaṁ — recommended; ghoraṁ — terrible; tapyante — tbey endure; ye — who; tapo = tapaḥ — austerity; janāḥ — people; dambhāhaṁkārasaṁyuktāḥ = dambha — deceit + ahaṁkāra — misplaced identity + saṁyuktāḥ — enthused with; kāmarāgabalānvitāḥ = kāma — craving + rāga — rage + bala — brute force + anvitāḥ — possessed with

People who endure terrible austerities which are not recommended in the scripture, people who are enthused with deceit and misplaced identity, who are possessed with craving, rage and brute force, (17.5)

कर्शयन्तः शरीरस्थं
भूतग्राममचेतसः ।
मां चैवान्तःशरीरस्थं
तान्विद्ध्यासुरनिश्चयान् ॥ १७.६ ॥

karśayantaḥ — torturing, troubling; śarīrasthaṁ — within the body; bhūtagrāmam — collection of elements; acetasaḥ — senseless; māṁ — me; caivantaḥ = ca — and + eva — indeed + antaḥ — within; śarīrasthaṁ — within the body; tān

karśayantaḥ śarīrasthaṁ
bhūtagrāmamacetasaḥ
māṁ caivāntaḥśarīrasthaṁ
tānviddhyāsuraniścayān (17.6)

— *them; viddhi — know; āsura — wicked; niścayān — intentions*

...those who torture the collection of the elements which comprise the body, who also trouble Me within the body, know that they have wicked intentions. (17.6)

Commentary:

In every case, a limited being is under the influence of persons and forces. None of us is free to do as we please. When we are happy about something, it means that we are favorably responsive to a particular influence. When we are distraught, we prefer not to be under that specific association. In kriyā yoga, we sort out the various influences and stick to preferences by positioning ourselves in certain psychological niches. There is deliberation in a human being but it is done under certain influences only. No one is so isolated that his deliberation is completely independent of everything else.

The austerities which are not recommended in the scriptures but which spring from ulterior motives, come from persons and forces which are positioned to defy the Universal Form. Śrī Krishna keynoted the life of Duryodhana, the opposing Kuru prince, who practiced yoga with ulterior motives. In the *Mahābhārata* it is described that once when he lay down to sleep, his subtle body was pulled into a parallel world where he met a horde of ghostly persons who were of a demonic clan. They wanted rights to enter into earthly wombs. Addressing Duryodhana as dear son, dear brother, they petitioned him to set up conditions for their entry into earthly wombs. This is what he was working for. That is why he opposed the Pandavas. At least that was the psychological basis for his objection to their rule.

With Prince Yudhiṣṭhira ruling, that horde of ghosts would get no chance of taking human forms in the Kuru territory, something they craved tremendously. Thus they empowered Duryodhana to fight on their behalf. With King Yudhiṣṭhira, a different group of spirits would take bodies. Those who were akin to him would bar entry to the group Duryodhana supported.

Warfare deals primarily with supernatural hassles between one horde of ghosts and another, all seeking predominance on earth. We interpret this as one race against the other or one nation versus the other. The real cause is supernatural. It appears that Śrī Krishna hurled a certain group of spirits into a cross world. He had no intentions of allowing them to escape from confinement. On the level of the Universal Form He fought all persons who wanted to assist them. He used barbaric methods of fighting to include, biting, chewing and blow—torching.

If we want to do karma yoga, we will have to get involved in such things either openly as warriors like Arjuna or covertly as nice-guy priests and philanthropists who help a particular group while neglecting others. In truth we have preferences. There will always be a group of departed souls who want to enter into the human world to displace and predominate others. Such is this existence.

Śrī Krishna mentioned that the demonic people trouble Him within their bodies. This means the subtle and causal forms, not the physical one. Śrī Krishna in His supersoul feature is not directly situated in the physical body. His influence filters down through the causal and subtle forms. Demonic people who trouble Him as He claims, do so instinctively and not consciously. When one is in such a state of mind, one does not have direct perception to know that God lives in the psyche. This is because the more demonic we are, the more darkness surrounds us in the sky of consciousness and the more unable we are to see supernaturally. Thus we focus more sharply on what we do see, which are the objects in the material atmosphere. We disavow that there is a God.

However from another angle, the denial is itself evidence of God. It is the force of God that causes a demon to deny Him, just as wayward teenagers do whatever is contrary to what their parents desire. In such cases, if the parents say no, the teenager says yes. If the parent says yes, the teenager says no. If the parents act indifferently, the juvenile embraces whatever it is. Thus in a demonic mentality, we instinctively do whatever is opposed to the Supersoul Personality.

That is the problem with karma yoga. To be a perfect karma yogi, one has to represent God in the cultural and political environments. This means that one will have to take the resentments and hostilities which are directed to God, just as Arjuna had to take the anger of the opposing Kurus. One must be courageous in sacrificing oneself for Śrī Krishna.

It is this facility of karma yoga, that has caused some spiritual masters in the disciplic succession from Śrī Krishna to label karma yoga as bhakti yoga. Actually karma yoga is not bhakti yoga but when we consider that a karma yogi has to sacrifice himself for the Universal Form it appears to be a kind of love for Krishna. And thus we may call it a type of devotional service, a type of affection for the Lord.

If one reads Śrīla Bhaktivedanta Swami's *Bhagavad Gītā* commentary, one will see that in almost every instance he converts karma yoga into bhakti yoga. This is because a great sacrifice is required of any karma yogi like Arjuna. However for the purpose of kriyā yoga, we are not much interested in that sort of sacrifice. It pertains to work in this world. It does not bring on spiritual perfection by itself. It must be transferred into more advanced kriyā practice. We see this in the life of Arjuna and his brothers. They had to resume the kriyā practice later on in their lives. Śrīla Bhaktivedanta Swami conveyed the idea that they just went back to Godhead. Exactly where he got that idea from, I do not know. The *Mahābhārata* does not say that. Śrīla Bhaktivedanta Swami, however, the god that he was, walking on this earth in human form, should not be neglected or disrespected. His intention was to make people conscious of the existence of Śrī Krishna and to make them know that Śrī Krishna is the Supreme Personality of Godhead, unrivaled and unparalleled.

Śrī Krishna is there in the psyche as the Supersoul but to see Him as such requires mystic clarity. This is gained by very advanced yoga practice when one can see into the sky of consciousness, when the supernatural darkness that surrounds one's spirit is dissipated.

आहारस्त्वपि सर्वस्य
त्रिविधो भवति प्रियः ।
यज्ञस्तपस्तथा दानं
तेषां भेदमिमं शृणु ॥ १७.७॥
āhārastvapi sarvasya
trividho bhavati priyaḥ
yajñastapastathā dānaṁ
teṣāṁ bhedamimaṁ śṛṇu (17.7)

āhāraḥ — food; tu — but; api — as well; sarvasya — of all; trividho = trividhaḥ — three kinds; bhavati — is; priyaḥ— likes; yajñaḥ— religious ceremony; tapaḥ — austerity; tathā— as; dānaṁ — charity; teṣāṁ — of them; bhedam — difference; imaṁ — this; śṛṇu — hear

But food as well, which is liked by all, is of three kinds, as are religious ceremony, austerity and charity. Hear of the difference between them. (17.7)

Commentary:

Our worship intentions, food, religious ceremony, austerity and charity are all sectioned off depending on the kind of energy we use. The energy which is available dictates what we will or will not do. It is in our interest to recognize the various influences to which we may be subjected in these transmigrations. One should be able to admit when one is in the lower mode. One should learn how to avoid the lower energies and how to maintain oneself on higher levels.

आयुःसत्त्वबलारोग्य—
सुखप्रीतिविवर्धनाः ।
रस्याः स्निग्धाः स्थिरा हृद्या
आहाराः सात्त्विकप्रियाः ॥ १७.८॥
āyuḥsattvabalārogya—
sukhaprītivivardhanāḥ
rasyāḥ snigdhāḥ sthirā hṛdyā
āhārāḥ sāttvikapriyāḥ (17.8)

āyuḥsattvabalārogya = āyuḥ — duration of life + sattva — spiritual well-being + bala — strength + ārogya — health; sukhaprītivivardhanāḥ = sukha — happiness + prīti — satisfaction + vivardhanāḥ — increasing; rasyāḥ — juicy; snigdhāḥ — milky; sthirā — sustaining; hṛdyā — palatable; āhārāḥ — foods; sāttvikapriyāḥ — dear to the clear-minded people

Foods which increase the duration of the life, the spiritual well-being, strength, health, happiness and satisfaction, which are juicy, milky, sustaining and palatable, are eatables which are dear to the clear-minded people. (17.8)

Commentary:

Food is related to consciousness. From food, subtle energy is derived. This subtle energy activates, supports and monitors our consciousness. The wrong type of foods produces a reduction in objectivity and a proportional dullness which causes us to miscalculate.

It may be said that today's food is tomorrow's consciousness. Or rather, what you ate in the morning influences how you think in the evening. Physical food has subtle counterparts which affect the subtle body. People who live on celestial planets use celestial food only, but so do the departed spirits who have left animal or human forms in the physical world. These ghostly creatures also procure subtle food according to their particular selections and habits.

Śrī Krishna gave a general classification of foods which promote clarity of consciousness. In kriyā yoga we take this guideline. We adjust our diet according to the level of practice. For the purpose of yoga there should be no animal bodies eaten. One may take milk from bovine creatures like cows, buffalo or goats, but one may not eat these creatures or any other type of animal or fish. A kriyā yogi should also not take peppered or spicy foods. The best diet is dairy products, vegetables, fruits and nuts. When preparing cooked foods, one should not mix up various items. It is preferred that each type of food be cooked separately, prepared in such a way as to bring out the natural flavor. Spices should be used sparingly. They should not predominate over the natural flavor of the particular foods to which they are added.

There is a rule for eating in kriyā yoga. It is this: One should eat to facilitate the practice of yoga. For instance, if one eats heavy meals at night or if one eats at night at all, then his yoga practice may be inefficient in the morning. Thus one should give up night eating to facilitate the practice.

Devotees of Krishna who do not do yoga, have this idea that so long as they take foods which were offered to the deity of Śrī Krishna, there is no harm. They feel that such foods may be taken at any time without interference to their spiritual life. These views stem mostly from the *Śrī Caitanya Caritāmṛta*, a text of Krishna das Kaviraj Goswami. In that text, there are many descriptions of the glories and spiritually—elevating properties of the food which is offered to the Deities.

However for those of us who do yoga, we cannot submit ourselves regularly to much late night eating, even of sanctified foods. On special occasions like the Appearance Days of the Deities and of the great spiritual masters, we should honor the official fasting and eating schedules but on other days night meals should be avoided totally.

A yogi should eat to facilitate the practice. That is the rule. It depends on his stage of advancement. For instance, when I first began doing Kuṇḍalinī yoga, I ate mostly during the day. Sometimes I ate at night but that was due to previous habit and mixing with Americans who considered a night meal as essential. Later on, with progression, I got rid of night eating but I increased the quantity of food I took during the day.

When I joined the Hare Krishna Society established by Śrīla Prabhupāda Bhaktivedanta Swami my yoga practice came to a standstill because yoga was prohibited by him. To remain in his ashram, I had to abandon my practice completely. His followers were highly critical of it and considered all yogis to be impersonalist rascals. After I left the society, I resumed the practice. Then I continued the daytime eating with no nighttime meals. After my practice accelerated, I reduced the daytime eating too. I ceased all late afternoon meals.

Later on with more advancement, I had a last meal for the day at around noon. Now I have only one main meal in the morning. This was all done to facilitate haţha yoga postures and prāṇāyāma breathing exercises. From those two practices, one can build a foundation for deep meditation, samādhi.

One's food should be sanctified but that does not mean that one should eat sanctified food at any and all times. I feel that Lord Caitanya's stress on the potency of sanctified food was given to highlight deity worship and its related procedures. I do not feel that He meant we should eat at any or all times. If on festival days, we are offered food at some odd hour of the night, then we should take it as Śrī Krishna's mercy on us but that does not mean that we should do this as a habit.

A yogi, if he is at all in his right mind, should never refuse sanctified food. It is a great insult to the Deity and to the devotees who endeavor to prepare it. One should take it promptly and appreciate the opportunity to eat it. However one should not make it a habit to eat large quantities in the late afternoon or at night.

Let us remember that according to the *Gītā*, yoga means isolation for serious practice. If you are isolated, you will not be in a place where you can get even sanctified food offered to you at any and every hour of the day or night. All the great yogi devotees of the past, took sanctified food but they also ate to facilitate the practice. Even Śrī Krishna and Arjuna who did the kriyā yoga practice to perfection, did stop eating during some strict austerities for the sake of entering the samādhi phase of practice. We should read in the *Mahābhārata* about this.

In this existence, food is a basic need but it is also a craving. Thus we have to be careful that we do not use prasadam sanctified food to further the craving or to legitimize it. If we do this, our spiritual life will pan out eventually. We will end up as rejected devotees. Śrī Krishna will not like to see any of us in that sorry condition. If one uses the holy name of the Lord and the holy food which is offered to Him, as a justification to continue sordid habits or greeds, one will be cast aside by the very same holy name and sanctified food. Sanat Kumāra once told King Dhṛtarāṣṭra that the holy name abandons a devotee who misuses it, just as birds fly away from a tree upon which they were disturbed.

कट्वम्लवणात्युष्ण-
तीक्ष्णरूक्षविदाहिनः ।
आहारा राजसस्येष्टा
दुःखशोकामयप्रदाः ॥ १७.९ ॥
kaṭvamlalavaṇātyuṣṇa-
tīkṣṇarūkṣavidāhinaḥ
āhārā rājasasyeṣṭā
duḥkhaśokāmayapradāḥ (17.9)

kaṭvamlalavaṇātyuṣṇa = kaṭv (kaṭu) — pungent + amla — sour + lavaṇa — salt; atyuṣṇa —peppery; tīkṣnarūkṣavidāhinaḥ = tīkṣṇa — acidic + rūkṣa — dry + vidāhinaḥ — overheated; āhārā — foods; rājasasyeṣṭā = rajasasya — of the passionate people + iṣṭā — desired; duḥkhaśokāmayapradāḥ = duḥkha — pain + śoka — misery + āmaya — sickness + pradāḥ — causing

Foods which are pungent, sour, salty, peppery, acidic, dry and overheated, are desired by the passionate people. These foods cause pain, misery and sickness. (17.9)

Commentary:

Pungent, sour, salty, peppery, and acidic foods have strong chemicals which affect the brain of the body. These foods have a slightly narcotic or stimulant effect. Peppers for instance, which are a favorite of Indians, have a stimulant chemical. One becomes addicted to peppers without knowing it. The addiction is mild, like the addiction to coffee or betel nuts. It is experienced that once a devotee becomes addicted to peppers he cannot live without them. Unfortunately if one took birth in an Indian family, he was more than likely addicted from infancy due to his mother's pepper addiction.

Some sour, pungent, and acidic fruits and herbs are good for medicinal purposes. These should not be confused with nourishing foods. For nutritional purposes one should stay away from such items, even though quantities of these are required for medicinal usage. One should be clear about the distinction between medicinal intake and nutritional foodstuffs.

Dry or overheated foods should not be taken. Dry foods make for a hard stool. Haṭha yoga practice is ruined by an intake of dry foods. Super—heated food taken at a temperature which burns the tongue, is obviously harmful to the very body which it is supposed to nourish.

Right now due to the rampant and indiscriminate but convenient use of chemical fertilizers, we have much pain and distress. We have to realize that our bodies are not designed to use those chemicals. We contaminate water supplies and affect the water dependent species. All such sordid activities which short—circuit the system of reciprocation established by Brahmā, the creator god, will bring adverse reactions in this and in succeeding lives.

We should make an effort to go back to animal manure and composting, abandoning the much easier method of chemical fertilizers. Otherwise we will ruin the body's health and jeopardize every other species.

यातयामं गतरसं
पूति पर्युषितं च यत् ।
उच्छिष्टमपि चामेध्यं
भोजनं तामसप्रियम् ॥ १७.१० ॥

yātayāmaṁ — stale; gatarasaṁ — tasteless; pūti — rotten; paryuṣitaṁ — left over; ca — and; yat = yad — which; ucchiṣṭam — rejected; api — also; cāmedhyam = ca — and

yātayāmaṁ gatarasaṁ
pūti paryuṣitaṁ ca yat
ucchiṣṭamapi cāmedhyaṁ
bhojanaṁ tāmasapriyam (17.10)

+ amedhyaṁ — unfit for religious ceremony; bhojanaṁ — food; tāmasapriyam.— cherished by the depressed people

Food which is stale, tasteless, and rotten, which was left over, as well as that which is rejected or unfit for religious ceremony, is cherished by the depressed people. (17.10)

Commentary:

It is established by Lord Śrī Caitanya Mahāprabhu that prasadam, sanctified food which was offered to Śrī Krishna's Deity, is never to be considered stale. Because of the sanctification, it is exempt from the ruling of this verse. Otherwise one should stay away from stale, tasteless or rotten food, as well as anything that is left over from persons who are not advanced.

Since our consciousness is, in a way, boosted or depressed by the type of food we eat, it is very counterproductive to eat stale, tasteless or rotten foods. The energy in such food would dull or sicken our psychology. Some other species have body types which are nourished by stale, tasteless or rotten foods but if a yogi eats these, it would lower his psychology.

There are exceptions, however. We heard of ancient yogis who ate questionable food. These were rare incidences, after those yogis became very advanced and after they manifested perfectional powers which nullified the adverse effects.

अफलाकाङ्क्षिभिर्यज्ञो
विधिदृष्टो य इज्यते ।
यष्टव्यमेवेति मनः
समाधाय स सात्त्विकः ॥ १७.११ ॥
aphalākāṅkṣibhiryajño
vidhidṛṣṭo ya ijyate
yaṣṭavyameveti manaḥ
samādhāya sa sāttvikaḥ (17.11)

aphalākāṅkṣibhiḥ = aphalā — no benefits + kāṅkṣibhiḥ — desiring; yajño = yajñaḥ — a religious discipline or ceremony; vidhidṛṣṭo — vidhidṛṣṭaḥ = vidhi — scripture + dṛṣṭaḥ — observing; ya — who; ijyate — is offered; yaṣṭavyam — to be sacrificed; eveti = eva — indeed + iti — thus; manaḥ — mind; samādhāya — concentrating; sa —it; sāttvikaḥ — realistic

A religious discipline or ceremony in observance of the scripture, by those who do not desire a benefit and who, while concentrating, think, "This is to be sacrificed," is a ceremony of the realistic type. (17.11)

Commentary:

This is the type of ceremony which Brahmā instructed his sons to perform. Nowadays it is difficult to do the procedure. We are bogged down with a reward—seeking mentality. We should make every endeavor to act in this detached duty—bound way where we do not desire a benefit from the religious activities, where we do it as a matter of course and to please Krishna and Brahmā, the affectionate creator—god.

अभिसंधाय तु फलं
दम्भार्थमपि चैव यत् ।
इज्यते भरतश्रेष्ठ

abhisandhāya — kept in mind; tu — but; phalam — benefit; dambhārtham — for the sake of outsmarting the deity; api — also;

तं यज्ञं विद्धि राजसम् ॥ १७.१२ ॥
abhisaṁdhāya tu phalaṁ
dambhārthamapi caiva yat
ijyate bharataśreṣṭha
taṁ yajñaṁ viddhi rājasam (17.12)

caiva — and indeed; yat = yad — which; ijyate — is offered; bharataśreṣṭha — best of the Bhāratas; tam — this; yajñaṁ — disciplined worship; viddhi — know; rājasam — impulsive

But when a benefit is kept in mind and when the motive is to outsmart the deity, know, O best of the Bharatas, that the disciplinary worship offered is based on impulsion. (17.12)

Commentary:

This is a key verse for understanding how to perform a religious ceremony, regarding what not to do and what attitude not to assume. This applies even to chanting the holy names. Even though one is encouraged to call on the name of the Lord in adversity to get help and relief and for other purposes, the plain truth is that these uses for the holy name are actually outlawed by the *Gītā*.

One should not use any sort of religious procedure for a cultural benefit. If one does this, one will in the course of time, be ruined.

We are under the pressure of many impulsions which come from here or there, but regardless, we should try to free ourselves from the numerous influences and stick to the guidelines in the *Gītā*. Religions that compromise or adjust the *Gītā*, should, in the course of time, be abandoned. This applies even to religions which have sprung up in the Vaishnava system of belief but which give us allowance to ignore the stipulations of the *Gītā*. Gradually one should shed the need for such allowances and take to the *Gītā* as it was delivered to Arjuna.

विधिहीनमसृष्टान्नं
मन्त्रहीनमदक्षिणम् ।
श्रद्धाविरहितं यज्ञं
तामसं परिचक्षते ॥ १७.१३ ॥
vidhihīnamasṛṣṭānnaṁ
mantrahīnamadakṣiṇam
śraddhāvirahitaṁ yajñaṁ
tāmasaṁ paricakṣate (17.13)

vidhihīnam — scripture neglected; asṛṣṭānnaṁ = asṛṣṭa — not offered + annam — food; mantrahīnam — Vedic hymn not recited; adakṣiṇam — no fee for the priest; śraddhāvirahitaṁ — confidence lacking; yajñaṁ — disciplinary worship; tāmasaṁ — depressive; paricakṣate — they regard

When scripture is neglected, food is not offered, Vedic hymns not recited, a fee not given to the priest, and confidence is lacking, regard that disciplinary worship as depressive. (17.13)

Commentary:

This applies directly to the religious way of life in the time of Śrī Krishna and Arjuna. We may apply it to own time and place as follows: A religion should not be created on the basis of our current opinions and needs. We should check with posterity to see what was done before.

As far as possible, one should try to adopt the ancient procedure for religious ceremonies. The modern culture of a technologically—advanced civilization does not have the proper basis for religion. Nowadays there is more dependence on man—made gadgets. Our minds are surcharged with media through newspapers, radio, television and computer communications. Even though we assume that we are freer than our ancestors, in a way, we are even more confined than they were. And of course, we ourselves were the very ancestors whom we denigrate.

This does not mean that we should be naive or superstitious or stubbornly cling to a belief of the past. We have to approach religion in a balanced way.

At religious ceremonies, scriptures should be recited, preferably Vedic scriptures. A priest should be invited. He should be given a fee. One should not call a priest if one cannot afford his fee or if one cannot give him the money without resentment. If one feels the fee is too high, one should not engage his services. Out of modesty some priests do not stipulate a fee. They leave it to the host to determine a suitable stipend. In that case one should give as much as one can afford and offer additional items like freshly—picked fruits or new pieces of fabric. One should facilitate the priest by offering transportation and by making sure that he is escorted to his home when the function is finished.

A preacher may be invited to preach at one's home or to explain the complexities of life. Such a person should be treated respectfully even if his body is younger in age. One should give that person the proper accommodations and should never ask him to lay down or to stay in an unclean place or in a place unsuitable for human habitation.

One should be mindful of the needs of a priest or preacher since such a person might have particular ways in which he prefers to be treated. Even if one is wealthy, one should afford the priest or preacher the option of staying in a well furnished or a very simple outfitted area of one's home. Some priests and preachers prefer a simple setting while others are at ease in luxurious surroundings. One should not force a priest or preacher to stay at a luxurious place. Sometimes one invites a priest in whom one has little or no confidence. One might do this under pressure from that priest or in a competitive mood to a neighbor. This is not a good tactic. One should not invite a religious leader, who one shuns or hates.

देवद्विजगुरुप्राज्ञ—
पूजनं शौचमार्जवम् ।
ब्रह्मचर्यमहिंसा च
शारीरं तप उच्यते ॥१७.१४॥
devadvijagurprājña—
pūjanaṁ śaucamārjavam
brahmacaryamahiṁsā ca
śārīraṁ tapa ucyate (17.14)

devadvijagurprājña = deva — supernatural ruler + dvija = those who are qualified by sacred thread ceremony + guru — spiritual teacher + prājña — wise man; pūjanaṁ — reverential respect; śaucam — purity; ārjavam — straightforwardness; brahmacaryam — celibacy; ahiṁsā — non — violence; ca — and; śārīraṁ — body; tapa — austerity; ucyate — is said to be

Reverential respect of the supernatural rulers, of those who are qualified by the sacred thread ceremony, of the spiritual teacher, and of the wise man, purity, straightforwardness, celibacy and non—violence, are said to be austerity of the body. (17.14)

Commentary:

At last, Śrī Krishna mentions pūjanam, reverential respects of the spiritual master. He itemizes others like the deva supernatural rulers, dvijas or twice—born individuals of the three higher castes in India, and of the wise man. We should note that Śrī Krishna does not go overboard here in respect to the worship of a spiritual master. Here he does not ridicule nor ban the worship of the deva supernatural rulers.

I say this because it has come down in some disciplic successions, that the worship of the devas is taboo. With this etiquette, one does not necessarily respect a brahmin unless he is a Vaishnava in one's succession of teachers. However that approach is not given in the *Gītā*.

For kriyā yoga, the *Gītā* is most important. We desire to follow these verses to the letter. Reverential respect should be offered to those teachers whom we regard as our gurus. We can have more than one guru. Our guru does not have to be a Vaishnava missionary. Anyone who gives us the techniques of kriyā yoga which effect psyche purification is one of our gurus.

A person may not be one of our gurus, initiated as a member of the three higher castes in India but if he is wise, we should respect him. We have to be free of prejudice so that we can see what is what. One should not disrespect anyone since that will cause harm to oneself in return.

Purity is purity of the psyche which is a tall order for any living being. It takes years of austerity in yoga practice to achieve that. Anyone can take a bath but to clean the mind, emotions and life force is a hard achievement. For ordinary religion, a bath and the effort to be truthful, is sufficient.

Straightforwardness like purity was listed before as one of the godly qualities. As far as possible one should be straightforward consistently. However for ordinary religion one should be polite in dealings.

In kriyā yoga, celibacy is an on—going quest. It must be achieved for success. It is done by haţha yoga, prāṇāyāma and mystic means. In ordinary religions, if a man stays with his wife and if he is able to refrain from over—indulgences, he is regarded as celibate. This is the minimum level of celibacy.

In Vedic functions, the yajnam or sacrificial performer is usually instructed by the priest to be celibate on some days prior to the functions. This is stipulated in the Vedic literature. The number of days varies according to the specific ceremony performed.

Non—violence here means refraining from killing any creatures physically. This includes small bugs, even nuisance insects like mosquitoes. On religious days one should refrain from any type of violence in the matter of killing other creatures. For a kriyā yogi this is a basic requirement for all time. Sometimes a yogi moves from a place in which he would be forced to commit violence. If a yogi goes to live in a forest, and if he is attacked by wild animals, he might have to relocate to avoid committing violence. As far as possible one should not kill other creatures. Yet one should not let them act violently to one's body since one's body is valuable because of its capacity to facilitate liberation.

अनुद्वेगकरं वाक्यं
सत्यं प्रियहितं च यत् ।
स्वाध्यायाभ्यसनं चैव
वाङ्मयं तप उच्यते ॥ १७.१५॥
anudvegakaraṁ vākyaṁ
satyaṁ priyahitaṁ ca yat
svādhyāyābhyasanaṁ caiva
vāṅmayaṁ tapa ucyate (17.15)

anudvegakaraṁ — not causing distress; vākyaṁ — speech; satyam — truthful; priyahitam — agreeable and beneficial; ca — and; yat = yad — which; svādhyāyābhyasanaṁ = svādhyāya — recitation of scripture + abhyasanaṁ — practice, regularity; caiva — and indeed; vāṅmayaṁ — speech — made; tapa — discipline; ucyate — is called

Speech which does not cause distress, and is truthful, agreeable and beneficial, as well as regular recitation of the scriptures is the discipline of speech. (17.15)

Commentary:

To honor this request of disciplined speech, one must be in an environment which does not evoke resentment and anger. Such a place is described as an ashram, a place where spiritual life is foremost. We have to create an environment that fosters spiritual life. To do this, we must abandon places and people who cause agitation. There is a technicality, however, in that if we do restrain ourselves but do not become purified in fact, the resentments and anger will remain dormant. That will not suit the objective of kriyā yoga.

The hermitage environment should be there and the purity should be astride so that resentments and anger exit our nature.

मनःप्रसादः सौम्यत्वं
मौनमात्मविनिग्रहः ।
भावसंशुद्धिरित्येतत्
तपो मानसमुच्यते ॥ १७.१६ ॥
manaḥprasādaḥ saumyatvaṁ
maunamātmavinigrahaḥ
bhāvasaṁśuddhirityetat
tapo mānasamucyate (17.16)

manaḥprasādaḥ = manah — mind + prasādaḥ — peace; saumayatvaṁ — gentleness; maunam —silence; ātmavinigrahaḥ — self—restraint; bhāvasaṁśuddhiḥ = bhāva — being + saṁśuddhiḥ — purity; iti — thus, etat = etad — this; tapo = tapaḥ — discipline; mānasam — of the mind; ucyate — is called

Peace of mind, gentleness, silence, self restraint, and purity of being, this is called discipline of mind. (17.16)

Commentary:

This is a description of the accomplishment of kriyā yoga. It yields peace of mind, gentleness, silence, self—restraint and purity of being. These are all results of advanced yoga practice. Self—restraint is the same as pratyāhār sense withdrawal. Purity of being is effected by kuṇḍalinī yoga and by purity of the psyche yoga. Silence is effected in the stage of yoga which is dhyāna, contemplation. It means that the buddhi organ in the mind of the subtle body has stopped its impulsive willy—nilly imaginings and subtle soundings. Gentleness comes when one has mastered his interaction with the social world. That happens when one gets a waiver from the Supreme Being so that one does not have to perform karma yoga on His behalf and one can completely step aside from the social scene. And lastly peace of mind comes when one masters samādhi practice. One cannot achieve these states without practicing yoga.

श्रद्धया परया तप्तं
तपस्तत्त्रिविधं नरैः ।
अफलाकाङ्क्षिभिर्युक्तैः
सात्त्विकं परिचक्षते ॥ १७.१७॥
śraddhayā parayā taptaṁ
tapastattrividhaṁ naraiḥ
aphalākāṅkṣibhiryuktaiḥ
sāttvikaṁ paricakṣate (17.17)

śraddhayā — with faith; parayā — with the highest; taptam — performed; tapaḥ — austerity; tat = tad — this; trividham — three — fold; naraih — by people; aphalākāṅkṣibhiḥ — by those who do not aspire for a benefit; yuktaiḥ — by those disciplined in yoga; sāttvikaṁ — realistic; paricakṣate — they consider

When this threefold austerity is performed with the highest faith by yogicly—disciplined people who do not aspire for a benefit, the authorities consider it to be realistic. (17.17)

Commentary:

The threefold austerity of the body, speech and mind is a tall order but some commentators took the liberal gesture of explaining these disciplines in a way which make them seem easy to attain even by an undisciplined person. Many commentators fail to realize that these three austerities cannot be completed without the use of yoga. They give audiences the idea that it can be done just as we are, without any type of yoga practice. This is a misrepresentation of these *Gītā* verses.

The Sanskrit word yukta pertains to the yogicly—disciplined people. Others can try to reach up to these requirements but they will not attain the completion, because the power of yoga is needed to achieve that, just as Arjuna needs to apply that power in his battlefield work as stipulated by Śrī Krishna.

सत्कारमानपूजार्थं
तपो दम्भेन चैव यत् ।
क्रियते तदिह प्रोक्तं
राजसं चलमध्रुवम् ॥ १७.१८ ॥
satkāramānapūjārthaṁ
tapo dambhena caiva yat
kriyate tadiha proktaṁ
rājasaṁ calamadhruvam (17.18)

satkāramānapūjārthaṁ = satkāra — reputation +māna — respect + pūjā — reverence + arthaṁ — for the sake of; tapo = tapaḥ — austerity; dambhena — with trickery; caiva — and indeed; yat = yad — which; kriyate — performed; tat — this; iha — in this world; proktaṁ — is declared; rājasaṁ — impulsive; calam — shifty; adhruvam — temporary

Austerity which, in this world is performed with trickery for the sake of reputation, respect and reverence, is declared to be impulsive, shifty and temporary. (17.18)

Commentary:

It is quite natural for most persons to try for this three—fold austerity of the body, speech, and mind for acquiring celebrity status, attracting the admiration of others, and getting reverence. Therefore we have to work hard with the yoga austerities to get the required purity. Then we could leave aside our insecurities which cause us to hound for fame, prestige and charismatic influence.

मूढग्राहेणात्मनो यत्
पीडया क्रियते तपः ।
परस्योत्सादनार्थं वा
तत्तामसमुदाहृतम् ॥ १७.१९ ॥
mūḍhagrāheṇātmano yat
pīḍayā kriyate tapaḥ
parasyotsādanārthaṁ vā
tattāmasamudāhṛtam (17.19)

mūḍhagrāheṇātmano = mūḍha — foolish + grāheṇa= by miṣṭaken ideas + ātmano (ātmanaḥ) — of the self; yat = yad — which; pīḍayā — with torture; kriyate — is performed; tapaḥ — austerity; parasyotsādanārthaṁ = parasya — of someone else + utsādana — harming + artham — purpose; vā — or; tat — that; tāmasam — depressive; udāhṛtam — said to be

Austerity performed with foolish, mistaken ideas, and with torture or for the purpose of harming someone else, is said to be depressive. (17.19)

Commentary:

This type of austerity is sponsored by resentment and the anger energy. It is created in and pushed by the energies of the depressive mode. One has to do his best to lift himself out of such conditions.

दातव्यमिति यद्दानं
दीयतेऽनुपकारिणे ।
देशे काले च पात्रे च
तद्दानं सात्त्विकं स्मृतम् ॥ १७.२० ॥
dātavyamiti yaddānaṁ
dīyate'nupakāriṇe
deśe kāle ca pātre ca
taddānaṁ sāttvikaṁ smṛtam (17.20)

dātavyam — to be given; iti — thus; yat — which; dānaṁ — gift; dīyate — is given; 'nupakāriṇe = anupakāriṇe — to one who has not done a prior favor; deśe — in proper place; kāle — at the proper time; ca — and; pātre — to a worthy person; ca — and; tat — that; dānaṁ — gift; sāttvikaṁ — virtuous; smṛtam — remembered as

A gift given to one who has not done a prior favor, in the proper place and time and to a worthy person, is remembered as being virtuous. (17.20)

Commentary:

This means that one should be a free spirit in the act of charity and in honored giving. Charity is usually offered to the needy. Honored giving is to someone who is not in need but who inspires one to give by his or her endearing nature.

यत्तु प्रत्युपकारार्थं
फलमुद्दिश्य वा पुनः ।
दीयते च परिक्लिष्टं
तद्दानं राजसं स्मृतम् ॥ १७.२१ ॥
yattu pratyupakārārthaṁ
phalamuddiśya vā punaḥ
dīyate ca parikliṣṭaṁ
taddānaṁ rājasaṁ smṛtam (17.21)

yat — which; tu — but; pratyupakārārthaṁ — for a compensation; phalam — a result; uddiśya — pointing to, hoping; vā — or; punaḥ — alternately; dīyate — is given; ca — and; parikliṣṭaṁ — grudgingly; tat — that; dānaṁ — gift; rājasaṁ — impulsive; smṛtam — mentally noted

But the gift which is given grudgingly for a compensation or alternately hoping for a reward, is mentally noted as being impulsive. (17.21)

Commentary:

The whole idea is ideal behavior. We should endeavor for purity in motive and a lack of assault in character dealings. Whatever is required to achieve this, should be done. Kriyā yoga really means a turning about so that we begin to see our faults and take up whatever reformatory methods effect their removal.

अदेशकाले यद्दानम्
अपात्रेभ्यश्च दीयते ।
असत्कृतमवज्ञातं
तत्तामसमुदाहृतम् ॥ १७.२२ ॥

adeśakāle — at the wrong place and time; yat — wbich; dānam — gift; apātrebhyaśca = apātrebhyaḥ — to an unworthy person + ca — and; dīyate — is given; asatkṛtam — without paying respect; avajñātaṁ — without due consideration; tat = tad — that;

adeśakāle yaddānam
apātrebhyaśca dīyate
asatkṛtamavajñātaṁ
tattāmasamudāhṛtam (17.22)

tāmasam — depressive mode; udāhrtam — is said to be

That gift which is given in the wrong place and time, to an unworthy person, without paying respect, without due consideration, is said to be of the depressive mode. (17.22)

Commentary:

There is really no point in giving such a gift. If we catch ourselves in such undesirable acts, we should stop and reconsider. The depressive or retardative mood is the most difficult to detect. When under its influence, we lose objectivity. Prāṇāyāma is the sure method to remove oneself from this lowest of modes. By prāṇāyāma also, we burn off the passionate energy and can use it constructively as guided by the clarifying feature. Yoga has such usage.

ओं तत्सदिति निर्देशो
ब्रह्मणस्त्रिविधः स्मृतः ।
ब्राह्मणास्तेन वेदाश्च
यज्ञाश्च विहिताः पुरा ॥१७.२३॥
oṁ tatsaditi nirdeśo
brahmaṇastrividhaḥ smṛtaḥ
brāhmaṇāstena vedāśca
yajñāśca vihitāḥ purā (17.23)

oṁ — Om; tat — Tat; sat = Sat; iti — pronouncement; nirdeśo = nirdeśaḥ — designation; brahmaṇaḥ — of spiritual reality; trividhaḥ — three-fold; smṛtaḥ — is known; brāhmaṇāḥ — by the brahmins; tena — by this; vedāsca = vedāh — of the Vedas + ca — and; yajnāśca = yajnāḥ — religious disciplines and ceremony + ca — and; vihitāḥ — prescribed; purā — ancient

The pronouncement *Om Tat Sat* is known as the threefold designation of spiritual reality. By this expression, the brahmins, the *Vedas*, and the prescribed religious disciplines and ceremonies were ordained in ancient times. (17.23)

Commentary:

Om Tat Sat was used by the ancient seers who used the *Vedas* as their primary scripture. In the times of the *Upanishads*, *Om Tat Sat* was used at every step especially in the consecration of brahmins, the recitation of the *Vedas* and the enactment of religious disciplines and ceremonies. We are not in the environment of those ancient sages. Everything changed considerably.

तस्मादोमित्युदाहृत्य
यज्ञदानतपःक्रियाः ।
प्रवर्तन्ते विधानोक्ताः
सततं ब्रह्मवादिनाम् ॥१७.२४॥
tasmādomityudāhṛtya
yajñadānatapaḥkriyāḥ
pravartante vidhānoktāḥ
satataṁ brahmavādinām (17.24)

tasmāt — hence; om — the sound Om; iti — thus; udāhṛtya — uttering; yajñadānatapaḥkriyāḥ = yajña — sacrifice + dāna — charity + tapaḥ — austerity + kriyaḥ — acts; pravartante — they begin; vidhānoktāḥ = vidhāna — prescription + uktāḥ — said; satatam — always; brahmavādinām — of the spiritual masters

Hence as prescribed in the *Vedic* scriptures, acts of sacrifice, charity, and austerity always begin by the spiritual masters while uttering the sound *Om*. (17.24)

Commentary:

Throughout the Vedic literature, especially in the *Vedas*, the *Upanishads* and the *Puranas*, the sound *Om* is stressed. Śrī Krishna used the terms brahmavādinām which means of the knowers of brahman.

One can chant *Om* properly if he is given it in a formal or informal initiation by a person who is a knower of brahman. Ultimately *Om* is heard in the supernatural world as a naturally occurring sound.

As kriyā yogins, we do not accept the instruction of modern Vaishnava teachers who ask us to hold a bias towards those who know of and advocate the brahman spiritual energy. Śrī Krishna did not condemn or express dislike for the brahmavādis. Therefore we have no bias against them.

तदित्यनभिसंधाय
फलं यज्ञतपःक्रियाः ।
दानक्रियाश्च विविधाः
क्रियन्ते मोक्षकाङ्क्षिभिः ॥ १७.२५ ॥
tadityanabhisaṁdhāya
phalaṁ yajñatapaḥkriyāḥ
dānakriyāśca vividhāḥ
kriyante mokṣakāṅkṣibhiḥ (17.25)

tat — Tat; iti — saying; anabhisaṁdhāya — without an interest; phalam — benefit; yajñatapaḥkriyāḥ= yajña — sacrifice + tapaḥ — austerity + kriyaḥ— actions; dānakriyāśca = dānakriyāḥ— acts of charity + ca — and; vividhāḥ— various types; kriyante — are performed; mokṣakāṅkṣibhiḥ — by those who desire liberation

While saying *Tat* without an interest in a benefit, acts of sacrifice, austerity and various types of charity are performed by those who are desirous of liberation. (17.25)

Commentary:

Tat means 'that' in English. It refers to what is being offered in the religious ceremony or what is being restrained or developed in the austerity.

सद्भावे साधुभावे च
सदित्येतत्प्रयुज्यते ।
प्रशस्ते कर्मणि तथा
सच्छब्दः पार्थ युज्यते ॥ १७.२६ ॥
sadbhāve sādhubhāve ca
sadityetatprayujyate
praśaste karmaṇi tathā
sacchabdaḥ pārtha yujyate (17.26)

sadbhāve = sad (sat) — reality + bhāve — in meaning; sādhubhāve = sādhu — excellence + bhāve — in meaning; ca — and; sat — reality, that which is productive of reality; iti — thus; etat = etad — this; prayujyate — is used; praśaste — is praiseworthy; karmāṇi — in action; tathā — also; sacchabdaḥ = sat + śabdaḥ — word; pārtha — son of Pṛthā; yujyate — is used

The word *Sat* is used to mean reality and excellence and also for a praiseworthy act, O son of Pṛthā. (17.26)

Commentary:

Sat means what is real, what is the best and what is praiseworthy. In kriyā yoga we strive for all that.

यज्ञे तपसि दाने च
स्थितिः सदिति चोच्यते ।
कर्म चैव तदर्थीयं
सदित्येवाभिधीयते ॥ १७.२७॥
yajñe tapasi dāne ca
sthitiḥ saditi cocyate
karma caiva tadarthīyaṁ
sadityevābhidhīyate (17.27)

yajñe — in sacrifice; tapasi — in austerity; dāne — in charity; ca —and; sthitiḥ — steady application; sat — realism; iti —thus; cocyate = ca —and + ucyate — is designated; karma — action; caiva —and indeed; tadarthīyaṁ — for the purpose of that; sat — realistic; iti — thus; evābhidhīyate = eva — indeed + abhidhīyate — is designated

Steady application in sacrifice, austerity and charity, is also called *Sat*. An action which is supportive of this purpose is also designated as *Sat*. (17.27)

Commentary:

Faith in the process of austerity as well as in religious ceremony, is necessary. It is confidence in those who give us or share with us, the techniques of psyche purification.

अश्रद्धया हुतं दत्तं
तपस्तप्तं कृतं च यत् ।
असदित्युच्यते पार्थ
न च तत्प्रेत्य नो इह॥ १७.२८॥
aśraddhayā hutaṁ dattaṁ
tapastaptaṁ kṛtaṁ ca yat
asadityucyate pārtha
na ca tatpretya no iha (17.28)

aśraddhayā — with a lack of faith; hutaṁ — oblation; dattaṁ —offered; tapaḥ — austerity; taptaṁ — performed; kṛtaṁ— done; ca — and; yat — which; asat — unrealistic; iti — thus; ucyate — is called; pārtha— son of Pṛthà; na —no; ca — and; tat — that; pretya — hereafter; no = naḥ— to us; iha — here

An oblation offered with a lack of faith and austerity performed in the same way is called asat, unrealistic, O son of Pṛtha. And that has no value to us here or in the hereafter. (17.28)

Commentary:

Regardless of whether one believes in religious ceremonies or in personal upliftment through austerities (tapas), one may judge an undertaking by the faith invested in it. If there is a lack of faith, even a valid process becomes unreliable.

CHAPTER 18

The Most Secret of All Information*

अर्जुन उवाच
संन्यासस्य महाबाहो
तत्त्वमिच्छामि वेदितुम् ।
त्यागस्य च हृषीकेश
पृथक्केशिनिषूदन ॥ १८.१ ॥
arjuna uvāca
saṁnyāsasya mahābāho
tattvamicchāmi veditum
tyāgasya ca hṛṣīkeśa
pṛthakkeśiniṣūdana (18.1)

arjuna — Arjuna; uvāca — said; saṁnyāsasya — of the rejection of opportunity; mahābāho — O strong-armed hero; tattvam — fact; icchāmi — I want; veditum — to know; tyāgasya — of the rejection of consequences; ca — and; hṛṣīkesa — O Hṛṣīkeśa; pṛthak — distinguish; keśiniṣūdāna — slayer of Keshi

Arjuna said: Regarding the rejection of opportunity, O strong—armed hero, I want to know the fact. And regarding the rejection of consequences, O Hṛṣīkeśa, distinguish these, O slayer of Keshi. (18.1)

Commentary:

This Chapter Eighteen is the last in the *Bhagavad Gītā*. Arjuna will ask questions to clear up whatever else he does not understand and to remove any doubts regarding what Śrī Krishna proposed. Arjuna still has not agreed to fight. He is still hesitant.

Arjuna asked about the rejection of opportunity. He wanted to know the facts. At first he wanted to reject the fighting opportunity which was placed before him. The key point is that Arjuna cannot turn away without consequence. The Central Figure in the Universal Form selected Arjuna to do the task. If Arjuna rejected that opportunity he would have lost Śrī Krishna's association and would have been confronted by Śrī Krishna's disciplinary energy. This is not what Arjuna really wants. The Kurus were dear to Arjuna but they were not as important as Śrī Krishna.

As I stated before, unless one has a waiver from cultural activity, one should not reject such an opportunity even if it is unpalatable. Come what may, do or die, we should maintain positive relations with the Universal Form. There is no benefit to us or to those we love if we gain His disapproval. It is a matter of getting our priorities in order. In this life there will always be times when we are faced with dilemmas or situations that put us to the test. Pleasing limited beings is never as important as pleasing the Supreme Personality or the parallel people in His Universal Form.

Honestly speaking, if I was Arjuna, I too would want to leave the battlefield but I would consider Śrī Krishna's view. Once I understood that He requested my services, I would harden my emotions, stand my ground and fight, even though I would sense the disapproval of relatives and friends. It would be an uneasy situation but considering myself as a limited being and considering my relatives and friends as such also, I would side with the Supreme Person, Śrī Krishna.

**The Mahābhārata contains no chapter headings. This title was assigned by the translator on the basis of verse 64 of this chapter.*

Arjuna asked about the rejection of consequences. If he fought, there would be consequences since that is the nature of violent acts. These acts always bring resentment, hatred and brooding energies which cause retaliations. Arjuna wanted to know if in fact one could reject or ward off such negative feedback. Was it a fact? Or was Śrī Krishna talking in a way to convince Arjuna to fight, knowing fully well that afterwards, Arjuna would become miserable.

I stated in the previous commentary that the *Bhagavad Gītā* is more like a legal document rather than a devotional talk. That is substantiated by Arjuna's questions in this final chapter. Despite the showing of the Universal Form which scared Arjuna, still he wants to get the legal clarification regarding the laws of nature in terms of what his fighting action would bring on him later.

Stated differently, suppose I do reject an opportunity to do undesirable service for the Universal Form, then what? How will His disapproval surface in my life? What reaction will He levy on me? When we look at it in this way, we shed sentiments and face Śrī Krishna square on. This is what Arjuna did here.

Supposing I serve the mission given by the Universal Form and perform acts that outrage humanity, then can I be sure that I will be able to reject the consequences when humanity reacts to me? Or is it that Śrī Krishna will shift my existence out of the human plane so that the negative dispositions never reach me? Would Śrī Krishna assign someone else to absorb them? These are the legal aspects implied by Arjuna's questions to Śrī Krishna.

The rejection of opportunity is the more advanced stage but Śrī Krishna did not want Arjuna to take it. Arjuna was to stay on the low road of working in karma yoga which consists of working in the world, taking opportunities and becoming insensitive to the good or bad consequences.

Why then did Śrī Krishna, the God that He is, and the friend of Arjuna which He was, not let Arjuna take the high road to spiritual life which is the way of rejection of social opportunities so that one can accelerate one's spiritual progress? Did Śrī Krishna think that Arjuna was just a mediocre yogin who could not safely and thoroughly reject opportunities, but who could only halfheartedly do so which is very dangerous?

Śrī Krishna virtually blocked the high road of sannyasa yoga. He pointed His dear friend Arjuna down the hell—hole of tyāga yoga which is the application of yoga maturity to working like a dog in the material world. And to boot, Śrī Krishna asked Arjuna not to be interested in benefits. Essentially Arjuna was to fight on the basis of the Universal Form's antagonism towards the opposing army.

This is the *Gītā* in its raw state.

Readers should be mindful that these are the last inquires of Arjuna. There will be no more questions.

Finally Arjuna wants to know point blank how he is covered by Śrī Krishna, if he does what Śrī Krishna suggests and what the Central Figure in the Universal Form enacted on the supernatural plane. This is the *Gītā*. Can we say that this is a treatise of devotion? I say not. This is a person doubting the validity of Śrī Krishna and wanting to be shown that Śrī Krishna knows exactly what He spoke of. This is Arjuna who does not follow Śrī Krishna blindly but who wants to be certain that Śrī Krishna is who He proclaims Himself to be. Arjuna is cautious.

Arjuna could have asked: "How can I be Your devotee, Śrī Krishna? How can I offer loving service unto You, my dear cherished Deity?" But no, Arjuna wants to know where he stands in truth if he follows Śrī Krishna's unpalatable suggestions about fighting and killing relatives and friends on the warfield.

श्रीभगवानुवाच
काम्यानां कर्मणां न्यासं
संन्यासं कवयो विदुः ।
सर्वकर्मफलत्यागं
प्राहुस्त्यागं विचक्षणाः ॥ १८.२ ॥
śrībhagavānuvāca
kāmyānāṁ karmaṇāṁ nyāsaṁ
saṁnyāsaṁ kavayo viduḥ
sarvakarmaphalatyāgaṁ
prāhustyāgaṁ vicakṣaṇāḥ (18.2)

śrī bhagavān — The Blessed Lord; uvāca — said; śrī kāmyānāṁ — prompted by craving; karmaṇāṁ — of actions; nyāsaṁ — renunciation; saṁnyāsaṁ — rejection of opportunity; kavayo = kavayaḥ — authoritative speakers; viduḥ — know; sarvakarmaphalatyāgaṁ = sarva — all + karma — action + phala — benefit + tyāgaṁ — abandonment; prāhuḥ — they declare; tyāgaṁ — rejection of consequences; vicakṣaṇāḥ — the clear-sighted person

The Blessed Lord said: The authoritative speakers know the rejection of opportunity as renunciation of actions which are prompted by craving. The clear—sighted seers declare the abandonment of the results of benefit—motivated action as the rejection of consequences. (18.2)

Commentary:

Śrī Krishna answered the first question about the rejections of opportunities in a totally different way in comparison to what He said in previous chapters. Now He explains it in terms of the critical attitude of the great authoritative speakers from the Upanishadic period. According to them, a yogin, if he has the power, should reject any opportunity which faces him if the situation is powered by passionate energy. In other words any opportunity which is presented by destiny but which was initially projected by the passionate energy, should be rejected. There is a technicality however, as Śrī Krishna explained before:

saṁnyāsastu mahābāho duḥkhamāptumayogataḥ
yogayukto munirbrahma nacireṇādhigacchati (5.6)

Renunciation of opportunities is difficult to attain without yoga practice, O mighty man. In the nick of time, a yoga—proficient sage reaches the spiritual plane. (5.6)

That means that even if one suspects that an action has the passionate energy as its source, still one should not renounce it unless one is fully proficient in yoga and has the waiver from the Supreme Being.

Some readers may realize that this indicates that even actions in which the Universal Form is involved, may have passionate energy within them. This is absolutely correct. This is why karma yoga is not the highest path. This is why we desire the waiver from it. Still it is not a good idea to reject karma yoga if one does not have the waiver from the Central Person in the Universal Form.

त्याज्यं दोषवदित्येके
कर्म प्राहुर्मनीषिणः ।
यज्ञदानतपःकर्म
न त्याज्यमिति चापरे ॥ १८.३ ॥

tyājyaṁ — to be abandoned; doṣāvat — full of fault; iti — thus; eke —some; karma — action; prāhur = prāhuḥ — they declare; manīṣiṇaḥ — philosophers; yajñadānatapaḥkarma = yajña — sacrifice + dāna — charity + tapaḥ — austerity +

tyājyaṁ doṣavadityeke
karma prāhurmanīṣiṇaḥ
yajñadānatapaḥkarma
na tyājyamiti cāpare (18.3)

karma — action; na — not; tyājyam — be abandoned; iti — thus; cāpare = ca — and + apare — others

Some philosophers declare that action is to be abandoned, since it is full of faults. Some others say that acts of sacrifice, charity and austerity are not to be abandoned. (18.3)

Commentary:

Seeing that all actions have inherent faults and will bring on some type of binding result whether for good or bad, some of the sages in the Upanishadic era said that all actions should be abandoned. Arjuna heard these views. These ideas ran through his mind substantiating the doubts about participation in the battle.

Some other sages said that even though there are faults in all actions, still one should be careful not to avoid acts of sacrifice, charity and austerity. They were of the opinion that if one abandoned these, one would regret it later on.

निश्चयं श्रृणु मे तत्र
त्यागे भरतसत्तम ।
त्यागो हि पुरुषव्याघ्र
त्रिविधः संप्रकीर्तितः ॥ १८.४॥
niścayaṁ śṛṇu me tatra
tyāge bharatasattama
tyāgo hi puruṣavyāghra
trividhaḥ saṁprakīrtitaḥ (18.4)

niścayaṁ — view; śṛṇu — hear; me — my; tatra — here, on this matter; tyāge — in the abandonment of consequences; bharatasattama — best of the Bharatas; tyāgo (tyāgaḥ) — abandonment of consequences; hi — indeed; puruṣavyāghra — tiger among men; trividhaḥ — three-fold; saṁprakīrtitaḥ — designated

Hear my view on this matter of abandonment of the consequences of action, O best of the Bharatas. The abandonment of consequences, O tiger among men, is designated as being threefold. (18.4)

Commentary:

Even though Arjuna's first question was about the rejection of opportunities, Śrī Krishna tactfully avoids speaking much about that. Instead Śrī Krishna focuses on what He wants Arjuna to do which is to take the path of karma yoga. This a path which was maneuvered successfully by King Janak by the use of yoga expertise in accepting opportunities, even dangerous and unpalatable ones, and sidestepping the consequences which resulted from participation.

Śrī Krishna is determined to make Arjuna fight. That is the issue here. We should know that in relating to Śrī Krishna, we are dealing with a very directive personality Who will have His way eventually. Unless a yogin has the waiver from cultural activities, his best course is to do what is suggested to Him by the Central Figure in the Universal Form. Such suggestions are manifested on this plane as opportunities to take up certain responsibilities. That is not kriyā yoga but the practice of kriyā yoga would better equip a person to perform successfully as an agent for the divine. And through such performance, he would eventually earn the waiver.

Śrī Krishna will elaborate about the abandonment of consequences because this is the path which Arjuna must take. Arjuna or any of us may reject that path but if we gain the disapproval of Śrī Krishna, then our rejection will be converted by destiny into even more responsibility. This is because Śrī Krishna will set up supernatural obstacles to our success in that course. Therefore it is best to work along with Śrī Krishna.

यज्ञदानतपःकर्म
न त्याज्यं कार्यमेव तत् ।
यज्ञो दानं तपश्चैव
पावनानि मनीषिणाम् ॥ १८.५॥
yajñadānatapaḥkarma
na tyājyaṁ kāryameva tat
yajño dānaṁ tapaścaiva
pāvanāni manīṣiṇām (18.5)

yajñadānatapaḥkarma = yajña — sacrifice + dāna — charity + tapaḥ — austerity + karma — action; na — not; tyājyaṁ — to be abandoned; kāryam — to be performed; eva — indeed; tat = tad — this; yajño = yajñaḥ — sacrifice; dānaṁ — charity; tapaścaiva = tapaḥ — austerity + caiva — and indeed; pāvanāni — purificatory acts; manīṣiṇāṁ — for the wise men

Acts of sacrifice, charity, and austerity are not to be abandoned but should be performed. Sacrifice, charity and austerity are purificatory acts even for the wise men. (18.5)

Commentary:

Acts of sacrifice, charity and austerity are purificatory acts even for the great yogins who may participate in them, what to speak of what such acts would do for any of us. We recall this verse:

kāyena manasā buddhyā kevalairindriyairapi
yoginaḥ karma kurvanti saṅgaṁ tyaktvātmaśuddhaye (5.11)

With the body, mind and intelligence, or even with the senses alone, the yogis, having discarded attachment, perform cultural acts for self purification. (5.11)

This means that there is something in it for us, for our purification, if we take up these cultural activities as supervised by Śrī Krishna. As I stated previously, one limitation we face is that Śrī Krishna has every intention of making us work hard in the material world to keep this place in order by His view of what that order should be. He does not intend to do the work by Himself. He wants to use us as agents, even for unpalatable tasks which He performs in the disciplinary role as God Supreme.

एतान्यपि तु कर्माणि
सङ्गं त्यक्त्वा फलानि च ।
कर्तव्यानीति मे पार्थ
निश्चितं मतमुत्तमम् ॥ १८.६॥
etānyapi tu karmāṇi
saṅgaṁ tyaktvā phalāni ca
kartavyānīti me pārtha
niścitaṁ matamuttamam (18.6)

etāni — these; api — also; tu — but; karmāṇi — actions; saṅgaṁ — attachment; tyaktvā — giving up; phalāni — results; ca — and; kartavyānīti = kartavyāni — to be done + iti — thus; me — my; pārtha — O son of Pṛthā; niścitaṁ — definitely; matam — opinion; uttamam — highest

But these actions are to be performed by giving up attachment to results, O son of Pṛthā. This is definitely My highest opinion. (18.6)

Commentary:

The boom fell on Arjuna's head. This is the last word by Śrī Krishna. Arjuna could take it or leave it. Either we do what He says and help Him with His preferences in the role He assigns us or be in His disfavor. It is a toss—up between pleasing Śrī Krishna and satisfying fellow limited beings. I must clarify that even though Śrī Krishna stressed this as His highest opinion for Arjuna, it is not Krishna's highest opinion for everyone else. It was not His highest opinion for Uddhava or many others who were not required by Śrī Krishna to fight. This applies to Arjuna and to those who do not have the waiver from social, cultural and political acts. Some persons, a few, do have the exemption from karma yoga.

नियतस्य तु संन्यासः
कर्मणो नोपपद्यते ।
मोहात्तस्य परित्यागस्
तामसः परिकीर्तितः ॥ १८.७॥
niyatasya tu saṁnyāsaḥ
karmaṇo nopapadyate
mohāttasya parityāgas
tāmasaḥ parikīrtitaḥ (18.7)

niyatasya — of obligation; tu — but; saṁnyāsaḥ — renunciation; karmaṇo (karmaṇaḥ) — of action; nopapadyate = na — not + upapadyate — it is proper; mohāt — from delusion; tasya — of it; parityāgaḥ — rejection; tāmasaḥ — influence of depression; parikīrtitaḥ — is said to be

But renunciation of obligatory actions is not proper. The rejection of it on the basis of delusion, is said to occur by the influence of depression. (18.7)

Commentary:

This is a catch phrase. The renunciation of obligations which are approved by the Supreme Being cannot be effectively renounced even by a great yogin. One has to fulfill such obligations even if they are not to one's liking.

If even a yogi rejects such obligations while influenced by ignorance, he will suffer the consequences. His quest for liberation will be delayed further.

दुःखमित्येव यत्कर्म
कायक्लेशभयात्त्यजेत् ।
स कृत्वा राजसं त्यागं
नैव त्यागफलं लभेत् ॥ १८.८॥
duḥkhamityeva yatkarma
kāyakleśabhayāttyajet
sa kṛtvā rājasaṁ tyāgaṁ
naiva tyāgaphalaṁ labhet (18.8)

duḥkham — difficult; ityeva = iti — thus + eva — indeed; yat = yad — which; karma — action; kāyakleśabhayāt = kāya — body + kleśa — suffering + bhayāt — from fear; tyajet — should abandon; sa — saḥ — he; kṛtvā — having performed; rājasaṁ — impulsive influence; tyāgaṁ — renunciation; naiva = na — not + eva — indeed; tyāgaphalam — result of renunciation; labhet — should obtain

He who abandons action because of difficulty or because of a fear of bodily suffering, performs impulsive renunciation. He would not obtain the desired result of that renunciation. (18.8)

Commentary:

Usually a good man tries to avoid unpalatable responsibilities which would cause him emotional suffering but Śrī Krishna stated that even so, that person will not get the benefit he desires. In fact he will be in more agony when the disapproval of the Supreme Being causes an upset in his life.

Indirectly Arjuna is warned that if he did not fight and if it was because he feared bodily harm or because the task was difficult, he would not get the peace of mind or satisfaction that he hoped for. The avoidance would bring to him reactions for a greater default.

कार्यमित्येव यत्कर्म
नियतं क्रियतेऽर्जुन ।
सङ्गं त्यक्त्वा फलं चैव
स त्यागः सात्त्विको मतः ॥ १८.९ ॥
kāryamityeva yatkarma
niyataṁ kriyate'rjuna
saṅgaṁ tyaktvā phalaṁ caiva
sa tyāgaḥ sāttviko mataḥ (18.9)

kāryam — to be done; ityeva = iti — thus + eva — indeed; yat — which; karma — action; niyataṁ — disciplinary manner; kriyate — is performed; 'rjuna = arjuna — Arjuna; saṅgaṁ — attachment; tyaktvā — abandoning; phalaṁ — result; caiva — and indeed; sa = saḥ — it; tyāgaḥ — renunciation; sāttviko = sāttvikaḥ — of the clarifying mode; mataḥ — is considered

O Arjuna, when an action is done in a disciplinary manner, because it is to be performed, and with renunciation of the attachment to the results, it is considered to be in the clarifying mode. (18.9)

Commentary:

This is where the practice of kriyā yoga is helpful in the performance of work or karma. To act in a disciplinary manner and rid oneself of the tendency for acquiring or enjoying results, requires some application of the emotional maturity gained by yoga practice. Just being determined is not enough because one's nature will prevail. One's emotions will force one to abandon destined actions, which would, in turn, incur the disfavor of the Supreme Personality.

Death of bodies is not a big issue with the Supreme Person. He does not see a person as the body or that saving a person's body means saving the person.

As indicated in this verse, attachment to results causes a human being to reject the plan of the Universal Form. One who makes the rejection may not understand that his attachment to results caused it. He may think that it was caused by his compassion and kindness to others. His intellect will, in turn, form justifications to support the attachment. Then he will go against the wishes of the Supreme Personality. He will not care about the divine will.

न द्वेष्ट्यकुशलं कर्म
कुशले नानुषज्जते ।
त्यागी सत्त्वसमाविष्टो
मेधावी छिन्नसंशयः ॥ १८.१० ॥
na dveṣṭyakuśalaṁ karma
kuśale nānuṣajjate
tyāgī sattvasamāvisṭo
medhāvī chinnasaṁśayaḥ (18.10)

na — not; dveṣṭi — hates; akuśalaṁ — disagreeable; karma — action; kuśale — is agreeable; nānuṣajjate = na — not + anuśajjate — is attached; tyāgī — renouncer; sattvasamāviṣṭo = sattva — clarity + samāviṣṭo (samāviṣṭah) — filled with; medhāvi — wise man; chinnasaṁśayaḥ = chinna — removed+ saṁśayaḥ — doubt

The renouncer who is filled with clarity, the wise man whose doubts are removed, does not hate disagreeable action, nor is he attached to agreeable performance. (18.10)

Commentary:

This person is free to act neutrally.

न हि देहभृता शक्यं
त्यक्तुं कर्माण्यशेषतः ।
यस्तु कर्मफलत्यागी
स त्यागीत्यभिधीयते ॥१८.११॥
na hi dehabhṛtā śakyaṁ
tyaktuṁ karmāṇyaśeṣataḥ
yastu karmaphalatyāgī
sa tyāgītyabhidhīyate (18.11)

na — not; hi — indeed; dehabhṛtā — by the body-supported; śakyaṁ — possible; tyaktuṁ — to abandon; karmāṇi — actions; aśeṣataḥ — completely; yaḥ — who; tu — but; karmaphalatyāgī = karma — action + phala — result + tyāgī — remover; sa = saḥ — he; tyāgīti = tyāgī — renunciate + iti — thus; abhidhīyate — is called

Indeed it is not possible for the body—supported beings to abandon actions completely. But whosoever is the renouncer of the results of actions is called a renunciate. (18.11)

Commentary:

The body—supported beings are those who cannot exist comfortably without a subtle body *and* without having that subtle form procure physical forms. Such persons are always turned in the direction of the material world. Some of these individuals are devotees of Śrī Krishna. Some are not. They all share the same determined focus into the gross material manifestation. For such a person, it is not possible to abandon mundane actions.

Thus, among such people, one who is practical, will renounce the results of actions, not the actions. It is different for those who are not body—prone. They are able to effectively renounce the opportunities for action.

Those of us who are crossing over from being body—supported beings to being non—body supported, will still have to do some destined activity, at least until we develop further in advanced yoga and can get the waiver from the Supreme Being.

अनिष्टमिष्टं मिश्रं च
त्रिविधं कर्मणः फलम् ।
भवत्यत्यागिनां प्रेत्य
न तु संन्यासिनां क्वचित् ॥१८.१२॥
aniṣṭamiṣṭaṁ miśraṁ ca
trividhaṁ karmaṇaḥ phalam
bhavatyatyāgināṁ pretya
na tu saṁnyāsināṁ kvacit (18.12)

aniṣṭam — undesired; iṣṭaṁ — desired; miśraṁ — mixed; ca — and; trividham — three types; karmaṇaḥ — of action; phalam — result; bhavati — it is; atyāgināṁ — of those who do not renounce results; pretya — departing; na — not; tu — but; saṁnyāsināṁ — of the renouncers; kvacit — any at all

Undesired, desired and mixed are the three types of results of actions that occur for the departing souls who do not renounce results. But for the renouncers of opportunity, there is no result at all. (18.12)

Commentary:

This explanation is technical because it does not deal with persons who perform karma yoga. Instead it deals with those who just perform karma or work, without yoga expertise. It pertains to those who have the exemption from karma yoga as well. This is the way the Sanskrit reads since Śrī Krishna did not discuss the tyāgis or persons like Arjuna who do karma yoga but rather the non—tyāgis (atyāginām) and also the extremists, the sannyasis who renounce the opportunities because they have a waiver to sidestep the social, cultural and political world.

Śrī Krishna did not discuss persons in Arjuna's class because their situation is only definite if they are able to follow the Universal Form's instructions completely. Most of the karma yogis are not like King Janak who did so. Most of them comply in part and deviate in part.

However, according to the information given, those who do not perform karma yoga will have accrued undesirable, desirable or mixed results all according to how their actions complemented or counteracted the Supreme Will.

On the other hand, those great personalities who had exemption from cultural activity, would not accrue any result. Subsequently they would experience liberation from the ways and means of this world.

पञ्चैतानि महाबाहो
कारणानि निबोध मे ।
सांख्ये कृतान्ते प्रोक्तानि
सिद्धये सर्वकर्मणाम् ॥ १८.१३ ॥
pañcaitāni mahābāho
kāraṇāni nibodha me
sāṁkhye kṛtānte proktāni
siddhaye sarvakarmaṇām (18.13)

pañcaitāni = pañca — five + tāni — these; mahābāho — O mighty-armed man; kāraṇāni — factors; nibodha — learn; me — from me; sāṁkhye — in Sāṁkhya philosophy; krtānte — in conclusion, in doctrine; proktāni — declared; siddhaye — in accomplishment; sarvakarmaṇām — of all actions

Learn from Me, O mighty—armed man, of the five factors declared in the Sāṁkhya doctrine for the accomplishment of all actions: (18.13)

Commentary:

Śrī Krishna is admirable in the way He dealth with His devotee Arjuna. Śrī Krishna addressed Arjuna as mighty—armed. Despite the acclaim, Arjuna fell apart when confronted with duties. One's might or one's skill is only one of the five factors required for an occurrence. Arjuna was not the all in all.

अधिष्ठानं तथा कर्ता
करणं च पृथग्विधम् ।
विविधाश्च पृथक्चेष्टा
दैवं चैवात्र पञ्चमम् ॥ १८.१४ ॥
adhiṣṭhānaṁ tathā kartā
karaṇaṁ ca pṛthagvidham
vividhāśca pṛthakceṣṭā
daivaṁ caivātra pañcamam (18.14)

adhiṣṭhānaṁ — location; tathā — as well as; kartā — the agent; karaṇaṁ — the instrument; ca — and; prthagvidham — various kinds; vividhāśca = vividhāḥ — various + ca — and; pṛthakceṣṭa — movements; daivam — destiny; caivātra = ca — and + eva — indeed + atra — here in this case; pañcamam — the fifth

The location, the agent, the various instruments, the various movements, and destiny, the fifth factor. (18.14)

Commentary:

The location: That must be there, otherwise even if the other factors are present, the action will not take place. Modern astronomers find this to be true. They send astronauts into space but they cannot find a suitable habitat. One may have desires, trained men, materials and technical means but if one does not find a suitable location, the plans will not be manifested.

The agent: At Kurukṣetra, Arjuna just happened to be the agent. At first he was reluctant to perform. The agent must be capable and willing to do the task assigned. If he buckles under pressure, he will not perform.

The various instruments: The agent must have tools. In Arjuna's case, he had a chariot, horses, a special driver (Śrī Krishna), as well as weapons. No matter the task there are always tools of the craft which must be acquired. Even if one has the skill he still needs tools. Except for yoga, where one uses his body as the tool, most other tasks involve instruments.

The various movements: The situation must be such that it is not at a standstill. There must be mobility in some way or other.

Destiny: And of course there must be destiny, something that is set on by supernatural force. This is the most important factor. Unless destined to do something, even the most capable individual cannot function. But if one is destined, even if not perfectly suited to the task, one will get the opportunity.

शरीरवाङ्मनोभिर्यत्
कर्म प्रारभते नरः ।
न्याय्यं वा विपरीतं वा
पञ्चैते तस्य हेतवः ॥१८.१५॥
śarīravāṅmanobhiryat
karma prārabhate naraḥ
nyāyyaṁ vā viparītaṁ vā
pañcaite tasya hetavaḥ (18.15)

śarīravāṅmanobhiḥ = śarīra — body + vān(vās) — speech + manobhiḥ — with mind; yat = yad — whatever; karma — project; prārabhate — he undertakes; naraḥ — a human being; nyāyyaṁ — moral; vā — or; viparītam — immoral; vā — or; pañcaite = pañca — five + ete — these; tasya — of it; hetavaḥ — factors

As for whatever project a human being undertakes with body, speech and mind, regardless of it being moral or immoral, these are its five factors. (18.15)

Commentary:

This is self evident.

तत्रैवं सति कर्तारम्
आत्मानं केवलं तु यः ।
पश्यत्यकृतबुद्धित्वान्
न स पश्यति दुर्मतिः ॥१८.१६॥
tatraivaṁ sati kartāram
ātmānaṁ kevalaṁ tu yaḥ
paśyatyakṛtabuddhitvān
na sa paśyati durmatiḥ (18.16)

tatraivaṁ = tatra — here, in this case + evam — thus; sati — in reality, correctly; kartāram — agent; ātmānaṁ — self; kevalam — only; tu — but; yaḥ — who; paśyati — he regards; akṛtabuddhitvāt = akṛta — undone, defective + buddhitvāt — due to intellect; na — not; sa = saḥ — he; paśyati — he perceives; durmatiḥ — idiot

In that case, whosoever regards himself as the only agent, does not perceive correctly. This is due to the defective intellect of the idiot. (18.16)

Commentary:

This is very clear.

यस्य नाहंकृतो भावो
बुद्धिर्यस्य न लिप्यते ।
हत्वापि स इमाँल्लोकान्
न हन्ति न निबध्यते ॥ १८.१७॥
yasya nāhaṁkṛto bhāvo
buddhiryasya na lipyate
hatvāpi sa imāṁllokān
na hanti na nibadhyate (18.17)

yasya — regarding who; nāhaṁkṛto = na — not + ahaṁkṛto (ahaṁkṛtaḥ) — falsely assertive; bhāvo = bhāvaḥ — attitude; buddhiḥ — intellect; yasya — of whom; na — not; lipyate — is clouded; hatvāpi = hatvā — having slain + api — even; sa = saḥ — he; imān — these; lokān — people; na — not; hanti — he slays; na — not; nibadhyate — is implicated

Regarding the person whose attitude is not falsely assertive, whose intellect is not clouded, even after slaying these people, he would not slay or be implicated. (18.17)

Commentary:

Śrī Krishna stressed his original point that the spirit does not perish when the body dies, and that the reality—perceptive person does not feel that he can kill anyone, even in instances where he has to be harsh to others. It is not that such a person commits a murder and justifies it on the basis of the spirit's eternality, but rather because he knows for sure that the act of displacing a spirit from his body would bear undesirable consequences, he acts cautiously. But if he is assigned disciplinary tasks by the Universal Form, he would honor the instructions rather than back out on the basis of emotions which charm his intellect.

Śrī Krishna said that Arjuna would not be implicated in the death of any of the soldiers whom Arjuna would be required to kill. This is because Arjuna was just an agent for the supreme power, the Central Figure in the Universal Form.

ज्ञानं ज्ञेयं परिज्ञाता
त्रिविधा कर्मचोदना ।
करणं कर्म कर्तेति
त्रिविधः कर्मसंग्रहः ॥ १८.१८॥
jñānaṁ jñeyaṁ parijñātā
trividhā karmacodanā
karaṇaṁ karma karteti
trividhaḥ karmasaṁgrahaḥ (18.18)

jñānaṁ — experience; jñeyaṁ — the item of research; parijñātā — the experiencer; trividhā — three aspects; karmacodanā = karma — action + codanā — impetus for; karaṇaṁ — instrument; karma — action; karteti = kartā — agent + iti — thus; trividhaḥ — three; karmasaṁgrahaḥ = karma — action + saṁgrahaḥ — parts

Experience, the item of research, and the experiencer are the three aspects which serve as the impetus for action. The instrument, the action itself, and the agent are three parts of an action. (18.18)

Commentary:

This is technical information given to us long ago by the expert yogis of the Samkhyas. In the Samkhya philosophy, the whole array of material existence is theoretically laid out on the basis of the mystic perception of the reality—perceptive seers.

Even though five factors, namely the location, agents, instruments, movements and destiny are required for an action to take place, these together are not parts of the impetus for action. The impetus is the actual driving force, the causative principle. That is a combination of experience to be gained, the subtle or gross item to be experienced and the experiencer himself. These three facets combined, produce an impetus which causes formation of the circumstances.

Once an action begins, time comes into play. Time affects the act by applying pressures on the way it is experienced, on the action itself and on the agent involved. Time may sometimes warp or twist a particular experience so that the repetition of it occurs in an entirely different way and baffles the observer. At other times, time allows the experience to occur as a recognizable repetition.

The time pressure is applied by supernatural beings. By sheer mystic force they can warp a person's life and frustrate his attempt to fulfill desires. In addition material nature is very subtle. It borders the spiritual world. It is a force to contend with. Many religious people mistake the subtle material and its influences to be spiritual reality. This is due to their lack of keen mystic perception, something that cannot be developed without yoga practice.

ज्ञानं कर्म च कर्ता च
त्रिधैव गुणभेदतः ।
प्रोच्यते गुणसंख्याने
यथावच्छृणु तान्यपि ॥१८.१९॥
jñānaṁ karma ca kartā ca
tridhaiva guṇabhedataḥ
procyate guṇasaṁkhyāne
yathāvacchṛṇu tānyapi (18.19)

jñānaṁ — experience; karma — action; ca — and; kartā — agent; ca — and; tridhaiva = tridha — three types + eva — indeed; guṇabhedataḥ — categorized by the influences of material nature; procyate — is stated; guṇasaṁkhyāne — in the Sāṁkhya analysis of the influences of material nature; yathāvat — correctly; śṛṇu — hear; tāni — these; api — as well

In the Sāṁkhya analysis of the influence of material nature, it is stated that experience, action, and the agent are of three types as categorized by the influence of material nature. Hear correctly of these as well. (18.19)

Commentary:

The experience itself, the action involved in producing it, as well as the agent operating those energies are of three types essentially, according to the mixture of varying amounts of mundane energy.

सर्वभूतेषु येनैकं
भावमव्ययमीक्षते ।
अविभक्तं विभक्तेषु
तज्ज्ञानं विद्धि सात्त्विकम् ॥१८.२०॥
sarvabhūteṣu yenaikaṁ
bhāvamavyayamīkṣate
avibhaktaṁ vibhakteṣu
tajjñānaṁ viddhi sāttvikam (18.20)

sarvabhūteṣu — in all beings; yenaikaṁ = yena — by which + ekam — one; bhāvam — being; avyayam — imperishable; īksate — one perceives; avibhaktaṁ — undivided; vibhakteṣu — in the divided; tat — that; jñānaṁ — experience; viddhi — know; sāttvikaṁ — clarifying

That experience by which one perceives one imperishable being in all beings, undivided in the divided, know it to be an experience in clarity. (18.20)

Commentary:

Śrī Krishna graciously taught Arjuna this because Arjuna had some doubts about Krishna's instruction. Just in case Arjuna or any of us would think that Krishna just wanted to force Arjuna to fight and thereby used smart arguments in order to outwit Arjuna and then leave Arjuna with the reactions for killing soldiers, Śrī Krishna now clarified that in fact, Arjuna could not see perfectly what to do in that situation. It all depends on the type of psychological perception we have at the time of our refusal to cooperate with a person like Śrī Krishna.

Each of us is predominantly clear—minded, passionate or dull—witted. By that, our decision is made. It is not merely a matter of knowing the right action. A person does not necessarily know what is in his or her best interest. In fact most of us do not know what is to our benefit. At the same time, whom should we trust? How do we know for sure that anyone else's selection is better than our own? Suppose we are misled by a spiritual master? Would it not be better to just follow one's intuition than to be misguided by others?

Here Śrī Krishna provided a tremendous amount of assistance by giving guidelines for determining under which energy we perceive when making decisions. If, for instance, we cannot at the time of making a decision, see one imperishable being in all the psyches, being undivided in what is actually divided, then we can know that we are not seeing in clarity.

But where does that leave us?

Only the very advanced persons can see that one imperishable being in all psyches. That is a keen mystic perception of advanced yoga practice. Such vision is not the day—to—day perception by which we function.

The conclusion is that usually we should not trust perception. We should be hesitant to think that we know what we are doing. The plain truth is that most of the time, we make the wrong selections.

पृथक्त्वेन तु यज्ज्ञानं
नानाभावान्पृथग्विधान् ।
वेत्ति सर्वेषु भूतेषु
तज्ज्ञानं विद्धि राजसम् ॥ १८.२१ ॥
pṛthaktvena tu yajjñānaṁ
nānābhāvānpṛthagvidhān
vetti sarveṣu bhūteṣu
tajjñānaṁ viddhi rājasam (18.21)

pṛthaktvena — with difference; tu — but; yat — which; jñānaṁ — experience; nānābhāvān = nānā — different + bhāvān — beings; pṛthagvidhān — of different kinds; vetti — realizes; sarveṣu — in all; bhūteṣu — in beings; tat — that; jñānaṁ — experience; viddhi — know; rājasam — of the impulsive mode

But that experience by which one realizes different beings of different kinds with differences in all beings, should be known as experience in the impulsive mode. (18.21)

Commentary:

This describes our normal experience as human beings. We see different beings of different kinds with differences in all beings. This is exactly what we normally perceive. This forms even our ideals for cooperative living and civil rights.

Śrī Krishna, following the Samkhya philosophy, assigns this to the impulsive mode. To His view our perception is stipulated to us by the passionate energy.

यत्तु कृत्स्नवदेकस्मिन्
कार्ये सक्तमहैतुकम् ।
अतत्त्वार्थवदल्पं च
तत्तामसमुदाहृतम् ॥ १८.२२ ॥

yat = yad — which; tu — but; kṛtsnavat — appears as the whole; ekasmin — in one; kārye — in order of action; saktam — attached; ahaitukam — without due cause; atattvārthavat — without a valid purpose;

yattu kṛtsnavadekasmin
kārye saktamahaitukam
atattvārthavadalpaṁ ca
tattāmasamudāhṛtam (18.22)

alpaṁ — petty; ca — and; tat = tad — that; tāmasam — of the depressive influence; udāhṛtam — is said to be

But that experience which appears to be the whole vision, being attached to one procedure without due cause, without a valid purpose, being petty, that is said to be of the depressive influence. (18.22)

Commentary:

This is also part of our experience where, on occasion, we feel as if we have the whole vision, where we become attached to one procedure without due cause, to a traditional way or to a new trend. Even though such a procedure has no valid purpose and is petty, we express it proudly and pawn it off on others as being the highest option before us. But Śrī Krishna said that this is caused by the depressive energy.

नियतं सङ्गरहितम्
अरागद्वेषतः कृतम् ।
अफलप्रेप्सुना कर्म
यत्तत्सात्त्विकमुच्यते ॥ १८.२३ ॥
niyataṁ saṅgarahitam
arāgadveṣataḥ kṛtam
aphalaprepsunā karma
yattatsāttvikamucyate (18.23)

niyatam — controlled; saṅgarahitam = saṅga — attachment + rahitam — free from; arāgadveṣataḥ — without craving or repulsion; kṛtam — performed; aphalaprepsunā = aphala — without result + prepsunā — desire to get; karma — action; yat = yad — which; tat = tad — such; sāttvikaṁ — of the clarifying influence; ucyate — is said

Action which is controlled, which is free from attachment, which is performed without craving or repulsion, without desire for results, such action is said to be of the clarifying influence. (18.23)

Commentary:

In human society, this type of action is considered to be callous and anti—social. In fact in family life I found that family members criticize and are irritated by this type of action. Even if such an act is enacted for their benefit, they resent it and verbally cut up the person who performs it. It is for this reason that it is believed that asceticism and householder life do not suit one another.

Śrī Bābāji Mahasaya asked many of his disciples like myself to stay on as householders. Such an instruction is difficult because of the rejection by family members when we act under the clarifying influence. This influence is not always to their liking. Sometimes they perceive it as a hostile destructive force. Śrī Bābāji Mahasaya understands this. Still he asked us to remain on as householder kriyā yogis.

When I ask male yogis to take wives and to keep a household, they sometimes cry out,

"O Swami, do not ask me to do this. I cannot do this. That will end my spiritual life. You know how women are. How can I live with a woman and be successful in the kriyā practice? This instruction will ruin me for life."

However I only give that instruction because of the orders of Śrī Bābāji Mahasaya and because Śrī Krishna is reluctant to award the waiver from cultural activity to neophytes. What can I do about it?

As far as possible, one should take a wife when his body reaches maturity. One should continue his kriyā yoga practice during the householder years. He should encourage his wife to take up the practice too. His actions should be controlled, being performed without craving and without desire for results. The power to act freely comes from a steady yoga practice.

Undoubtedly family members will dislike it, but that is the consequence we must accept in householder life. It is the pain of householder life for a kriyā yogi. It is a grim reminder that human existence is a serious matter. What sort of place is this where when one makes the best selection, he is resented by his own family?

यत्तु कामेप्सुना कर्म
साहंकारेण वा पुनः ।
क्रियते बहुलायासं
तद्राजसमुदाहृतम् ॥ १८.२४॥
yattu kāmepsunā karma
sāhaṁkāreṇa vā punaḥ
kriyate bahulāyāsaṁ
tadrājasamudāhṛtam (18.24)

yat = yad — which; tu — but; kāmepsunā = kāma — craving + ipsunā — desiring to get; karma — action; sāhaṁkāreṇa — with false assertion; vā — or; punaḥ = punar — alternatively; kriyate — is performed; bahulāyāsaṁ = bahula — much + āyāsaṁ effort; tat — that; rājasam — of the impulsive influence; udāhṛtam — is said to be

But that action which is performed with a wish for cravings, with false assertion or alternately with much effort, that is said to be of the impulsive influence. (18.24)

Commentary:

Usually family life is conducted under the passionate mode as described. It is filled with one craving after the other, with the father, if responsible, working many hours to provide money for the fulfillment of the desires. Socially this is considered to be the ideal family life. It is, in fact, faulty.

A human being cannot guarantee which family he will enter in the next birth. He cannot be certain when his investments in a family will return to him in the future. He cannot be sure that his grandchild will be his father in the next life.

He does not know for sure that his wife today will be his wife in a new body a hundred years hence. Thus the whole impulsive scheme for family life is unreliable. It gives a person a chance to invest his innate tendencies by capitalizing on opportunities for fulfillments. But that is not the sensible way to live, because that involves much emotional suffering in the long run. Such agony is welcomed by many living entities who are accustomed to it and who cannot see it for what it really is.

Our modern civilization is based on fulfillments. Our universities are there to create youths who will be ready to do whatever scientific research is necessary to create gadgets for fulfillments. But a kriyā yogi can never be happy in such a world. He is simply not suited to it.

अनुबन्धं क्षयं हिंसाम्
अनपेक्ष्य च पौरुषम् ।
मोहादारभ्यते कर्म
यत्तत्तामसमुच्यते ॥ १८.२५॥

anubandhaṁ — consequence; kṣayaṁ — damage; hiṁsām — violence; anapekṣya — regardless of; ca — and; pauruṣam — practical power; mohāt — from

anubandhaṁ kṣayaṁ hiṁsām
anapekṣya ca pauruṣam
mohādārabhyate karma
yattattāmasamucyate (18.25)

misconception; ārabhyate — is undertaken; karma — action; yat — which; tat — that; tāmasam — of the depressive mode; ucyate — is said to be

That action which is undertaken from a misconception, regardless of the consequence, the damage and the violence, and without considering one's practical power, is said to be of the depressive mode. (18.25)

Commentary:

This is another general basis for human action where we do not care about consequences, so long as we get immediate fulfillments. In householder life, a kriyā yogi is sometimes appalled at the desires that family members ask him to sponsor. In the developed countries, we see that regardless of the consequences, damage and violence, people see to it that their desires are fulfilled. The scientific community endeavors to provide every possible convenience. Even though the environment is ruined and our health is threatened, still because of the passionate force and depressive urges, hardly a person can resist. It is for this reason that a kriyā yogi is forced to step off from human civilization to live in isolation.

मुक्तसङ्गोऽनहंवादी
धृत्युत्साहसमन्वितः ।
सिध्यसिध्योर्निर्विकारः
कर्ता सात्त्विक उच्यते ॥१८.२६॥
muktasaṅgo'nahaṁvādī
dhṛtyutsāhasamanvitaḥ
siddhyasiddhyornirvikāraḥ
kartā sāttvika ucyate (18.26)

muktasaṅgo = muktasaṅgaḥ — freed from attachment; 'nahaṁvādi = anahaṁvādi — free from self praise, free from vanity; dhṛtyutsāhasamanvitaḥ = dhṛty (dhṛti) — consistence + utsāha — perseverance + samanvitaḥ — possessed with; siddhyasiddhyoḥ — in success or failure; nirvikāraḥ — unaffected; kartā — performer; sāttvika — in the clarifying mode; ucyate — is rated to be

A performer who is free from attachment, free from vanity, who is consistent and perseverant, and who is unaffected in success or failure, is rated to be in the clarifying mode. (18.26)

Commentary:

Though true, this does not mean that he will be liked by family members. A kriyā yogi acting like this must be prepared to be resented. He must accept such rejection as a normal response from human beings. If he acts in this way and wants to be appreciated, he may be frustrated. He must know beforehand that such actions which are in the clarifying mode, are considered to be hostile, callous and impersonal by most human beings, even by family members who are still dominated by the passionate and depressive influences.

रागी कर्मफलप्रेप्सुर्
लुब्धो हिंसात्मकोऽशुचिः ।
हर्षशोकान्वितः कर्ता
राजसः परिकीर्तितः ॥१८.२७॥

rāgī — prone to impulsiveness; karmaphalaprepsuḥ = karma — action + phala — result + prepsuḥ — craving; lubdho = lubdhaḥ — greedy; hiṁsāmako = hiṁsāmakaḥ — violent nature; 'śuciḥ = aśuciḥ —

rāgī karmaphalaprepsur
lubdho hiṁsātmako'śuciḥ
harṣaśokānvitaḥ kartā
rājasaḥ parikīrtitaḥ (18.27)

unclean; harṣaśokānvitaḥ = harṣa — joy + śoka — sorrow + anvitaḥ — prone to; kartā — performer; rājasaḥ — of the impulsive mode; parikīrtitaḥ — is declared

A performer who is prone to impulsiveness, who craves the results of action, who is greedy, violent by nature, unclean and prone to joy or sorrow, is declared to be under the impulsive mode. (18.27)

Commentary:

This is the average human being. He is best liked by human society.

अयुक्तः प्राकृतः स्तब्धः
शठो नैष्कृतिकोऽलसः ।
विषादी दीर्घसूत्री च
कर्ता तामस उच्यते ॥ १८.२८॥
ayuktaḥ prākṛtaḥ stabdhaḥ
śaṭho naiṣkṛtiko'lasaḥ
viṣādī dīrghasūtrī ca
kartā tāmasa ucyate (18.28)

ayuktaḥ — undisciplined; prākṛtaḥ — vulgar; stabdhaḥ — stubborn; śaṭho = śaṭhaḥ — wicked; naiṣkṛtiko = naiṣkṛtikaḥ — deceitful; 'lasaḥ = alasaḥ — lazy; viṣādī — depressed; dīrghasūtrī — neglectful; ca — and; kartā — performer; tāmasa — in the depressive mood; ucyate — is said to be

A performer who is undisciplined, vulgar, stubborn, wicked, deceitful, lazy, depressed and neglectful, is said to be in the depressive mode. (18.28)

Commentary:

This is a description of some modern youths who take pride in rejecting traditional values and moral restraints. Unfortunately some of these youths will become leaders of human society.

बुद्धेर्भेदं धृतेश्चैव
गुणतस्त्रिविधं शृणु ।
प्रोच्यमानमशेषेण
पृथक्त्वेन धनंजय ॥ १८.२९॥
buddherbhedaṁ dhṛteścaiva
guṇatastrividhaṁ śṛṇu
procyamānamaśeṣeṇa
pṛthaktvena dhanaṁjaya (18.29)

buddheḥ — intellect; bhedaṁ—difference; dhṛteḥ — determination; caiva — and indeed; guṇataḥ — according to the influences of material nature; trividham — three types; śṛṇu —hear; procyamānam — explained; aśeṣena — thoroughly; pṛthaktvena — distinctly; dhanaṁjaya — a conqueror of wealthy countries

Now, O conqueror of wealthy countries, hear of the three types of intellect and also of determination, explained thoroughly and distinctly, according to their distinctions under the influences of material nature. (18.29)

Commentary:

In the beginning of this chapter, Arjuna asked Lord Krishna about the rejection of opportunity and the rejection of consequences. Arjuna had still not decided what to do. Śrī Krishna answered with much detail. It is because the questions to be asked are these: Who should reject an opportunity? Who should accept it but sidestep its consequences?

To answer these questions, Śrī Krishna gives details about the person and his psychological equipment. The decision should be based on the person's psychology.

Śrī Krishna already said that Arjuna should accept the opportunity and sidestep the consequences. Arjuna was to be confident and fight without attachment since the Universal Form positioned him as the agent in this case. Still Arjuna had doubts. Śrī Krishna gave the final arguments so that Arjuna could make up his mind once and for all.

The condition of the intellect is important because the spirit decides to act or not to act according to what he is shown by the intellect. Even determination is based on the mood of the intellect.

प्रवृत्तिं च निवृत्तिं च
कार्याकार्ये भयाभये ।
बन्धं मोक्षं च या वेत्ति
बुद्धिः सा पार्थ सात्त्विकी ॥१८.३०॥
pravṛttiṁ ca nivṛttiṁ ca
kāryākārye bhayābhaye
bandhaṁ mokṣaṁ ca yā vetti
buddhiḥ sā pārtha sāttvikī (18.30)

pravṛttiṁ — endeavor; ca — and; nivṛttiṁ — non-endeavor; ca — and; kāryākārye = kārya — what should be done + akārya — what should not be done; bhayābhaye — what is dangerous and what is safe; bandhaṁ — restriction; mokṣaṁ — freedom; ca — and; yā — which; vetti — discerns; buddhiḥ — intellectual insight; sā — if, partha — son of Pṛthā; sāttvikī — in the clarifying mode

That intellectual insight which discerns when to endeavor and when not to strive, what should be done and what should not be done, what is dangerous and what is safe, what brings restrictions and what gives freedom, that O son of Pṛthā, is in the clarifying mode. (18.30)

Commentary:

This is the type of intellectual insight that is accurate. It sees in the long range. It is not concerned with immediate fulfillments. It does not focus on what gives the person immediate happiness.

यया धर्ममधर्मं च
कार्यं चाकार्यमेव च ।
अयथावत्प्रजानाति
बुद्धिः सा पार्थ राजसी ॥१८.३१॥
yayā dharmamadharmaṁ ca
kāryaṁ cākāryameva ca
ayathāvatprajānāti
buddhiḥ sā pārtha rājasī (18.31)

yayā — by which; dharmam — right; adharmaṁ — wrong; ca — and; kāryam — duty; cākāryam = ca — and + akāryam — neglect; eva — indeed; ca — and; ayathāvat — mistakenly; prajānāti — is identified; buddhiḥ — intellectual insight; sā — it; pārtha — son of Pṛthā; rājasī — in the impulsive mode

That intellectual insight by which right and wrong, duty and neglect, are mistakenly identified, is, O son of Pṛthā, in the impulsive mode. (18.31)

Commentary:

When right and wrong, duty and neglect, are confused, one for the other, then it is to be concluded that the intellect uses the passionate energy, a force which shuffles the perception of reality in order to facilitate enjoyment. Unfortunately, most human beings are guided by the passionate mode. To move out of this mode, one has to perform yoga austerities.

अधर्मं धर्ममिति या
मन्यते तमसावृता ।
सर्वार्थान्विपरीतांश्च
बुद्धिः सा पार्थ तामसी ॥ १८.३२ ॥
adharmaṁ dharmamiti yā
manyate tamasāvṛtā
sarvārthānviparītāṁśca
buddhiḥ sā pārtha tāmasī (18.32)

adharmaṁ — wrong method; dharmam — right method; iti — thus; yā — which; manyate — it considered; tamasāvṛtā = tamasa — ignorance + āvṛtā — absorbed by; sarvārthān — all values; viparītāṁśca = viparītān — perverted + ca — and; buddhiḥ — intellectual insight; sā — it; pārtha — son of Pṛthā; tāmasī — in the depressive mode

That intellectual insight which is absorbed by ignorance, which considers the wrong method as the right one and perceives all values in a perverted way, is, O son of Pṛthā, of the depressive mode. (18.32)

Commentary:

Most human beings are guided in part by the depressive mode and in part by the passionate energy. To move away from either influence, one has to perform austerities. The idea that one could be lifted from these modes, merely by the adoption of a certain religion, is a farce. A living being's psychology does not change merely by religious affiliation. He has to work on the mystic plane to alter his demeanor and to change out his diet of subtle energies. He cannot do this without practicing advanced yoga.

When a human being gets an uplifting experience that lifts him away from his normal psychology, he does not remain on that higher plane. He returns to the normal level after the experience passes. Thus unless he works for a permanent relocation to higher levels, he resumes the lower phase. I will give an example. In the month of March of the year 2002, the Siddha Swami Muktananda came to see me. He wanted to see how my yoga practice progressed. After reviewing my success in Kuṇḍalinī yoga and celibacy yoga, he said a few words to me. He felt that I was ready for samādhi practice. After stating that, Swami Muktananda went away. A few days after, he came again with his spiritual master Swami Nityananda, who is an extremely advanced person, but who is so humble and modest that his progression cannot be gauged. I was glad to see Swami Nityananda. After sometime he sent Swami Muktananda away. Swami Muktananda instead of going away stood nearby in a parallel dimension listening to everything his spiritual master said to me.

Suddenly as if he was late for an important appointment, Swami Nityananda got up and touched the top of my head. This was in the astral world. He said, "Look here, you just develop this body. This point should be focused on and tendered. This point should be eliminated completely. This scar should be made to disappear."

Right then he left in a haste. He was intercepted by Swami Muktananda, who said to him, "Guruji, you have never shown me those kriyās." Swami Nityananda replied, "You were not a householder. You had not contacted females. What would you have done with that sort of kriyā which is for a man who experienced sexual indulgence?" After that they both went away.

At the time I felt that I had switched over and out of my kuṇḍalinī chakra astral body. For two days after, I was aware of the bubble—shaped subtle body which has a hole at the top of it. After those two days I was again in the kuṇḍalinī astral form. In other words, I again resumed what was natural for me. I would have to work hard with the austerities to make the permanent change.

A human being can certainly get a flash vision or momentarily experience a higher state but he or she will not remain there. The person will again resume what is normal. If one wants permanent relocation, one must work for it. It cannot be bestowed permanently at the time of death or at any other time. One earns it by austerities. If you do not work for it, no one will be able to bestow it permanently. Your nature will resume its normal routine.

It is not so with degradation. That is why we are fooled into thinking that if we are graced we will go higher and stay there. The procedure for degradation is such that one can go down once and stay there for a long, long time, adopting that level permanently. One does not have to work to become degraded. My present life shows this. I did not have to work to get the vice-prone, lust-seeking body which I got from my parents. My nature was altered automatically just by the association. But I had to work to reverse it. I could not reverse it just by associating with great yogis, except that through their association, I got the disciplines for reform. It takes endeavor to go upwards. It only requires association to go downwards. That is the gist of it.

If I have to work for salvation, then I know for sure that most human beings will surely have to endeavor for it. I cannot endorse slogans which say that one can be permanently elevated by grace or religious affiliations alone.

धृत्या यया धारयते
मनःप्राणेन्द्रियक्रियाः ।
योगेनाव्यभिचारिण्या
धृतिः सा पार्थ सात्त्विकी ॥१८.३३॥
dhṛtyā yayā dhārayate
manaḥprāṇendriyakriyāḥ
yogenāvyabhicāriṇyā
dhṛtiḥ sā pārtha sāttvikī (18.33)

dhṛtyā — by determination; yayā — by which; dhārayate — it holds; manaḥprāṇendriyakriyāḥ = manaḥ — mind + prāna — energizing breath + indriyakriyāḥ — senses; yogenāvyabhicāriṇyā = yogena — by yoga practices + avyabhicāriṇyā — unwavering, constant; dhṛtiḥ — determination; sā — it; pārtha — son of Pṛthā; sāttvikī — of the clarifying influence

The determination which holds the mind, the energizing breath, and the senses by constant yoga expertise, that, O son of Pṛthā, is of the clarifying influence. (18.33)

Commentary:

Readers should check the Sanskrit to see the term yogenāvyabhicārinyā. Śrī Krishna is the one who stressed this.

When someone speaks of holding the mind, the energizing breath (prāṇa) and the senses with determination, he speaks of advanced yoga practice in the states of prāṇāyāma, pratyāhār, dhāraṇa, dhyāna and samādhi. Śrī Krishna labeled that as being under the clarifying influence, exactly so, because that cleans up the buddhi organ and stops absorption of mundane objects.

यया तु धर्मकामार्थान्
धृत्या धारयतेऽर्जुन ।
प्रसङ्गेन फलाकाङ्क्षी
धृतिः सा पार्थ राजसी ॥१८.३४॥
yayā tu dharmakāmārthān
dhṛtyā dhārayate'rjuna
prasaṅgena phalākāṅkṣī
dhṛtiḥ sā pārtha rājasī (18.34)

yayā — by which; tu — but; dharmakāmārthān = dharma — duty + kāma — pleasure + arthān — wealthy; dhṛtyā — with determination; dhārayate — it holds; 'rjuna = arjuna — Arjuna; prasaṅgena — with attachment; phalākāṅkṣī — desiring results; dhṛtiḥ — determination; sā —it; pārtha — son of Pṛthā; rājasī — impulsion

But the determination by which one holds duty, pleasure, and wealth with attachment and with desire for results, is an impulsion, O son of Pṛthā. (18.34)

Commentary:

This includes when such things are done for religious purposes. Even though one might be told that one can act with attachment if done for missionary purposes or that one may desire results so long as one engages the rewards in Krishna's service, the endeavors are still contaminated. It is merely a way of using one's impure psyche to imitate purity. Such acts are good but they are not pure. They will not be regarded as purity by the Krishna who spoke the *Gītā* to Arjuna. He will see them as productions of the impulsive energy.

यया स्वप्नं भयं शोकं
विषादं मदमेव च ।
न विमुञ्चति दुर्मेधा
धृतिः सा पार्थ तामसी ॥१८.३५॥
yayā svapnaṁ bhayaṁ śokaṁ
viṣādaṁ madameva ca
na vimuñcati durmedhā
dhṛtiḥ sā pārtha tāmasī (18.35)

yayā — by which; svapnaṁ — sleep; bhayaṁ — fear; śokaṁ — sorrow; viṣādaṁ — despair; madam — pride; eva — indeed; ca — and; na — not; vimuñcati — abandons; durmedhā — idiot; dhṛtiḥ — determination; sā — it; pārtha — son of Pṛthā; tāmasī — of the depressive mode

That determination by which an idiot does not abandon sleep, fear, sorrow, despair and pride, is of the depressing mode. (18.35)

Commentary:

Such a person is held fast by sluggish energies. Usually he has no choice but to continue under their influences. He is like a man who made contact with a high voltage wire. It will not release him until it has fried every cell in his body.

Many women are prone to sorrow and despair. A woman can spend days being absorbed by distraught emotions. Sometimes an entire week or month passes and a woman's attention is occupied with incidences which cause agony or some degree of emotional pain. How they do it, I do not know. I can tell you that they have an automatic mechanism which focuses on this. A kriyā yogi can learn much by observing the mood changes in women. Their focusing power is tremendous. It is the type of focusing power we are endeavoring to develop so we can enter into samādhi practice.

Male devotees should be wary of the emotional states of their wives. If one stays close to a woman, one will come down into sorrow and despair. One's practice will be ruined. A yogin should keep a safe distance from the emotional nature of women. Their status in existence should be respected but one should not get too close to it, otherwise one will have to spend years upgrading oneself. Those of us who already made the mistake of getting too close to the emotional psyche of women, know exactly what I discussed here. Others can spare themselves the psychological clean—up task by keeping a safe distance. Śrīla Yogeshwarananda, that great yogin said this to me. "As for women, I never understood them. It was never necessary for me to understand them either."

It may be that he understands them all too well. He saved himself from having to do extra work in cleaning up his psychology of emotionalism. Because the males and females have affinity for each other, it is a mishap when they associate too close to each other. My advice to all of you is to keep a safe distance. Do not disrespect women. Swami

Muktananda, even though he is a brahmachari siddha, and even though his subtle body has no evidence of female contact, showed me a woman. It was Srimati Kuṇḍalinī Shakti Ma.

If one practices sincerely he will not have to chase women. He has in his own subtle body the most sexually appealing woman in this creation. By the grace of Swami Muktananda, I give this hint to the kriyā yogis.

सुखं त्विदानीं त्रिविधं
शृणु मे भरतर्षभ ।
अभ्यासाद्रमते यत्र
दुःखान्तं च निगच्छति ॥ १८.३६ ॥
sukhaṁ tvidānīṁ trividhaṁ
śṛṇu me bharatarṣabha
abhyāsādramate yatra
duḥkhāntaṁ ca nigacchati (18.36)

sukhaṁ — happiness; tu — but; idānīṁ — now; trividhaṁ — types; śṛṇu — hear; me — from me; bharatarṣabha — O strong man of the Bharatas; abhyāsāt — from habit; ramate — enjoys; yatra —where, through which; duḥkhāntaṁ — end of sorrow; ca — and, or; nigacchati — one comes to

But now hear from Me, O strong man of the Bharatas, regarding the three types of happiness which one either enjoys from habit or through which one comes to the end of sorrow. (18.36)

Commentary:

Kriyā yoga lets one come to the end of sorrow and eliminate the tendency of enjoying from habit. It is a funny thing to find someone who sits daily in the half lotus posture and meditates with his eyes closed or half open with a broad smile on his face. What? Yes, that is not kriyā yoga.

Kriyā yoga is more about dukhānatam, the end (antam) of sorrow (dukha). It is not about the continuation of enjoying through habit. For going into samādhi, one does not powder his face, sit in half lotus and assume a broad pleasing smile.

यत्तदग्रे विषमिव
परिणामेऽमृतोपमम् ।
तत्सुखं सात्त्विकं प्रोक्तम्
आत्मबुद्धिप्रसादजम् ॥ १८.३७॥
yattadagre viṣamiva
pariṇāme'mṛtopamam
tatsukhaṁ sāttvikaṁ proktam
ātmabuddhiprasādajam (18.37)

yat = yad — which; tat — that; agre — initially; viṣam — poison; iva — like; pariṇāme — in changing; 'mṛtopamam = amṛtopamam = amṛta — nectar + upamam — likeness; tat = tad — that; sukham — happiness; sāttvikaṁ — of the clarifying mode; proktam — is said to be; ātmabuddhiprasādajam = ātmabuddhi — spiritual discernment + prasāda — clarity + jam — produced by

That which initially is like poison but which changes into an experience like nectar, and which is felt through the clarity of spiritual discernment, is said to be happiness in the clarifying mode. (18.37)

Commentary:

This happiness comes in the wake of action which is approved by the Universal Form. Such action may not be pleasurable to perform. It is more like the one Arjuna was reluctant to do at Kurukṣetra. This is why initially, it had a distaste. It is because the performer has to turn away from human views which are averse to the Universal Form. Once the action is taken, the distaste passes. It is replaced by a sure happiness in the clarifying mode. This is a sober type of happiness, not an enjoying type.

विषयेन्द्रियसंयोगाद्
यत्तदग्रेऽमृतोपमम् ।
परिणामे विषमिव
तत्सुखं राजसं स्मृतम् ॥ १८.३८॥
viṣayendriyasaṁyogād
yattadagre'mṛtopamam
pariṇāme viṣamiva
tatsukhaṁ rājasaṁ smṛtam (18.38)

viṣayendriyasaṁyogāt = viṣaya — attractive objects + indriya — sense organs + saṁyogāt — from contact; yat — which; tat — that; agre — in the beginning; 'mṛtopamam = amṛtopamam = amṛta — nectar + upamam — likeness; pariṇāme — changes into; viṣam — poison; ivā — like; tat — that; sukham — happiness; rājasaṁ — impulsion; smṛtam — recognized as

That happiness which in the beginning seems like nectar and which comes from the contact between the sense organs and attractive objects, which changes as if it were poison, is recognized as an impulsion. (18.38)

Commentary:

This is the usual happiness for human beings. People want to get this happiness continually. This is why they become prone to sexual indulgence and other enjoying arts of human association. People come to yoga practice wanting to enhance this sort of happiness. Yoga is not for giving this type of happiness. When people do not get it, they go away from yoga condemning it as being dry of sense fulfillment.

Invariably, the happiness which comes from contact between the sense organs and the attractive objects converts into suffering. Instead of realizing this, we conspire to escape from the suffering by indulging the senses in more contacts.

This tricky way of escaping destroys spirituality and causes the psyche to be further degraded. If for instance, I have sexual intercourse with a woman, there will undoubtedly be enjoyment, especially if the woman has a young body which is flushed by sexual maturity. But if such intercourse produces a child, I will be stuck with responsibility. I might have to live with the woman for a mandatory 16 or 18 years. Even though the woman's body gave me pleasure and drew pleasure from my form, still the woman's personality may cause me agony. Some of her habits might irritate me. Thus for the 16 years I will have to live with that. To escape this, I might get some inspiration from the impulsive mode to the effect that I can have more intercourse and thus blank out most of the irritations and agony. However by more intercourse, I would produce more children and so create more complexity.

It would be tricky because in the years ahead, the woman's body would begin to age and so would my form. The sexual intercourse would not be as pleasurable as it was in the beginning. I would be frustrated in that regard.

If on the other hand, I did not have children, I would still have to relate to the woman's personality, of which certain parts would irritate me. The impulsive relationship which began like honey, would end like a bitter syrup. If passion shares with me, its positive side, I would not be able to escape from its negative aspects.

यदग्रे चानुबन्धे च
सुखं मोहनमात्मनः ।
निद्रालस्यप्रमादोत्थं
तत्तामसमुदाहृतम् ॥ १८.३९॥

yat — which; agre — in the beginning; cānubandhe = ca — and + anubandhe — in consequence; ca — and; sukham — happiness; mohanam — bewildering; ātmanaḥ — of the person; nidrālasyapramādotthaṁ = nidrā — sleep + ālasya — laziness + pramāda —

yadagre cānubandhe ca
sukhaṁ mohanamātmanaḥ
nidrālasyapramādotthaṁ
tattāmasamudāhṛtam (18.39)

confusion + uttham — comes from; tat = tad — that; tāmasam — depressive mode; udāhṛtam — said to be

And that happiness which in the beginning and in consequence is bewildering to the person, which comes from sleep, laziness and confusion, is said to be of the depressive mode. (18.39)

Commentary:

When one is stunned and when one experiences happiness in a dazed state, it is to be assumed that one was overtaken by the depressive mode.

न तदस्ति पृथिव्यां वा
दिवि देवेषु वा पुनः ।
सत्त्वं प्रकृतिजैर्मुक्तं
यदेभिः स्यात्त्रिभिर्गुणैः ॥ १८.४० ॥
na tadasti pṛthivyāṁ vā
divi deveṣu vā punaḥ
sattvaṁ prakṛtijairmuktaṁ
yadebhiḥ syāttribhirguṇaiḥ (18.40)

na — not; tat— that; asti — there is; pṛthivyāṁ — on earth; vā — or; divi — in the supernatural world; deveṣu — among the supernatural rulers; vā — or; punaḥ = punar — even; sattvaṁ — something substantial; prakṛtijaiḥ — produced by material nature; muktaṁ — freed, without; yat — which; ebhiḥ — by these; syāt — it can exist; tribhiḥ — by three; guṇaiḥ — by influence

There is no object on earth or even in the subtle mundane domains, that can exist without these three modes which were produced from material nature. (18.40)

Commentary:

This means even the sanctified Deity forms in the temple, as well as Śrī Krishna's mundane body which He used. We have to accept this. The implication is that we have to strive for a complete removal from the mundane energy.

ब्राह्मणक्षत्रियविशां
शूद्राणां च परंतप ।
कर्माणि प्रविभक्तानि
स्वभावप्रभवैर्गुणैः ॥ १८.४१ ॥
brāhmaṇakṣatriyaviśāṁ
śūdrāṇāṁ ca paraṁtapa
karmāṇi pravibhaktāni
svabhāvaprabhavairguṇaiḥ (18.41)

brāhmaṅakṣatriyaviśāṁ = brāhmaṇa — priestly teacher + kṣatriya — ruling sector + viśāṁ — productive managers; śudrāṇāṁ — of the working class; ca — and; paraṁtapa — scorcher of the enemy; karmāṇi — activities; pravibhaktāni — allotted; svabhāvaprabhavaiḥ = svabhāva — own nature + prabhavaiḥ — by being produced; guṇaiḥ — by the modes of material nature

The activities of the priestly teachers, the ruling sector, the productive managers and the working class, are allotted by the modes of material nature which arise from natural tendencies. (18.41)

Commentary:

At present our svabhava or natural tendencies are mostly aspects of material nature. How material nature has infiltrated into our psychology was explained before in the *Gītā*. At this point it is important to note that our activities are being conditioned by material nature. Denial of this will not change the fact. The denial will set us off-guard and cause us to lose whatever percentage of true perception we may have. We must understand the thoroughness of the influence of material nature.

शमो दमस्तपः शौचं
क्षान्तिरार्जवमेव च ।
ज्ञानं विज्ञानमास्तिक्यं
ब्रह्मकर्म स्वभावजम् ॥ १८.४२ ॥
śamo damastapaḥ śaucaṁ
kṣāntirārjavameva ca
jñānaṁ vijñānamāstikyaṁ
brahmakarma svabhāvajam (18.42)

śamo = śamaḥ — tranquility; damaḥ — restraint; tapaḥ — austerity; śaucaṁ— cleanliness; kṣāntiḥ — patience; ārjavam — straightforwardness; eva — indeed; ca — and; jñānaṁ — knowledge; vijñānaṁ — discrimination; āstikyaṁ — a belief in God; brahmakarma — work of a priestly teacher; svabhāvajam — based on natural tendencies

Tranquility, restraint, austerity, cleanliness, patience, straightforwardness, knowledge, discrimination and a belief in God, are the work of a priestly teacher based on his natural tendencies. (18.42)

Commentary:

These are positive qualities of a superior human being. Still, they are all, to a degree, conditioned by material nature. Only by higher yoga can one transfer out of nature's domain. These qualities are preferred, but nonetheless, they are conditioned by subtle material nature.

शौर्यं तेजो धृतिर्दाक्ष्यं
युद्धे चाप्यपलायनम् ।
दानमीश्वरभावश्च
क्षात्रंकर्म स्वभावजम् ॥ १८.४३ ॥
śauryaṁ tejo dhṛtirdākṣyaṁ
yuddhe cāpyapalāyanam
dānamīśvarabhāvaśca
kṣātraṁkarma svabhāvajam (18.43)

śauryaṁ — heroism; tejo = tejaḥ — majesty; dhṛtiḥ — determination; dākṣyaṁ — expertise; yuddhe — in battle; cāpi — and also; apalāyanam — lack of cowardice; dānam — charitable disposition; īśvarabhāvaśca = īśvarabhāvaḥ — governing tendency + ca — and; kṣātraṁ — of the ruling human being; karma — action; svabhāvajam — based on natural tendency

Heroism, majesty, determination, expertise, lack of cowardice in battle, charitable disposition, and governing tendency are the actions of a ruling human being, based on natural tendency. (18.43)

Commentary:

This was Arjuna's psychology. Śrī Krishna stated that a person has to function according to his acquired psychology, at least until he can get it changed. Arjuna could not suddenly adopt the position of a priestly man, because Arjuna had the governing tendency. But the Universal Form has uses for all types of tendencies. Thus Śrī Krishna directed Arjuna to surrender to that Form.

कृषिगोरक्ष्यवाणिज्यं
वैश्यकर्म स्वभावजम् ।
परिचर्यात्मकं कर्म
शूद्रस्यापि स्वभावजम् ॥ १८.४४ ॥
kṛṣigorakṣyavāṇijyaṁ
vaiśyakarma svabhāvajam
paricaryātmakaṁ karma
śūdrasyāpi svabhāvajam (18.44)

kṛṣigaurakṣyavāṇijyaṁ = kṛṣi — agriculture + gaurakṣya — cow tending + vāṇijyaṁ — trading; vaiśyakarma — action of the productive manager; svabhāvajam — based on natural tendency; paricaryātmakaṁ = paricaryā — service + ātmakaṁ — of natural tendency; karma — action; śudrasyāpi = śudrasya — working class + api — also; svabhāvajam — based on natural tendency

Agriculture, cow-tending and trading are the productive manager's activity based on natural tendency. Service actions are produced of a working class person based on natural tendency. (18.44)

Commentary:

One must use his current tendency while he tries to upgrade himself to the next higher caste. Only those in the highest caste are usually given the exemption from work. All others are required to work and to try to upgrade themselves in their spare time. Human beings usually want to indulge in vices in their free time. This is the human fall down. Basically speaking a man wants to drink liquor and indulge sexually in his spare time. That is the normal way of life. A woman wants to eat sweet foods and get romantic in her spare time. This is more or less the sum and substance of human existence. We should curb ourselves morally and practice the yoga austerities for self purification:

tatraikāgraṁ manaḥ kṛtvā yatacittendriyakriyaḥ
upaviśyāsane yuñjyād yogamātmaviśuddhaye (6.12)

...being there, seated in a posture, having the mind focused, the person who controls his thinking and sensual energy, should practice the yoga discipline for self purification. (6.12)

When we work, when it is not our spare time, we should tend to the concerns of the Universal Form as stipulated in the following verse:

kāyena manasā buddhyā kevalairindriyairapi
yoginaḥ karma kurvanti saṅgaṁ tyaktvātmaśuddhaye (5.11)

With the body, mind and intelligence, or even with the senses alone, the yogis, having discarded attachment, perform cultural acts for self—purification. (5.11)

स्वे स्वे कर्मण्यभिरतः
संसिद्धिं लभते नरः ।
स्वकर्मनिरतः सिद्धिं
यथा विन्दति तच्छृणु ॥ १८.४५ ॥
sve sve karmaṇyabhirataḥ
saṁsiddhiṁ labhate naraḥ
svakarmanirataḥ siddhiṁ
yathā vindati tacchṛṇu (18.45)

sve sve — his own, his own, consistent; karmaṇi — in action; abhirataḥ — content; saṁsiddhiṁ — perfection; labhate — attain; naraḥ — human being; svakarmanirataḥ = svakarma — own duty + nirataḥ — satisfied; siddhiṁ — perfection; yathā — of the means; vindati — finds; tat — that; śṛṇu — hear

A human being attains perfection by being content in the consistent execution of his duty. Hear of the means through which a duty-satisfied person finds perfection. (18.45)

Commentary:

Attaining perfection means getting the approval for a waiver from the Central Person in the Universal Form. With that sanction, one gets the opportunity to proceed to advanced yoga practice, otherwise one is doomed to take birth after birth in a mundane life form somewhere somehow. One has to train himself or herself to be content and happy in a sober mood when serving the Universal Form as described in so many places in the *Bhagavad Gītā*. It is, from the enjoying perspective, a grim outlook, but it is the most efficient way to get out of material existence.

As far as Śrī Krishna was concerned Arjuna or any of us without the waiver from cultural acts, from karma yoga, has no alternative but to work steadily in getting the continuous approval of the Universal Form.

यतः प्रवृत्तिर्भूतानां
येन सर्वमिदं ततम् ।
स्वकर्मणा तमभ्यर्च्य
सिद्धिं विन्दति मानवः ॥ १८.४६ ॥
yataḥ pravṛttirbhūtānāṁ
yena sarvamidaṁ tatam
svakarmaṇā tamabhyarcya
siddhiṁ vindati mānavaḥ (18.46)

yataḥ — from whom; pravṛttiḥ — origin; bhūtānāṁ — of beings; yena — by whom; sarvam — all; idam — this; tatam — is pervaded; svakarmaṇā — through his duty; tam — his; abhyarcya — worshipping; siddhiṁ — perfection; vindati — he finds; mānavaḥ — human being

Through the performance of his own duty, a human being finds perfection by worshipping the Person from Whom the beings originate and by Whom all this is pervaded. (18.46)

Commentary:

According to what Arjuna saw in the Universal Form, that person is the same Śrī Krishna who spoke the *Bhagavad Gītā*. One's duty, the svakarmaṇā, is the duty dictated by the Central Figure in the Universal Form. Initially, Arjuna did not agree with Śrī Krishna. It means that at times the actor will disagree with Śrī Krishna and will feel that Śrī Krishna misleads him or gives him tasks which are against his very nature.

If we could get in touch with Krishna to actually know His preferences, and if we completed the tasks assigned, we would find perfection by honoring His requests. In His association the path for perfection would be revealed.

श्रेयान्स्वधर्मो विगुणः
परधर्मात्स्वनुष्ठितात् ।
स्वभावनियतं कर्म
कुर्वन्नाप्नोति किल्बिषम् ॥ १८.४७॥
śreyānsvadharmo viguṇaḥ
paradharmātsvanuṣṭhitāt
svabhāvaniyataṁ karma
kurvannāpnoti kilbiṣam (18.47)

śreyān — better; svadharmo = svadharmaḥ — own duty; viguṇāḥ — imperfectly; paradharmāt — then another's duty; svanuṣṭhitāt = su + anuṣṭhitāt — well performed, perfectly; svabhāvaniyataṁ = svabhāva — own nature + niyatam — restricted; karma — action; kurvan — performing; nāpnoti = na — not + āpnoti — he acquires; kilbiṣam — sin, fault

Better to attend to one's own duty imperfectly than to heed another's perfectly. By performing actions which are restricted by one's own nature, one does not acquire fault. (18.47)

Commentary:

Everyone has a particular duty which should be completed before he departs from his present body. That completed task is called svadharma, the righteous duty, for the proper use of the present body. One person's duty is different from another's even though there might be similarities.

One should stick to his own duty by staying attuned to the Universal Form. Even though a group of souls may work together, still there is individual accountability. If one sticks to his duty, even if one makes a mistake now and again, even if he is unable to do it efficiently, he will not acquire any faults which would send him downwards in the mundane evolutionary cycle. We are asked to fear the disapproval of the Universal Form because His disgust with noncompliance will be costly in terms of our descent into a lower species.

सहजं कर्म कौन्तेय
सदोषमपि न त्यजेत् ।
सर्वारम्भा हि दोषेण
धूमेनाग्निरिवावृताः ॥ १८.४८ ॥
sahajaṁ karma kaunteya
sadoṣamapi na tyajet
sarvārambhā hi doṣeṇa
dhūmenāgnirivāvṛtāḥ(18.48)

sahajaṁ — inborn; karma — action; kaunteya — son of Kunti; sadoṣam — with fault; api — even; na — not; tyajet — should abandon; sarvārambhā — all undertakings; hi — indeed; doṣeṇa — with defect; dhumenāgniḥ = dhumena — with smoke + āgniḥ — fire; ivāvṛtaḥ = iva — like + āvṛtaḥ — is shrouded

One should not abandon inborn duty, O son of Kuntī, even if it is faulty. Indeed, all undertakings are with defect, even as fire is shrouded with smoke. (18.48)

Commentary:

This means that even the assignment given by the Universal Form, by the Supreme Being, has defects. Nothing is perfect in the material world, because we are dealing with the mundane energy in conjunction with the divine will which supervises it. Karma yoga is defective but that does not mean that we can find a better alternative. We cannot. Whatever else we might do in the social, cultural and political fields will be even more defective. Karma yoga is the best way to act in this world, until at least we get the exemption so that we can step aside from the world.

Śrī Krishna indicated that we should still complete the duty He assigned, even if we are perceptive enough to realize that it has defects. As some philosophers concluded, there are faults in all actions. However that does not mean that we can attain perfection without actions. We must act regardless. God is supreme, regardless of whether we can prove that He gave us an instruction which was imperfect. That is the situation. The technicality is to be sure that we have His approval.

When a certain Swami was implicated in the murder of a Hare Krishna devotee, he left the United States to avoid trial. He did not murder the devotee but he helped to transport the person who did. When he was traveling in self—exile through other countries, he was questioned about the incidence. The fugitive explained that what he did in transporting the suspect was authorized. But the person who questioned him had the sense to ask the question. "By whom was your participation authorized?"

Actually the person who authorized it was another senior swami who became famous as a pure devotee of Śrī Krishna. That does not mean that the Central Person in the Universal Form had authorized the activity. We have to be sure that Krishna personally authorizes an activity. We should not take it for granted that our spiritual master is correct in all cases. We should not think that he can do no wrong. He should be respected. His views should be given precedence but we have to be sure that in any situation, his instructions are coming from the Universal Form.

Spiritual masters who have many disciples and are preoccupied in making many more, and with building huge missions with many temples, will invariably be distracted by influences other than the Universal Form. They are prone to giving the wrong instructions which we might mistake for rulings coming down from the Universal Form. Such mistakes will be costly for both disciples and the spiritual master concerned.

असक्तबुद्धिः सर्वत्र
जितात्मा विगतस्पृहः ।
नैष्कर्म्यसिद्धिं परमां
संन्यासेनाधिगच्छति ॥ १८.४९ ॥
asaktabuddhiḥ sarvatra
jitātmā vigataspṛhaḥ
naiṣkarmyasiddhiṁ paramāṁ
saṁnyāsenādhigacchati (18.49)

asaktabuddhiḥ = asakta — unattached + buddhiḥ — intellect; sarvatra — in all applications; jitātmā — self-conquered; vigataspṛhah = vigata — disappeared + spṛhaḥ — yearnings; naiṣkarmyasiddhiṁ = naiṣkarmya — exemption from activities + siddhim — perfection; paramāṁ — supreme; saṁnyāsenādhigacchati = saṁnyāsena — by renunciation of opportunities + adhigacchati — he attains

He whose intellect is unattached in every application, who is self—controlled, whose yearnings disappeared, by the renunciation of opportunities, attains supreme perfection of being exempt from action. (18.49)

Commentary:

Śrī Krishna spoke of higher issues in this verse. He already stressed that Arjuna was to practice karma yoga as a tyāgi, a person who declines the consequences of action but who takes opportunities.

Śrī Krishna now described the condition of the advanced yogis who got the exemption from karma yoga. Such people are naiṣkarma or exempt from social, cultural and political involvement. To be like this, one's intellect must be unattached in all applications. One must be self—controlled by virtue of mastership of advanced yoga practice. One's yearnings for mundane life in all its phases, must cease. Naiṣkarma does not mean selfless or philanthropic work.

सिद्धिं प्राप्तो यथा ब्रह्म
तथाप्नोति निबोध मे ।
समासेनैव कौन्तेय
निष्ठा ज्ञानस्य या परा ॥ १८.५० ॥
siddhiṁ prāpto yathā brahma
tathāpnoti nibodha me
samāsenaiva kaunteya
niṣṭhā jñānasya yā parā (18.50)

siddhiṁ — perfection; prāpto = prāptaḥ — attained; yathā — as; brahma — spirituality; tathāpnoti = tathā — thus + āpnoti — attains; nibodha — learn; me — from me; samāsenaiva = samāsena — in brief + eva — indeed; kaunteya — son of Kuntī; niṣṭhā — state; jñānasya — of experience; yā — which; parā — highest

Learn from Me briefly, O son of Kuntī, how a person who attained perfection, also reaches a spirituality which is the highest. (18.50)

Commentary:

Śrī Krishna will now summarize the *Gītā* discourse. From verse 51 through verse 66, Śrī Krishna will give a synopsis of his most important points. This is a summary of the *Gītā*, given by Śrī Krishna Himself. It is important because from this summary Arjuna had to make up his mind, either to accept or reject Śrī Krishna's suggestion about fighting on the battlefield.

We should look at this information too and make up our minds if we are going to follow Śrī Krishna and if we want to cooperate with the Universal Form.

बुद्ध्या विशुद्धया युक्तो
धृत्यात्मानं नियम्य च ।
शब्दादीन्विषयांस्त्यक्त्वा
रागद्वेषौ व्युदस्य च ॥ १८.५१ ॥
buddhyā viśuddhayā yukto
dhṛtyātmānaṁ niyamya ca
śabdādīnviṣayāṁstyaktvā
rāgadveṣau vyudasya ca (18.51)

buddhyā — with intellect; viśuddhayā — with purified; yukto = yuktaḥ — yogically disciplined; dhṛtyātmānaṁ = dhṛtyā — with firmness + ātmānaṁ — self; niyamya — controlling; ca — and; śabdādīn = śabda — sound + ādīn — beginning with, and others; viṣayān — attractive sensations; tyaktvā — abandoning; rāgadveṣau= rāga — craving + dveṣau — hatred; vyudasya — rejecting; ca — and

Being yogically-disciplined with purified intelligence and controlling the soul, firmly abandoning sound and other attractive sensations, rejecting craving and hatred, (18.51)

Commentary:

This is a description of what a yogi would accomplish before he enters samādhi. He must have a purified intellect which is an organ in the head of the subtle body. One must control his soul by not allowing it to become familiar with the subtle body any more. The familiarity with the subtle body makes the soul a stooge for that form causing the spirit to take numerous gross bodies helplessly. One must abandon sound and other attractive sensations both grossly and subtly by the practice of pratyāhār sense withdrawal. This is a mystic process which is accelerated by haṭha yoga and prāṇāyāma. One must reject cravings and hatred, doing so because one has the psychological strength from consistent yoga practice.

विविक्तसेवी लघ्वाशी
यतवाक्कायमानसः ।
ध्यानयोगपरो नित्यं
वैराग्यं समुपाश्रितः ॥ १८.५२ ॥
viviktasevī laghvāśī
yatavākkāyamānasaḥ
dhyānayogaparo nityaṁ
vairāgyaṁ samupāśritaḥ (18.52)

viviktasevī = vivikta — is isolated + sevī — living at; laghvāśī = laghv (laghu) — lightly + āśī — eating; yatavākkāyamānasaḥ = yata — controlled + vāk (vāc) — speech + kāya — body + mānasaḥ — mind; dhyānayogaparo = dhyāna — meditation + yoga — yoga + paro (paraḥ) — devoted to; nityam — always; vairāgyam — dispassion; samupāśritaḥ — resorting to

...living in isolation, eating lightly, controlling speech, body and mind, always being devoted to yogic meditation, resorting to dispassion, (18.52)

Commentary:

In so many of these verses the system of the eightfold yoga practice is given. It is repeated here again and again. Thus it is no wonder that those who use the *Gītā* without doing yoga practice, become baffled. It is not that the *Gītā* cannot be made practical to our modern situation but we should understand that it was not originally designed to accommodate a spiritual practice which was devoid of yoga expertise. Even senior warriors in Śrī Krishna's time were required to have yoga proficiency.

Here Śrī Krishna spoke of yogic meditation. This is different to meditation without yoga but we find that nowadays people feel that they can meditate and attain perfection without yoga. And what happens is that the majority of these people imagine peacefulness and reduction of stress and consider that to be spiritual perfection.

Even though I have highlighted yoga in this *Bhagavad Gītā* commentary, which is meant for kriyā yogins, still I am surprised at Śrī Krishna's continuous hawking about yoga as the basic requirement. This is very encouraging to those of us who do yoga. Hearing this from Śrī Krishna, we will not be disheartened by those preachers who blacklist or try to abolish the art of it.

अहंकारं बलं दर्पं
कामं क्रोधं परिग्रहम् ।
विमुच्य निर्ममः शान्तो
ब्रह्मभूयाय कल्पते ॥ १८.५३ ॥
ahaṁkāraṁ balaṁ darpaṁ
kāmaṁ krodhaṁ parigraham
vimucya nirmamaḥ śānto
brahmabhūyāya kalpate (18.53)

ahaṁkāraṁ — without a misplaced initiative, without a false assertion; balaṁ — brute force; darpaṁ — arrogance; kāmaṁ — cravings; krodhaṁ — anger; parigraham — possessions; vimucya — freeing oneself; nirmamaḥ — unselfish; śānto = śāntaḥ — peaceful; brahmabhūyāya = brahma — spirit + bhūyāyā — to that level, existential; kalpate — is suited

...freeing oneself from a false assertion, from the application of brute force, from arrogance, from craving and from possessiveness, being unselfish and peaceful, one is suited to the spiritual level. (18.53)

Commentary:

One must free himself from false assertion, which means that one should become detached from the sense of initiative which is known as ahamkara in Sanskrit. This means one must be able to see inside the causal body to find that sense of initiative and to separate oneself from it. This is mystic procedure.

One must be free from the application of brute force. This is attained by becoming resistant to the desire energy which oozes out of the causal form. So long as we are under the influence of the pleasure—seeking subtle body with its kuṇḍalinī survival mechanism, we cannot be free from brute force. We can speak of peace and human rights or whatever, but still, we will be under the dominance of the survival impulse. Kriyā yoga is the key to psyche purification.

We must realize that we are messed—up. We must understand that we should work to change this. The impurities will not go away by flash enlightenments, unless such graces influence us to apply powerful austerities upon ourselves for a sufficient period to effect the necessary purification and elevation.

ब्रह्मभूतः प्रसन्नात्मा
न शोचति न काङ्क्षति ।
समः सर्वेषु भूतेषु
मद्भक्तिं लभते पराम् ॥ १८.५४ ॥
brahmabhūtaḥ prasannātmā
na śocati na kāṅkṣati
samaḥ sarveṣu bhūteṣu
madbhaktiṁ labhate parām (18.54)

brahmabhūtaḥ — being absorbed in spiritual existence; prasannātmā = prasanna — peaceful + ātmā — self, spirit; na — not; śocati — laments; na — no; kāṅkṣati — hankers for something; samaḥ — impartial; sarveṣu — in all; bhūteṣu — in the beings; madbhaktiṁ — devotion to me; labhate — attains; parām — supreme

One who is absorbed in the spiritual existence, who has a peaceful spirit, who does not lament or hanker for anything, who is impartial to all beings, attains the supreme devotion to Me. (18.54)

Commentary:

Śrī Krishna again presented devotion to Himself, madbhaktim. Here He indicated that such devotion, the supreme type of it, is developed naturally in a person who is absorbed in spiritual existence, who has a peaceful spirit and who does not lament or hanker for anything. Such a person must be impartial to all beings. This, of course, pertains to those who have the exemption from karma yoga.

It means that even if a person perfects yoga without taking to Krishna consciousness as it is described in the *Gītā* in Chapter Ten, that person, by absorption in spiritual existence and by the completion of yoga disciplines, will gravitate towards being a devotee of Śrī Krishna. He will not be mediocre devotee but one of the greatest souls, developing causelessly the supreme devotion to Śrī Krishna. There is an example of this in Shuka, the son of Śrīla Vyāsadeva. In fact, there was a question asked, regarding how it was that Shuka, a mahāyogīn, an absorber in spiritual existence, took to Krishna consciousness and developed the supreme devotion, even though Shuka was unemotional and indifferent to affectionate energies.

Some leaders in the disciplic succession, however, do not trust the process. They are of the view that if one practices yoga, one will never become a devotee. They deny this verse of the *Gītā*.

भक्त्या मामभिजानाति
यावान्यश्चास्मि तत्त्वतः ।
ततो मां तत्त्वतो ज्ञात्वा
विशते तदनन्तरम् ॥ १८.५५॥
bhaktyā māmabhijānāti
yāvānyaścāsmi tattvataḥ
tato māṁ tattvato jñātvā
viśate tadanantaram (18.55)

bhaktyā — by devotion; mām — to me; abhijānāti — he realizes; yāvān — how great; yaścāsmi = yaḥ — who + ca — and + asmi — I am; tattvataḥ — in reality; tato = tataḥ — then; mām — me; tattvato = tattvataḥ — in truth; jñātvā — having known; viśate — enters; tadanantaram — immediately

By devotion to Me, he realizes how great I am and who I am in reality. Then having known Me in truth, he enters My association immediately. (18.55)

<u>*Commentary:*</u>

Śrī Krishna admirably explained that one who is successful in psyche purification by yoga process, will develop devotion and will realize how great Krishna is in reality. Such a person is there in the example of Markandeya, who explained his realization to King Yudhiṣṭhira.

Another person was Maitreya Rishi who functioned as the spiritual master of Vidura. He mastered yoga and then became attached to Śrī Krishna and entered into Krishna's association.

सर्वकर्माण्यपि सदा
कुर्वाणो मद्व्यपाश्रयः ।
मत्प्रसादादवाप्नोति
शाश्वतं पदमव्ययम् ॥ १८.५६ ॥
sarvakarmāṇyapi sadā
kurvāṇo madvyapāśrayaḥ
matprasādādavāpnoti
śāśvataṁ padamavyayam (18.56)

sarvakarmāṇi — in all actions; api — furthermore; sadā — always; kurvāṇo = kurvāṇaḥ — performing; madvyapāśrayaḥ — taking reliance in me; matprasādāt — from my grace; avāpnoti — gets; śāśvataṁ — eternal; padam — abode; avyayam — imperishable

Furthermore, know that while performing all actions, he whose reliance is always on Me, gets by My grace, the eternal imperishable abode. (18.56)

Commentary:

This pertains to persons in Arjuna's status; those who do not yet have the exemption from karma yoga. They, by performing all actions, and by being reliant on Śrī Krishna for the inspirations to complete the tasks put before them by destiny, eventually acquire by Śrī Krishna's grace, the eternal imperishable abode. They no longer have to serve Krishna in tasks in this material world.

चेतसा सर्वकर्माणि
मयि संन्यस्य मत्परः ।
बुद्धियोगमुपाश्रित्य
मच्चित्तः सततं भव ॥१८.५७॥
cetasā sarvakarmāṇi
mayi saṁnyasya matparaḥ
buddhiyogamupāśritya
maccittaḥ satataṁ bhava (18.57)

cetasā — by thought; sarvakarmāṇi — all actions; mayi —on Me; saṁnyasya — devoted to me; matparaḥ — devoted to Me; buddhiyogam — disciplining the intellect by yoga practice; upāśritya — relying on; maccittaḥ — thinking of Me; satataṁ — constantly; bhava — be

Renouncing by thought, all actions to Me, being devoted to Me, relying on the process of disciplining the intellect by yoga, be constantly thinking of Me. (18.57)

Commentary:

This has to do with our relationship to the Universal Form. It is not based on the relation to Śrī Krishna as a cowherd boy in Vṛndāvana. It is strictly in terms of the Universal Form's interactions in approving and disapproving human activity.

One has to divest personal concern for this world, shed desires as they were, and take up the mission of the Universal Form in so far as one is assigned to complete tasks stipulated by Him. Sometimes it is palatable work; sometimes it is disagreeable, but it should be done regardless.

One has to renounce his own thoughts or as Jesus Christ indicated, a person may deny his own self in order to do what God requests. One has to do karma yoga if one does not have an exemption from cultural life but one must do buddhi yoga simultaneously because it is buddhi yoga which gives one the upper hand emotionally. It is by the perfection of buddhi yoga that one develops the required detachment from relatives and friends, something that Arjuna did not have when his knees buckled and told Krishna that he would not fight.

Make no mistake about it. Let no one fool you into thinking that buddhi yoga is bhakti yoga. Buddhi yoga concerns curbing the buddhi organ in the head of the subtle body by means of pratyāhār sense withdrawal which is the 5th stage in the practice of yoga.

One must be constantly thinking of Śrī Krishna also but this refers to thinking of what He, as the Central Figure in the Universal Form, wants one to do as one's duty in the social, cultural or political fields.

This does not mean thinking of Śrī Krishna's Vṛndāvana pastimes which are an entirely different practice in spiritual life.

मच्चित्तः सर्वदुर्गाणि
मत्प्रसादात्तरिष्यसि ।
अथ चेत्त्वमहंकारान्
न श्रोष्यसि विनङ्क्ष्यसि ॥१८.५८॥
maccittaḥ sarvadurgāṇi
matprasādāttariṣyasi
atha cettvamahaṁkārān
na śroṣyasi vinaṅkṣyasi (18.58)

maccittaḥ — thinking of Me; sarvadurgāṇi — all difficulties; matprasādāt — from my grace; tariṣyasi — you will surpass; atha — but; cet = ced — if; tvam — you; ahaṁkārān — false assertion; na — not; śroṣyasi — you will listen; vinaṅkṣyasi — you will be lost

Thinking of Me, you will, by My grace, surpass all difficulties. But if by false assertion, you do not listen, you will be lost. (18.58)

Commentary:

Śrī Krishna was not asking Arjuna to think of Vṛndāvana pastimes with the cowherd boys or with the gopis, even though these are the highest activities of the Lord. This refers to thinking of the mission as assigned by the Universal Form and as well as the most effective way of accomplishing it to His satisfaction. This is serious business. Arjuna has before him, the task of fighting a battle and wielding dangerous weapons for killing those who opposed Śrī Krishna's view about righteous living and saintly conduct.

As stated, if Arjuna or any of us do not comply with the Universal Form, we will be lost. Of course we might be appreciated by fellow human beings. Still, in terms of our spiritual aspirations we will have lost out for the time being.

यदहंकारमाश्रित्य
न योत्स्य इति मन्यसे ।
मिथ्यैष व्यवसायस्ते
प्रकृतिस्त्वां नियोक्ष्यति ॥१८.५९॥
yadahaṁkāramāśritya
na yotsya iti manyase
mithyaiṣa vyavasāyaste
prakṛtistvāṁ niyokṣyati (18.59)

yat — which; ahaṁkāram — false assertive attitude; āśritya — relying on; na — not; yotsya — I will fight; iti — thus; manyase — you thing; mithyaiṣa = mithya — mistaken + eṣa — this; vyavasāyaḥ — determination; te — your; prakṛtiḥ — material nature; tvāṁ — you; niyokṣyāti — you will be forced

While relying on a false assertive attitude, you may think, "I will not fight." But that determination is mistaken. Your material nature will force you. (18.59)

Commentary:

This is an alert. If we do not comply with Him, then taking help from other persons, relying on them, being inspired by them, we will reject the idea of the Universal Form. We will be mistaken about duty. Material nature itself, the very force that we are so trusting of, which is embedded in our psyche, will force us to become responsible for the same action which the Universal Form placed before us previously.

स्वभावजेन कौन्तेय
निबद्धः स्वेन कर्मणा ।
कर्तुं नेच्छसि यन्मोहात्
करिष्यस्यवशोऽपि तत् ॥१८.६०॥

svabhāvajena — of your own natural tendencies; kaunteya — son of Kuntī; nibaddhaḥ — bound; svena — by your own; karmāṇa — obligation; kartuṁ — to perform; necchasi = na — not + icchasi — you want; yan = yad — which; mohāt —

svabhāvajena kaunteya
nibaddhaḥ svena karmaṇā
kartuṁ necchasi yanmohāt
kariṣyasyavaśo'pi tat (18.60)

from delusion; kariṣyasi — you will do; avaśo = avaśaḥ — against your own will; 'pi = api — also, even; tat = tad — that

By your natural tendencies, being bound by obligations, O son of Kuntī, that which you do not want to perform due to delusion, you will do even if it is against your will. (18.60)

Commentary:

A person is placed in certain situations because of specific movements of providence. It is not as some teachers say that in all circumstances we end up doing something because it is our karma or because it is developed out of our past actions. That is true only in some situations. A person might end up doing something which did not develop out his past actions but which is forced into his venue by providence. In other words, the limited beings are regularly victimized by providence. But that is the way it is. We can just cope with this.

Some situations arise out of our previous actions. Some do not. The obligations are there as soon as we appear in any given environment. We experience this when we keep track of dreams. Sometimes a yogin is transferred in a parallel world. Immediately after, he fits in and begins to function as if he was always a part of that scene. It may be that he was never manifested in that world so how is it that he may fit in so suddenly? It is because the obligations latch on to a person. That energy finds a good or bad use for him.

Thus Arjuna or any of us, being bound by obligations which latch on to us in any given environment, are induced to act even against our will. The best course if we can take it, is to link up with the Universal Form as an agent. That is the highway out of these places in the material world. He is the only One who can free us from having to participate here. Others can engage us but they do not have the power or divine interest to free us.

ईश्वरः सर्वभूतानां
हृद्देशेऽर्जुन तिष्ठति ।
भ्रामयन्सर्वभूतानि
यन्त्रारूढानि मायया ॥ १८.६१ ॥
īśvaraḥ sarvabhūtānāṁ
hṛddeśe'rjuna tiṣṭhati
bhrāmayansarvabhūtāni
yantrārūḍhāni māyayā (18.61)

īśvaraḥ — Lord; sarvabhūtānām — of all beings; hṛddeśe = hṛd — central psyche + deśe — in the place; 'rjuna = arjuna — Arjuna; tiṣṭhati — is situated; bhrāmayan — cause to transmigrate; sarvabhūtāni — all beings; yantrārūḍhāni = yantra — machine + ārūḍhāni — fixed to; māyayā — by mystic power

The Lord of all beings is situated in the central psyche, O Arjuna, causing all beings to transmigrate by His mystic power, just as if they were fixed to a spinning machine. (18.61)

Commentary:

Now we get some inside information. Even though immediately we transmigrate on the basis of the energies and desires in the subtle body and the overall configuration at any given time, still there is another more important principal involved. That is the Supersoul, the Lord of all these psyches. It is His mystic power which energizes or restricts the subtle bodies. As this planet earth remains in an orbit around the sun and cannot escape by its own accord, so we remain at a certain mystic distance from the Supersoul. By His power we transmigrate here and there on the basis of the energy in the subtle body.

तमेव शरणं गच्छ
सर्वभावेन भारत ।
तत्प्रसादात्परां शान्तिं
स्थानं प्राप्स्यसि शाश्वतम् ॥ १८.६२ ॥
tameva śaraṇaṁ gaccha
sarvabhāvena bhārata
tatprasādātparāṁ śāntiṁ
sthānaṁ prāpsyasi śāśvatam (18.62)

tam — to him; eva — only; śaraṇaṁ — shelter; gaccha — go; sarvabhāvena — with all your being; bhārata — O descendant of Bharata; tatprasādāt — from that grace; parāṁ — supreme; śāntiṁ — security; sthānaṁ — place; prāpsyasi — you will attain; śāśvatam — eternal

With your whole being, go only to Him for shelter, O descendant of Bharata. You will attain the supreme security and the eternal place by His grace. (18.62)

Commentary:

Because we are so attuned to the subtle form and because our gross bodies are formed on the basis of its energy, we should pay attention to the Supersoul Personality. However, that cannot be done unless we have mystic perception. The advice in this verse cannot be used by someone who has not mastered advanced yoga practice. Arjuna had the proficiency. He applied this advice of Śrī Krishna.

इति ते ज्ञानमाख्यातं
गुह्याद्गुह्यतरं मया ।
विमृश्यैतदशेषेण
यथेच्छसि तथा कुरु ॥ १८.६३ ॥
iti te jñānamākhyātaṁ
guhyādguhyataraṁ mayā
vimṛśyaitadaśeṣeṇa
yathecchasi tathā kuru (18.63)

iti — thus; te — to you; jñānam — information; ākhyātaṁ — was explained; guhyāt — than secret; guhyataraṁ — more secret; mayā — by me; vimṛśyaitat = vimṛśya — having considered + etat — this; aśeṣena — fully; yathecchasi = yathā — as + icchasi — you desire, you please; tathā — in the way; kuru — act

The information that is more secret than secret was explained by Me to you. Having considered this fully, you may act as you please. (18.63)

Commentary:

Śrī Krishna concluded the discourse. Arjuna had to think it over and decide whether to fight or run away.

सर्वगुह्यतमं भूयः
श्रृणु मे परमं वचः ।
इष्टोऽसि मे दृढमिति
ततो वक्ष्यामि ते हितम् ॥ १८.६४ ॥
sarvaguhyatamaṁ bhūyaḥ
śṛṇu me paramaṁ vacaḥ
iṣṭo'si me dṛḍhamiti
tato vakṣyāmi te hitam (18.64)

sarvaguhyatamaṁ — of all, the most secret; bhūyaḥ — again; śṛṇu — hear; me — of me; paramaṁ — supreme; vacaḥ — discourse; iṣṭo = iṣṭaḥ — loved; 'si = asi — you are; me — of me; dṛḍham — surely; iti — this; tato = tataḥ — hence; vakṣyāmi — I will speak; te — your; hitam — benefit

Hear again of My supreme discourse, the most secret of all information. You are surely loved by Me. Hence I speak for your benefit. (18.64)

Commentary:

Out of sheer love for Arjuna, Śrī Krishna will give more information.

मन्मना भव मद्भक्तो
मद्याजी मां नमस्कुरु ।
मामेवैष्यसि सत्यं ते
प्रतिजाने प्रियोऽसि मे ॥ १८.६५॥
manmanā bhava madbhakto
madyājī māṁ namaskuru
māmevaiṣyasi satyaṁ te
pratijāne priyo'si me (18.65)

manmanā — be mindful of me; bhava — be; madbhakto = madbhaktaḥ — be devoted to me; madyājī — sacrifice to Me; māṁ — to me; namaskuru — do bow; mām — to me; evaiṣyasi = eva — in this way + eṣyasi — you will come; satyaṁ — in truth; te — to you; pratijāne — I promise; priyo = priyaḥ — dear; 'si = asi — you are; me — of me

Be mindful of Me, be devoted to Me. Sacrifice to Me. Do bow to Me. In this way you will in truth come to Me. I promise, for you are dear to Me. (18.65)

Commentary:

This is purely an instruction about Arjuna's personal relation with Śrī Krishna. The love between them flowed. We can feel the intensity of it as we read the discourse.

Adopting the suggestions of their spiritual master, many devotees apply this verse to themselves personally. They substitute themselves here for Arjuna. However for us as kriyā yogis, that is not the proper method. We stand by and feel that energy of love flow from Śrī Krishna to Arjuna, and from Arjuna to Śrī Krishna, the pretty but dangerous Supreme Person.

सर्वधर्मान्परित्यज्य
मामेकं शरणं व्रज ।
अहं त्वा सर्वपापेभ्यो
मोक्षयिष्यामि मा शुचः ॥ १८.६६ ॥
sarvadharmānparityajya
māmekaṁ śaraṇaṁ vraja
ahaṁ tvā sarvapāpebhyo
mokṣayiṣyāmi mā śucaḥ (18.66)

sarvadharmān — all traditional conduct; parityajya — abandoning; mām — in me; ekam —alone; śaraṇaṁ — refuge; vraja — take; aham — I; tvā — you; sarvapāpebhyo = sarvapāpebhyaḥ — from all sins, of faults; mokṣayiṣyāmi — I will cause you to be freed; mā — not; śucaḥ — worry

Abandoning all traditional conduct, take refuge in Me alone. I will cause you to be freed of all faults. Do not worry. (18.66)

Commentary:

This is the final appeal of Śrī Krishna for Arjuna to fight. Arjuna is to abandon all his attachments to traditional conduct, something he argued for in Chapter One of the *Gītā*. He is to take refuge in Śrī Krishna alone, leaving his friends and relatives aside. Śrī Krishna promised to create energies which would cause Arjuna to be free from ghastly acts Arjuna would commit on the battlefield. Arjuna was not to be sorry about the consequences. The Central Person of the Universal Form, Śrī Krishna Himself, would cover the liabilities.

इदं ते नातपस्काय
नाभक्ताय कदाचन ।
न चाशुश्रूषवे वाच्यं
न च मां योऽभ्यसूयति ॥१८.६७॥
idaṁ te nātapaskāya
nābhaktāya kadācana
na cāśuśrūṣave vācyaṁ
na ca māṁ yo'bhyasūyati (18.67)

idaṁ — this; te — of you; nātapaskāya = na — not + atapaskāya — to one who does not perform austerity; nābhaktāya = na — not + abhaktāya — to one who is not devoted; kadācana — at any time; na — not; cāśuśrūṣave = ca — and + aśuśrūṣave — one who does not desire to hear; vācyaṁ — what is to be said; na — not, ca — and; mām — me; yo — yaḥ — who; 'bhyasūyati = abhyasūyati — he is critical

This should not be told by you to anyone who does not perform austerity or is not devoted at anytime, or does not desire to hear what is said or is critical of Me. (18.67)

Commentary:

This applies to verses 65 and 66. Śrī Krishna seems to want to bar this information from being given to persons who might try to exploit it but who will be ruined if they attempt that and then discover that they are not covered by Śrī Krishna. In other words, such persons will be left with the liabilities for reckless actions, even though they believed that Śrī Krishna would protect them and save them from implications. Śrī Krishna prohibited that they should be given the information.

य इदं परमं गुह्यं
मद्भक्तेष्वभिधास्यति ।
भक्तिं मयि परां कृत्वा
मामेवैष्यत्यसंशयः ॥१८.६८॥
ya idaṁ paramaṁ guhyaṁ
madbhakteṣvabhidhāsyati
bhaktiṁ mayi parāṁ kṛtvā
māmevaiṣyatyasaṁśayaḥ (18.68)

ya — who; idam — this; paramam — supreme; guhyam — secret; madbhakteṣu — to my devotees; abhidhāsyati — he will explain; bhaktiṁ — devotion; mayi — to me; parām — highest; kṛtvā — having performed; mām — me; evaiṣyati = eva — indeed + eṣyati — he will come; asaṁśayaḥ — without a doubt, certainly

Whosoever, having performed the highest devotion to Me, will explain this supreme secret to My devotees, will certainly come to Me. (18.68)

Commentary:

Here Śrī Krishna placed a limitation that unless one has the highest devotion to Him, one should not explain the supreme secret of how to follow the instructions of the Universal Form as described in verses 65 and 66 in this chapter. If one tries to explain without being so qualified, then one will undoubtedly explain it in the wrong way and will ruin the hearers.

No one, unless he is qualified by this verse, should give out this guarantee to human beings; otherwise they will be misled into thinking that whatever they do will be covered by Śrī Krishna. We should recall the disclaimer:

nādatte kasyacitpāpaṁ na caiva sukṛtaṁ vibhuḥ
ajñānenāvṛtaṁ jñānaṁ tena muhyanti jantavaḥ (5.15)

The Almighty God does not receive from anyone, an evil consequence or a good reaction. The knowledge of this is shrouded by ignorance through which the people are deluded. (5.15)

न च तस्मान्मनुष्येषु
कश्चिन्मे प्रियकृत्तमः ।
भविता न च मे तस्माद्
अन्यः प्रियतरो भुवि ॥ १८.६९ ॥
na ca tasmānmanuṣyeṣu
kaścinme priyakṛttamaḥ
bhavitā na ca me tasmād
anyaḥ priyataro bhuvi (18.69)

na — not; ca — and; tasmān — than this person; manuṣyeṣu — among human beings; kaścit — anyone; me — of me; priyakṛttamaḥ = priyaḥ — pleasing + kṛttamaḥ — more in performance; bhavitā — he will be; na — not; ca — and; me — to me; tasmāt — than this person; anyaḥ — other; priyataro = priyataraḥ — more dear; bhuvi — on earth

And no one among human beings is more pleasing to Me in performance than he. And no one on earth will be more dear to Me than he. (18.69)

<u>*Commentary:*</u>

Arjuna was definitely dear to Śrī Krishna, but this verse described a person who is even dearer. By the indication in the previous verse, we can deduce that this dearest of devotees would not be a warrior like Arjuna but would be a brahmin spiritual master. One should go over the Sanskrit in these verses very carefully.

अध्येष्यते च य इमं
धर्म्यं संवादमावयोः ।
ज्ञानयज्ञेन तेनाहम्
इष्टः स्यामिति मे मतिः ॥ १८.७० ॥
adhyeṣyate ca ya imaṁ
dharmyaṁ saṁvādamāvayoḥ
jñānayajñena tenāham
iṣṭaḥ syāmiti me matiḥ (18.70)

adhyeṣyate — he will study; ca — and; ya — who; imaṁ — this; dharmyaṁ — sacred; saṁvādam — conversation; āvayoḥ — of ours; jñānayajñena — by the sacrifice of his knowledge; tenāham = tena — by him + aham — I; iṣṭaḥ — loved; syām — I should be; iti — thus; me — my; matiḥ — opinion

I would be loved by the devotee who by sacrifice of his knowledge, will study this sacred conversation of ours. This is My opinion. (18.70)

<u>*Commentary:*</u>

This is self explanatory. Those of us who can take shelter of this verse, can be relocated into the affectionate energies of Śrī Krishna. This is one way to initiate ourselves into being devotees.

श्रद्धावाननसूयश्च
शृणुयादपि यो नरः ।
सोऽपि मुक्तः शुभाँल्लोकान्
प्राप्नुयात्पुण्यकर्मणाम् ॥ १८.७१ ॥
śraddhāvānanasūyaśca
śṛṇuyādapi yo naraḥ
so'pi muktaḥ śubhām̐llokān
prāpnuyātpuṇyakarmaṇām (18.71)

śraddhāvān — with confidence; anasūyaśca = anasūyaḥ — without ridiculing + ca — and; śṛṇuyāt — he should hear; api — even; yo = yaḥ — who; naraḥ — the person; so = saḥ — he; 'pi = api — also; muktaḥ — freed; śubhān — happy; lokān — worlds; prāpnuyāt — he should attain; puṇyakarmaṇām = punya — pious + karmaṇām — of actions

Even the person who hears with confidence, without ridiculing is freed. He should attain the happy worlds where persons of pious actions reside. (18.71)

Commentary:

This is self explanatory. It does not say that such a person would go to the kingdom of God. It only promises that he will go to heavenly places where the celestial people live. And it does not say that he will live there permanently.

कच्चिदेतच्छ्रुतं पार्थ
त्वयैकाग्रेण चेतसा ।
कच्चिदज्ञानसंमोहः
प्रनष्टस्ते धनंजय ॥ १८.७२ ॥
kaccidetacchrutaṁ pārtha
tvayaikāgreṇa cetasā
kaccidajñānasaṁmohaḥ
pranaṣṭaste dhanaṁjaya (18.72)

kaccit — has it?; etat — this; śrutaṁ — was heard; pārtha — son of Pṛthā; tvayaikāgreṇa = tvayā — by you + ekāgreṇa — by one-pointed; cetasā — by mind; kaccit — has it?; ajñānasaṁmohaḥ = ajnāna — ignorance + saṁmohaḥ — confusion; pranaṣṭaḥ — removed; te — your; dhanaṁjaya — conqueror of wealthy countries

Was this heard by you, O son of Pṛthā, with a one—pointed mind? Was your ignorance and confusion removed, O conqueror of wealthy countries? (18.72)

Commentary:

Śrī Krishna now concludes the discourse. All glories to Him! At last He gave us a glimpse of His love which flowed to Arjuna. That is sufficient to increase our faith in Him!

अर्जुन उवाच
नष्टो मोहः स्मृतिर्लब्धा
त्वत्प्रसादान्मयाच्युत ।
स्थितोऽस्मि गतसंदेहः
करिष्ये वचनं तव ॥ १८.७३ ॥
arjuna uvāca
naṣṭo mohaḥ smṛtirlabdhā
tvatprasādānmayācyuta
sthito'smi gatasaṁdehaḥ
kariṣye vacanaṁ tava (18.73)

arjuna — Arjuna; uvāca — said; naṣṭo = naṣṭaḥ — removed; mohaḥ — confusion; smṛtiḥ — memory; labdhā — retrieved; tvat prasādān = tvat — your + prasādān (prasādāt) — from grace; mayācyuta = mayā — by me + acyuta — O unaffected one; sthito = sthitāḥ — standing; 'smi = asmi — I am; gatasaṁdehaḥ = gatā — gone, cleared away + saṁdehaḥ — doubt; kariṣye — I will execute; vacanaṁ — instruction; tava — your

Arjuna said: Through Your grace, the confusion is removed, memory is retrieved by Me, O unaffected one. I stand clear of doubts. I will execute Your instruction. (18.73)

Commentary:

For Arjuna it was that easy. After hearing the *Gītā*, he decided in Śrī Krishna's favor.

संजय उवाच
इत्यहं वासुदेवस्य
पार्थस्य च महात्मनः ।
संवादमिममश्रौषम्
अद्भुतं रोमहर्षणम् ॥ १८.७४ ॥

saṁjaya — Sanjaya; uvāca — said; iti — thus; aham — I; vāsudevasya — of the son of Vasudeva; pārthasya — of the son of Pṛthā; ca — and; mahātmanaḥ — great souled one; saṁvādam — talk; imam — this; aśroṣam — I heard; adbhutaṁ —

saṁjaya uvāca
ityahaṁ vāsudevasya
pārthasya ca mahātmanaḥ
saṁvādamimamaśrauṣam
adbhutaṁ romaharṣaṇam (18.74)

amazing; romaharṣaṇam — causing hair to stand on end

Sanjaya said: In this way, I heard this talk of the son of Vasudeva and the great—souled son of Pṛthā. It is amazing. It causes the hairs to stand on end. (18.74)

Commentary:

Definitely so! Our hairs may not stand on end, but this talk between Śrī Krishna and Arjuna is mind boggling, something which we need to consider again and again. It is a very serious discourse touching on our response to the Supreme Being.

From one perspective, Śrī Krishna left us aside. He took Arjuna into His affections. But we are unfortunate to have seen and felt that loving action of this Supreme Lord.

व्यासप्रसादाच्छ्रुतवान्
एतद्गुह्यमहं परम् ।
योगं योगेश्वरात्कृष्णात्
साक्षात्कथयतः स्वयम् ॥ १८.७५ ॥
vyāsaprasādācchrutavān
etadguhyamahaṁ param
yogaṁ yogeśvarātkṛṣṇāt
sākṣātkathayataḥ svayam (18.75)

vyāsaprasādāt = vyāsa — Vyasa + prasādāt — from grace; śrutavān — one who heard; etad — this; guhyam — secret; aham — I; param — supreme; yogaṁ — yoga; yogeśvarāt = yoga — yoga + īśvarāt — from the Lord; kṛṣṇāt — from Krishna; sākṣāt — directly; kathayataḥ — explaining; svayam — himself

By the grace of Vyasa, I am the one who heard this secret information of the supreme yoga from the Lord of yoga, Krishna, who Himself explained it directly. (18.75)

Commentary:

Sanjaya appreciates His spiritual master, Śrīla Vyāsadeva, who did not restrict him but who freed him so that he could feel the relationship between Śrī Krishna and Arjuna.

राजन्संस्मृत्य संस्मृत्य
संवादमिममद्भुतम् ।
केशवार्जुनयोः पुण्यं
हृष्यामि च मुहुर्मुहुः ॥ १८.७६ ॥
rājansaṁsmṛtya saṁsmṛtya
saṁvādamimamadbhutam
keśavārjunayoḥ puṇyaṁ
hṛṣyāmi ca muhurmuhuḥ (18.76)

rājan — king; saṁsmṛtya saṁsmṛtya — remembering repeatedly; saṁvādam — talk; imam — this; adbhutam — amazing; keśavārjunayoḥ — of Keśava and Arjuna; puṇyaṁ — holy; hṛṣyāmi — I rejoice; ca — and; muhuḥ muhuḥ — again and again

O King, remembering repeatedly, this amazing and holy talk between Keśava and Arjuna, I rejoice again and again. (18.76)

Commentary:

Who could disagree with this?

तच्च संस्मृत्य संस्मृत्य
रूपमत्यद्भुतं हरेः ।
विस्मयो मे महान्राजन्
हृष्यामि च पुनः पुनः ॥ १८.७७॥
tacca saṁsmṛtya saṁsmṛtya
rūpamatyadbhutaṁ hareḥ
vismayo me mahānrājan
hṛṣyāmi ca punaḥ punaḥ (18.77)

tat — this; ca — and; saṁsmṛtya saṁsmṛtya — remembering repeatedly; rūpam — form; atyadbhutaṁ — super-fantastic; hareḥ — of Hari; vismayo = vismayaḥ — astonished; me — my; mahān — great; rājan — O King; hṛṣyāmi — I excitedly rejoice; ca — and; punaḥ punaḥ — again and again

And remembering repeatedly that super—fantastic form of Hari, my astonishment is great, O King, and I excitedly rejoice again and again. (18.77)

Commentary:

This is related to the Universal Form as well as to the four—handed divine Form but specifically to the Universal Form which was described as being super—fantastic (atyadbhutam).

यत्र योगेश्वरः कृष्णो
यत्र पार्थो धनुर्धरः ।
तत्र श्रीर्विजयो भूतिर्
ध्रुवा नीतिर्मतिर्मम ॥ १८.७८॥
yatra yogeśvaraḥ kṛṣṇo
yatra pārtho dhanurdharaḥ
tatra śrīrvijayo bhūtir
dhruvā nītirmatirmama (18.78)

yatra — wherever; yogeśvaraḥ — the Lord of yoga; kṛṣṇo = kṛṣṇaḥ — Kṛṣṇa; yatra — wherever; pārtho = pārthaḥ — son of Pṛthā; dhanurdharaḥ — bowman; tatra — there; śrīḥ — splendor; vijayo = vijayaḥ — victory; bhūtiḥ — prosperity; dhruvā — surely; nītiḥ — morality; matiḥ — opinion; mama — my

Wherever there exists the Lord of yoga, Krishna, wherever there is the son of Pṛthā, the bowman, there would surely be splendor, victory, prosperity and morality. This is my opinion. (18.78)

Commentary:

What else can be said about this?

OM TAT SAT

END

Author's Notation on Kriyā Yoga

Sriman Rāmanand Prasad brought to my attention that this commentary does not actually give out kriyā yoga techniques. His view is that without doing so I may not be completing the task set out by writing this commentary. He cited my purports to nine verses, namely *Bhagavad Gītā* verses 4.29, 4.30, 5.27, 6.13, 8.10, 8.12, 8.13, 8.24 and 8.25. However the title of this book is ***Kriyā Yoga Bhagavad Gītā***. It is an exposition on kriyā yoga which mimics whatever Śrī Krishna told Arjuna about the practices.

Under obligation I could not expand on anything which Śrī Krishna did not elaborate. We must understand that both Śrī Krishna and Arjuna were practicing kriyā yogins. Therefore an elaboration on details of the practice was not necessary since both had expertise. In addition, there was a crisis, since two armies confronted each other. The soldiers on either side could not be held off much longer than it took for Śrī Krishna to expound the *Gītā*. These men were armed for combat, ready to vent their grievances in war.

I will however go through the nine verses which Dr. Rāmanand Prasad singled out:

अपाने जुह्वति प्राणं
प्राणेऽपानं तथापरे ।
प्राणापानगती रुद्ध्वा
प्राणायामपरायणाः ॥४.२९॥
apāne juhvati prāṇaṁ
prāṇe'pānaṁ tathāpare
prāṇāpānagatī ruddhvā
prāṇāyāmaparāyaṇāḥ (4.29)

apāne — in exhalation; juhvati — they offer; prāṇam — inhalation; prāṇe — in inhalation; 'pānaṁ = apāṇaṁ — in exhalation; tathāpare = tathā — similarly + apare — others; prāṇāpāna gatī = prāṇa — energizing air + apāna — de—energizing air + gatī — channel; ruddhvā — restraining; prāṇāyāmaparāyaṇāḥ = prāṇa — inhaling + āyāma — regulating + parāyaṇāḥ — intent

Some offer inhalation into the exhalation channels; similarly others offer the exhalation into the inhalation channels, thus being determined to restrain the channels of the energizing and de—energizing airs. (4.29)

Details:

This concerns mastery of prāṇāyāma practice, particularly alternate breathing for specific durations. It can be mastered more rapidly by doing bhastrika or kapalabhati rapid breathing. Śrī Harbhajan Singh Yogiji popularized bhastrika as the breath—of—fire or as the process for rapidly awakening the Kuṇḍalinī chakra. One has to learn prāṇāyāma from a teacher who mastered it sufficiently. One has to practice. As for a short cut, I found none besides doing bhastrika or kapalabhati rapid breathing in combination with haṭha yoga postures.

अपरे नियताहाराः
प्राणान्प्राणेषु जुह्वति ।
सर्वेऽप्येते यज्ञविदो
यज्ञक्षपितकल्मषाः ॥४.३०॥

apare — others; niyatāhārāḥ — persons restrained in diet; prāṇān — fresh air; prāṇeṣu — into the previous inhalations; juhvati — impel; sarve — all; 'pyete (apyete) = apy (api) — also + ete — these; yajñavido = yajñavidaḥ — those who know the value of an act of

apare niyatāhārāḥ
prāṇānprāṇeṣu juhvati
sarve'pyete yajñavido
yajñakṣapitakalmaṣāḥ (4.30)

sacrifice; yajñakṣapitakalmaṣāḥ = yajña — austerity and religious ceremony + kṣapita — destroyed, removed + kalmaṣāḥ — impurities

Others who were restrained in diet, impel fresh air into the previously inhaled air. All these ascetics whose impurities were removed by austerity and religious ceremony understand the value of an act of sacrifice. (4.30)

Details:

This verse concerns a restraint in diet which comes about through past mastery of prāṇāyāma. It is not just a diet control scheme. It is a diet control which comes on by virtue of the advancement made in prāṇāyāma practice.

The bit about the value of an act of sacrifice is a key statement, in which Śrī Krishna tactfully and secretly gives approval and assistance to those who follow the restraint process by yoga practice. If one just restrains himself without yoga, he will either fail or will have partial success and then regress considerably. In another verse of the *Gītā*, Śrī Krishna asked Arjuna about the value of restraint as if to say that it was useless, since the restrained energy will be held in reserve for expression at some other opportunity. But for the yogi, the restrained energy goes through transformation. That is the value of the yogi's sacrificing of lower experiences for higher ones.

स्पर्शान्कृत्वा बहिर्बाह्यांश्
चक्षुश्चैवान्तरे भ्रुवोः ।
प्राणापानौ समौ कृत्वा
नासाभ्यन्तरचारिणौ ॥५.२७॥
sparśānkṛtvā bahirbāhyāṁś
cakṣuścaivāntare bhruvoḥ
prāṇāpānau samau kṛtvā
nāsābhyantaracāriṇau (5.27)

sparśān — sensual contact; kṛtvā — having done; bahir = bahiḥ — external; bāhyāṁś = bāhyān — excluded; cakṣuścai 'vāntare = cakṣuś — visual focus + ca — and + iva (eva) — indeed + antare — in between; bhruvoḥ — of the two eyebrows; prāṇāpānau — both inhalation and exhalation; samau — in balance; kṛtvā — having made; nāsābhyantaracāriṇau = nāsa — nose + abhyantara — within + cāriṇau — moving

Excluding the external sensual contacts, and fixing the visual focus between the eyebrows, putting the inhalation and exhalation in balance, moving through the nose... (5.27)

Details:

The exclusion of the external sensual contacts is the process of pratyāhār which is the 5th stage of yoga. There is really no set way of doing this because each person has to work with his own psyche to conquer its outward—going or extroverted tendencies. Thus each person should have a tailored process suited to curb the particular interest of the untamed nature. Fixing the visual focus between the eyebrows is a two—fold method. One is the elementary stage when one focuses through the space at the center of the eyebrows. The advanced stage is when one finds that, effortlessly, the practice is performed.

Putting the inhalation and exhalation in balance is done by prolonged prāṇāyāma practice and by subtle meditation, positioning the buddhi organ in a balanced way in reference to the sensual orbs in the subtle body.

समं कायशिरोग्रीवं
धारयन्नचलं स्थिरः ।
संप्रेक्ष्य नासिकाग्रं स्वं
दिशश्चानवलोकयन् ॥६.१३॥
samaṁ kāyaśirogrīvaṁ
dhārayannacalaṁ sthiraḥ
saṁprekṣya nāsikāgraṁ svaṁ
diśaścānavalokayan (6.13)

samam — balanced; kāyaśirogrīvaṁ = kāya — body + śiro (śiraḥ) — head + grīvam — neck; dhārayan — holding; acalam — without movement; sthiraḥ — steady; saṁprekṣya — gazing at; nāsikāgraṁ = nāsikā — nostril + agram — tip; svam — own ;diśaścānavalokayan = diśaḥ — the directions + ca — and + anavalokayan — not looking.

Holding the body, head and neck in balance, steady without movement, gaze at the tip of the nose, not looking in any other direction. (6.13)

Details:

This holding of the body, head and neck in balance is ideally done in the lotus posture, the famous padmāsana sitting pose. One has to do this for hours if one is to learn how to enter samādhi. It may be asked why there is a stress on that posture. The answer is that ancient yogis found that to be the most conducive posture for meditation and samādhi.

The gazing at the tip of the nose is related to the breath tracking technique in which the yogi tracks the movement of subtle air through the nose down to the base chakra and then up through the sushuma subtle spinal channel out of the subtle body. Some yogis recommend focusing between the eyebrows while doing this. Others say it is a focus at the tip of the nose and not at its bridge. It is not a contention because ultimately one has to practice. The yogi learns all relevant techniques as he advances.

प्रयाणकाले मनसाचलेन
भक्त्या युक्तो योगबलेन चैव ।
भ्रुवोर्मध्ये प्राणमावेश्य सम्यक्
स तं परं पुरुषमुपैति दिव्यम् ॥८.१०॥
prayāṇakāle manasācalena
bhaktyā yukto yogabalena caiva
bhruvormadhye prāṇam āveśya samyak
sa taṁ paraṁ puruṣamupaiti divyam (8.10)

prayāṇakāle — at the time of death; manasācalena = manasā — by the mind + acalena— by unwavering; bhaktyā — with devotion; yukto = yuktaḥ — connected; yogabalena — with psychological power developed through yoga practice; caiva = ca — and + eva — indeed; bhruvor = bhruvoḥ — of the two eyebrows; madhye — in the middle; prāṇam — energizing breath; āveśya— having caused to enter; samyak — precisely; sa = saḥ — he; tam — this; param — supreme; puruṣam — person; upaiti — he goes; divyam — divine

...and that meditator who even at the time of death, with an unwavering mind, being connected devotedly, with psychological power developed through yoga practice, and having caused the energizing breath to enter between the eyebrows with precision, goes to the divine Supreme Person. (8.10)

Details:

This is only true for persons who mastered this before leaving their bodies. This does not happen to others. This practice is part of the dhāraṇa 6th stage. If one has mastered that before death, then he can do this.

The practice of this hinges on mastery of prāṇāyāma. One should mastered kuṇḍalinī chakra by doing kuṇḍalinī yoga. And then one should mastered yogic celibacy. Therefore one must take help from perfected yogis who give hints and help one to curb the buddhi organ; otherwise one cannot do this.

सर्वद्वाराणि संयम्य
मनो हृदि निरुध्य च ।
मूर्ध्न्याधायात्मनः प्राणम्
आस्थितो योगधारणाम् ॥८.१२॥
sarvadvārāṇi saṁyamya
mano hṛdi nirudhya ca
mūrdhnyādhāyātmanaḥ prāṇam
āsthito yogadhāraṇām (8.12)

sarvadvārāṇi = sarva — all + dvārāṇi — entrances; saṁyamya — controlling; mano = manaḥ — mind; hṛdi — in the core of consciousness; nirudhya — confining; ca — and; mūrdhny = mūrdhni — in the brain; ādhāyātmanaḥ = ādhāya — situating + ātmanaḥ — of the soul; prāṇam — energizing breath; āsthito = āsthitaḥ — remain fixed; yogadhāraṇām — yoga concentration

Controlling all openings of the body, and restricting the mind in the core of consciousness, situating the energizing energy of the soul in the brain, remaining fixed in yoga concentration, (8.12)

Details:

This cannot be done at the time of death or in the hereafter after leaving a body, unless one has mastered it before. These verses, even though they gave details of advancing kriyā yoga practice, pertain to those who have practiced this repeatedly for many years and who have definitely mastered this. These procedures are mystic. They are practiced in isolation with help from mahāyogīns on the astral planes.

ओमित्येकाक्षरं ब्रह्म
व्याहरन्मामनुस्मरन् ।
यः प्रयाति त्यजन्देहं
स याति परमां गतिम् ॥८.१३॥
omityekākṣaraṁ brahma
vyāharanmāmanusmaran
yaḥ prayāti tyajandehaṁ
sa yāti paramāṁ gatim (8.13)

om — the uttered sound om; ity = iti — thus saying; ekākṣaram — one syllable; brahma — spiritual reality; vyāharan — chanting; mām — Me; anusmaran — meditating on; yaḥ — who; prayāti — passes on; tyajan — renouncing; deham — body; sa = saḥ — he; yāti — attains; paramām — supreme; gatim — objective

...uttering *Om,* the one-syllable sound which represents the spiritual reality, meditating on Me, the yogi who passes on, renouncing the body, attains the highest objective. (8.13)

Details:

This will only work for somebody who is a yogi by lifestyle and who practiced the samādhis. If one just utters *Om* at the time of death, it will not help him if he has not mastered yoga beforehand. He must do so by completing the course for the 5th, 6th, 7th and 8th stages of practice. The success of these hinges on mastership of the āsana postures and the prāṇāyāma breath—charging techniques, which are the 3rd and 4th stages.

अग्निर्ज्योतिरहः शुक्लः
षण्मासा उत्तरायणम् ।
तत्र प्रयाता गच्छन्ति
ब्रह्म ब्रह्मविदो जनाः ॥८.२४॥

agnir = agniḥ — summer season; jyotir = jyotiḥ — bright atmosphere; ahaḥ — daytime; śuklaḥ — bright moonlight; saṇmāsā — six months; uttarāyaṇam — the time when the sun appears to

agnirjyotirahaḥ śuklaḥ
ṣaṇmāsā uttarāyaṇam
tatra prayātā gacchanti
brahma brahmavido janāḥ (8.24)

move north; tatra — at that time; prayātā — departing; gacchanti — they go; brahma — to the spiritual location; brahmavido = brahmavidaḥ — knowers of the spiritual dimension; janāḥ — people

The summer season, the bright atmosphere, the daytime, the bright moonlight, the six months when the sun appears to move north; if at that time, they depart the body, those people who know the spiritual dimension, go to the spiritual location. (8.24)

Details:

This is only applicable to yogins. Others cannot use this course because their subtle bodies will be too heavy to take advantage of the subtle solar energy. Someone might doubt this and might think that it is not possible to weigh the subtle body. But it is possible. In fact the subtle body is light or heavy all depending on the type of mental and emotional energy it ingests. You may have heard of the tan mātras or the subtle material elements. These constitute energies. If one's subtle body is habituated to heavier subtle force, it will not be able to make use of the sun's northern course. Śrī Bhiṣmadeva is the person who became famous for taking this course but he was a practicing mahāyogīn. He was a warrior too but he was an expert at prāṇāyāma techniques.

धूमो रात्रिस्तथा कृष्णः
षण्मासा दक्षिणायनम् ।
तत्र चान्द्रमसं ज्योतिर्
योगी प्राप्य निवर्तते ॥८.२५॥
dhūmo rātristathā kṛṣṇaḥ
ṣaṇmāsā dakṣiṇāyanam
tatra cāndramasaṁ jyotir
yogī prāpya nivartate (8.25)

dhūmo = dhūmaḥ — smoky, misty or hazy season; rātris — night time; tathā — as well as; kṛṣṇaḥ — the dark moon time; saṇmāsā — six months; dakṣiṇāyanam — the time when the sun appears to move south; tatra — at that time; cāndramasam — moon; jyotir = jyotiḥ — light; yogī — yogi; prāpya — attaining; nivartate — is born again

The smoky, misty or hazy season, as well as in the night—time, the dark—moon time, the six months when the sun appears to move south; if the yogi departs at that time, he attains moonlight, after which he is born again. (8.25)

Details:

Please note the word yogi. Please do not take out this word in your effort to understand this and other such verses.

Even though Śrī Rāmanand Prasad has graciously requested that I elaborate on these techniques, the truth is that I cannot elaborate on anything without the permission of Śrī Bābāji Mahasaya. He said that each yogi has to practice and by the practice, a yogi finds his way by a method which suits his nature. Śrī Bābāji Mahasaya seems to think that if one practices sincerely the eightfold yoga process, the ashtanga yoga system, then that person will reach the perfections by a method of deliberance that is suitable.

He wanted me to tell Dr. Rāmanand Prasad this:

There is no set practice for any yogi until one reaches the 6th stage of dhāraṇa focusing. Before that one has to work to get rid of one's particular sensual addictions, according to the particular sensual pursuits to which one's nature is habituated. One yogi might be more addicted to sound more than anything else; another to vision and yet another to the touching sense. One may be addicted to odors, and another to colors. Thus until one has perfected the 5th stage, one cannot follow any standard method. Before the completion of the 5th stage, each yogi has to get a tailored method that suits him.

When one reaches the 6th stage, then I usually come to the person or I send someone else. Alternately, Lord Śrī Krishna or Śrī Mahādeva will send someone, or another mahāyogī will send someone to give the first kriyā for the dhāraṇa process.

From then on, there are standard kriyas but it is not necessary to discuss these, since the yogi will get them automatically as he advances through the various stages. The standard kriyās for higher yoga are not hidden. They are not secretive, but all the same they cannot be practiced until one completes the 5th stage of pratyāhār sense withdrawal, which is the stage in which one struggles to control the psyche and to cause it to become introverted.

Concluding Remarks:

I am grateful to several great yogins for permitting me to approach the Śrīmad *Bhagavad Gītā* from the kriyā yoga perspective. Foremost is Lord Shiva. If it were not for Him, I would not have made such steady progress or received from so many great yogins, instructions in kriyā yoga. I must thank Śrī Bābāji Mahasaya, the Bābā who was made famous by Śrī Paramhansa Yoganandaji in that stunning book, *Autobiography of a Yogi*. It was Śrī Bābāji Mahasaya who stood over me as I typed the commentary. He was constantly by my side in his sunlight yoga—siddha body. To estimate, I would say that more than 75% of this book is his. I was only a literary agent because I happen to have a physical body which proved to be useful to get this information to kriyā yogins.

I must thank Yogiraj Śrīla Yogeshwarananda because for some years now he resided in my brahmarandra. He showed me many kriyās and caused me to advance considerably on the path of kriyā yoga, a path which caused my supernatural vision to develop far enough to follow along behind Arjuna as Śrī Krishna stressed one point after the other.

There were many other yogins who assisted me. Some of them did not even reveal their names. These were persons whom I met on the astral planes. Overall I was lucky to have retrieved myself in yoga. When I got this body, I took a risk. I was saved by the mercy of my spiritual masters. Last but not least I must thank Śrīla Bhaktivedanta Swami, the founder of the International Society for Krishna Consciousness. He did bring to my attention the importance of the *Bhagavad Gītā*. And though this translation and commentary does not follow his vision line for line and word for word, I still appreciate him considerably. As he always told us:

CHANT:

HARE KṚṢṆA HARE KṚṢṆA KṚṢṆA KṚṢṆA HARE HARE

HARE RĀMA HARE RĀMA RĀMA RĀMA HARE HARE

Indexed Names of Arjuna

anagha — blameless one, good man, 3.3
anagha — sinless one, 14.6
Arjuna —— third son of King Pāndu and Queen Kuntī, cousin of Lord Krishna, 1.4; 2.1,4,54; 2.68; 3.1,7,36; 4.4,5,9,37; 5.1; 6.16,32,33,37; 6.46; 7.16; 8.1,16; 10.32,37,39,42; 11.1,36,50,51,54; 13.1; 18.73,76
bhaktaḥ — devoted person, 4.3
bhārata — man of the Bharata family, descendant of Bharata, 2.18,30; 3.25; 4.7,42; 7.27; 11.6; 13.3,34; 14.3,8,9,10; 15.19,20; 16.3; 17.3; 18.36,62
bharatarṣabha — powerful son (strong man) of the Bharatas, bullish man of the Bharata family, 7.11,16; 8.23; 13.27; 14.12
bharataśreṣṭha — best of the Bharatas, 17.12
dehabhṛtām vara — best of the embodied souls, 8.4
dhanaṁjayaḥ — conqueror of wealthy countries, 1.15; 7.7; 11.14; 18.29,72
dhanurdharaḥ — bowman, 18.78
guḍākeśa — the thick—haired baron, conqueror of sleep, 1.24, 11.7
kapidhvajaḥ — the man with a monkey insignia (Hanuman), 1.20
kaunteya — son of Kuntī (Pṛthā), 1.27; 2.14,21,60; 3.37; 5.22; 6.35; 7.8; 8.16; 9.7,10,23,27,31; 13.2; 14.4; 16.20,22; 18.50,60
kurunandana — dear son of the Kurus, 2.41,48; 6.43, 14.13
kurupravīra — great hero of the Kurus, 11.48
kurusattama — best of the Kurus, 4.31
kuruśreṣṭha — best of the Kuru clan, 10.19
mahābāho — powerful man, 3.28,43; 5.3; 10.1; 14.5; 18.13
pāṇḍava — son of Pāndu, 1.14; 4.35; 6.2; 11.13,55; 12.1; 14.21,22; 16.5; 17.1, 18.1,9,34,61
paraṁtapa — burner of enemy forces, scorcher of enemies, 4.2,5; 11.51
pārtha — son of Pṛthā (Kuntī), 1.25,26; 2.3,32,39,42,55,72; 3.16,22,23; 4.11,33; 6.40; 7.1,10; 8.8,14,19,22,27; 9.32; 10.24; 11.5,9; 12.7; 16.4,6; 17.26,28; 18.6,31,33,72,78
puruṣarṣabha — bull among men, 2.15
puruṣavyāghra — tiger among men, 18.4
sakhā — friend, 4.3
savyasācin — ambidextrous archer, 11.33
tāta — ideal one, 6.40

Indexed Names of Krishna

acyuta, infallible one, 11.42
adhyātma, Supreme Spirit, 15.5
ādidevaḥ, first God, 11.38
ādidevamajaṁ, Primal God, 10.12
ādikartre, original creator, 11.37
ādyaṁ, primal person, 11.31
ajam, birthless, 10.12
akṣaraṁ, imperishable basis of energies, 11.37
akṣaraṁ paramaṁ, indestructible Supreme Person, 11.18
anādimadhyāntam, Person without beginning, middle or ending, 11.19
ananta deveśa, infinite Lord of the gods, 11.37
anantabāhuṁ, Person with unlimited arms, 11.19
anantarūpa, Person of lnfinite Form, 11.38
anantavīryam, Person with infinite manly power, 11.19
anumantā, permitter, 13.23
aprameyam, one who is boundless, 11.42
apratimaprabhāva, person of incomparable splendor, 11.43
asat, sum total temporary existence, 11.37
atyadbhutaṁ hareḥ, super—fantastic form of Hari, 18.77
bhagavān (śrī bhagavān), the Blessed Lord, 2.2,11,55; 3.3,37; 4.1,5; 5.2; 6.1,35,40; 7.1; 8.3; 9.1; 10.1,14,17,19; 11.5,32,47,52; 12.2; 13.2; 14.1,22; 15.1; 16.1; 17.2; 18.2
bhartā, supporter, 13.23
bhavantam, Your lordship, 11.31
bhavānugrarūpo, respected person of terrible form, 11.31
bhoktā, experiencer, 13.23
bhūtabhāvana, one who sustains the existence of all others, 10.15
bhūteśa, Lord of created beings, 10.15
caturbhujena, person with four arms, 11.46
devadeva, God of the gods, 10.15
devam, God, 11.11,14,15,44,45
devavara, best of the gods, 11.31
deveśa (deva + īśa), Lord of all lords, 11.25,45
dīptahutāśavaktraṁ, Person with the blazing oblation—eating mouth, 11.19
govinda, chief of cowherds, 1.32, 2.9
hariḥ, Hari, the God Vishnu, 11.9; 18.77
hṛṣīkeśa, Master of the sense organs, 1.15,18,24; 18.1
īśam īḍyam, Lord who is to be praised, 11.44
īśvaraḥ, Lord, 4.6

jagannivāsa (jagat—nivāsa),
refuge of the worlds, 11.25
resort of the world, 11.37
shelter of the world, 11.45
jagatpate, Lord of the universe, 10.15
janārdana, motivator of human beings, 1.38;43; 3.1; 11.51
kālo (kālah), time—limit, 11.32
kamalapatrākṣa, Person whose eyes are shaped like lotus petals, 11.2
keśava, pretty—haired one, 2.54; 10.14; 11.35; 13.29; 15.17;18.61,75,76
keśiniṣūdāna, slayer of Keshi, 18.1
kṛṣṇa, person with blackish complexion, 1.28,31; 6.34,37,39; 11.35,41; 17.1; 18.75,78
kṣetrajñam (sarva), experiencer of all living spaces, 13.3
mādhava, descendant of Madhu, 1.36
madhusūdana, slayer of Madhu, 1.34; 2.1; 6.33; 8.2
mahābāho, mighty—armed Person, 11.23
mahātma, great personality, 11.20,37
mahātmanaḥ, great personality, 11.12
mahāyogeśvaro, the great master of yoga, 11.9
maheśvara, Supreme Lord, 5.29,13.23
mahīpate, Lord of the earth, 1.21
paraṁ brahma, supreme reality, 10.12
paraṁ dhāma,
supreme refuge, 10.12
ultimate sanctuary, 11.38
paraṁ nidhānam, ultimate shelter, 11.18
paramātmā, Supreme Soul, Supreme Spirit, 13.32,15.17
parameśvara, Supreme Lord, 11.3; 13 28
pavitraṁ paramaṁ, 10.12
prabho (prabhuḥ), respected Lord, 5.14; 11.4; 14.21
prapitāmahaḥ, father of Brahmā, 11.39
pūjyaḥ guruḥ garīyān, gravest spiritual master, 11.43
puruṣaḥ paraḥ, highest spirit, 13.23
puruṣaḥ purāṇaḥ, most ancient spirit, 11.38
puruṣaṁ śāśvataṁ divyam, eternal divine person, 10.12
puruṣottama, Supreme Person, 11.3; 10.15; 15.18,19
rūpaṁ, God—form, 11.45
sahasrabāho, O thousand—armed person, 11.46
sanātanas puruṣo, most ancient person, 11.18
śaśisūryanetram, Person who has sun and moon as eyes, 11.19
śāśvatadharmagoptā, eternal guardian of law, 11.18
sat, sum total permanent life, 11.37
svatejasā viśvamidaṁ tapantam,
Person heating this universe with splendor, 11.19
tatparaṁ, that which is beyond, 11.37
upadraṣṭā, observer, 13.23
vārṣṇeya, clansman of the Vṛṣṇis, 1.40

vāsudevasya, of the son of Vasudeva, 7.19; 11.50; 18.74
vibhum (vibhuḥ), Almighty God, whose influence spreads everywhere, 5.15; 10.12
viṣṇo, Lord Viṣṇu, 11.24,30
viśvamūrte,person of universal dimensions, 11.46
viśvarūpa, form of everything, 11.16
viśvasya paraṁ nidhānam, supreme refuge of all the worlds, 11.38
viśveśvara, Lord of all, 11.16
yādava, family man of the Yadus, 11.41
yogeśvara,
    Lord of yoga disciplines, 18.75,78
    Master of yoga technique, 11.4
yogin, mystic master, 10.17

Names, Places and Things

Ādityas, 10.21
Agni, 10.23; 11.39
Airāvata, 10.27
Ananta, 10.29
Anantavijaya, 1.16
Arjuna,
——see Indexed Names of Arjuna
Aryamā, 10.29
Ashvattha, 10.26
Asita, 10.13
Aśvatthāmā, 1.8
Bhīma, 1.4,10,15
Bhishma, 1.8,10,25; 2.4; 11.26,34
Bhrigu, 10.25
Brahmā, 3.10; 8.16—19; 9.7; 10.33; 11.15,37,39
Brihaspati, 10.24
Cekitāna, 1.5
Chitraratha, 10.26
Dānavāḥ, 10.14
Danu, 10.14
Devadatta, 1.15
Devala, 10.13
Dhātā, 10.33
Dhṛṣṭadyumna, 1.17
Dhṛṣṭaketu, 1.5
Dhṛtarāṣṭra, 1.1,19,20,23
Dhṛti, 10.34
Diti, 10.30
Draupadi,1.6,18
Droṇa, 1.25; 2.4; 11.26,34
Drupada, 1.3,4,18
Duryodhana, 1.2,12
dvijottama, 1.7
Gāṇḍīva, 1.29
Gayatri, 10.35
Hanuman (kapi), 1.20
Hari, 11.9; 18.77
Himalayas, 10.25
Ikṣvāku, 4.1
Indra, 10.22
Jahnu, 10.31
Jayadratha, 11.34
Kamadhuk, 10.28
Kandarpa, 10.28
kapi, 1.20
Kapila, 10.26
Karṇa, 1.8; 11.34
Kāśi, 1.5,17
Kīrti, 10.34
Krishna,
— see Indexed Names of Krishna
Kṣamā, 10.34
Kubera, 10.23
Kuntī, 1.16; 13.2
Kuntibhoja, 1.5
Kuru, 1.12,25
kurukṣetre, 1.1
Manipushpaka, 1.16
Manu, 4.1
Marīci, 10.21
Medhā, 10.34
Meru, 10.23
Nakula, 1.16
Narada, 10.13
narapuṁgavaḥ, 1.5
Pāñcajanya, 1.15
Pandava, 1.2
Pāndu, 1.1,3
Paundra, 1.15
Pavāka, 10.23
Prahlāda, 10.30
Purujit, 1.5
Rāma, 10.31
Rudra, 10.23
Sādhya, 11.22
Sahadeva, 1.16
Śaibya, 1.5
Sāma Veda chants, 10.35
Sāṁkhya, 5.5
Sanjaya, 1.1,2,24; 18.74
Śāśaṅka, 11.39
Sātyaki, 1.17
Shankara, 10.23
Shiva, 10.23
Śikhandī, 1.17
Skanda, 10.24
Smṛti, 10.34
Somadatta, 1.8
Śrī, 10.34
Subhadrā, 1.6,18
Sughosha, 1.16
Uccaihśrava, 10.27
Ushana, 10.37
Uttamauja, 1.6
Vaiśvāanara, 15.2
Vajra, 10.28
Vāk, 10.34
Varuṇa, 10.29; 11.39
Vasava, 10.22
Vasudeva, 7.19; 10.37
Vasuki, 10.28
Vasus, 11.22
Vāyu, 11.39
Vikarṇa, 1.8
Vinata, 10.30
Virāṭa, 1.4,17
Vishnu, 10.21; 11.9,24,30
Vishvadevas, 11.22
Vitteśaḥ, 10.23
Vivasvat, 4.1,4
Vṛṣṇis, 1.40, 10.36
Vyasa, 10.13
Vyasa, 10.37; 18.75
Yakshas, 10.23
Yama, 10.29, 11.39
Yudhamanyu, 1.6
Yudhishthira, 1.16
Yuyudhāna, 1.4

Index To Verses: Selected Sanskrit Words

A

ā, 8.16
abhāvayataḥ, 2.66
abhāvo, 2.16
abhipravṛttaḥ, 4.20
abhyāsena, 6.35,44; 8.8;12.9
abhyasūyanto, 3.31
abhyutthānam, 4.7
abuddhayaḥ, 7.24
acalapratiṣṭhaṁ, 2.70
ācaratyātmanaḥ, 16.22
ācāryam, 1.2
ācāryopāsanaṁ, 13.8
acchedyo, 2.24
acetasaḥ, 3.32
acintya, 2,25; 8.9
acireṇādhigacchati, 4.39
adharma, 1.39,40; 4.7; 18.32
ādhāyātmanaḥ, 8.12
adhibhūtaṁ, 8.1,4
adhidaivaṁ, 8.1
adhipatyam, 2.8
adhiṣṭhānam, 3.40; 18.14
adhiṣṭhāya, 4.6
adhiyajñaḥ, 7.30; 8.2,4
adhyātma, 7.29; 13.12
adhyeṣyate, 18.70
ādidevamajaṁ, 10.12
ādityavaj, 5.16
ādityavarṇaṁ, 8.9
ādyantavantaḥ, 5.22
agatāsūṁś, 2.11
aghāyurindriyārāmo, 3.16
āgnidagdha, 4,19
agnirjyotirahaḥ, 8.24
ahaṁ sarvasya, 10.8
ahaṁkāraṁ, 16.18
ahaṁkāraṁ balaṁ, 18.53
ahaṁkāravimūḍhā, 3.27
āhārāḥ, 17.8
ahiṁsā, 10.5; 16.2
ahoratra, 8.17
ajānantaḥ, 7.24
ajñānāṁ, 3.26
ajñānasaṁbhūtaṁ, 4.42
ajñānenāvṛtaṁ, 5.15
ajo, 4.6
akarmakṛt, 3.5
akarmaṇi, 4.18
akartāram, 4.13
ākāśaṁ, 13.33
akhilam, 7.29
ākhyāhi me ko bhavānugrarūpo, 11.31
akīrtikaram, 2.2
akṣara, 3.15; 8.3,11,21; 15.18
akṣayam, 5.21
alpamedhasām, 7.23
ambhasi, 2.67
amṛta, 2.15; 9.19
anabhisnehas, 2.57
anādimatparaṁ, 13.13
anāditvānnirguṇa, 13.32
anahaṁkāra, 13.9
anāmayam, 2.51
anantaṁ, 11.11
ananyacetāḥ, 8.14
ananyamanasaḥ, 9.13
anapekṣya, 18.25
anāryajuṣṭam, 2.2
anāśino, 2.18
anasūyantaḥ, 3.31
anāvṛttim, 8.23
anekacittavibhrāntā, 16.16
anekajanma, 6.45
anekavaktra, 11.10
aniṣṭamiṣṭaṁ, 18.12
anīśvaram, 16.8
aṇīyāṁsam, 8.9
annādbhavanti, 3.14
antakāle, 8.5
antarātmanā, 6.47
anubandhaṁ, 18.25
anucintayan, 8.8
anudvegakaraṁ, 17.15
anusmaran, 8.13
anuśocanti, 2.11
anuśocitum, 2.25
anuśuśruma, 1.43
apahṛta, 2.44
apāne juhvati, 4.29
aparaṁ bhavato, 4.4
apare niyatāhārāḥ, 4.30
apareyamitastvanyāṁ, 7.5
aprameyasya, 2.18
apratiṣṭho, 6.38
apunarāvṛttiṁ, 5.17
āpūryamāṇam, 2.70
arāgadveṣataḥ, 18.23
ārjavam, 16.1
arpitamanobuddhir, 8.7
ārurukṣormuner, 6.3
asaktir, 13.10
asaṁśayaṁ, 6.35; 7.1; 8.7
asaṁyatātmanā, 6.36
asaṅgaśastreṇa, 15.3
asatas, 2.16
asito devalo vyāsaḥ, 10.13
aśraddadhānāḥ, 4.40; 9.3
aśraddhayā, 17.28
aśru, 2.1
asvargyam, 2.2
aśvinau, 11.6
atīndriyam, 6.21
ātiṣṭhottiṣṭha, 4.42
atisvapna, 6.16
ātmabuddhiprasāda, 18.37
ātmānaṁ mat, 9.34
ātmanātmānaṁ, 6.5; 13.29
ātmanyevātmanā, 2.55
ātmasaṁbhāvitāḥ, 16.17
ātmasaṁsthaṁ, 6.25
ātmasaṁyamayogā, 4.27
ātmaśuddhaye, 5.11
ātmatṛptaśca, 3.17
ātmaupamyena, 6.32
ātmavān, 2.45
ātmavantaṁ, 4.41
ātmavaśyair, 2.64
ātmikā, 2.43
avabodhasya, 6.17
avadhyaḥ, 2.30
avaśaṁ, 9.8
avaśiṣyate, 7.2
avatiṣṭhate, 6.18
avibhaktaṁ, 13.17; 18.20
avidhipūrvakam, 9.23
avidvāṁsa, 3.25
avināśi, 2.17
āvṛtam, 3.38,39
āvṛttiṁ, 8.23
avyaktaḥ, 2.25,28; 7.24; 12.3

avyaktāsaktacetasām, 12.5
avyavasāyinām, 2.41
avyaya, 2.17; 7.24
avyayātmā, 4.6
ayajñasya, 4.31
āyuḥsattvabalārogya, 17.8
ayuktasya, 2.66

B

bahumataḥ, 2.35
bahūnāṁ janma, 7.19
bahūni me vyatītāni, 4.5
bahuśākhā, 2.41
bahuvidhā, 4.32
balavaddṛḍham, 6.34
balavānsukhī, 16.14
bandhurātmātmanas, 6.6
bhagavanmayā, 10.17
bhagavanvyaktiṁ, 10.14
bhaikṣyam, 2.5
bhakta, 9.23,31; 12.1,20
bhaktiṁ mayi, 18.68
bhaktimānme, 12.19
bhaktimānyaḥ sa, 12.17
bhaktiyogena, 14.26
bhakto'si me sakhā, 4.3
bhaktyā, 8.10,22; 9.29; 11.54; 18.55
bhartā bhoktā, 13.23
bhāṣā, 2.54
bhasmasātkurute, 4.37
bhāvamāśritāḥ, 7.15
bhavantaḥ, 1.11
bhavārjuna, 2.45; 6.46
bhavato, 4.4
bhāvayatā, 3.11
bhinnā, 7.4
bhogā, 1.32; 2.5
bhogaiśvarya, 2.44
bhojanaṁ, 17.10
bhoktā, 9.24
bhoktāraṁ, 5.29
bhoktṛtve, 13.21
bhrāmayansarva, 18.61
bhraṁśāt, 2.63
bhruvoḥ, 5.27; 8.10
bhūmirāpo'nalo, 7.4
bhuñjānaṁ, 15.10
bhuñjate, 3.13
bhuñjīya, 2.5
bhuṅkte, 3.12; 13.22
bhūtabhartṛ, 13.17
bhūtabhāvana, 9.5; 10.15
bhūtabhāvodbhava, 8.3
bhūtabhṛnna, 9.5
bhūtagrāmaḥ, 8.19
bhūtagrāmamimaṁ, 9.8
bhūtamaheśvaram, 9.11
bhūtānāmīśvaro'pi, 4.6
bhūtaprakṛti, 13.35
bhūtapṛthag, 13.31
bhūtasargau, 16.6
bhūteśa, 10.15
bhūtvā, 3.30; 8.19
bījaṁ, 7.10
bījamavyayam, 9.18
boddhavyaṁ, 4.17
brahma, 8.13
brahma brahma, 8.24
brahmabhūto, 5.24
brahmabhuvanāl, 8.16
brahmabhūyāya, 14.26; 18.53
brahmacārivrate, 6.14
brahmacaryaṁ, 8.11
brahmacaryama, 17.14
brahmāgnau, 4.24,25
brahmakarma, 18.42
brahmākṣarasamud, 3.15
brahmaṇaḥ, 6.38
brāhmaṇakṣatriya, 18.41
brahmāṇamīśaṁ, 11.15
brahmaṇastri, 17.23
brahmanirvāṇaṁ, 2.72; 5.24—26
brahmaṇo hi, 14.27
brahmaṇo mukhe, 4.32
brahmaṇyādhāya, 5.10
brahmārpaṇaṁ, 4.24
brahmasaṁsparśam, 6.28
brahmavādinām, 17.24
brahmavidbrahmaṇi, 5.20
brāhmī sthitiḥ, 2.72
brahmodbhavaṁ, 3.15
buddhibhedaṁ, 3.26
buddhigrāhyamatī, 6.20
buddhiḥ, 2.44
buddhimānmanuṣyeṣu, 4.18
buddhimānsyāt, 15.20
buddhimatām, 7.10
buddhināśo, 2.63
buddhi, 2.41,66; 13.6
buddhirbuddhimatām, 7.10
buddhirjñānama, 10.4
buddhirvyatitariṣyati, 2.52
buddhisaṁyogaṁ, 6.43
buddhiyoga, 2.49; 18.57
buddhiyuktā, 2.50,51
buddhvā, 3.43
budhā, 4.19; 10.8

C

cakraṁ, 3.16
calamadhruvam, 17.18
cañcalatvātsthitiṁ, 6.33
cāndramasaṁ, 8.25
caratāṁ, 2.67
caturbhujena, 11.46
cāturvarṇyaṁ mayā, 4.13
caturvidhā, 7.16
cendriyagocarāḥ, 13.6
cetasā, 8.8
chandāṁsi, 15,1
chinna, 5.25; 18.10
cintayet, 6.25

D

daiva, 4.25; 16.6
daivī, 7.14
dakṣiṇāyanam, 8.25
dambha, 16.17; 17.5
daṁṣṭrākarālāni, 11.25, 27
dānakriyāśca, 17.25
dānavāḥ, 10.14
darśanakāṅkṣiṇaḥ, 11.52
darśayātmānamavyayam, 11.4
dehabhṛtāṁ, 8.4
dehasamudbhavān, 14.20
devabhogān, 9.20
devadvijaguru, 17.14
devān, 3.11; 7.23
devarṣirnāradas, 10.13
dhāma, 8.21
dhārayāmyaham, 15.13
dhārayan, 5.8; 6.13
dhārayate, 18.33
dharma, 1.39; 2.7
dharmakṣetre, 1.2
dharmamadharmaṁ, 18.31
dharmasaṁsthā, 4.8
dharmātmā, 9.31
dharmyaṁ, 9.2; 12.20
dhāryate, 7.5
dhātāhaṁ viśvato, 10.33
dhātāram, 8.9
dhīmatām, 6.42
dhṛtigṛhītayā, 6.25
dhruva, 2.27; 12.3; 18.78
dhūmena, 3.38; 18.48
dhūmo rātristathā, 8.25

dhyānātkarma, 12.12
dhyānenātmani, 13.24
dhyāyanta, 12.6
dhyāyataḥ, 2.62
dīpaḥ, 6.19
dīrghasūtrī, 18.28
diśaścānavalokayan, 6.13
divya, 1.14 ; 11.5
doṣa, 1.42; 2.7
dravyas, 4.28, 33
dṛḍhavratāḥ, 7.28, 9.14
dṛṣṭvā lokāḥ, 11.23
dṛṣṭvā rūpaṁ, 11.49
dṛṣṭvādbhutaṁ, 11.20
dṛṣṭvedaṁ, 11.51
duḥkhadoṣā, 13.9
duḥkhahā, 6.17
duḥkhālayam, 8.15
duḥkhaśokāmaya, 17.9
duḥkheṣvanudvigna, 2.56
durāsadam, 3.43
duratyayā, 7.14
durbuddher, 1.23
durgatiṁ, 6.40
durlabhataraṁ, 6.42
durmatiḥ, 18.16
durnigrahaṁ, 6.35
duṣkṛtino, 7.15
duṣprāpa, 6.36
duṣpūreṇānalena, 3.39
dvaṁdvamoha, 7.27,28
dvaṁdvātīto, 4.22
dvārāṇi, 8.12
dveṣṭyakuśalaṁ, 18.10
dvividhā, 3.3
dvijottama, 1.7

E

ekabhaktirviśiṣyate, 7.17
ekākī, 6.10
ekākṣaram, 8.13
ĕśvaraṁ, 11.3

G

gahanā karmaṇo, 4.17
gāmāviśya, 15.13
gandharva, 10.26; 11.22
gāṇḍīvaṁ, 1.29
garbhas, 3.38
garīyase, 11.37
gatāḥ, 8.15
gataprāṇā, 10.9
gatasaṅgasya, 4.23
gatāsūn, 2.11
gatim, 8.13,21
gāyatrī, 10.33
glānirbhavati, 4.7
grasiṣṇu, 13.17
guhyādguhyataraṁ, 18.63
guhyamadhyātma, 11.1
guhyamahaṁ, 18.75
guhyatamam, 9.1; 15.20
guṇabhedataḥ, 18.19
guṇabhoktṛ, 13.15
guṇakarma, 3.28,29; 4.13
guṇamayī, 7.14
guṇasaṁkhyāne, 18.19
guṇātītaḥ, 14.25
gurūn, 2.5

H

hānir, 2.65
hantāraṁ, 2.19
hanyamāne, 2.20
hareḥ, 18.77
hariḥ, 11.9
hatam, 2.19
hitakāmyayā, 10.1
hṛdayadaurbalyaṁ, 2.3
hṛddeśe'rjuna, 18.61
hṛtsthaṁ, 4.42
hutam, 4.24

I

icchā dveṣa, 7.27; 13.6
īkṣaṇam, 2.1
indriyāgniṣu, 4.26
indriyagrāmaṁ, 6.24
indriyāṇi mano, 3.40
indriyāṇīndriyā, 2.58, 68
indriyārāmaḥ, 3.16
indriyārtheṣu, 13.9
indriyasyendriyasy, 3.34
iṣṭakāmadhuk, 3.10
iṣṭānbhogānhi, 3.12
īśvaraḥ sarvabhūtānāṁ 18.61
ivāmbhasi, 2.67

J

jagadavyaktamūrtinā, 9.4
jagadbhāsayate, 15.12
jagadviparivartate, 9.10
jagannivāsa, 11.25,45
jāgarti, 2.69
jagataḥ, 8.26
jagatkṛtsnaṁ, 11.7,13
jagatpate, 10.15
jaghanyaguṇa, 14.18
jāgrato, 6.16
janakādayaḥ, 3.20
jānan, 8.27
jānāti, 15.19
janma, 2.27
janmabandha, 2.51
janma karma ca me, 4.9
janmakarmaphala, 2.43
janmamṛtyujarā, 13.9
janmāni, 4.5
jarāmaraṇamokṣāya, 7.29
jātidharmāḥ, 1.42
jijñāsurapi, 6.44
jitasaṅgadoṣā, 15,5
jitātmanaḥ, 6.7
jīvabhūta, 7.5; 15.7
jñānacakṣuṣa, 13.35; 15.10
jñānadīpena, 10.11
jñānadīpite, 4.27
jñānāgnidagdha, 4.19
jñānāgniḥ, 4.37
jñānaṁ jñeyaṁ, 13.18
jñānamāvṛtya, 3.40; 14.9
jñānamupāśritya, 14.2
jñānamuttamam, 14.1
jñānanirdhūta, 5.17
jñānārthadarśanam, 13.12
jñānasaṅgena, 14.6
jñānāsinātmanaḥ, 4.42
jñānatapasā, 4.10
jñānavānmāṁ, 7.19
jñānāvasthitacetasaḥ, 4.23
jñānavijñāna, 3.41; 6.8
jñānayajña, 4.33; 9.15; 18.70
jñānayoga, 3.3; 16.1
jñānī, 3.38,39; .6.46; 7.18
jñāninastattva, 4.34
jñātavyamavaśiṣyate, 7.2
jñeyo'si niyatātmabhiḥ, 8.2
juhvati, 4.26,27
jvaraḥ, 3.30
jyotir, 8.24

K

kālena, 4.2, 38
kalevaram, 8.5
kalmaṣāḥ, 4.30; 5.17
kalpakṣaye, 9.7
kalyāṇakṛtkaścid, 6.40
kāmabhoga, 16.12,16
kāma, 2.5,62; 7.22
kāmahaitukam, 16.8
kāmaistaistairhṛta, 7.20
kāmakāmā, 2,70; 9.21
kāmakārataḥ, 16.23

kāmakāreṇa, 5.12
kāmakrodhaṁ, 5.26
kāmamāśritya, 16.10
kāmarūpa, 3.39,43
kāmātmānaḥ, 2.43
kāmopabhoga, 16.11
kāmyānāṁ, 18.2
kāṅkṣantaḥ, 4.12
kapidhvajaḥ, 1.20
kāraṇaṁ guṇasaṅgo, 13.22
kāraṇamucyate, 6.3
karmabandhaṁ, 2.39
karmabandhana, 3.9; 9.28
karmabhirna sa, 4.14
karmajā, 4.12
karmajaṁ, 2.51
karmajānviddhi, 4.32
karmākhilaṁ, 4.33
karmānubandhīni, 15.2
karmaṇyabhirataḥ, 18.45
karmaṇyakarma, 4.18
karmāṇyaśeṣataḥ, 18.11
karmaṇyatandritaḥ, 3.23
karmaphala,
4.14; 6.1; 18.27
karmaphalahetur, 2.47
karmaphala, 5.14
karmaphalāsaṅgaṁ, 4.20
karmasamādhinā, 4.24
karmasaṁgrahaḥ, 18.18
karmasaṁjñitaḥ, 8.3
karmasaṁnyāsāt, 5.2
karmasaṅga, 3.26; 14.7,15
karmayoga,
3.3'7; 13.24; 5.2
kārpaṇya, 2.7
karśayantaḥ, 17.6
kartāraṁ, 14.19
kāryakāraṇa, 13.21
kāryākārye, 18.30
kaśmalam, 2.2
kauśalam, 2.50
kavim, 8.9
kāyakleśabhayāt, 18.8
kāyaśirogrīvaṁ, 6.13
keśavārjunayoḥ, 18.76
kevalairindriyairapi, 5.11
khaṁ mano buddhir, 7.4
kiṁ tadbrahma, 8.1
kirīṭinaṁ, 11.17,46
kīrtayanto, 9.14
klaibyaṁ, 2.3
kleśo'dhikataras, 12.5
kraturahaṁ, 9.16
kriyā, 1.41
kriyābhirna, 11.48
kriyamāṇāni, 3.27; 13.30
kriyāviśeṣabahulāṁ, 2.43
krodho, 2.62
kṛpaṇāḥ, 2.49
kṛpayāviṣṭam, 2.1
kṛṣigorakṣya, 18.44
kṛṣṇaḥ, 8.25
kṛtāñjalirabhāṣata, 11.14
kṛtsnakarmakṛt, 4.18
kṛtsna, 7.6,29
kṛtsnavin, 3.29
kṣāntirārjavam, 13.8
kṣaraścākṣara, 15.16
kṣātraṁkarma, 18.43
kṣayāya jagato'hitāḥ, 16.9
kṣetrajña iti tadvidaḥ, 13.3
kṣetrakṣetrajña, 13.,27
kṣetrakṣetrajñayor, 13.3,35
kṣetraṁ kṣetrajñam, 13.1
kṣetraṁ kṣetrī tathā, 13.34
kṣīṇakalmaṣāḥ, 5.25
kṣipraṁ hi mānuṣe, 4.12
kṣudraṁ, 2.3
kuladharmāḥ, 1.39,42,43
kulaghnānāṁ, 1.41,42
kulasya, 1.41
kurukṣetre, 1.1
kurunandana, 2.41
kutaḥ, 2.66
kūṭastho, 6.8; 15.16

L

lāghavam, 2.35
lipyate, 5.6
loka, 2.5; 7.25
lobhopahata cetasaḥ, 1.37
lokamaheśvaram, 10.3
lokasaṁgraham, 3.25
lokastadanuvartate, 3.21
lokatrayamāviśya, 15.17
loke janma, 6.42
luptapiṇḍodaka, 1.41

M

madarpaṇam, 9.26
madasrayah, 7.1
madbhakta, 7.23; 11.55;
12.14; 13.19
madbhakteṣu, 18.68
madbhaktiṁ, 18.54
madbhāva, 4.10; 10.6;
14.19
mādhavaḥ, 1.14
madvyapāśrayaḥ, 18.56
madyājī, 9.25,34; 18.65
madyogamāśritaḥ, 12.11
mahadyonir, 14.4
mahāpāpmā, 3.37
mahārathāḥ, 2.35
maharṣī, 10.2,6
mahāśano, 3.37
mahatā, 4.2
mahātmā, 7.19; 8.15;
9.13; 11.12; 18.74
mahatpāpaṁ, 1.44
mahāyogeśvaro, 11.9
maheśvara, 9.11; 13.23
mama māyā, 7.14
mama yo vetti, 10.7
māmāśritya, 7.29
māmevānuttamāṁ, 7.18
māmupāśritāḥ, 4.10
manaḥ, 6.26; 15.7,9; 17.16
mānasa, 1.46; 17.16
mānāvamānayoḥ, 6.7
manave, 4.1
manīṣiṇām, 18.5
manmanā, 9.34; 18.65
manmayā, 4.10
manogatān, 2.55
mantra, 9.16; 17.13
manuṣya, 3.23; 7.3; 15.2
manyate, 3.27
mārdavaṁ, 16.2
martyalokaṁ, 9.21
matkarma, 11.54; 12.10
matparaḥ, 6.14; 18.57
matparāyaṇaḥ, 9.34
matprasādāt, 18.58
mātrāsparśās, 2.14
matsaṁsthām, 6.15
matsthāni, 9.4
matvā, 3.28
maunamātmaḥ, 17.16
mayādhyakṣeṇa, 9.10
māyayā, 4.6; 7.15
mayi buddhiṁ, 12.8
mayi saṁnyasya, 12.6;
18.57
mayyarpitamano, 8.7
mayyāveśitacetasām, 12.7
mayyāveśya, 12.2
mitrāripakṣayoḥ, 14.25
modiṣya, 16.15
moghaṁ, 3.16
moghāśā, 9.12
mohādārabhyate, 18.25

mohakalilaṁ, 2.52
mohanaṁ, 14.8; 18.39
mohayasi, 3.2
mohinīṁ, 9.12
mohitam, 7.13
mokṣakāṅkṣibhiḥ, 17.25
mokṣaparāyaṇaḥ, 5.28
mokṣayiṣyāmi, 18.66
mokṣyase, 9.1,28
mriyate, 2.20
mṛtyusaṁsāra, 9.3
mucyante, 3.31
mūḍhā, 9.11
mūḍhagrāheṇā, 17.19
mūḍhayoniṣu, 14.15
muhurmuhuḥ, 18.76
muhyati(-yanti), 5.15; 8.27
mukhe, 4.32
mukta, 5.28
muktasaṅga, 3.9; 18.26
muktasya, 4.23
mukto yaḥ, 12.16
mumukṣubhiḥ, 4.15
muniḥ, 2.56
munirbrahma, 5.6
munirmokṣa, 5.28
mūrdhny, 8.12
mūrtayaḥ, 14.4

N

nābhaktāya, 18.67
naiṣkarmya, 3.4; 19.49
naiṣṭhikīm, 5.12
namaskṛtvā, 11.35
namaskuru, 9.34
nānāvarṇākṛtīni, 11.5
narādhama, 7.15; 16.19
narakāya, 1.41,42
nāsābhyantara, 5.27
nāsikāgraṁ, 6.13
nāśitamātmanaḥ, 5.16
nātyaśnatastu, 6.16
navadvāre, 5.13
nāvam, 2.67
nibaddhaḥ, 18.60
nibadhnanti, 4.41
nibadhyate, 4.22
nibandhāyāsurī, 16.5
nibodha, 18.13
nidhanaṁ, 3.35
nidhanāni, 2.28
nidrālasyapramād, 18.39
nigrahaṁ, 6.34
niḥspṛhaḥ, 2.71; 6.18
niḥśreyasakarāv, 5.2
nirahaṁkāraḥ, 2.71; 12.13
nirāhārasya 2.59
nirāśīr, 3.30; 4.21; 6.10
nirāśrayaḥ, 4.20
nirdeśo, 17.23
nirdhūta, 5.17
nirdoṣaṁ, 5.19
nirdvandvo, 2.45; 5.3
nirguṇaṁ, 13.15
nirmamo, 2.71; 12.13
nirmānamohā, 15.5
nirmuktā, 7.28
nirudhya, 8.12
nirvāṇam, 2.72; 6.15
nirvedaṁ, 2.52
niryogakṣema, 2.45
niścayena, 6.23
niṣṭhā, 3.3
nistraiguṇyaḥ, 2.45
nītirmatirmama, 18.78
nityābhiyuktānāṁ, 9.22
nityajātaṁ, 2.,26
nityaśaḥ, 8.14
nityasaṁnyāsī, 5.3
nityasattvastho, 2.45
nityatṛpto, 4.20
nityavairiṇā, 3.39
nityayukta, 7.17; 8.14; 12.2
nivartate, 2.59; 8.25
nivṛttāni, 14.22
niyamya, 3.7,41;
6.26; 18.51
niyatāhārāḥ, 4.30
niyata, 6.15; 8.2;18.7,9
niyojitaḥ, 3.36
niyokṣyati, 18.59
nyāyyaṁ, 18.15

O

Om, 8.13

P

pacantyātmakāraṇāt, 3.13
padmapatram, 5.10
paṇḍitāḥ, 2.11; 4.19; 5.4,18;
pāpakṛttamaḥ, 4.36
pāpayonayaḥ, 9.32
pāpmānaṁ, 3.41
paradharmā, 3.35; 18.47
paradharmo, 3.35
paraṁ bhūyaḥ, 14.1
paraṁ brahma, 10.12
parāṁ gatim, 6.45
paraṁ janma, 4.4
paramāṁ, 8.13
paramāpnoti, 3.19
paramātmā, 6.7
paramātmety, 15.17
paramavyayam, 7.13
parameśvara, 11.3; 13.28
paramparāprāptam, 4.2
parāṇyāhur, 3.42
parastasmāttu, 8.20
parastāt, 8.9
parataraṁ, 7.7
parāyaṇāḥ, 4.29; 5.17
paricakṣate, 17.17
paridevanā, 2.28
parigrahaḥ, 4.21
parijñātā, 18.18
parikīrtitaḥ, 18.7,27
pariṇāme, 18.38
paripanthinau, 3.34
paripraśnena, 4.34
parisamāpyate, 4.33
paritrāṇāya, 4.8
parjanyāt, 3.14
paryavatiṣṭhate, 2.65
paśya me yogam, 11.8
paśyāmi devāṁ, 11.15
paśyāmi viśveśvara,
11.16
paśyañśṛṇvan, 5.8
paśyantyātmany, 15.11
paśyato, 2.69
patanti, 1.41
patraṁ puṣpaṁ, 9.26
paurvadehikam, 6.43
pavitraṁ, 4.38; 9.2; 10.12
phalahetavaḥ, 2.49
phala, 2.47; 7.23; 17.21
piṇḍa, 1.41
pitāmahaḥ, 9.17
pitaro, 1.41
pitāsi, 11.43
pitṝnyānti, 9.25
prabhāṣeta, 2.54
prabhavaḥ, 7.6
prabhureva, 9.24
prahasann, 2.10
prāhu, 18.2,3
prajāḥ, 3.10
prajahihyenaṁ, 3.41
prajāpatiḥ, 3.10
prajñā, 2.11,57,58,61,67,68
prakāśa, 7.25,14.6,11,22
prakāśayati, 5.16; 13.34
prakṛteḥ, 3.27,29,33; 9.8
prakṛtijair, 3.5; 18.40

prakṛtiṁ, 9.8; 13.1
prakṛtiraṣṭadhā, 7.4
prakṛtisaṁbhavā,
13.20; 14.5
prakṛtisthāni, 15.7
pralayaṁ, 14.14
pralaya, 7.6; 14.2
pralīyante, 8.18,19
pramāda, 11.41; 14.9,17
pramāṇaṁ, 3.21
pramāthīni, 2.60
prāṇakarmāṇi, 4.27
prāṇam, 1.33; 8.12
praṇamya, 11.14
prāṇānprāṇeṣu, 4.30
prāṇāpāna, 5.27; 15.14
pranaṣṭaste, 18.72
praṇaśyāmi, 6.30
praṇaśyati, 2.63; 9.31
praṇavaḥ, 7.8
prāṇāyāma, 4.29
prāṇendriyakriyāḥ, 18.33
prāṇe'pānaṁ, 4.29
praṇipātena, 4.34
prapadyante, 4.11; 7.19,20
prapadyate, 7.19
prapannam, 2.7
prasāda, 2.64,65; 11.43
prasaktāḥ, 16.16
prasaṅgena, 18.34
prasannacetaso, 2.65
prasannātmā, 18.54
praśānta, 6.7,14,27
prasīda deveśa, 11.45
pratiṣṭhita, 2.57,58,61;
3.15; 6.11
pratyavāyaḥ, 2.40
pravakṣyāmi, 4.16
pravakṣye, 8.11
pravartante'śuci, 16.10
pravartitaṁ, 3.16
praveṣṭuṁ, 11.54
pravilīyate, 4.23
pravṛtti, 14.12;15.4;
16.7; 18.30,46
prayāṇakāle, 7.30; 8.2
prītamanāḥ, 11.49
prītiḥ, 1.35
priya, 5.20; 9.29; 10.1;
11.44;17.15; 18.69
priyaḥ priyāyārhasi, 11.44
priyo hi jñānino, 7.17
proktavān, 4.4
pṛthagvidham, 18.14
pūjanaṁ, 17.14
pūjārhāu, 2.4
punarāvartino'rjuna, 8.16
punarbrāhmaṇāḥ, 9.33
punardhanam, 16.13
punarjanma, 4.9; 8.15,16
punaryogaṁ, 5.1
puṇyakarmaṇām, 7.28
puṇyakṛtām, 6.41
puṇyaphalam, 8.28
puṇyo gandhaḥ, 7.9
purāṇamanuśāsitāram, 8.9
purātanaḥ, 4.3
pūrṇa, 2.1
puruṣaḥ, 8.4,22
puruṣottama, 8.1; 15.18,19
pūrvābhyāsena, 6.44
pūrvaiḥ, 4.15
puṣpitāṁ, 2.42

R

rādhanamīhate, 7.22
rāgadveṣau, 2.64,
3.34; 18.51
rahasi, 4.3; 6.10
rajaḥ karmaṇi, 14.9
rājarṣayaḥ, 4.2
rājavidyā, 9.2
rajoguṇa, 3.37
ramanti, 10.9
ramate, 5.22
ratāḥ, 5.25, 12.4
rātri, 8.17,18,25
ripurātmanaḥ, 6.5
ṛksāma, 9.17
romaharṣa, 1.29; 18.74
ṛṣibhirbahudhā, 13.4
ruddhvā, 4.29
rudhirapradigdhān, 2.5
rūpaṁ paraṁ, 11.47
rūpamaiśvaram, 11.9
rūpamatyadbhutaṁ, 18.77

S

śabdabrahm, 6.44
śabdādīnviṣayān, 4.26
śabdaḥ khe, 7.8
sacarācaram, 9.10
sacchabdaḥ, 17.26
sadbhāve, 17.26
sādharmyamāgatāḥ, 14.2
śādhi, 2.7; 7,30
sādhu, 4.8; 6.9
sadityevābhidhīyate, 17.27
sahasra, 7.3; 11.5,46
sahayajñāḥ, 3.10
śakyo'vāptum, 6.36
samabuddhirviśiṣyate, 6.9
samadarśana, 5.18; 6.29
samādha, 2.43,53;
12.9; 17.11
samādhisthasya, 2,54
samaduḥkha, 2.15; 14.24
samagraṁ, 4.23
samāhitaḥ, 6.7
samantataḥ, 6.24
samatītāni, 7.26
saṁbhavaḥ, 3.14; 14.3
saṁbhavāmi, 4.6,8
saṁchinna, 4.41
saṁgraham, 3.20,25
saṁgrāmaṁ, 2.33
samīkṣya, 1.27
saṁjāyate, 2.62
saṁjñake, 8.18
saṁjñārthaṁ, 1.7
saṁkalpa, 6.2,24
saṁkara, 1.41,42; 3.24
sāṁkhya, 2.39; 3.3;
5.4,5; 13.25
saṁmohaṁ, 7.27
sammūḍha, 2.7
saṁniyamyendriya, 12.4
saṁnyāsa, 3.4; 5.1;
9.28, 18.1
saṁnyāsī, 6.1; 18.12
saṁnyasyādhyātma, 3.30
saṁpadvimokṣāya, 16.5
saṁpadyate, 13.31
saṁpaśyan, 3.20
saṁprekṣya, 6.13
samṛddhavegāḥ, 11.29
śaṁsasi, 5.1
saṁśaya, 4.40; 8.5,6
saṁsiddhi, 3.20; 6.43; 8.15
saṁsparśajā, 5.22
saṁstabhyātmānam, 3.43
saṁsthāpana, 4.8
saṁśuddhakilbiṣaḥ, 6.45
saṁtariṣyasi, 4.36
saṁtuṣṭa, 3.17; 4.22; 12.14
samupāśritaḥ, 18.52
saṁvādamimamad, 18.76
saṁyamī, 2.69
saṁyamya, 2.61; 3.6; 4.26;
6.14;8.12
saṁyatendriyaḥ, 4.39
śanaiḥ śanair, 6.25
sanātana, 2.24; 4.31;

7.10; 8.20
sanātanastvaṁ, 11.18
saṅgavivarjitaḥ, 12.18
sañjayatyuta, 14.9
śānti, 2.66; 4.39
śaraṇaṁ, 18.62,66
śarīravāṅmano, 18.15
sarvabhāvena, 15.19
sarvabhūtānāṁ, 5.29; 12.13
sarvabhūtāni, 7.27; 9.7
sarvadharmānpari, 18.66
sarvajñāna, 3.32
sarvakāmebhyo, 6.18
sarvakarma, 12.11; 18.2
sarvaloka, 5.29
sarvāṇīndriya, 4.27
sarvasaṁkalpa, 6.4
sarvatokṣiśiro, 13.14
sarvayoniṣu, 14.4
śaśisūryayoḥ, 7.8
śāśvataṁ, 18.56
śāśvate, 8.26
sasvato, 2.20
sataḥ, 2.16
satataṁ, 9.14
satkāramānapūjā, 17.18
śatruvat, 6.6
sattvamityuta, 14.11
sāttvikaṁ nirmalaṁ, 14.16
sāttvikapriyāḥ, 17.8
saukṣmyād, 13.33
saumyavapur, 11.50
siddhānāṁ, 7.3
siddhasaṁghāḥ, 11.36
siddhāvasiddhau, 4.22
siddhi, 3.4; 4.12; 12.10
siddhyasiddhyoḥ, 2.48; 18.26
śiṣyas, 2.7
śītoṣṇasukha, 2.14; 6.7
smaran, 8.5,6
smarati, 8.14
smṛti, 2.63; 15.15; 18.73
somapāḥ, 9.20
sparśanaṁ, 15.9
sparśānkṛtvā, 5.27
śraddhā, 7.20; 17.3
śraddhāvāṁ, 4.39; 6.47
śraddhāvirahitaṁ, 17.13
śraddhayānvitāḥ, 17.1
śraddhayopeto, 6.37
śreya, 3.11; 4.33; 12.12; 18.47
śrīmatāṁ, 6.41
śrīrvijayo, 18.78
sṛjāmyaham, 4.7
śrotavyasya, 2.52
śrotrādīnīndriyāṇy, 4.26
sṛtī, 8.27
śrutiparāyaṇāḥ, 13.26
śrutivipratipannā, 2.53
srutva, 2.29; 13.26
stena, 3.12
sthāne hṛṣīkeśa, 11.36
sthāvarajaṅgamam, 13.27
sthirabuddhira, 5.20
sthiramāsanam, 6.11
sthitadhīḥ, 2.54, 56
sthitaprajña, 2.54,55
sthitaścalati, 6.21
striyo vaiśyāstathā, 9.32
stutibhiḥ, 11.21
śubhāśubha, 2.57; 9.28
śubhāṁllokān, 18.71
śucīnāṁ, 6.41
sudurlabhaḥ, 7.19
suduṣkaram, 6.34
suhṛnmitrāryudāsīna, 6.9
sukhaduḥkha, 2.14; 13.21; 15.5
sukhamātyantikaṁ, 6.20
sukhasaṅgena, 14.6
sukhī, 5.23
śuklaḥ, 8.24
śuklakṛṣṇe, 8.26
sukṛtaduṣkṛte, 2.50
sukṛtino'rjuna, 7.16
sūkṣmatvāttada, 13.16
sulabhaḥ, 8.14
suniścitam, 5.1
surendralokam, 9.20
susukhaṁ, 9.2
sūtre maṇigaṇā, 7.7
suvirūḍhamūlam, 15.3
svabāndhavān, 1.36
svabhāva, 2.7; 5.14; 18,41,42,47,60
svacakṣuṣā, 11.8
svadharmam, 2.31
svādhyāyā, 17.15
svādhyāyajñāna, 4.28
svajanaṁ, 1.36, 44
svakaṁ rūpaṁ, 11.50
svakarmanirataḥ, 18.45
svāmavaṣṭabhya, 9.8
svanuṣṭhitāt, 3.35
śvapāke, 5.18
svargadvāram, 2.32
svargalokaṁ, 9.21
svargaparā, 2.43
svasyāḥ, 3.33
svatejasā viśvam, 11.19
svayamevātmanā, 10.15

T

tadbhāvabhāvitaḥ, 8.6
tadviddhi, 4.34
tamasaḥ, 8.9
tapasvibhyo, 6.46
tapobhirugraiḥ, 11.48
tapoyajñā, 4.28
tasmādyogī, 6.46
tatraikāgraṁ, 6.12
tattvadarśinaḥ, 4.34
tattvataḥ, 4.9; 6.21; 7.3
tattvavit, 3.28
tejasvinām, 7.10
tejobhirāpūrya, 11.30
tejomayaṁ, 11.47
tejorāśiṁ sarvato, 11.17
titikṣasva, 2.14
traiguṇya, 2.45
trailokya, 1.35
tribhiḥ, 7.13
trīnguṇānativartate, 14.21
trividhaṁ,16.21
tulyanindāstutir, 12.19
tulyapriyāpriyo, 14.24
tyāgaphalaṁ, 18.8
tyāgītyabhidhīyate, 18.11
tyajatyante, 8.6
tyaktasarva, 4.21
tyaktvātmaśuddhaye, 5.11

U

udaka, 1.41
udbhava, 8.3
uddharedātmanā, 6.5
upadhāraya, 7.6
upahata, 2.7
upāyataḥ, 6.36
ūrdhvaṁ, 14.18; 15.1
utkrāmantaṁ, 15.10
utsīdeyurime lokā, 3.24
uttamam, 4.3
uttaram, 6.11
uttarāyaṇam, 8.24

V

vādinaḥ, 2.42
vahnir, 3.38

vairāgya, 6.35; 13.9
vakṣyāmyaśeṣataḥ, 7.2
varṇasaṁkaraḥ, 1.40,42
vartamāno, 6.31
vartmānuvartante, 3.23; 4.11
vāsudevastathoktvā, 11.50
vaśyātmanā, 6.36
vedāntakṛdvedavid, 15.15
vedavādaratāḥ, 2.42
vibhāga, 4.13
vibhuḥ, 5.15
vibhūti, 10.7,16
vicālayet, 3.29
viddhy, 3.37; 4.13
vidheyātmā, 2.64
viduryānti, 13.35
vidvān, 3.26
vidyādduḥkha, 6.23
vidyāvinaya, 5.18
vigatajvaraḥ, 3.30
vigatakalmaṣaḥ, 6.28
vigataspṛhaḥ, 2.56; 18.49
viguṇaḥ, 3.35
vijānataḥ, 2.46
vijānīto, 2.19
vijitātmā jitendriyaḥ, 5.6
vijitendriyaḥ, 6.8
vijñāna, 9.1; 18.42
vijñātumicchāmi, 11.31
vimohayati, 3.40
vimokṣaṇāt, 5.23
vimokṣyase, 4.32
vimūḍho, 6.38
vimuñcati, 18.35
vināśam, 2.17
vināśastasya, 6.40
vinaśyati, 4.40; 13.28
vindatyātmani, 5.21
viniyamya, 6.24
viniyataṁ, 6.18
vipaścitaḥ, 2.60
vipratipannā, 2.53
visargaḥ, 8.3
viṣayān, 2.62,64
viṣayapravālāḥ, 15.2
viṣayendriya, 18.37
viṣīdantam, 2.1,10
viśiṣṭā, 1.7
viśiṣyate, 3.7; 6.9
visṛjāmyaham, 9.7
vistareṇātmano, 10.18
viśuddhātmā, 5.6,7
viśuddhayā, 18.51
viśuddhaye, 6.12
viśvamanantarūpa, 11.38
viśvatomukham, 9.15; 10.33; 11.11
vītarāgabhaya, 2.56; 4.10
vitatā brahmaṇo, 4.32
vivasvataḥ, 4.4
viviktadeśa, 13.11
vivṛddha, 14.11,13
viyogaṁ, 6.23
viyuktānāṁ, 5.26
vratāḥ, 4.28
vṛjinaṁ, 4.36
vyāharan, 8.13
'vyakto'vyaktāt, 8.20
vyāmiśreṇeva, 3.2
vyapāśrayaḥ, 3.18
vyatitariṣyati, 2.52
vyavasāyātmikā, 2.41,43,44

Y

yadā yadā hi, 4.7
yadrājyasukha, 1.44
yadṛccha, 2.32; 4.22
yajanta iha devatāḥ, 4.12
yajjñātvā, 13.13;14.1,12,16,35
yajjuhoṣi, 9.26
yajñabhāvitāḥ, 3.12
yajñakṣapita, 4.30
yajñānayajñāśca, 4.28
yajñārthāt, 3.9
yajñaśiṣṭāmṛtabhujo, 4.31
yajñaśiṣṭāśinaḥ, 3.13
yajñatapasāṁ, 5.29
yajñavido, 4.30
yajñenaivopajuhvati, 4.25
yaṁ yaṁ vāpi, 8.6
yānti devavratā, 9.25
yantrārūḍhāni, 18.61
yatacetasām, 5.26
yatacitta, 4.21; 6.19
yatamānas, 6.45
yatātmānaḥ, 5.25
yatendriyamano, 5.28
yathaidhāṁsi, 4.37
yatīnāṁ, 5.26
yoga, 2.48; 4.1,2; 6.2
yogabalena, 8.10
yogabhraṣṭo, 6.41
yogāccalitamānasaḥ, 6.37
yogadhāraṇām, 8.12
yogāgnau, 4.27,28
yogaḥ proktaḥ, 4.3
yogakṣemaṁ, 9.22
yogaṁ yogeśvarāt, 18.75
yogamaiśvaram, 9.5; 11.8
yogamātmanaḥ, 6.19
yogamavāpsyasi, 2.53
yogamāyāsamāvṛtaḥ, 7.25
yogārūḍha, 6.3,4
yogasaṁjñitam, 6.23
yogasaṁnyasta, 4.41
yogasaṁsiddhaḥ, 4.38
yogasaṁsiddhiṁ, 6.37
yogasthaḥ, 2.48
yogasya, 6.44
yogavittamāḥ, 12.1
yogayukta, 5.6; 6.29; 8.27
yogenāvyabhicāriṇyā, 18.33
yogeśvara, 11.4; 18.75,78
yogī, 3.3; 4.25; 5.11; 6.15,19,32,42,47; 8,14,23
yogī vigatakalmaṣaḥ, 6.28
yogī yuñjīta satatam, 6.10
yonijanmasu, 13.22
yonirmahadbrahma, 14.3
yudhyasva, 2.18; 3.30
yuga, 8.17
yugasahasrāntāṁ, 8.17
yujyasva, 2.50
yukta āsīta matparaḥ, 6.14
yuktacetasaḥ, 7.30
yuktaḥ, 3.26
yuktāhāravihārasya, 6.17
yuktatamo, 6.47
yuñjan, 6.15; 7.1

Index to Translation

A

A——letter, 10.33
abandonment of consequences, 18.4
Abode of Universe, 11.25
absorber God, 13.17
absorption, 14.26
abusive language, 16.4
accomplishment, factors, 18.3
action/activity,
abandonment?, 18.5, 11
appropriate, 4.17
clarity type, 18.23
conclusion, 4.33
consequence, 5.14
controlled, 18.23
craving, 18.24
deferred to Krishna, 12.6
desireless, 18.23
disciplined, 4.32
distressful, 14.16
essential, 3.8
factors, 18.13—15,18
faulty, 18.3
forceful, 18.60
God created?, 5.14
ignorant, 14.16
implication transcended, 5.7
impulsion, 14.9
impulsive, 18.24
inappropriate, 4.17
incomprehensible, 4.17
Krishna, 4.14
material nature, 3.33; 13.28, 15.2; 18.41
misconception, 18.25
modes, 14.16
mundane energy, 3.27, 28
action/activity,
nature-produced, 5.14
necessary, 6.1
non-action, 4.18,20
non-defective, 14.16
non-defiling, 5.10
obligatory, 6.1
offering to Krishna, 9.27
parts of, 18.18
performance required, 16.24
questioned, 4.16
reduced, 4.37
regulation, 3.3
results, 2.51
Sat type, 17.27
seer's, 2.54
spiritual, 4.24
transcending, 9.28
types, 18.9,19,23—25
unmotivated, 18.23
yoga mood, 2.48
acts of sacrifice, charity, austerities, 17.24
Ādityas, 10.21
affections,
crippling, 2.57
yogic type, 14.26
agency, 13.21
agent,
factor, 18.14,18
Krishna's, 11.33
types, 18.19,26—28
Agni, 11.3
agreeable / disagreeable, 12.17
agriculture, 18.44
air regulation, 4.30
Airāvata, 10.27
airs, 4.29
all—pervasive Form, 11.20
Almighty God,
consequence free, 5.15
Krishna, 6.38; 9.11; 10.3
alone, yogi, 6.10
alphabet, 10.33
alternatives, Arjuna's, 2.6
ambidextrous, 11.33
Ananta, 10.29
anantavijayam, 1.16
ancestors, 9.25
ancient person, 8.9
ancient spirit, 11.38
angel, 11.22
angelic kingdom,
king, 9.20
paradise, 9.21
sovereignty, 2.8
warriors attain, 2.35
anger,
absence of, 16.2
cause, 2.62,63; 5.28
cherished, 16.12
eliminated, 4.10
endured, 5.23
hell, 16.21
tendency, 16.4,18
animals, 10.30
antelope skin, 6.11
anxieties, 2.56,57; 12.16
aquatics, 10.29
Arjuna,
—Also see ***Indexed Names of Arjuna***
agent, 11.33
amazed, 11.14
ambidextrous, 11.33
appreciations, 11.1
bowing, 11.14
bowman,1.4; 18.78
conch blown, 1.14
confusion, 18.73
death preferred, 1.45
depression, 2.8
devotion, 9.33

Arjuna continued,
disoriented, 11.25
fear—free, 11.49,50
frightened, 11.35
God vision, 11.45
hopelessness, 2.1
instructed, 2.37
intimidation, 2.35
Krishna, 10.37
liberated, 11.1
lost?, 18.58
loved, 18.64,65
majestic form, 11.3
material nature, 18.59
monkey insignia, 1.20
normalized, 11.51
obeisance, 11.39,40
ordered, 11.33,34
overwhelmed, 1.27,46
past birth, 4.5
refuses to fight, 2.9
repulsed, 1.35
request, 1.21,22; 4.42
sense of duty, 2.7
shifty vision, 6.33,34
sickly emotion, 2.2
sinless one, 14.6
sits down, 1.46
stunned, 1.28
submits, 2.7; 18.73
trembles, 1.29, 11.45,48
Universal Form seen, 11.15
work, 4.15
armored warriors, 11.32,34
arms, 11.19, 23
army, destroyed, 11.32,34
arrogance, 16.4,17,18
Aryamā, 10.29
asana, 6.11—13
ascetic,
Krishna related, 7.9
sacrifice, 4.30
temptations, 2.59
yogi superior, 6.46
Asita, 10.13
assertion, false type, 18.52
assertive attitude, 18.17
assurance, 12.8
astral region, 9.20
aśvattha tree, 10.26; 15.1—3
Aśvatthāmā, 1.8
atmosphere, 7.8
attachment,
as Cause, 13.22
cause, 2.62; 11.55
conquered, 15.5
discarded, 5.10,11
finished, 4.23
freedom from, 3.9; 12.18
idleness, 2.47
attack, superiors, 2.4
attainment, 6.22, 8.21
attention,
drift / restraint, 6.26
Krishna absorbed, 7.1
attractive objects,
addictive, 15.9
detachment, 6.4
living space, 13.6
senses interlocked, 5.9
audiences, 18.67
austerities, enjoyer, 5.29
austerity,
abandoned?, 18.3
asat, 17.28
categories, 17.7—10
faith in, 17.17
godly nature, 16.1
impulsive type, 17.18
ineffective, 11.48,53
invented ones, 17.1
Krishna derived, 7.9; 10.5
mistaken type, 17.19
motivation, 4.23
purificatory, 4.10,30; 18.5
rain, 3.14
realistic type, 17.17
religion, 3.14; 4.23
sacrifice, 4.25
tendency, 18.42
terrible type, 17.5
tricky type, 17.18
types, 17.14—17
Universal Form, 11.48
authority, besides Krishna, 9.30; 10.38
avenues of depression, 16.22
axe, 15.3

B

battle formation, 1.33; 2.31
beasts, 10.30
begetting, 10.28
begging, 2.5
beginning of creation, 7.27
beginningless, Krishna, 10.3
behavior, codes of, 12.20
beings,
disintegration, 13.28
independent, 9.4
influenced, 7.27
Krishna produces, 9.7
Krishna's energy sustains, 9.4
origin / ruination, 11.2
production, 9.8
psychological supremacy, 9.5
relation, 4.35
Supreme Lord inhabits, 13.28
types, 16.6
belief in God, 18.42
belief in Krishna, 3.31
belief in others, 7.21
beliefs of wicked people, 16.8,13—15
bellies, 11.16,23
benefit,
abandoned, 12.11
detachment from 4.20,22; 17.17
disinterest in, 17.25
luck, 4.22
types, 17.11—23; 18.12
best of gods, 11.31
bewitching energy, 7.14
Bhagavad Gītā,
hearing of, 18.67,71
preachers, 18.67
study, 18.70
Bhīma, 1.4,10,15
Bhishma, 1.8,10—12,25;. 2.4; 11.26,34
Bhṛgu, 10.25
Bhṛhat Sama Melody, 10.35
birds, 10.30
birth,
certain, 2.27
rebirth, 4.4,5
liberation from, 5.19; 7.19; 14.20
birthless, Krishna, 10.3,12

blockheads, 16.20
body,
acquirement / departure from, 2.13; 15.8
assumption of, 2.22
detachment, 14.23
head—neck balance, 6.13
living space, 13.2
maintenance, 3.8
purification usage, 5.11
restriction, 3.7
terminal, 2.18
bondage tendencies, 16.5
boys, 10.6
Brahma Sūtras, 13.5
Brahmā,
day / night, 8.17—19; 9.7
instructed, 3.10,11,12
Krishna as father, 11.39
Krishna greater, 11.37
Krishna identity, 10.33; 11.39
procreator, 3.10
Universal Form, 11.15
world of, 8.16
brahmin,
compared, 5.18
ordained, 17.23
perceptive, 2.46
praised, 9.33
respected, 17.14
branches of imperishable tree, 15.2
breathing, nature function, 5.8
Bṛhaspati, 10.24
brilliant consciousness, 5.24
brothers, 1.26
brow chakra, 8.10
brute force, 16.18, 17.5
buddy, 11.41,44
business men, 9.32

C

cakes, 1.41
cannibals, 17.4
cardinal points, 11.25
career categories, 4.13
caste, 4.13; 18.41
categories of elements, 13.6
cause,
non—deteriorating, 9.18
destruction, 11.32
elaborated, 13.21
series of, 16.8
Cekitāna, 1.5
celebrity, 3.21
celestial body, 9.19
celestial delights, 9.20
celestial musicians, 11.22
celestial regions, 6.40,41
celestial sea, 10.27
celibacy,
austerity, 17.14
destination, 8.11
yogi's, 6.14
celibate boys, 10.6
ceremonial articles, 4.24
ceremonial rites, 2.43 —see religious ceremony
cessation, 5.25,26
changes of living space, 13.20
chaos, 3.24
chariot, Arjuna's, 1.21
charitable disposition, 18.43
charity,
abandoned?, 18.3
categories, 16.1; 17.7—10
ineffective, 11.48,53
Krishna derived, 10.5
purificatory, 18.5
Universal Form, 11.48
yogi bypasses, 8.28
cherish the imperishable, 12.3
choice, Arjuna's, 2.6
chum, 11.44
circular process, 3.16
Citraratha, 10.26
clan, 1.37—42
clarity,
captivating, 14.6
disease—free, 14.6
expertise, 14.6
happiness produced by, 14.6,9
illuminating, 14.6
influence, 14.5
clarity continued,
lack of, 14.13
predominating, 14.10,11
class, 1.40,41,42
clay, 6.8; 14.24
cleanliness, 16.7; 18.42
cleansers, 10.31
clear—minded people, 17.8
cloud comparison, 6.38
club, 11.17, 46
cold, 2.14; 6.7
colors, 11.5
command, 2.47
commerce, 18.44
common factor, 5.18
comparative view, 6.33
comparison,
lamp, 6.19
mind / wind, 6.34
yoga methods, 12.1,2,3
compassion, 1.27; 12.13; 16.2
compensation, 17.21
competence, 12.16
compulsion to act, 3.36, 37
conceit, 16.3
concentrated mental focus, 7.30
concentration, lacking, 2.66
concepts, discipline, 9.15
conclusion, 4.33;10.32; 13.1,2
condemnation, resisted, 12.19; 14.24
conditions, 2.15
conduct, 14.21
confidence, 12.10; 17.3,13
confidential teaching, 4.3
confusion,
devoid of, 15.5
impulsion, 14.17
production, 14.13
congratulations, 14.24
consciousness,
detachment, 14.22
Krishna, 10.22
living space, 13.7
purifier, 9.2

consequence,
abandonment, 16.2
aftermath, 2.47
Almighty God, 5.15
freedom from 3.31; 9.28
rejection, 18.1,2,4
types, 18.12
contact, happiness, 18.37
contentment, 2.71; 10.5; 12.14
continuation, 10.32
controller, I, 16.14
conviction, 13.7
coping, 2.14
core self, 6.18; 8.12
cosmic destroyers, 10.23
couch, 11.42
cow, 5.18; 10.28; 18.44
cowardice, 2.3; 18.43
craving,
abandoned, 2.55
cause, 2.62; 3.37
cherished, 16.12,16
degrading, 16.18,21
eliminated, 4.10; 8.11; 12.17
endured, 5.23
freedom from, 3.30; 6.18; 16.2
impulsion, 14.11
possession of, 17.5
resisted, 2.70
transcended, 2.70,71
created being, 10.39; 16.6
creation, 10.32; 14.2
creative power, 8.3
creator, 9.17
creature,
disintegrated, 8.20
evolution, 10.6
Krishna knows, 7.26
Krishna related, 7.9
nourishment, 3.14
origination, 7.6
spirit habitat, 6.29
crippling emotions, 2.48, 57
criticism, 16.2
crowds, 13.11
crown, 11.46
culprit, 4.36
cultural activity,
cause of, 3.15
creative power, 8.3
cultural activity con't,
exemption, 3.17; 18.49
inferior, 2.49
Krishna, 4.13,14; 9.9
mandatory, 4.15
mental / physical, 3.1
perfection related, 3.20
production, 3.14
purification usage, 5.11
questioned, 4.16
religious type, 3.9
rewards abandoned, 5.12
social affairs, 3.4
transcended, 4.41
value, 7.29
yoga method, 6.3
cultured man, 2.2
cumulative intellectual interest, 6.43
cutting instrument, 4.42
cycles of rebirth, 16.19
cynical, 9.1

D

dairy farming, 18.44
damage, 18.25
danger of birth/death, 13.9
danger, avoidance, 2.56
Danu, 10.14
dark moon, 8.25
darshan, 11.53
day / night, 8.17—19,24
death,
attainments, 2.72
certainty, 2.27
devotee, 12.7
devotion applied, 8.10
duty, 3.35
eyebrow focus, 8.10
Krishna, 4.9; 8.5; 9.19; 10.34; 15.8
liberation, 7.29; 8.25; 14.20
modes influence, 14.14,15
psychology, 15.8
rebirth, 9.3
repetitive, 8.16
supervisor, 11.39
death continued,
texture of existence recalled, 8.6
deceit, 13.8; 16.4; 17.5
deceiver, 3.6
December, 10.35
decision, 9.30
deeds of Krishna, 4.9
defeat, victory, 2.38
defect universal, 18.48
deity worship, 7.21
deity, outsmarting, 17.12
deliverer, 12.7
delusion,
banished, 4.35
cause / production, 2.63
experience, 18.22
overpowering, 16.16
saturated mind, 2.52
demigods, 7.23; 11.52; 16.20
—also see supernatural rulers
demons, 11.36; 16.20
— also see wicked people
departed spirits, 1.41; 7.26; 9.25
departure of yogis, 8.23
depressed people, 17.10
depression,
detachment from, 14.22
predominating, 14.10,12
release from, 16.22
desire,
abandoning, 6.24
contrary ones, 7.20
desire for pay—off, 4.14
eliminated, 5.28
freedom from, 6.18
impulsive type, 2.5
living space, 13.7
motivated action, 5.12
productions, 14.8
resistance, 5.20
restrained, 4.19
satisfaction, 2.70
desireless, 6.10
despair, 18.35

destination, highest, 18.50
destiny, factor, 18.14
destroyers, 11.6
destruction, 7.6
detachment,
axe, 15.3
conditions resisted, 6.7
recommended, 3.7,9; 12.19
detection device, 15.7
determination,
tendency, 18.43
types, 18.29, 33—35
yoga practice, 6.23
Devadatta, 1.15
Devala, 10.13
devas,
—see supernatural rulers
deviation, 6.37
devilish people, 9.12
devotee,
categorized, 7.16—18; 12.17
dear, 12.20
delivered, 12.7
guarantees, 18.68—70
Krishna attraction 9.28
Krishna enlightens, 10.11
Krishna protects, 9.22
Krishna's favorite, 9.29
Krishna's proximity, 13.19
offerings, 9.26
ruination, 9.31
yogi, 12.14
devotion,
dear to Krishna, 12.18
extolled, 12.17
great soul's, 9.14
Krishna, 4.3; 11.55; 18.65
offerings related, 9.26
opportunity, 9.33
required, 12.20; 13.11
supreme type, 18.54,55
unique, 11.54
yogic type, 14.26
devotional practice, 12.8—11
devotional relationship, requirement, 8.22
devotional service, 9.27
devotional worship, 9.29
dharmakṣetre, 1.1
Dhātā, 10.33
Dhṛṣṭadyumna, 1.17
Dhṛṣṭaketu, 1.5
Dhṛtaraṣṭra, 1.1,18,35,45; 2.9; 11.26
Dhṛti, 10.34
diet restraint, 4.30
differences, 18.21
digestive heat, 15.14
dimensions beyond, 4.40
dining, 11.42
direction, 11.25
directive self, 6.7
disc, 11.46
discernment,
adjusted, 3.39
constant type, 2.68
maintained, 3.41
senses affected, 2.67
uncontrolled person, 2.66
disciplic succession, 4.34
discipline,
accomplishment, 4.32
body, 17.14
concepts, 9.15
continuous, 6.15
mind, 17.16
offering to Krishna, 9.27
speech, 17.15
types, 17.11—13
disciplined behavior, 3.26
disciplined person, 6.36; 9.26
discredit Krishna, 3.32
discrimination, 2.52; 18.42
discus, 11.17
discussion, 10.10
disease, 13.9
disgrace, 2.2
disgusted / tradition, 2.52
disintegration, 13.28
dislikes / likes, 3.34; 4.22
dispassion, 12.18,19; 18.52
dissolution, 14.2
distinction, 6.9
distress,
cessation, 2.57,65
happiness, 2.38
remover, 6.17
transcended, 12.15; 14.20
distressed person, 7.16
Diti, 10.30
divine form, 11.52, 54
Divine Supreme Person, 8.8,10
divinity, 2.72
doctors, 11.22
dog, 5.18
doubt, 4.40; 6.39
Draupadī, 1.6,18
Droṇa, 1.7,25;2.4; 11.26,34
Drupada, 1.3,4,18
dry food, 17.9
duality, 2.14; 6.7,32
duration of life, 17.8
Duryodhana, 1.2,12
duty,
abandoned?, 18.48
alternatives, 2.31
another's, 3.35
discipline, 6.17
necessary, 3.35; 6.1
neglect, 2.33
perfection, 18.45—48
preferred, 3.19
sin—resistant, 2.38
dying person, 8.5

E

earth, resonated, 1.19; 7.9; 8.15; 15.13
easy to practice, 9 .2
eatables, 17.7—10
eating, yoga method, 5.8; 6.16,17; 9.27
educated people, 3.39
education,
purificatory, 4.10
ineffective, 11.48,53
Krishna, 9.17; 13.18
elements, categories, 13.6
elephant, 5.18; 10.27
embodied soul,
—see also Spirit
nine—gate city, 5.13
embryo, 3.38
emotional detachment, 13.10
emotional distress, 2.65

emotional stability, 2.66
emotional weakness, 2.3
emotions, 1.19; 2.38,48
endeavor,
intention free, 4.19
Krishna, 10.36
righteous type, 2.40
ending, 10.32
enemy killed, 16.14
enemy, passion, 3.37
energizing airs, 4.29
energizing breath, 8.10,12
energy, 7.4—6; 14.13
enjoyable aspects, 1.32
enjoyer, I, 16.14
enjoyment, 2.43,57,58
enlightened parents, 6.42
enlightenment, 14.22
enthusiasm, 14.22
environment of psyche, 13.4
envy—free person, 4.22
equally—disposed, 12.13; 14.25
equanimity, 12.18,19; 14.24,25
era to era, 4.8
essential nature, 17.3
eternal divine person, 10.12
eternal abode, 18.56
eternal life, 9.19; 13.13
eternal peace, 9.31
evacuation, 5.9
even—minded, 12.4; 13.10
everlasting principle, 2.17
evil action forced, 3.36,37
evil—doers, 7.15
evolution, 14.18
example, 3.21
excitement, 2.56,57; 5.20; 12.15; 14.23
exclusive worship, 9.30
exemption, 18.49
exertion, 14.11
exhalation, inhalation, 4.29; 5.27
existence,
ceaseless, 2.12
enduring/ non—enduring, 2.16; 4.24
Krishna originates, 10.5,41
Krishna upholds, 7.7
existential arrangement, 6.29
existential conditions, 10.5
existential residence, 9.18
expectations, 16.12
experience,
depression obscures, 14.9
explained, 13.13
ignorance, 5.16
illuminating, 4.27
impetus, 18.18
incomparable, 4.38
Krishna gave, 7.2
overshadowed, 7.20
spirit's, 13.22
Supreme Spirit, 13.15
types, 7.2; 18.19—22
experiencer, 13.1,2,23,27
expertise, 18.43
eye movement, 5.9
eyebrows, 5.27
eyes, 11.2,10,16,19

F

faces, 11.16
facilities of species, 6.32
factors, five, 18.13—15
failure/ success, 2.48; 4.22
faith,
experience yielding, 4.39
Krishna awards, 7.21
nature based, 17.3
persons, 6.37
required, 9.3
undisciplined
faithfulness, 10.34
faithless person, 4.40; 9.3
fallen yogi, 6.37,41
fame, 10.5,34
familiarity, 11.41
family duties, 1.42
family, fallen yogi, 6.41—43
fantasy, 16.13
father, Krishna, 9.17; 11.43; 14.4
fathers, 1.26,33
faults, 3.13; 4.21; 5.17,25; 6.28; 10.3
fear, 2.56; 4.10; 5.28; 10.5; 12.15; 17.20; 18.35
fearlessness, 10.5; 16.1
features, 14.21
fee, 17.13
feelings, 10.34; 13.7
feet, 11.23
feverish mood, 3.30
fickleness, absence of, 16.2
fig tree, 10.26
financial assets, 1.33
fire ceremony, 6.1
fire controller, 11.39
fire,
comparison, 18.48
Krishna, 9.16
lust compared, 3.39
universal destruction, 11.25
spirit resists, 2.23
splendor, 15.12
supreme residence 15.6
five factors, 18.13—15
flame, 7.4
flower, Krishna accepts, 9.26
focus on Krishna, 12.2
food, categories, 17.7—10,13
foolish people, 9.11
forbearance, 16.3
forced action, 3.36,37
forgiveness, 11.42
Form of everything, 11.16
Form of Mine, 11.47
formation, 10.32
forms,
Krishna inhabits, 6.30
unlimited, 11.5
womb produced, 14.4
fortune, 10.34
foundation,
material nature, 9.8
future, 10.34
singular, 13.31
yogi compared, 6.38
four celibate boys, 10.6
four kinds/people, 7.16
four—handed Form, 11.52
fresh air, 4.30
friend, 1.26; 3.21; 9.18; 11.41,44; 12.13
friendship, with Krishna, 4.3
fright, 11.35
fruit, 9.26

fulfillments, 7.22
functional work, 4.15
future productions, 10.34

G

gain, 3.18
gambling, 10.36
Gāṇḍīva, 1.29
garlands, 11.11
garments, 2.22; 11.11
Garuḍa, 10.30
gas, 7.4
Gāyatrī, 10.35
geniuses, 7.10
gentleness, 16.2, 17.16
ghastly form, 11.49
ghee, Krishna, 9.16
ghosts, 9.25; 17.4
gift, 17.20—22
glorification, resisted, 12.19
glory, 11.41
goal of invisible reality, 12.5
God form, 11.45
God of gods, 11.13
god of romance, 10.28
God Vishnu, 11.24, 30
God,
 action free, 5.14
 described, 10.12; 11.11; 18.46
 Krishna, 10.15
 location in body, 8.2
 near / far, 13.16
 pervader, 9.4
goddess of counsel, 10.34
goddess of faithfulness, 10.34
goddess of fame, 10.34
goddess of fortune, 10.34
goddess of patience, 10.34
goddess of recollection, 10.34
goddess of speech, 10.34
godly nature, 16.1—3
gods, 7.22
 —see also supernatural rulers
gold, 6.8, 14.24
good feelings, 1.31
good people, 7.18
governing tendency, 18.43
Govinda, 2.9
grace, 11.47
grandfather Krishna, 9.17
grandfathers, 1.26,33
grandsons, 1.26
grasping, 2.45; 4.21
great person, 3.21
Great Personality, 11.12
great soul,
 rare, 7.19
 rebirth exemption, 8.15
 reliance, 9.13
greed, mental obsession, 1.37; 14.11,17; 16.21
grossness, free of, 8.9
grudge, 17.21

H

habits, 4.12
hairs on end, 18.74
Hanuman, 1.20
happiness,
 achievement, 2.66
 detachment, 5.23
 distress, 2.38
 endless type, 6.28
 non—fluctuating, 5.21
 production of, 14.6,9
 spiritual type, 5.24
 superior type, 6.27
 types, 18.36—39
 ultimate, 5.2
Hari, 11.9; 18.77
harmony, 6.31
hatred, 16.3
hazy season, 8.25
head posture, 6.13
health, 17.8
hearing
 about soul, 2.29
 austerity, 4.26
 perception, 13.26
 nature function, 5.8
 valid method, 13.26
heat, 2.14; 9.19
heaven,
 attainment, 9.20,21
 material nature, 18.40
 open, 2.31
 sickly emotion, 2.2
hell, avenues, 1.43; 16.16,21
hereafter, 4.31; 14.14,15,18
heroes, 1.9
heroism, 18.43
highest living state, 6.15
highest reality, 5.17
highest well—being, 3.11
Himālaya, 10.25
holding, 5.9
home, 13.10
honor / dishonor, 6.7
honored man, 2.34
hope, 2.41; 4.21
hordes of ghost, 17.4
horses, 10.27
hostility, 11.55; 16.20,21
Hṛṣikeśa, 1.15,21,24; 11.36
human being,
 Brahman realization, 12.5
 creation of, 3.10
 Krishna affects, 4.11
 material nature, 15.2
 perfection, 7.3
 regard for Krishna, 10.3
 world of, 11.48
 worship gods, 4.12
human body of Krishna, 9.11
hygiene, 12.16
hymns, 10.35
hypocrisy, 16.10

I

idea of Krishna, 3.31
ideas, overpowering, 16.16
identity—confusion, 3.27
idiot, 15,1018.16
idleness, 2.47
ignorance,
 defined, 13.12
 doubt, 4.42
 impulsion, 14.17
 knowledge shrouded, 5.15
 Krishna banishes, 10.11
ignorant person, 4.40
Ikṣvāku, 4.1
illusion, 7.14
immortality, 14.20
impartiality, 5.19; 10.5; 12.16; 14.24,25; 18.54
impatience, 12.15

imperishable destination, 8.11
imperishable invisible existence, 12.1,3
impersonal existence, 12.1,3
impetus, 18.18
implication, avoidance, 4.22; 5.3; 9.28
impulsion,
activity produced by, 14.6
attachment, 14.6
desire, 14.6
endured, 5.23
influence, 14.5,10,13
mentality adjusted, 2.60
passion, 14.6
impulsiveness, 2.71
impure objectives, 16.10
impurities, 4.30; 9.1
inattentiveness, 14.8,13,17
inconceivable reality, 12.3
independence, 4.20
indestructible factor, 2.17
indetermination, 3.26
indifference, 5.3;6.9,35; 12.16; 13.9
individual existence, 2.12
individualized
conditioned beings, 15.7
infamy, 10.5
inferior energy, 7.4,5
influence, 10.12; 17.2
information,
God, 13.18
highest, 11.1; 14.1
informed person, 7.16
Krishna's, 7.2; 10.42
liberating, 14.1
secret, 15.20; 18.63,64
Supreme Spirit, 13.12
ultimate, 9.2; 10.1
inhalation, 4.29; 5.27
inherent nature, 18.47
initiate action, 5.8
initiative, 7.4; 13.6,9
innate tendency, 17.2
inner peace, 2.66
inquisitive person, 7.16
insensibility, cause, 14.8
insight,
Arjuna's, 11.8
blocked, 3.38,40
Krishna gives, 10.11
protects, 2.40
reaction—resistant, 2.39
reality—piercing, 2.50
steady type, 2.55
view different, 2.41
instruments, 18.14,18
intellect,
controlled, 5.28
defective type, 18.16
detached type, 18.49
grasped, 6.25
living space, 13.6
self—focused type, 2.44
spiritual happiness, 6.21
types, 18.29—32
intellectual discipline, 2.49
intelligence,
compared, 3.42
grasped, 6.25
Krishna anchored, 8.7
Krishna derived, 10.5
Krishna related, 7.10
mundane, 7.4
passion fostered, 3.40
purification, 5.11
stable, 2.65
intelligent statements, 2.11
intentions,
Krishna's, 11.31
restrained, 4.19
wicked ones, 17.6
interaction, 2.68
interim, 2.28
intoxication, 16.10
introspection, 8.11
intuitive perception, 10.35
invisible existence, 8.18,21;.12.1,3,5;
isolation, 6.10; 13.11; 18.52
item of research, 18.18

J

Jāhnavī, 10.31
Jahnu's daughter, 10.31
Janaka, 3.20
Janārdana, 11.51
japa, 10.25
Jayadrath, 11.34
jinxed, 3.32
joke, 11.42
joy, 5.25
judgment, 6.9

K

Kāmadhuk, 10.28
Kandarpa, 10.28
Kapila, 10.26
karma yoga, 3.7; 4.2
Karṇa, 1.8; 11.26,34
Kaśi, 1.5,17
Keshava, 2.54; 10.14; 13.1; 18.76;
Keśi, 18.1
Killed/ killer, 2.19
killing, Arjuna repulsed, 1.34; 18.17
kinfolk, Arjuna, 1.31
king, 4.2; 10.27
king's son, 2.31
Kīrti, 10.34
knower of reality, 5.8
knowledge
clarity produces, 14.17
control, 4.33
defined, 13.8—12
derived, 12.12
experience, 9.1
fiery force, 4.19
Krishna produced, 10.5; 15.15
Krishna represented, 10.38
lack of, 16.4
of Krishna, 4.14
Krishna, Lord,
—also see ***Indexed Names of Krishna***
A – letter, 10.33
actions of, 4.11
Ādityas, 10.21
Agni, 11.39
Airāvata, 10.27,29
Almighty God, 10.3
ancient person, 11.18
appeasers of, 9.25
approach to, 8.15,16
aquatics, 10.29
Arjuna and, 18.78
Arjuna identity, 10 37
Arjuna loved by, 18.64,65
Arjuna's welfare, 10.1

Krishna continued,
armies shown, 1.25
Aryamā, 10.29
ascetics, 7.9
aspiration—free, 3.22
association, 18.55
Aśvattha, 10.26
atmosphere, 7.8
austerity, 7.9
authority, 10.38
basis supreme, 11.37; 14.27
beasts identity, 10.30
beautiful-haired, 1.30
begetting, 10.28
beginningless, 11.19
beings caused by, 9.5
best of gods, 11.31
beyond range, 7.24
birds identity, 10.30
birth transcended, 7.25
birthless, 4.6; 10.12
births, 4.5
body situated, 13.32
Brahmā compared, 10.33; 11.37,39
Bṛhaspati, 10.21
Bṛhgu identity, 10.25
cause of integration, 9.18
cause ultimate, 7.6
celestial sea, 10.27
chanting, 10.25
chariot driver, 1.24
chief of cowherds, 1.32; 2.9
Chitraratha, 10.26
clansman of Vrishnis, 1.40
cleansers, 10.31
commanders, 10.21
conch blown, 1.14
conclusion, 10.32
condition of existence, 8.5
consciousness, identity, 10.22
constant factor, 9.13
continuation, 10.32
contrasting, 11.26
cows identity, 10.28
creations, 10.32
creator, 9.17

Krishna continued,
creatures, 7.9
death producer, 9.19
December, 10.35
dependence on, 7.1,29; 11.55
descendant of Madhu, 1.14 ,36
detachment, 9.9
devoted to, 6.14
devotee approaches, 9.28
devotee delivered by, 12.7
devotee guarantee, 9.31
devotee yogi, 12.16
devotion to, 9.14; 13.11; 18.55
devotional worship 9.29
Dhātā, 10.33
digestion, 15.14
disciplines, 10.25
disliked, 16.18
Diti identity, 10.30
divine form, 11.50
divine glory, 10.7
duty—free / duty—bound, 3.22
earth, 7.9; 15.13
easy to reach, 8.14
education, 9.17
elephants, 10.27
endeavor, 9.27; 10.36
ending identity, 10.32
endless, 11.16
enjoyer, 5.29
entered, 15.15
equally—disposed, 9.29
eternal life, 9.19
everything, 7.19; 11.40
exclusive worship, 9.30
exemplary, 3.23
existential level, 4.10
existential residence, 9.18
exists in body, 8.4
eyes, 11.2,19
fame, 11.36
father, 9.17
father of world, 11.43

Krishna continued,
favorites, 9.29
fig tree identity, 10.26
fire, 9.16
First God, 11.38
focus on, 4.10; 7.30; 8.7; 11.38; 12.8
Form Infinite, 11.16,38
formation, 10.32
foundation, 9.18
four—armed Form, 11.46
fraction, 10.42
friend, 5.29 ; 9.18
gambling, 10.36
garlands, 11.11
garments, 11.11
Garuḍa, 10.30
Gāyatrī, 10.35
geniuses, 7.10
ghastly Form, 11.49
ghee, 9.16
glorified, 9.14; 11.2,9
God of gods, 10.15; 11.13
god of romance, 10.28
Govinda, 2.9
grace, 18.56,58
grandfather, 9.17
great souls, 9.13
handsome—haired, 3.1; 11.35
happiness, 14.27
heat producer, 9.19; 11.19
herb, 9.16
higher existence, 7.24; 9.11
highest reality, 7.7
Himalaya, 10.25
honored, 11.39
horses identity, 10.27
Hṛṣikeśa, 1.15
human—like Form, 11.49,51
hurls the wicked, 16.19
hymns identity, 10.35
idea, 3.31
impartial, 9.29
important, 12.6
indifference, 9.9
infallible, 11.42

Krishna continued,
infinite Lord of gods, 11.37
infinite, 11.11,16
influence, 9.6; 10.12
intelligence, 7.10
items accepted, 9.26
Jāhnavī, 10.32
Jahnu's daughter, 10.32
Janārdana, 11.51
japa identity, 10.25
Kāmadhuk, 10.28
Kandarpa, 10.28
Kapila, 10.26
killer of Madhu, 2.1
king identity, 10.27
king of beasts, 10.30
knower, 11.38
knowledge, 10.38
knowledge of, 4.14
known, 7.1
known at death? 8.2
knows Himself, 10.15
Kuvera identity, 10.23
law guardian, 11.18
liberated, 9.9
liberation offered, 18.66
life energy focus, 10.9
life, 7.9
light, 10.21
limitless, 10.19
lion identity, 10.30
logicians, 10.32
longevity, 9.19
Lord of created beings, 10.15
lord of creatures, 4.6
Lord of gods, 11.37
Lord of beings, 7.30
Lord of supernatural rulers and powers, 7.30
Lord of the earth, 1.21
Lord of universe, 10.15
Lord of yoga, 18.75,78
maintainer, 10.15
manifestation, 4.7; 10 40
manliness, 7.9
Marīci, 10.21

Krishna continued,
master of religious ceremony, 9.24
master, 9,18
medicinal herb, 9.16
meditation upon, 8.12; 10.8; 12.6
men, 7.9
mental productions, 10.6
Meru identity, 10.23
mind, identity, 10.22
monitors, 10.30
monsters, 10.31
moon, 7.8; 10.21; 15.13
morality, 7.11; 10.38
mother, 9.17
motivator of humans, 1.38
motivator, 1.38; 10.18
mountain, 10.23
mystic discipline, 10.7
mystic master, 7.25; 10.7,17
Nārada, 10.26
nature of, 14.2
non—dependent, 7.12
non—deteriorating cause, 9.18
not fruitive, 4.14
not recognized, 7.26
not visible, 7.25
November, 10.35
obeisance to, 11.37, 39
objective, 9.18
oblation, 9.16
observer, 9.18
ocean, 10.21
odor, 7.9
offering, 9.27
ointments, 11.11
Oṁ, 7.8; 9.17
omni vision, 9.15
omni—directional, 11.11
one—syllable sound 10.25
opinion, 18.6
opponents, 3.32
opulences, 10.40
origin, 9.18; 10.39
originator, 9.13; 10.8
ornaments, 11.10
Pāṇḍavas, 10.37

Krishna continued,
partner, 15.7
Pāvaka, 10.23
penetrates, 11.40
perfected souls, 10.26
perfumes, 11.11
Person of incomparable splendor, 11.43
Person of universal dimensions, 11.46
plants, 15.13
poets identity, 10.37
Power Infinite, 11.40
Prahlāda, 10.30
praised, 11.44
prayers, 10.25
priests identity, 10.21
Primal God, 10.12
Primal Person, 11.31
primeval cause, 7.10
priority, 12.20
procreators, 10.6
punishment, 10.38
purifier, 9.17
rainfall control, 9.19
Rakṣas identity, 10.23
Rāma identity, 10.31
rarely known, 7.3
recalled at death, 8.5
reciprocates, 4.11
recognizing, 5.29
refuge, 11.38
relation to, 4.35
reliance effective, 9.32
reliance on 4.10; 7.14; 18.56
remembered, 8.7
reproduction, 10.28
research of, 10.17
reservoir of energies, 9.18
residence, 15.6
resort of world, 11.37
respected, 11.31
responsibility, 3.24; 10.20
Rig Veda, 9.17
rivers identity, 10.32
romance, 7.11; 10.28
rulers identity, 10.38
rules of social conduct, 14.27

Krishna continued,
sacrificial ceremony, 9.16
Sāma Veda, 9.17; 10.22,35
sanctified offering, 9.16
sanctuary ultimate, 11.38
Śaśāṅka, 11.39
sciences, 10.32
sea identity, 10.21,27
sea monsters, 10.31
season identity, 10.35
secrets identity, 10.38
self disciplinary, 10.18
self-declaration, 10.13
self-sufficient, 7.12
senses, identity, 10.22
serpents, 10.28
service to, 14.26
shark identity, 10.31
shelter, 9.18; 11.18,43
shielded, 7.25
Shiva identity, 10.23
silence identity, 10.38
Singular Basis, 9.15
Skanda identity, 10.21
slayer of Madhu, 1.34
smiling, 2.10
snakes identity, 10.29
sound, 7.8; 9.16; 10.25
speech about, 10.9
spirits identity, 10.29
spiritual master, 11.43
splendor, 7.10; 10.36,41; 11.19,43
spring identity, 10.35
stars, 10.21
strength, 7.11
subduers, 10.29
sum total, 11.37,40
sun, 10.21
sunlight, 7.8,9
supernatural power, 4.6
supernatural rulers, 10.2,22
supervisor, 9.10
supporter, 9.18
Supreme Being, 9.9
Supreme Form, 11.9
Supreme God, 5.29

Krishna continued,
Supreme Master, 7.30; 8.4
Supreme Objective, 6.14
Supreme Person, 10.15; 15.18,19
Supreme Reformer, 10.12
Supreme Refuge, 10.12
supreme residence, 8.21
Supreme Soul, 10.32
sustains, 9.5
swindlers, 10.36
taste, 7.8
thick-haired, 1.24
think about, 10.10
thinking of, 6.14; 18.57,58
thousand-armed, 11.46
thunderbolt, 10.28
thunderstormers, 10.21
time, 10.30,33
titan identity, 10.30
trend-setter, 3.23
troubled in psyche, 17.6
Uccaiḥśrava, 10.27
unaffected, 1.21; 7.13,25
unbiased, 9.29
uncontaminated, 13.32
under-estimated, 7.24
unique, 11.43
universal father, 9.17
Universal Form, 11.7
universal, 10.12
universal influence, 4.11; 10.39
universally available, 6.30
universe reality, 11.13
unrecognized, 7.13; 9.24
Usana identity, 10.37
Vaiśvānara, 15.13
Vajra identity, 10.28
variety, 9.15
Varuṇa, 10.29; 11.39

Krishna continued,
Vāsava Indra, 10.22
Vāsudeva, 10.37
Vāsuki identity, 10.28
Vasus identity, 10.23
Vāyu, 11.39
Vedas, 7.8; 9.17; 10.22; 15.18
Vedic ritual, 9.16
victory, 10.36,38
Vinata identity, 10.30
Vishnu, 10.21; 11.9,24
Vitteśa identity, 10.23
Vṛṣṇis identity, 10.37
Vyāsa identity, 10.37
water, 7.8
weapon, 10.28,31; 11.10
wind identity, 10.31
wise men, 10.38
word, 10.25,33
work of, 11.55; 12.10
worship, 7.28; 9.14,15,20,22,23,29; 12.6; 15.19
Yajur Veda, 9.17
Yakṣas identity, 10.23
Yama, 10.29; 11.39
yoga master, 11.4,9
yoga process, 12.10
yogi attainment, 12.4
yogi dear, 7.17; 12.14
yogi sages, 10.2,25,26,37
yogi sages' cause, 10.6
Kṣamā, 10.34
Kuvera, 10.23
Kuntī, 1.16,27; 2.14,37,60; 3.9,39; 5.22; 8.16; 9.7; 13.2; 14.4
Kuntibhoja, 1.5
Kuru, 1.25; 2.41; 4.31; 6.43
kurukṣetre, 1.1
kuśa grass, 6.11

L

laborers, facilitated, 9.32
lamentation, 2.25; 12.17
lamp, 6.19
language, 16.4
lawlessness, 1.40
laziness, 14.8
leaf, 9.26

left—over food, 17.10
leisure, 6.17
letters, 10.33
levels of reality, 9.15
liberated person, 4.23; 14.2,23—26
liberation,
dedication to, 5.28
knowers of, 10.35
many births, 6.45
perpetual type, 5.28
described, 13.24
godly talent, 16.5
status, 14.2
life, Krishna, 7.9
life—duration, 9.21
life—giving codes, 12.20
light of luminaries, 13.18
light, 7.8; 10.21; 15.12
liking, 3.34; 4.22; 7.27
lion, 10.30
liquids, 7.4
listeners, 18.67
lives, sacrificed, 1.33
living beings, 2.28; 9.8
living space, 13.1,2,6,7,20,27,35
location of yogi, 6.11
location, 18.14
logic, 13.5
logicians, 10.32
Lord of all beings, 18.61
Lord of gods, 11.25,37,45
Lord of supernatural rulers and powers, 8.4
Lord of yoga, 18.75,78
lotus leaf, 5.10; 11.2
lover, 11.44
low opinion, 9.11
luck, warrior's, 2.32
lust, resistance, 2.71
lusty enjoyment, 16.11
lusty urge, 3.39; 16.10
luxuries, 2.5; 9.21

M

Madhu, 1.14,34; 2.1; 6.33; 8.2
majesty, 18.43
managers, 18.41,44
manifestations, 10.16,19
manifested energies, 4.6; 8.18,19
Maṇipuṣpaka, 1.16
manliness, 7.8
Manu, 4.1
Marīci, 10.21
mass of splendor, 11.17
masses, 2.69
master, Krishna, 8.4; 9.18
master, spirit is, 15.8
masters of philosophical theory, 6.46
material energy, 4.6; 7.14
material existence, cessation, 5.25,26
material nature,
–also see modes of material nature
action bound, 3.9
actions, 9.12
as cause, 13.21
beginningless, 13.20
forces, 18.59
foundation, 9.8
imperceptible, 15.3
influence banished, 10.11; 18.19
inquiry, 13.1
Krishna's womb, 14.3,4
Krishna's, 9.7
moods, 13.20
overpowering, 9.8
performer, 14.19
producer, 9.10
productions, 13.27
reliance on, 9.12
restrictive, 7.20
retrogression into, 9.7
spirit transcends, 14.20
sponsors hopes, 9.12
submission to, 3.33
supernatural level, 9.13
Supreme Spirit, 13.15
universal, 18.40
Medhā, 10.34
meditation,
compared, 12.12
death method, 8.10
deep type, 8.8
energization, 8.10
God as subject, 8.9
on Krishna, 2.61; 9.22; 10.17; 12.8
meditation continued,
pleasure—prone people, 2.44
power—seeking people, 2.44
scriptural information, 2.53
steady type, 2.55—56
superficial type, 3.6
valid type, 3.7
meditator, inquiry of, 2.54
memory,
Krishna produced, 15.15
indulgences, 2.59
men, 7.8; 10.27
mental approach, 3.1
mental concepts, 16.1
mental dominance, 2.54
mercy, 11.1, 25,31,44,45
merit—based world, 9.20
Meru, 10.23
mind,
6th device, 15.7
compared, 3.42
control absolute, 8.14
control difficult, 6.34,35
controlled, 5.28; 6.35
drift / restraint, 6.26
impulsive, 6.34
interiorized, 8.8
Krishna anchored, 8.7
passion fostered, 3.40
purification, 5.11
regulation, 3.3
resistant, 6.34
restricted, 8.12
troublesome, 6.34
unsteady, 6.35
wanderings, 6.26
mindal energy, 7.4
minute factor, 8.9
mirror, 3.38
miserable conditions, 2.56
misery—free place, 2.51
misfortune, 6.40
misplaced self identity, 16.18; 17.5
misty season, 8.25
moderation, 6.16,17
modes of material nature, 14.10,23
modesty, 16.2

money, 16.12,17
monitor, 10.30
monkey insignia, 1.20
month, 10.35
moods,
detachment, 14.22
extraction, 2.58
hindrance, 3.34
like / dislike, 3.34
material nature's, 13.20
motivation, 3.29
phases, 2.45
yogic, 5.2
moon,
death, 8.24,25
eye, 11.19
Krishna, 7.8; 10.21
lord, 11.39
mundane, 15.6
sap, 15.13
splendor, 15.12
moral action, 3.8
morality, 7.11; 10.38; 18.78
mother, 9.17
motivation, 2.47; 6.4
mountain, 10.23
mourning, 2.11
mouth, 11.10,25
mouth of spiritual existence, 4.32
mouth of Universal Form, 11.19
movement, 18.14
multiplicity, 18.21
multitude of beings, 8.19
mundane affinity, 6.15
mundane energy, 3.5; 7.4
mundane influences, 15.2
musical instruments, 1.13
musicians, 11.22
mystic seers, 2.16

N

Nakula, 1.16
Nārada, 10.13,26
Narāyana Form, 11.46,52
natural resources, 11.22
Nature,
Krishna's, 14.2
producer, 5.14
types, 16.3,4
neck posture, 6.13
nectar, 18.37
needy person, 7.16
negligence, 14.9
nervousness, 3.30
night of Brahmā, 8.17—19
nighttime, death, 8.25
nine—gate city, 5.13
no possessions, 6.10
non—acting factor, 4.18
non—attachment, 3.28; 6.4; 15.3
non—existence, 10.5
non—reliance, 3.18
non—violence, 10.5; 13.8; 16.2; 17.14
northern sun passage, 8.24
nose, breath, 5.27
nose—tip gazing, 6.13
nourishment, 3.14
November, 10.35

O

obeisance, 11.21,35,39,44; 18.65
objective, Krishna, 9.18
oblation, 9.16; 11.19; 17.28
obligatory action, 6.1; 18.7
observer of reality, 14.19
observer, 13.23
ocean, absorption, 2.70
ocean, Krishna, 10.24
odor, Krishna related, 7.9
offering, 3.12; 9.16
ointments, 11.11
old age, 13.9, 14.20
Oṁ, 7.8; 8.13; 9.17; 17.24
Oṁ tat sat, 17.23
one imperishable being, 18.20
oneness, 18.20
openings of body, 8.12
opinion of Krishna, 9.11
opportunity,
devotion, 9.33
rejection, 18.1,2
renunciation, 18.49
usage, 5.2
opposite features, 5.3
opulences, 10.40
origin, 9.18; 10.39; 11.2; 14.3
ornaments, 11.10
overheated food, 17.9

P

pacified mind, 2.65
pain,
Krishna derived, 10.5
periodic, 2.14
pleasure related, 5.22
spirit cause, 13.21
pancajanya, 1.15
Pandava, 6.2; 10.37
pandit, 4.19
Pāndu, 1.1,3,14; 4.35; 11.55; 14.22; 16.5
parentage, 9.32
partial insight, 3.29
partner, 15.7
passion,
avoidance, 2.56
emotion, 3.37
insight blocked, 3.38
rooted out, 3.43
ruins discernment, 3.41
squelched, 3.41
warehouse, 3.40
past life impetus, 6.43,44
paths, hereafter, 8.26,27
patience, required, 10.5,34; 12.13; 13.8; 18.42
Pauṇḍra, 1.15
Pāvaka, 10.23
pay—off, 4.20
peace, 5.12; 12.12; 17.16
pearls, 7.6
peer pressure, 2.34,35
penance, 4.28
people,
deluded, 5.15
four kinds, 7.16
peppery food, 17.9
perception,
clear type, 14.11
dangers, 13.9
hearing method, 13.26
mystic, 13.25; 15.10,11
spiritual, 15.10,11
Supreme Lord, 13.28
perceptive impurities, 14.6
perceptive person, 10.3
perceptive speakers, 5.4
perfected souls, 11.36
perfection,
supreme, 8.15
work, 12.10

performance,
detachment from, 6.4
recommended, 3.8
types, 18.10
performer,
confusion, 3.27
types, 18.19,26—28
perfumes, 11.11; 15.8
permitter, 13.23
Person of universal dimensions, 11.46
Person, knowing everything, 8.9
personal energies,
controlled, 3.43
friend / enemy, 6.6
yoga control, 4.1
personal existence, Supreme Soul, 8.3
personal initiative, 13.6,9
personal undertakings, 12.16
personality, 2.12; 13.1,2
Personified Veda, 3.15
philosophers, 6.3,46
physical activity, 6.1
pious merits, 9.21
pious person, 6.40
piously—departed spirits, 10.29
plants, 15.13
pleasure
cause sin, 1.44
family, 1.32
Krishna derived, 10.5
objective, 9.21
pain, 6.7
poetic quotation, 2.42
sensual contact, 5.22
spirit cause, 13.21
terminal, 5.22
poets, poetry, 10.35,37
poison, 18.37,38
political affairs, 1.1
political power, 1.31,32; 2.43
population, 7.25
possessions,
absent, 6.10
austerity, 4.28
detachment towards, 12.13
freedom from, 2.45
indifference, 2.71
potential, 13.4
power, anger, 3.37
practice, mind control, 6.35
Prahlāda, 10.30
pranayama, 18.33
pratyāhar, 8.11
prayers, 10.25; 11.14
predominating influences, 14.10
pressure of change, 7.25
pride, 13.8; 15.5; 16.10,17; 18.35
priest, 4.24; 11.22
priestly teachers, 18.41,42
Primal God, 10.12
Primal Person, 11.31; 15.4
primeval unmanifested states, 8.20
priority, 3.2
Procreator Brahmā, - see Brahmā
procreators, 10.6
producer God, 13.17
production, 7.6; 13.27
property control, 4.33
proposal, two—way, 3.2
prosperity, 18.78
prosperous parents, 6.41
prostrations, 11.35
Pṛthā, 1,25,26; 2.3,21,39,42,55,72; 3.16; 4.11; 6.40; 7.1; 8.8,14,19; 9.32; 10.24; 12.7; 18.6
psyche,
described, 13.6,7
directive part, 6.7
friend / enemy, 6.6
God inhabits, 18.61
Krishna entered, 15.15
perceiver different, 10.35
spirit powered, 10.34
psychological core, 13.18
psychological environment, 13.19
psychological perfection, 7.3
psychological power, 8.10
psychological results of sacrifice, 4.31
psychological supremacy, 9.5
psychologically pacified, 6.27
pungent food, 17.9
punishment, 10.38
purificatory acts, 18.5
purified parents, 6.41
purifier,
consciousness, 9.2
experience, 4.38
Krishna, 9.17
purity of being, 16.1; 17.16
purity, 13.8; 17.14
Purujit, 1.5

Q,R

questions, 4.34; 5.1
radiance, 8.9; 11.17
rage, 17.5
rain, 3.14; 9.19
Rakṣas, 10.23
Rāma, 10.31
range of Supreme Spirit, 13.14—18
reactionary work, 4.19
realism, 16.7
Reality,
Krishna highest, 7.7
Krishna represented, 10.36
Krishna's womb, 14.3,4
One, 11.7,13
perceiving person, 3.28
reality—piercing vision, 2.57,58
science, 13.12
undefinable, 12.3
realized knowledge, 4.37,42
reasoning, 15.15
rebels, 11.22
rebirth,
avoidance, 5.17
cessation, 15.4,6
exemption, 4.9; 8.15,16
faithless person, 9.3
formula for, 8.6
freedom from, 2.51
heaven prior, 9.21
planetary effect, 8.25
promised, 2.43
repetitive, 8.16
transcended, 13.24

rebirth continued,
wicked peoples', 16.19
yogi's, 6.41
recitation of scripture, 16.1; 17.15
reciters, 2.42,43
recognition of reality, 10.34; 16.2
reference, 5.17
reference, senses, mind, intelligence, spirit, 3.42
reform, 9.31
reformed persons, 9.20
Refuge Supreme, 11.38
regulation,
——see mind regulation,
——see action regulation
reincarnation,
devotee, 12.7
formula for, 8.6
Krishna, 7.26
resisted, 5.17
rejection of consequences, 18.1,2,4
rejection of opportunity, 18.1,2
relation, 5.7
relatives, war field, 1.26
reliance on Krishna, 9.32
religion, 9.24
religious ceremony,
—see also ritual action
austerity, 4.28
categories, 17.7—10
enjoyer, 5.29
false type, 16.17
invented ones, 17.1
Krishna / master, 9.24
ordinances, 3.9,10; 17.23
prescribed, 17.25
purifies, 4.30
sacrifice, 4.25
types, 17.11—13
unapproved type, 9.23
yogi bypass, 8.28
religious fulfillment, 3.9,10
remembering, objects, 3.6
renouncer,
charity, 18.10
consistent type, 5.3
defined, 6.1
renunciation,
compared, 12.12
cultural activity, 5.2
defined, 18.11
insufficient, 3.4
mental type, 5.13
social activity?, 5.1
social opportunities, 5.2
to Krishna, 18.57
types, 18.7—9
yoga applied, 6.2
renunciation of opportunities, 5.6
reproduction, 10.28
repulsion, 12.15
reputation, 2.34—36; 17.18
research, 18.18
reservoir of energies, 9.18
residence, supreme, 15.6
resident of body, 5.13
resort of the world, 11.37
Respected Person, 11.31
restlessness, 14.11
restraint,
bodily limbs, 3.6
questioned, 3.33
tendency, 18.42
result,
best one, 3.2
giving up, 18.6
motivation resisted, 2.47
transcended, 6.1
types, 18.12
yogi bypass, 8.28
retardation, 14.5
retarded people, 14.18; 17.4
retrogression, 9.7
revelation, 11.53
reverence, 11.40,44
reversion, 8.18
reward, 17.21
Rig Veda, 9.17
righteous behavior, 9.3
righteous duty, 3.35
——also see duty
righteous lifestyle, 9.21
righteous method, 9.2
righteous practice, 2.40
righteousness, 4.7
ritual action,
conditional, 4.12
results rapid, 4.12
Universal Form, 11.48
ritual performers, 6.46
ritual regulation, 4.33
rivers, Krishna represented, 10.31
romance, 7.11; 10.28
rotten food, 17.10
ruination, 11.2
rulers, 10.38
ruling sector, 18.41,43

S

sacred thread, 17.14
sacrifice,
abandoned?, 18.3
purificatory, 18.5
results, 4.31
to Krishna, 18.65
types, 17.11—13
value, 4.30
sacrificial ceremony, 9.16; 11.48,53
sacrificial fire, 3.38
sacrificial ingredients, 4.24
Sādhyā, 11.22
Sahadeva, 1.16
Śaibya, 1.5
saint / wicked person, 9.30
saintly people, 4.8
salty food, 17.9
Sāma Veda, 9.12; 10.22,35
sāṁkhya philosophy, 2.39; 13.25; 18.3,19
sāṁkhya, yoga practice, 5.4,5
sanctification, 3.13
sanctified offering, 9.16
sanctuary, 11.38
sanity, 10.5
Sanjaya, 1.1,2,24; 2.1,9; 18.74,76
sannyāsa, 18.2
Śaśaṅka, 11.39
sat, 17.26,27
satisfaction, 2.70; 4.20; 10.18
Sātyaki, 1.17
science of reality, 13.12
sciences, 10.32
scriptural injunctions, 16.23,24; 17.1

scripture, 2.53
sea, 10.24,27
sea monsters, 10.31
seasons, 10.35
seat of yogi, 6.11,12
seclusion, 13.11
secret, 9.1,2; 10.38
security, 6.15; 16.2; 18.62
seeing what was never seen, 11.45,47
seeing, 5.8
seer,
attainment, 5.25,26
common factor, 5.18
destination, 2.51
inquiry of, 2.54
self,
concentration on, 6.10
core, 6.18
enemy, 6.5
evaluation, 6.5
fixed on, 6.25
friendship, 6.5
pacified, 6.14
self—composed, 4.41
self—conceited, 16.17
self—content, 2.55
self—control, 5.7; 6.7; 10.5
self—denial, 4.28
self identity, 16.18, 17.5
self—image, 18.16
selfishness, 3.30
self—perception, 6.20
self—purification, 6.12
self—realization, 4.38
self—restraint, 12.11; 13.8; 16.1; 17.16
self—satisfaction, 6.20
self—situated, 3.17
sensations,
alternating, 2.14
coping, 2.14
detachment, 5.21
sense control, 2.69
senseless, 3.32
senses,
attractive objects, 5.9
compared, 3.42
death baggage, 15.8
Krishna represented, 10.22
like / dislike, 3.34
living space, 13.6
mind affected, 2.67
senses continued,
passion fostered, 3.40
purification usage, 5.11
regulating, 3.41
restraint, 2.61
torment ascetic, 2.60
withdrawn, 2.58
sensual activity, withdrawal, 6.25
sensual contacts, 5.27
sensual energy control, 5.28; 6.12; 12.4
sensual energy, restraint, 4.39; 6.24
sensual feelings, retraction, 2.68
sensual objects, 2.62
sensual potency, 13.21
sensual powers, 4.26
sensual pursuits, 4.26
sensual range, 7.24
sensuality, controlled, 2.61; 5.24
sensuality, perpetual, 7.27
separation, from emotion, 6.23
serpents, 10.28; 11.15
service sector, 18.44
serving, 4.34
sexual intermixture, 1.40
sexual restraint, 6.14
sexual urge, 16.8
Shankara, 10.23
shark, 10.31
shelter, 9.18; 18.62
ship, 2.67
Shiva, 10.23
sickness, 17.9
Śikhandī, 1.17
silence, 10.38; 17.16
simpletons, 3.26; 5.4
sin,
considered, 1.36,38
God's resistance, 5.15
sinful propensities, 7.28
singers, 10.26
sins terminated, 5.25
situations, 13.22
sixth device, 15.7
Skanda, 10.24
skills destroyed, 1.42
sky resonated, 1.19
sleep regulator, 10.20
sleep, 5.8; 6.16,17; 14.8; 18.35
smelling, 5.8
smoke, 18.48
smoky season, 8.25
Smṛti, 10.34
snakes, 10.29
social circumstance, 6.41
social life, 13.10
social values, 18.34
society, maintenance, 3.25
solids, 7.4
soma drinkers, 9.20
Somadatta, 1.8
son of charioteer, 11.26
son, 1.26,33; 11.44
sorcerers, 17.4
sorrow, 18.35
soul, embodied, adaptations, 2.13
soul, see spirit
soul—situated, 2.45
sound,
austerity, 4.26
Krishna related, 7.8; 10.25
Oṁ, 17.24
sour food, 17.9
space,
comparison, 9.6; 10.33
mundane, 7.4
pervaded, 11.20
species,
as facility, 6.32
comparison, 5.18
ignorant type, 14.15
Krishna inhabits, 6.30; 7.26
rebirth, 14.15
spirit caused, 7.6
spirits inhabit, 15.8
speech,
control, 18.51,52
disciplined, 17.15
Krishna, 10.34
spinning machine, 18.61
spirit,
addicted, 15.9
affected, 15.16
amazing, 2.29
beginningless, 13.20
body energizer, 10.34
cannot be killed, 2.19
cannot kill, 2.19
captivated, 14.5

spirit continued,
compared, 3.42
condition—resistant, 2.23
confused, 3.40
considered temporary, 2.26
creature habitat, 6.29
death impossible, 2.20,21
degradation, 16.21
dry—less, 2.23
elevate self, 6.5
eternal, 2.20; 15.7
experience, 13.22
fantastic, 2.29
faultless, 5.19
going to Krishna, 4.9
governor of psyche, 15.9
higher energy, 7.5; 13.23; 15.17
immeasurable, 2.18
imperishable, 2.21
impulsion captivates, 14.6
incombustible, 2.23
indestructible, 2.17
individual, 15.7
Krishna represented, 10.29
Krishna's partner, 15.7
master of body, 15.8
material nature captivates, 14.5
material nature transcended, 14.20
mourning unworthy, 2.30
movements, 15.10
non—actor, 5.13
non—doer, 13.28
non—killable, 2.30
not born, 2.26
not killed, 2.26
origin of species, 7.6
perception, 13.25,28
permanent, 2.24
primeval, 2.20
seen / unseen, 15.11
self upliftment, 13.28
sensation cause, 13.21
stable type, 15.16

spirit continued,
stable, 2.24; 15.16
transcendental, 13.33
types, 15.16
unaffected ones, 10.33; 15.16
undetected, 2.28
undisplayed, 2.25
unimaginable, 2.25
universe sustained by 7.5
unknown, 2.29
wet—less, 2.23
wonderful, 2.29
spiritual core self, 6.18
spiritual delight, 5.24
spiritual discernment, 18.37
spiritual existence,
known, 7.29
mouth of, 4.32
sacrifice support, 4.24,25
spiritual level, 5.10
spiritual master, 4.34; 11.43; 17.24; 18.68,69
spiritual peace, 5.29
spiritual perfection, 3.4
spiritual plane, 5.19,20
spiritual reality,
description, 6.44
designation, 17.23
question of, 8.1
unaffected, supreme, 8.3
spiritual religion, 4.31
spiritual self, 2.55
spiritual teacher, 17.14
spiritual world, 8.20,21,24
spirituality, 5.24—26
spiritually content, 3.17
spiritually—pleased, 3.17
splendor, 7.10; 10.36; 18.78
spring, 10.35
Śrī, 10.34
stability, 13.8
stale food, 17.10
standard position, 6.33
standard, two—fold, 3.3
stars, 10.21
states of being, 7.12; 13.31
status of next life, 8.6
stone, 6.8; 14.24

stormers, 11.22
straightforwardness, 13.8; 16.1; 17.14; 18.42
strength, 7.11
string comparison, 7.6
strong—mindedness, 16.3
stubborn, 16.17
student, 4.34
stupified at death, 2.72
subduers, 10.29
Subhadrā, 1.6,18
substantial things, 2.16
subtle body, 9.19
success/ failure, 2.48; 4.22
suffering, 13.9
Sughoṣa, 1.16
sum total, 8.1,4
summer season, 8.24
sun,
comparison, 5.16; 10.34
death affected by, 8.25
eye, 11.19
Krishna related, 7.8,9; 10.21
Krishna's splendor, 15.12
mundane, 15.6
thousands, 11.11
super-fantastic form, 18.77
Supermost Personality, 8.1
supernatural destroyers, 11.6
supernatural manifestations, 10.40
supernatural rulers,
appeasers of, 7.4,.20,23; 9.23,25
Divine Form not seen, 11.52
human relation, 3.11,12
Krishna represented by, 10.22
Krishna unknown to, 10.2,14
respect, 17.14
source, 10.2
Universal Form, 11.6,15,21
supernatural sight, 11.8
supernatural stormers, 11.6
supernatural wondrous manifestations, 10.16,19

supernatural, material nature, 9.13
supernaturally disposed, 11.33,34
Supersoul,
beings inhabited by, 13.28
described, 13.14-18,23
disliked, 16.18
transmigration, 18.61
troubled, 17.6
supporter, 9.18
Supreme Being, 9.4—6,9; 18.62
—see also Krishna
supreme destination, 13.28; 16.23
Supreme Form, 11.9,47
supreme goal, 6.45; 9.32
Supreme God, 5.29; 16.18
supreme information, 10.1
Supreme Lord, 13.23,28,32; 16.8
supreme objective, 6.14; 7.18; 8.21
supreme peace, 4.39
supreme perfection, 8.15; 14.1
Supreme Person,
action free, 5.14
cause of all causes, 8.22
defined, 15.18
described, 8.9
Krishna, 10.15
reached, 8.8
Supreme Primal State, 8.28
Supreme Reality, 10.12; 11.18; 13.13—18
Supreme Reformer, 10.12
Supreme Refuge, 10.12
Supreme Regulator of religious ceremonies and disciplines, 8.2,4
Supreme Soul / Spirit,
association, 15.5
austerity, 3.15
described, 15.17
explained, 11.1
information, 13.12
known, 7.29
Krishna, 10.32
meditate upon, 3.30
Supreme Soul / Spirit, continued,
mundane world producer, 8.3
permitter, 13.23
personal existence, 8.3
Personified Veda, 3.15
question of, 8.1
religious ceremony, 3.15
supporter, 15.17
Supreme Supernatural Person and Power, 8.1
Supreme Supervisor, 8.9
Supreme truth, 5.16,17
supreme yoga, 18.75
supreme destination, 10.35
Supreme, pure world, 14.14
Surendra, 9.20
surrender, 18.62
sustainer, God, 13.17
svarga angelic world, 2.43
swindlers, 10.36
syllable, 10.25
synthesis, 13.27

T

take note of it, 9.31
talents, 16.3
talking, 5.9
taste, 7.8
tat, 17. 25
teachers,
Gītā, 18.68,69
lineage, 4.2
reality—conversant, 4.34
social, 1.26,33
teaching, best, 4.3; 15.20
teeth, 11.23,25
temptation, 2.59
tendencies,
elaborated, 18.42—44
eliminated, 6.27
innate, 17.2
overcome, 4.36
texture of existence, 8.6
thief, 3.12
thighs, 11.23
thinking,
controlled, 6.10,12
restrained, 5.26
stoppage, 6.20,25
wicked people, 16.13,14
thought controlled, 6.18
thoughts on Krishna, 12.9
threefold influence, 16.21
thunderbolt, 10.28
time, 10.30,33; 11.32
time cycle, 8.17—19
titan, 10.30
tortoise, 2.58
torture, 17.6,19
touching, 5.8
trading, 18.44
tradition,
abandoned, 18.66
Arjuna considers, 1.39
destroyers of, 1.43
disgust with, 2.52
trance, 6.22
tranquility, 10.5; 18.42
transcendent person, 14.21
transformation of psyche, 14.2
transmigration, 18.61
tree, 10.26; 15.1—3
trend, 17.3
trickery, 17.18
truth, 9.1
truthfulness, 10.5
truths of existence, 2.16
tyāga, 18.2

U

Uccaiḥśrava, 10.27
unavoidable circumstance, 2.27
uncles, 1.26
uncontrolled person, 2.66
undisciplined person, 6.36
undivided God, 13.17
unintelligent person, 7.24
universal destruction, 11.25
Universal Form,
displayed, 11.3,5—47
Sanjaya, 18.77
supernatural rulers terrified, 11.21
viewers listed, 11.22
universal integration, 9.18
Universal Soul, 13.14—18

universe,
Krishna supports, 10.42; 11.38
one reality, 11.7
operations, 9.9
production / destruction, 7.6
rejoices, 11.36
spirit sustained, 7.5
three partitions, 11.43
unmanifested energy, 13.6
unmanifested states, 8.20
unpleasant things, 5.20
Upanishads, 13.5
upper class, 16.15
Uśanā, 10.37
Uttamauja, 1.6

V

Vaiśvānara, 15.14
vajra, 10.28
Vāk, 10.34
vanity, 18.26
vapor bodies, 11.22
variations, 3.28,29
variety, 9.15
Varuṇa, 10.29; 11.38
Vāsava, 10.22
vast existence of death, 12.7
Vāsudeva, 7.19; 10.37; 11.50
Vāsuki, 10.28
Vasus, 10.23
Vāyu, 11.39
Veda knower, 8.11; 9.20; 15.1
Veda,
Krishna knows / known, 15.15
Krishna related, 7.8; 10.22
offers of, 2.45
ordained, 17.23
Personified, 3.15
spoken description, 6.44
surpassed, 6.44
Vedānta, 15.15
worth, 2.46
yogi beyond, 8.28
Vedic education, Universal Form, 11.48
Vedic hymns recited, 13.5; 15.1; 17.13
Vedic injunction, 9.21; 16.17
Vedic ritual, 9.16
Vedic ceremonies, 11.48
Vedic study, 11.53
Vedic verses, 2.42
vibration, necessary, 3.5
vices, terminated, 5.25
victory,
defeat, 2.38
Krishna represented, 10.36,38; 18.78
not desired, 1.31
viewers, 2.19
vigor, 16.3
Vikarṇa, 1.8
Vinata, 10.30
violence, 5.10; 18.25
Virāṭa, 1.4,17
virtue, deviation, 9.24
virtuous acts, 6.40
virtuous character, 9.31
virtuous people, 3.13
Vishnu, 10.21
visible world, 8.18,19
vision of reality, 15.10,11
vision of yogi, 2.61
vision, Arjuna given, 11.8
visitation of Krishna, 4.9
visual focus, 5.27
Viśvadeva, 11.22
Vitteśa, 10.23
Vivasvāt, 4.1,4
void, 2.69
vows, ascetics of, 4.28; 7.28; 9.14
Vṛṣṇis, 1.40; 3.36; 10.37
Vyāsa, 10.13,37; 18.75

W

walking, 5.8
war, 2.33,34
warriors,
battle hungry, 1.22
heaven, 2.32
supernaturally disposed, 11.33
water,
Krishna accepts, 9.26
Krishna related, 7.8
lotus leaf, 5.10
master of, 11.39
psychic type, 1.41
weapon carriers, Krishna represented, 10.31
weapons, 2.23; 10.28,31; 11.10
weather, 2.14
welfare of all, 12.4
well (water), 2.46
what to do, 16.7
whole multitude, 9.8
wicked persons, 4.8; 16.7
wickedness, 4.7
wife, 13.10
will power, 18.60
wind
Krishna compared, 9.6; 10.31
mind compared, 6.34
regulator, 11.39
ship, 2.67
spirit compared, 15.8
wise person,
condition-resistant, 2.15
duty, 3.25
immortality, 2.15
Krishna represented, 10.38
realization, 2.13
womb, Krishna's, 14.3,4
wombs of wicked people, 16.20
women, 1.40; 9.32; 10.34
wonders, 11.6
wood, 4.37
word compound, 10.33
work,
discarded, 2.50
material nature, 13.21
tendency, 4.13
working power, 3.30
work-prone people, 14.15
world,
action bound, 3.9
God pervades, 9.4
maintenance, 3.20
other, 4.31
production, 8.18,19
spirit pervaded, 2.17
stupefied, 7.13
trembles, 11.20,23
types, 14.14,15
utilized, 4.31
worries, 2.56; 16.10,11
worship,
ceremony, 16.1
exclusive, 9.22
God, 18.46

worship continued,
Krishna's, 7.16,28; 12.2
procedure, 3.10—12
supernatural rulers', 9.23
types, 17.4,11—13
worshippers of gods, 7.23
worshippers of Krishna, 7.23
worshippers rated, 9.25
worthless person, 3.16

Y

Yadu family man, 11.41
Yajur Veda, 9.17
Yakṣas, 10.23
Yama, 10.29; 11.38
yearning, 3.39; 18.49
yoga practice,
application lost, 4.2
application, 5.1; 6.2,28; 16.1
austerity, 4.28
celibacy required, 8.11
concentration, 8.12
controlling force, 4.1
cultural activities, 3.7; 4.41
determination, 18.33
deviation, 6.37
distress-remover, 6.17
exertion, 12.5
expertise, 6.3
harmonized, 10.7
indifference, 2.48
insight applied, 2.39
intellectual discipline, 2.49; 18.57
interiorization, 8.8
Krishna worship, 9.22
Krishna's, 11.47; 12.11
mastery, 2.53; 6.23,36
methods, 6.3
moderation, 6.16
mood, 2.48,50
perfected, 4.38; 6.43
performance skill, 2.50
preliminary, 12.9
proficiency, 5.7,8,12; 6.4,18,29
purpose, 6.12
yoga practice continued,
recommended, 7.1;.8.27; 12.9
renunciation, 9.28
required, 13.11
requirements, 12.4
sāṁkhya, 5.4
spiritual plane, 5.21
skill described, 4.18
technique, 4.3,42; 12.2
undistracted, 12.6
yogi,
action austerity, 4.27
actions antiseptic, 5.10
Arjuna, 6.46
attainment, 8.23
austerities bypassed, 8.28
baffled, 6.38
births end, 7.19
breath, 4.27
charity, 8.28
death, 8.10,13,24
defined, 6.1
destination, 4.31; 8.28
deviant, 6.37
devotee, 12.14,17
discipline, 6.8; 18.51
distinguished, 7.17
Divine Supreme Person, 8.10
existential position, 6.15
experience, 6.8
faults ended, 6.28
fond to Krishna, 7.17
happiness, 5.21; 6.28
hearing, 4.26
highest type, 6.32
informed type, 7.17
inquiry, 2.54
intention, 6.2
isolation, 6.10
kings, 4.15; 9.33
knowledge, 4.28
Krishna / everything, 7.19
Krishna attracts, 6.47
Krishna contact, 6.30; 8.14
Krishna devoted, 6.47
Krishna remembrance, 8.13
yogi continued,
Krishna seen, 6.30
Krishna worship, 6.47; 12.6
Krishna's representative, 7.18
Krishna—knowing, 7.30
lamp, 6.19
liberation, 5.26—28; 6.15
meditation, 6.12
memory, 3.6
methods, 12.1,2,3
non—actor, 5.13
past life impetus, 6.43,44
perfection, 6.43
philosophers, 10.37
philosophical / non—philosophical, 3.3
planetary influence, 8.26
possessions, 4.28
proficiency, 6.4
psychologically pacified, 6.27
purification, 5.11
release, 7.29
religion, 4.25
religious ceremonies, 8.28
seat, 6.11
sensual austerity, 4.26
sound austerity, 4.26
spiritual plane, 5.6
steadiness, 6.21
supernatural authority, 4.25
supreme primal state, 8.28
tendencies, 6.45
two standards, 3.3
valid type, 3.7
Veda austerity, 4.28
Veda bypassed, 8.28
vision of species, 6.29
yoga austerity, 4.28

yogi sages,
aśvattha tree, 15.1—3
Krishna praised, 10.13; 11.21
Krishna represented, 10.25,26
Krishna unknown, 10.2
seven, 10.6
source, 10.2
Universal Form, 11.15
Yudhāmanyu, 1.6
Yudhiṣṭhira, 1.16
Yuyudhāna, 1.4

Index to Commentary

A

abandonment of consequences, 459, 460
Abhimanyu, 471
Abhyāsena, 216
aborigine, 162
absence of anger, 458
absence of destructive criticism, 460
absence of fickleness, 468
absoluteness, 103
abstract, 380
abusive language, 472
accountability, 106, 530
acidic foods, 493
acintabhedābheda tattva, 353
actions,
——see also cultural activities
  clarifying mode, 425
  contradictions, 109
  divinely inspired?, 422
  impetus, 514
  implications avoided, 65
  intracacies, 45,131,132
  material nature creates, 10
  motivation, 110
  yogic mood, 74
Adam, 313
addiction, 463
adhyakṣena, 285
ādideva, 365
Aditī, 326
Ādityas, 326
ādyam puruṣam, 436
Africa, 313
Agastya Muni, 40,213,300,392
agent, 512, 513
aggression,
  political, 28
  sexual type, 427
Agni, 92,328
ahankar, 174
ailments, 55
Airāvata, 331
akṣara, 269,446
akṣaram avyaktam, 378
aksharam brahma, 255
alcoholic, 162
A—letter, 336
allowances, religious, 495
alternatives, 63
Ananta, 332
anantarūpa, 365
ancestors,
  deprived, 38
  lusty urge, 476
  money, 478
  piety, 38
  sex personified, 478
  sexual attraction as, 15
  subtle support, 19
  support of, 19
angelic realm,
  residential status, 295
  warrior's, 63
anger,
  absence of, 458
  God's?, 457
  lust converted, 472
Aṅgirā, 313
animals,
  dream, 185
  human birth desired, 429
  subtle body, 272
  supernatural, 330
Aniruddha, 222
antar jyotih, 169
Antaryami, 210
antelope skin, 189
anthropology, 313
antlers, 232
anus, 393
ape, 313
apology, 367
application,
  Arjuna's, 181
  yoga to concepts, 452
approved conducts, 26
Approver, 297
aquatics, 92
Archa Vigraha, 214
Arjuna,
  apology, 367
  application unknown, 181
  austerities, 320
Arjuna continued,
  beloved of Krishna, 308
  childhood, 33
  dimension transfer, 361
  face of Universal Form, 452
  foremost desire, 369
  forgot self, 25
  jñāna yoga, 105
  karma yoga, 149
  Krishna as, 338
  Krishna's friend?, 357
  Krishna friendship perpetual, 123
  kriyā yogi, 319
  mercy—prone, 46
  mystic vision lacking, 215
  refresher course, 173
  respected practitioner, 28
  shifted, 29
  siddhas observed by, 366
  sleep conquered, 325
  spiritual form, 373
  spiritual sight, 427
  student, 46
  Universal Form relevant, 371
  Universal Form vision, 351
  yoga boost, 206, 207
  yoga practice, 20
  yoga proficient, 149
astral travel, 320
arrogance energy, 49,472
Arundhatī, 467
Aryamā, 326, 327
āsana, incomplete, 96
ascetics, Upamanyu's, 93
ashram, 82, 83
Ashvattha, 329
Asita Devala, 319
association,
  astral type, 26
  control, 75
  purpose, 27
associative thinking, 325
astral plane/world,
  ancestors, 38
  residents, 295

astral projection/travel,
pioneer of, 332
sun effects, 272
yogi's, 273
astrology, 448
astronauts, 512
astronomers, 360, 512
asuric nature, 474
Aśvatthāmā, 16
Atharva Veda, 447
Atlantic Ocean, 272, 274
ātma, brahma, 164
ātmaśuddhaye, 155
ātmaviśuddaye, 190
Atri, 313
attachment,
discarded, 155
gross existence, 425
attraction, material nature, 244
Aurobindo, Śrī, 213, 352
austerity,
anger sponsored, 499
body, 499
described, 455
mind, 499
necessary, 181
resentment sponsored, 499
speech, 499
author,
annotation, 147
Bābāji's association, 461
birth environment, 398
birth mistake, 464
childhood, 162
children, 459
commissioned, 212, 213
cultural resistance, 39
degradation, 475
disciples, 194
experience of God, 311
householder advice, 90
inspired, 200
lower birth, 480
Muktananda assists, 425
Nityananda's kriyās, 522
notation, 546
parents, 162
past life, 461, 464
puberty, 477
rebirth, 466
author continued,
revelation Universal Form, 347
sexual exposure deity, 426
sexual nature, 476
Shiva seen, 465
sister of, 463
theft of, 463
vision of God's form, 374, 375, 376
waiver granted, 438
yoga background, 461
authority, 339
authorized, 531
Autobiography of a Yogi, 551
avaktya, 265
Avatar, 370
avekṣe, 25— 26
axis, 295
Axis Supreme, 295, 442
ayati, 218

B

Bābāji, Śrī Mahāsaya
Bloom's association, 438
commissioned author, 212, 243
critical energy, 461
donations, 397
expedite instruction, 29
grace on author, 464
householder encourage, 299, 300
inspiration, 200,233
knife objection466
liberation method, 549, 550
naad sound, 174
orphan comparison, 279
sunlight body, 29, 223
yoga siddha body, 29
bad feelings, 62
Baladeva, see Balarāma 213, 332
Balarāma, Lord,
14.93, 173, 233, 279, 347, 392, 436
Balarāmā Deity, 173
Bali, 326
bath, 497
battery comparison, 58
battle, forced on, 359
battlefield, 10
bed—couch, 332
begetting, 331
beginningless Supreme Reality, 405
belief,
misconception, 293
powerless, 203
reincarnation, 57
believer, 165
Beloved, Bloom, 438
benefits,
absurd, 32
influence causes, 425
Bengal, 298
Bengali scriptures, 198
betel nut, 493
Beverford, Arthur, 461
Bhaga, 326
Bhagavad Gītā,
legal document, 505
author, 11
curriculum, 90
kriyā yoga application, 44
kriyā yoga document, 73
symbolic?, 201
Bhagavan, 77
Bhāgavat Purana
——see Śrīmad
Bhāgavatam
Bhāgavatam
——see Śrīmad
Bhāgavatam
bhakti,
false type, 93
not main idea, 65
bhakti yoga,
bhakti + yoga, 402
buddhi yoga development, 91, 92
different, 536
karma yoga, 490
not mentioned, 121
Bhaktipada,
--see Kirtanananda Swami
Bhaktisiddhānta Sarasvati, Śrīla, 303,335
bhaktisiddhanta theology, 342

Bhaktivedanta Swami, Śrīla Prabhupada, 20,21,228,291,297, 298,300,304,325,327, 329,334,335,345,348, 399,439,454,470,490,551
bhakto, 122
bhārah, 183
Bharat Patel, Śrīman, 213
bhastrika, 140
bhastrika, 274
bhastrika, 318
bhasvara agni, 318,444
Bhavān, 16
Bhīma, 21,471,472
Bhīṣma,
death route, 550
elderly, 17
kriya teacher, 46
protected, 18
statesman, 19
superior, 16
supernaturally hurt, 363
vision of Vishnu, 373
vow, 9
yogi of repute, 273
bhoktā, 296
Bhṛgu, 329
Bhrihaspati, 328
big cat, 480
birth control, 477
birth, death, old age and disease, 400
birth,
great soul's, 222
work-prone people, 425
black holes, 360
blemish in psyche, 278
blindness, 27
Bloom Beloved, 438
bluish sky, 202
boar, 232
body,
light type, 370
sequential, 50
supernatural residents of, 409
types, 368
value, 50,457
body—supported beings, 511
Bolivia, 273
boosts, 207
bovine creatures, 491
boys, ashram life, 84
brahma yoga, 167,476
brahma, 164
brahma, questions on, 253
Brahmā—Creator God,
advisory, 92,453
bound, 407
Brahmā, 453
creative monoply, 98
creator sub—god, 312
father of, 366
knowledgeable, 98
Krishna compared, 309
psychological grip, 266
reliance on, 268
superior to supernatural rulers, 99
territory, 264, 265
Upamanyu saw, 93
Veda Person, 101
brahmarandra, 244,476
brahmavādis, 502
brāhmī stithih, 88
brahmins, discussed, 162
brain injury, 210
breast area cleaning, 476
breast nourishment, 426
brilliant consciousness, 169
British domination, 397
brooding energies, 505
brow chakra, 406,426
bubble—shaped subtle body, 522
Buddha,182,183,379, 381,383,397,407
buddhi līlā, 16
buddhi organ-see intellect
buddhi vision, 138
buddhi yoga,
defined, 16,73,317
insufficient, 192
budhah, 168
buffalo, 491
bulb, 296
bull comparison, 117
buttocks, 476

C

Caitanya Caritāmṛta, 242, 243,491
Caitanya Mahaprabhu, Lord Śrī Kṛṣṇa, 198,242,243,259,298, 342,353,433,491
cakṣusā, 416
Canada, 272
carrion birds, 480
caste,
body type, 163
change of, 470
compared, 306
prejudice, 188
traditional, 162
causal body, contents, 393
causal body/form,
content, 163
elimination, 164
hunger, 394
potent, 395
root, 179
subconscious reserve, 232
subtle one affected by, 201
subtle one caused by, 391
subtle one controlled by, 395
Supersoul, 210
transcending it, 469
causal existence, 234
causal territory, 312
Cause of all causes, 339
cause, 293
cave men, 91
celibacy yoga, 261,465,476
celibacy,
essential, 421
sexual attraction, 14
shaktipat, 345
celibate boys, 312
cells, 395
Central Personality, 347
chakra, 233
chakra regulator, 395
chakra vision, 393
change of tendency, 166
chant Hare Krishna and be happy, 292
chanting, 214,317,329
chants, 210
charisma,
greed for, 499
law, 106
charismatic leaders, 488
charity,
described, 452
limited, 375
types, 500, 501

chemicals, 493
chest, 476
chidakash, 287
Chidvilasananda, 431
Chief of cowherds, 33
children, 13
China, 50
Chitraratha, 330
chitta,
--see also mento-emotional energy
described, 203
motivates, 160
unmanifest energy, 393
chloroform, 282
chocolate bars, 463
Christian God, 314
Christians, 295
Christ—see Jesus Christ
cities, 395
citta, — see chitta
city of nine gates, 156
civil rights, 516
civil war, 33
clairvoyance, 11,27
clans, 489
clarifying energy, 420
cleanliness, 188
coffee, 493
collages, 312
colon, 393
Colorado, 461
comparitive similar view, 212—215
compassion,
divine state compared, 88
necessary, 465
reviewed, 212
compensation, next life, 453
compressed impression, 182
conceit, 470,472
concepts, 290
conclusion, 141,390
confidence, 487,503
congregation, 188
conscience, 82,483
consciousness,
conventional type, 395
research into, 283
consequence,
abandonment, 459, 460
forced, 465
rejection, 505
contemplation, 26
contrasting others, 359
convention, birth, 122
conviction, 395
Core Personality, 297
cosmic dissolution, 15
cosmic emotions, 165
cosmic energy reserve, 233
cosmic material nature, 418
Cosmic Person, 365,366
coveteousness, 463
cow, 117,297,491
cowherd boys, 373
creation, 91
Creator God, 268
creator, 292
creature forms, 234
crimes, supernatural type, 228
criminal credit, 304
critical energy, 484
criticism, absence of, 460
crowd consciousness, 20
cruelty, 42
cultural activities,
——see also action
clarifying mode, 425
disciplined in, 148
exemption, 94
near absolute, 155
required, 155
cultural personality, 211,312
cushion, 189

D

dairy products, 256
dairy farm, 297
daivam prakṛtim, 287
Dānavas, 320
danger,
great, 66
worldly life, 148
darkness in the head, 468
darkness, supernatural type, 490
Dasharatha, 332,408
death,
danger of, 400
Krishna as, 336
name of God, 257
recall during, 257
rites, 38
scary, 284
struggle within, 18
sun/ moon influence, 272—274
texture of existence, 257
deceit, 397,471
deceiver, meditator, 95
deer, 480
degradation, 220,523
Deity, 214,373
Deity Form, 291
Deity remnants, 492,494
Deity Worship,
advancement beyond, 173
ancient, 82
compared, 81
described, 138
elementary, 173
Kapila's opinion, 203
offering to, 300
purpose, 202
Vaishnava, 381
deliberation, 489
Denver, 461
desire,
contrasting, 359
cosmic pool, 394
energy fosters, 435
psyche possessions, 188
seed, 201
destiny,
compulsions, 49
enforced, 235, 236
necessary factor, 513
detachment,
development of, 401
discouragement, 110
non—absolute, 135
reasons for, 110
required, 189
deva persons, 295
deva rishi, 329
Devahūti, 330,407
Devakī, 286,301,351, 373,379,447
Devala Rishi, 319
Devi Purāṇa, 448

devotee of Krishna,
—see also pure devotee
bias harmful, 62
casualty, 418
exemption lacking?, 102
spiritual view of, 51
types, 47
yogi?, 385
devotion to Krishna,
described, 534
formula, 244
kriyā practice, 71
necessary, 121, 122
necessary, 270
questioned, 505
recommended, 225
undistracted, 376
unswerving, 402
yoga reconciled?, 378,381
devotional service, 93,490
Dewaki, — see Devakī
dhāma paramam mama 439
dhāraṇa, 26
dharma,
——see also responsibility
duty, 60
misery, 438
responsibility, 10,183
dharmasetra, 10
Dhatā, 326
dhīmatām, 221
dhira, 51
Dhṛtarāṣṭra,
blindness, 27
ruler, 23
Universal Form, 349
yoga postponed, 9, 10
Dhṛti, 336
Dhruva, 203
dhyāna, 26,202
diaspora, 329
diet
practice regulates, 197
restraint, 140
yogi's, 255,491
diet of energies, 256
digestion, 192
digestive heat, 444
dimension,
adjacent, 283
culture affected, 367
transfer, 361
dingy dirty psychology, 481
dinosaur, 92,313
discernment, 85
disciples,
acceptance of, 194
Bābāji's view, 467
causal region of limits, 439
disempowered, 206
family compared, 438
requirements, 142
disciplic succession, 121
disease, 400
disembodied souls,
enter emotions, 11
passion empowered, 421
disgust, 189
dispassion, 394
dispositions, 165
dividend, 158
divine being, 187,223
divine eyesight, 372
divine grace, 94,198
Divine Hierarchy, 364
Divine Life Society, 399
divine state, 88
divine work, 94
divorce, 37
donations, 397
dormancy,
anger/resentment, 498
doubts, 171,234
Draupadī, 14,23
dream,
animal's, 185
transcendence, 183
vision in, 288
Droṇa,
consulted, 10
dear teacher, 16
Drupada offended by, 14
fooled, 471
military skill sold, 12-13
priest, 454
supernaturally hurt, 363
unfulfillments, 11
used, 17
drugs, 210,283,288,289
Drupada, 14,23
duhkhahā, 197
Durgā,Goddess,
——see also Umā
418,448,464,467
Durgā/Mahavishnu, 418
Duryodhana,
consulted Droṇa, 10
dream with ghosts, 489
Krishna disbelieved by, 247, 248
unchanged, 457
dust particles, 272
duty,
another's risky, 114
detachment, 45
relevant, 42
restrictive, 61
yoga excuse, 176
yoga facilitated, 198
dvijottama, 15

E

East Indians, 38
eating urge, 444
edge—light, 85
education, 292,336,479
efforts, required, 124
ekākī, 188,216
elders, 44,45
elements, 393
elephant, 330,471,480
elevation, earned, 523
embryo, 58
emotion,
cosmic type, 165
crippling, 72
disembodied souls enter, 11
intellect used by, 49
powerful, 114
sickly type, 43
subtle energy, 390
emotional body, 66
emotional cleanliness, 497
emotional nature, 205
empowerment, explained, 472
end of sorrow, 525
endeavor, Krishna as, 338
enemy of the psyche, 116,250
energies,
decisive type, 229
intellectual type, 229
mental type, 229
enjoying propensity, 134
environment body, 390, 391
escape, 178

essential nature, 487
European country, 465
Eve, 313
evidence, 227
evolution of scriptures, 165
example, 109
excitement, 78,206
excretion, 192
exemption,
explained, 94
God awards, 95
retracted, 178
existence, suspension, 282
existential arrangement, 210
existential backdrop, 354
expedite, 29
experience,
categories, 515
enjoyments, 13
essential, 115
evidence, 391
final, 143
inducement, 403
motivates, 185
senses require, 13
suffering, 13
experiencer, 391
expertise, 420
exploitation, engrained, 228
exposure, 426
eye of knowledge, 246
eyebrows, center, 260, 261
eyes,
psychic, 27
subtle body's, 288
types, 426

F

fabric of being, 487
factory comparison, 213
faith,
experience?, 281
expression, 487
required, 503
Universal Form increases, 389
faithfulness, 336
fame,
embodied, 336
feared, 106
greed for, 499
fame continued,
modesty destroyed by, 467
yogi flaw, 407
family life, 518
family,
disciples compared, 438
influence, 34
fasting, 196,398
fate, twist of, 168
Father of Jesus Christ, 297
father, 292,518
fault, 61,171
fearlessness, 452
fees, 397
fellowship of yogin, 193
females,
center of life, 448
exposure, 426
modes magnified, 425
psyche, 279
supernatural, 336
fertilizer, 493
fickleness, 468
fifth caste, 306
film, mystic, 27
Final Sampler, 297
fire, 148
fire sacrifices, 91
First God, 365
flash visions, 523
flashlight, 58
flavor, 393
focal point of impact, 480
focus of soul, 174
focus, 26,186
focusing power, women, 524
food,
consciousness affected by, 491
dry, 493
greed, 463
overheated, 493
rotten, 494
subtle type, 38,491
tasteless, 494
foot, 393
forebearance, 469
formality of ritual, 129
fortune, 336
fossil, 313
foundation, 293
four celibate boys, 312
franchise, Brahma's, 98
freedom from conceit, 470
freedom from craving, 463
frequencies of consciousness, 283
friend, 293
friendship with Krishna, 121
fright, 369
fruitarian diet, 256
fulfillments, 408

G

Gada, 93
galaxies, 360
Gambhiranatha, 438
gambling, 338
Gandhārī, 43
Gandhi, 397
Ganesha, Śrī, 222,233,279,465
Ganges River, 333
Gangotri, 231
Garbhodakaśāyī Viṣṇu, 312,366
garments, 55
Garuḍa, 332
Gaudīya Math Sampradāya, 304
Gauri, 309
Gautama Buddha, 182,183,379,383,400
genetic structure, 162
genital, 393,465
genius, supreme, 234
gentleness, 466,498
geography, 279
ghastly superbeing, 359
Gherwal, Rishi Singh, 461
gift of nature, 479
gift, types, 500, 501
Gītā Govinda, 242
glow in the distance, 461
goat, 491
God
Brahmā, 266
influenced? 447
interest of, 235
sin acceptance, 158
Vishnu, 362,365
yogi recognizes, 98
goddesses, 336

Godhead,
——see also God,
——see also Supreme Person
cited, 87
lay—out, 442
godly nature, 452
gopis, 198,227,242, 259,342,433
Gorakshnath, Mahayogin 298,438,465
grace, 207,290
grace of providence, 83, 84,399
grand delusion, 432
grand escape, 178
grandfather, 292
grandparent, 163
greed, 427,463
Greek, 454
groin area, 465,476
gross existence, 425
group security, 85
guarantees, applicants, 302
guardian of law, 354
guru—see spiritual master
gurukulas, 454

H

habits, 455
Haidakan Bābā, 461
hallucinations of yogis, 233
hallucinogenic drugs, 283,334
hallucinogenic mushrooms, 294
hand, 393
Hanumān, 24,40,213,300
happiness,
non—fluctuating, 167
objective, 34
sensual, 526
superior type, 208
types, 525
Hare Krishna, 138,292,399,551
Hari, Śrī, 375
harṣam, 19
haṭha yoga,
condemned, 298
Gorakshnath, 465
haṭha yogi, 92
hatred, 394
health, 197
hearing, 59,65,143,412—414
heat, 294,354
heaven, 221,273,295
hell, 221
hell—hole, 505
herbs, 334, 335
herbs, medicinal, 493,476
hereafter, 279,427
Himalaya, 93,207,320, 328,329
Hindi, 454
Hindu God, 314
Hindus, 329,465
His Divine Grace, 297
hocus pocus initiation, 345
honesty, 458
hope, 203
horns, 232
horse, 330
hospitality, 496
householder life,
practice continued in, 518
suggested, 299, 300
unfavorable effects, 89
yogis distrusted, 465
human being,
mediocre, 486
passion inspired, 4290
personality components, 212
purpose, 255
spare time, 529
undecisive, 486
vices, 529
human body, 457
humility energy, 49
hurricane, 326
hyenas, 480

I

Icon, 214,291
Ikṣvāku, 120,377
imagination instrument,
buddhi focus, 75
orb, 81,350
explained, 75
inverted vision, 288
perception tool, 288
curbed, 246
impact, focal point, 480
impartiality, 164
impersonal existence, 380
impersonalist,
aspiration, 378
branded, 488
Krishna observes, 261
impetus for action, 514
impressions, 408
impulsions, 80,114
impulsive influence, described, 421
Incarnation of passion, 427
Incarnations, 87,267
inconceivable oneness and difference, 353
indescribable beauty, 363
indestructible factor, 52
India, 397
indifference,
development of, 216
necessary, 133
unnatural, 64
Indra, 93,160,207, 320,327,330
I—ness, 325
infancy, absent in other worlds, 264
inherent nature, 157,487
initiation, 345
initiative, 204,212,393
inner nature, 18
insight,
application, 65
development, 77
priests lack, 68
types, 521
insight yoga visions, 202
institutions, restricting, 438
instruments, 512, 513
integration, 293
intellect organ,
component, 212
conspiracy, 463, 464
control of, 73
decisive part, 85
described, 393
emotions use, 49
eye of, 238
focus, 68
imagination, 75
insight, 521
lowered, 32
purified, 158
shrouded, 115,116

intentions, 179
internalization, 204
International Society for Krishna Consciousness, 551
intoxicant, 476
introspection, 26
introversion, 551
invisible existence, 380
invisible world, 266
irresponsibility, 401
ishtadeva, 373
isolation,
problems, 102
psychological, 194
required, 169,402

J

jagat—guru, 407
Jahnavī, 332
Jahnu, 332
Jamadagni, 332
Jāmbhavatī, 93,454
Janaka, 105
Janaka, 151,179,194
japa, 329
Jayadratha, 363,471
Jesus Christ, Lord, 295—297,311,429,482,536
jitah, 180
jñāna, 92
jñāna yoga,
Arjuna bared, 105
Arjuna discouraged, 149
brahmins, 306
described, 452
Uddhava, 149
jñānacakṣuh, 441
jñānadipa, 27
jñānayajñena, 290
judge of the dead, 332

K

Kailash, 465
kalyāṇakṛts, 220
kāma, 117, 118
Kāmadhuk, 331
kandarpa, 331
Kansa, 482
Kapila Muni, 203,330,392,407
Karanadakashayi Vishnu, 340
Kardama, 330
karma yoga
bhakti yoga, 490
defined, 65,96
described, 121
details, 104
faulty, 531
Gita subject, 473
Gītā textbook, 339
kings practiced, 120
limited, 185
resentments shared, 490
rulers learnt, 121,306
skill, 103
yogi practices, 120
Karṇa, 16,17,359,363
kārpanya, 46
Kartikeya, Śrī, 222
Kaśmalan, 43
Keshava, 363
kevala, 103
kindness, yogi's, 458
Kīrtānanda Swami, Bhaktipāda, 285,325
knife, 466
knowledge, Krishna defines, 396
Kratu, 313
Krishna Consciousness
course, 325, 326
scope, 291
self discovery in, 198
sketch, 292
Krishna das Kaviraj Gosvami, 491
Krishna Dvaipāyana Vyāsadeva
——see Vyāsadeva
Krishna, Lord Śrī,
attraction to, 436
Axis Supreme, 442
body type?, 57,248
Center of divinities, 442
chief of cowherds, 33
claims, 297
contradictions, 109
Core Personality, 297
cosmic producer, 233
dangerous, 344
disliked, 482
excuses yogi?, 176
existential backdrop, 354
ghost hurled by, 489
God Himself?, 254
guardian of law, 354
Krishna, Lord Śrī con't,
human body?, 286
indifferent, 158
infallible, 42
kingdom of, 427
knowing Him, 226
kriyā yogi, 20
kundalini removal, approval, 233
student, 92
multi—dimensional, 126
Murti, 382
partners of, 439
penances, 94
physical form, 259
prefaced in everyone, 353
promise explained, 124
residence, 439
self recommendation, 81
Shiva, 94,455
Shiva Sahasranama, 92
spirit body focus, 81
spirits compared, 123
spirits deliverance, 267
spiritual form, 373
Supersoul association, 483
Supervising Universal Lord, 111
tricks, 471
ultimate man, 354
ultimate motivator, 233
ultimate shelter, 354
unaffected, 25
unique individual, 467
unknown?, 228
Veda, 445
Vedic rituals, 292
world located?, 268
yoga master, 345
yoga power, 371
yoga practice, 319
yogi, 349
Kṛṣṇa—Balarāma Deities, 200,375
kriyā ceremonies, 68
kriyā master
—see spiritual master

kriyā yoga practice,
1st stage, 26
application, 72
battle unusual, 21
complication, 148
concerns of, 9
consistency required, 159
cultural activities, 176
curriculum, 173
desired, 12
devotion reconciled, 381
diet, 491
distress—remover, 197
eight stages, 26
excuse of, 176
faulty idea removal, 172
five chapters, 227
gopis admired by, 242
integrated, 118, 119
intensity, 236
introspective, 14
involvement, 22
irreplaceable, 150—151
Krishna—teacher, 46
last resort, 80
lessons, 397
limited, 348
main course, 226
mixed?, 148
objective, 88
perspective, 26
political usage, 181
practice essential, 16
proficiency requirements, 153,201
psyche observation, 11
questioned, 473
recommended, 216
sāṁkhya compared, 151
Sanjaya's boosted, 11
self—effort, 17
social usage, 27
stability, 399
summary of, 196
teacher, 195
threatening, 43
waste of time?, 262
yogis attracted to, 461

kriyā yogi,
accomodations, 189
advanced type, 128,379
application training, 65
astral transfer, 294
battlefield?, 21
best devotee type, 225
birth importance, 221
body used by advanced yogis, 465
causal existence, 234
compared, 224
cooperation with providence, 236
cultural life, 89
destined duty, 60
devotional type, 261
dimensional perception, 74
efforts limited, 233
example, 109
excuses, 176
fame resistant, 47
female type, 467
fortunate birth, 222
genetic body, 221
heavenly degradation, 220
highest, 214
householder opportunity, 60
instinct for practice, 221
karma yoga necessary, 381
lessons from senses, 279
liberation forestalled, 236
limited, 98
location in psyche, 207
mistakes allowed, 246
objective, 34
perceptions, 49
reactions transmitted, 133
rebirth conditions, 220
responsibility, 34
sensual addiction, 551
sex overpowers, 15
sour attitude, 150
spiritual path, 149
subconscious entry, 232
sunlight form, 232
Supreme Person focus, 260

kriyā yogi continued,
teaching livelihood, 397
travel restrictions, 271, 272
types, 137
undisciplined one, 218
unstable?, 64
waiver retracted, 178
yoginis, 467
Kriyānanda, Swami, 437
Kṣama, 336
kṣara, 269,446
kṣetra, property, 10
kṣetri, 416
kuladharmah, 35
kuṇḍalinī chakra,
anger, 458
elimination, 233
limited, 275
purification, 452
residents of, 396
third—eye related, 427
Yogananda's interpretation, 273
Kuṇḍalinī Mātā, 426
Kuṇḍalinī Shakti Ma, 525
kuṇḍalinī yoga,
brain energization, 262
breath energization, 261
chakra cleaning, 476
elementary, 444
necessary, 269
raising of, 192
visions, 336
Kuru, dynasty, 10
Kurukṣetra, 10
kusha grass, 189
Kuvera, 328

L

lack of knowledge, 472
lack of pride, 396
Lahiri Mahasaya, Mahayogin, 299,467
Lakṣmī-Nārāyana, Śrī-Śrī, 233
lamp, 199
landscape of light, 233
language, 454
Lankā, 24
laughter, 63
law court, 10
leaders, 127,488

legal document, 505
letter A, 336
liabilities, 106
liberated souls, 417, 418
liberation,
achievement, 436
attainment elusive, 153
cosmic dissolution, 15
permissions required, 99
qualifications, 175
quantam leap, 94
reversal, 394
life force,
component, 212
food greed, 464
kundalini yoga, 197
purification, 192
sexual interest sacrificed, 17
life's complexity, 91
life's purpose, 44
light body, 232,370
light of luminaries, 406
light, in meditation, 202
light—emitting form, 353
light—emitting orbs, 393
lion, 19,332,479
liquor, 476,529
live electric wire, 482
livelihood, 397
Living Mundane Existence, 436
living space, 390
location,
dimensional, 204
important, 512
in meditation, 206
psychological, 204
logicians, 335
lokasamgraham, 108
lord of creation, 480
lord of psyche, 538
Lord of the earth, 25
lotus leaf, 155
love of Krishna, 244
love, Krishna-Arjuna, 540
LSD, 335

M

Mā Durgā,
——see Durgā
Mā Sarasvati, 467
madbhaktim, 534
Madhusūdana, 42
maha brahma, 418
Mahābhārata, 9,11,20,21, 274,286,294,320
Mahādeva, 20,279,429,551
——see also Shiva
Maharshis, 309
Mahatma Gandhi, 40,397, 398
MahaVishnu, 340
Mahavishnu/ Durga, 418
Maheśvarah, 92,409
Maitreya Muni, 242,330,536
mantra, 135
Manu, 120,313,377
mānuṣīm, 285
map, 290
Marīci, 313,326
marijuana, 334,335
Markandeya, Rishi, 231, 233,334,370,536
marriage, 37
Martin Luther King, Rev. Dr., 40
martyr, 40
Marutas, 326
master, 293
mat, 81
Matali, 320
Matanga Rishi, 40,392
material existence
bondage/ liberation, 435
cut down, 436
ended, 74
perception difficult, 436
tree, 434
material nature,
action forced by, 95
capable, 160
cosmic womb, 418
diversified, 228
encompassing, 212
reactions, 477
relationship with, 246
renunciation blocked by, 94
sexual, 435
subtle constituents, 228
supernatural, 287
material world, purpose, 255
matter, dead force?, 419
maya, 287
meals, 492
Medhā, 336
meditation,
deception in, 95
psychological bombardment, 63
shifts in, 172
memorization, 454
memory,
compressed, 182
conscious grip, 220
controller of, 445
other's penetrated, 232
spasms, 183
spirit different, 182
subconscious, 134
mental cleanliness, 497
mental movements cease, 169
mento—emotional energy, 272
mercy, 207
mercy—prone person, 46
Meru, 328
messiah image, 196
milk checker, 297
milk, serpent analogy, 449
mind,
chamber, 207
compartment, 212,445
contents, 173
control without diversions, 216
described, 393
energy intake, 215
imprints, 174
jumpy, 468
loss of, 445
monitored, 217
sensual interest sacrificed, 17
sky of, 452
stringent control, 216
misfit, 465
missionary work, 432
missionary yogi, 452
Mitra, 326
mobility, 192
modesty, 14,467
Mohammed, 294
mokṣaparāyaṇah, 175
money, 139,478
moon, 272-274,326,442
moonlight, death affected, 274

morality,
Buddha taught, 400
preliminary, 118
self restraint, 453
subtle type, 118
upset of, 39
victory, 340
mosquitoes, 497
mother,
breast, 426
comparison, 311
Krishna as, 292
mother's body, 58
motivation,
causal form, 179
limited, 179
motivations, source, 463
mourning, tendency, 59
mouth of the Supreme, 141
mouth, attack on, 360
movements, 513, 513
Muktānanda,
author interview, 345
divine sight method, 375
female exposure, 425,426,431
Nityananda, 436,452,522
mūlādhāra, 276
multi—personality, 311
murder, 53,531
Murti Icon, 81,81,214
mushrooms, 294,334,335
Muslims, 295
mystics, 448

N

naad sound, 174
Nachiketa, 50,332
naiṣkarma, 104,532
Name of God, 257,329
Nanda Gopa, 160
Nandī, 93
nanny, 441
Nārada Muni, 20,40,203,266,319,332, 334,370,390,392,407
Narasingha, 332
Nārāyaṇa, 93,309
narcotics, 288,289,335,493
nāsikāgram, 192
natal qualities, 470
Nath yogi, 438
national culture, 36
nationality, 488
Neem Karoli Baba, 452
neti neti, 465
Nevada City, 437
nine—gate city, 156
nirvāṇa, 88,436
nirveda, 189
nirvritti, 469
Nityananda, Siddha Swami, 436, 452,522
niyama, 26,96,117
non—attachment, 436
noncompliance, 531
non—interference, 111
non—violence, 397,457,497
northern hemisphere, 272
nose gazing, 192
notation, 147
nourishment, 101

O

objectiveness, 293, 442
obligatory actions, 176
observer, 293
ocean comparison, 87
Ocean of Nectar, 330
odor, 393
offerings, 300,492
old age, 400
Om, 138,231,262,263, 292,329,502
Om Tat Sat, 502
oneness, 103
oneness and difference, 353
opinions, 62
opium, 334,335
opportunity, rejection, 504
optic nerves, channel, 27
oral system, 454
orbs, 393
organ of psychic vision, 27
origin, 293,339
Over—lord, 467

P

Pacific Ocean, 272,274
pacifist, 397, 398,457
Padmanabha, Lord, 233,374,376
padmāsana, 548
Pandavas, 268
pandit, criticized, 67,133
Pandu, 43,338
Paramātmā, 210,409
paramātmā, directive self, 181
parambrahma, 403
Paramhansa Yogananda, ——see Yogananda
paramparā, 449
——see also disciplic succession
Parāśar Muni, 233
Paraśurāma, 332,454
paravairāgya, 394, 458
parents, 44
partners, 439
parts, 212
passion,
control of, 118
embodied, 427
forceful, 114
negative aspects, 526
spirit affected by, 116
usefulness, 427
past lives, 250
Patañjali Maharshi, Śrī, 26,170,174,199, 203,250,289,468
Patel, Bharat, 213,438
path of no return, 436
patience, 336,398
Paul Castagna, Sir, 473
Pāvaka, 328
peace of mind, 498
pearls, 230
peep, 195
peer pressure, 396
peering, 204
pepper, 493
perception, 288
perfection, 91
performers?, 156
perplexity, 26
person, 390
person source, 296
personal energies, 118,180
Personality Spread, 364
personality,
composite parts, 283
multiple, 311
segmented, 312
peyote mushrooms, 335
pig, 232
pinpoint of initiative, 204

pity, 42
place, body, 389, 390
plant bulb, 296
pleasing others, 504
pleasure, celestial type, 427
pleasure/ pain, 394
policeman, 32,123
politeness, 472
political power, ceremonial rites, 67
Pondicherry, 352
popularity, 106
possessions, 188
poverty, 13
Prabhupada, ——see Bhaktivedanta Swami
Prachinabarhi, 390
practice, —see kriya yoga practice
Pradyumna, 93,222
Prahlāda, 332
prakāśam, 430
prāṇa, 215,393
prāṇa vision, 138,233, 334,426,442
prāṇāyāma,
4th stage, 26
described, 173
Gorakshnath, 465
passion removed, 501
retardation removed, 501
prasadam, 492
pratiṣṭha, 433
pratyāhār,
5th stage, 144
buddhi yoga, 73
observations, 26
psychic perception, 58
pravritti, 9,469
prayer, 210,329
preacher, 402,496
preaching, 429
predictions, 448
pre—existence source, 265
preferences, 489
pregnancy, diet, 38
prehistoric creatures, 283
prehistoric man, 313
prejudices, 165
prenatal qualities, 470
President, 330
prestige, 420,499
pride, 13,396
priest, 67,496
primal instinct, 440
Primal Person, 436
printing press, 454
privacy, 403,472
privilege, duty, 70
procreators, 313
professors, 335
prohibited activities, 26
propensities, sinful type, 251
property control, 139
Prophet Mohammed, 295
prostitute, 467
providence,
consequences forced, 465
pressure, 220
supreme, 398
victimizes, 538
yogi agrees with, 276
proximity, 311
Pṛtha, 43
psilocybin, 335
psyche,
changes, 77
components, 393
described, 180
details, 118
observations, 26
recognized, 17
segments, 310
spirit different, 117
undivided, 516
psyche yoga, 344
psychedelic drugs, 287, 288
psychiatry, 334
psychic objects, 212
psychic parts, 212
psychic vision, 27
psychological control, 371
psychological maze, 26
psychological possessions, 188
psychological purification, 231
psychology, 334,440
puberty, 477
public, non—interference, 111
puja, 496
Pulaha, 313
Pulastya, 313
puma, 480
pungent food, 493
punishment, 339
puppets, 407
Purana, 203
Puranas, 165,202
pure devotee, 171
purgatory, 332
purifier, experience, 143
purity of being, 452,498
purity of psyche, 498
purity yoga, 476
purity, 225,398,469
Puruanjan, 390
puruṣa, 390
puruṣah parah, 409
Puṣa, 326
Pushti Ma, 426
puzzle of conjunction, 234

Q,R

Radha—Krishna Deities, Śrī Śrī,466
rainfall, 101,294
Rājarṣayo, 121
Rāma, Lord Śrī, 24,91, 296,332,408,438
Ramana Maharshi, 379
Rāmanand Prasad, Dr., 546
Ramananda Raya, 342
Rāmāyana, 24,327, 332,392,448
Rampa, T. Lobsang, 426
rapid breathing, 318
Rāvaṇa, 24,482
reaction,
divine supervision, 160
material nature's, 477
questioned, 505
reading, 454
realism, 338
reasoning, 115,445
rebels, 356
rebirth,
animal form, 480
cancellation, 161
family orientation, 19
recall absent, 57
recitation of scriptures, 453
recluse, 102
recognition of reality, 458
recollection, 336

reform, 304
reformatory energies, 407
refresher course, 173
regression, 221
reincarnation,
——see also transmigration
compensation, 453
risky, 507
uncontrolled, 391
rejection of consequences, 505
rejection of opportunity, 504
relationship with God, 314
relationship with Krishna, 304,342
reliance, 135,355
religion ceremony, 101
religious affiliation, 522
religious leaders, 396,478
religious ministers, 44
reluctance, 70
removal of faults, 171
Renukā, 332
renunciation,
confusion about, 148
defined, 177
insufficient, 94
mood of, 150
psychological attitude, 177
total, 149
repeated birth, 18
repossession of consciousness, 283
reputation, 61
resentment,
avoidance of, 498
feared, 62
Krishna targeted, 360
next life's, 19
Supreme Being as target, 482
reservoir, 293
response, 256
responsibility,
controls, 183
defence for, 24
developed, 54
enforced, 150—151
instructions on, 12
misery, 438
pleasure sponsors, 169
responsibility continued,
pressed in, 235, 236
sensuality promotes, 79
resting place, 324
restraint, questioned, 113
retaliations, 505
retarded psychic, 488
retarding force, usage, 421
return, no return, 204
revelation, 198,523
revivalist, 245
reward, 183,453
Ṛg Veda, 292,447
Riddhi, 465
rim, 296
Rishikesh, 461
risk, 113
ritual, 129
ritual mystics, 434
robots, 156
romance, 526
root, 434
ṛṣayah, 171
ṛtambhāra buddhi, 448
Rudras, 328
Rukmiṇī, 93

S

Sacramento, 437
sacrifical ceremony, 376
sacrifice of life, 17
sacrifices, 91
sadhanā bhakti, 301
sadhusaṅga, 193
Sahara Desert, 272
saintly credit, 304
sakho, 122
salty food, 493
salvation, 169
Sāma Veda, 292,327,447
samādhi, 26,76,324
Sambara, 93
sambhavah, 418
Samkhya philosophy,
application, 65
nature's usage, 45, 154
synthesis, 154, 413
theory insufficient, 65
yoga compared, 151
sampradāya, 20,376
——see also disciplic succession
samyama, 81
samyamī, 86
samye, 164
Sanaka, 313
Sanandan, 313
Sanātana, 313
Sanat—kumāra, 313
sanctification, 68
Sanjaya, 9,11,349
sannyasa,
Arjuna discouraged, 149
blocked, 505
modern type, 152
non—yogi type, 177
requirements, 153
Sanskrit, 454
Sanskrit literature, 336
Sanskrit sounds, 135
śāntim, 88,196
supernatural vision, 349
Sarasvatī, 467
Sat, 502
Śatru, 326
satsaṅga, 193
satyam, 458
Satyeshwarananda, 213
savior,
fallen yogi?, 234
fame basis, 407
image, 196
liberated entities, 418
pledges, 296
Savior-of-Humanity role, 438
Savita, 326
scholarship, 234
scientific research, 283
scriptural injunctions, 486
security, 56,460
seeking, 183
seers, 171
segmentations, 310
self analysis, 465
self consciousness reliance, 268
self critical energy, 465
self purification, 278
Self Realization Fellowship, 243
self—conviction, 234
self—critical energy, 461
self—critique, 208
self—denial, 536
self—focused intellect, 68
selfless service, 104
selfless work, 94
self—purification, 29,155

self—restraint, 453,498
sensations, 51
sense of initiative, 174,212
sense organs,
controlled, 13
detailed listing, 393
edge—lights, 85
information procurement, 13
nitpicking, 279
spiritual type, 440
torment seeker, 80
wind force, 85
sensual equipments,
——see sense organs
sensual withdrawal, 26,78
sensuality, 82,88
serpent, milk analogy, 449
serpent divinity, 332
seva, 94,104
seven great sages, 312
sexual aggression, 427
sexual association, 526
sexual attraction, 14
sexual connection, cosmic, 435
sexual energy vigor, 468
sexual exposure deity, 426
sexual intercourse,
sacred, 236
world cause, 475
sexual intermixture, 38
sexual lust, 463
sexual relationship, 497
sexual urge, 476
sexual, grace energy, 236
sexuality, kundalini, 192
sexually-disciplined procreators, 313
shakipat, 207,345,371
Shankara Shiva, 328
shantim, 88
shark, 333
Shatarupa, 313
shelter, 293
ship, 85
Shiva Deity, 173
Shiva Purāṇa, 448
Shiva, Lord,
advanced instructions, 164
Arjuna saw, 322
author avoided by, 465
author inspired by, 213
author saw, 465
authority, 392
cosmic energy producer, 233
disciplinary violence, 398
disquised, 93
glories of, 92
initiation by, 194
inspiration, 200
inspires incompetents, 430
Krishna called, 92
Krishna relationship, 94
Krishna saw, 319
Krishna worshipped, 309
kundalini removal approval, 233
nature conflicts in, 300
reliance on, 269
returns here, 407
revelation, 436
shelter, 80
sons, 222
Supreme Person?, 297
tridents, 438
Upamanyu worship, 93
yogis sent by, 551
Shivananda, 233,399, 431,461
Shivasahasranama, 92
short cut, 546
shrouding action, 158
Shuka, 40,222,242, 300,482,535
Shukracharya, 338
siddha—body, 427
Siddhi, 465
siddhis, 10
silence, 339,498
sincerity, 22
sins, 171
śiṣya, 46
Skanda Kumāra, 93,279,299,328,465
skills, 220
sky, 202
sleeping, yogi's, 197
small supernatural figures, 396
smell aspect, 232
Smṛti, 336
social affairs, continue, 9
social liberators, 40
soldiers, Gītā, 121
soma beverage, 294
Somadatta, 16
sound, 174,393
sour attitude, 150
sour food, 493
source, 265
southern hemishpere, 273
spare time, 529
species of life,
advantages, 165
origin, 234
passion—urged, 421
similarity, 164
speck, 358
speech, 336,498
spirit,
accessories, 325
categorical situation, 284
conjunction with causal energy, 234
connected to equipments, 71
dependence on material nature, 419
eternal, 49
exploitive, 439
focus, 204
Krishna compared, 123
lower nature, 446
material nature affinity, 246
material nature relationship, 237
objectivity lacking, 117
partners, 439
person source, 296
property? 229
psyche different, 117
psychic equipments, 214
psychology, 440, 441
resting place, 324
seen, 210
self—fascination, 59
sexual connection, 435
sustain world, 229
types, 445

spirit continued,
undetected, 58
unworthy of sympathy, 56
user of living space, 416
spiritual body,
Arjuna's, 373
development, 269
Krishna's, 81
spiritual master,
Bābāji's critique, 467
causal level, 334
chased, 91
description, 142
disciple's expectations, 31
disciples retard, 195
fake, 77
fallen yogi, 234
figurehead, 467
flattered, 15
gravest, 368
ideal one, 243
incompetent ones, 430
indispensible?, 307
instruction faulty?, 531
Krishna's representative, 243
many, 46,497
pretender, 168
protection limited, 90
puppet, 407
purity partial?, 111
questioned, 125
rare, 168
relationships, 168
respect/ disrespect, 15
respects for, 495
similar to Krishna, 30
spiritual peace, 175
spiritual security, 460
spiritual sight, Arjuna, 427
spiritual sky, 195,259
spiritual vision, 216
spiritual world transference, 266,267,269
spiritual, description, 186
spoke, 296
squirrel, 468
Śrī, 336
Śrīdhara Deva Gosvami, 313
Śrīmad Bhāgavatam, 20,149,198,242,286,301, 316,330,366,418,448
śrutiparāyaṇāh, 413
śrutvānyebhya, 413
stability, defined, 400
star, internal vision, 202
status,
not required, 48
risky, 130
spirits', 445
Vedic, 306
stooges of irresponsibility, 13
stool, 493
straight—forwardness, 455
string, 230
struggles, 135
students, 90
subconscious, 232,393
Subhadrā, 14
subtle body,
bubble—shaped, 522
desire—prone, 394
dispositions of, 163
disturbed, 418
elderly, 18
eyes of, 288
fault of, 428
foundation, 55
heavy, 550
influence of, 163
life duration of, 394
life span, 407
misleading, 18
observed, 18
prejudices, 407
spasms, 183
subconscious parts, 232
sun/ moon effect, 272
transmigration caused by, 391
usage described, 442
subtle elements, 393
subtle existence, 11
subtle objects, 201,331
subtle world, 185,256
succession of teachers, 449
sūkṣma, 404
summary, 533
Sum—total Reality, 366
sun energy, 442
Sun God, 447
sun planet civilization, 233
sun, influences yogi, 232,272,273
sunlight body, 232
sunset, 471
superbeing, 359
SuperGod, 340
super—imposition, 297
supernatural beings, 346
supernatural heat, 354
supernatural people, miniature, 233
supernatural perception, 288, 289
supernatural rulers, 99,352
supernatural warfare, 320
super—people, 297
Supersoul, 210, 211,256,538
superstition, 38
Supervising Universal Lord, 90,94,109
supporter, 293
Supreme Being, 142,236,282,446
Supreme Cause, 143,232,260,446
Supreme Energy, 142
Supreme God Vishnu, 379
Supreme Lord, 49,409
Supreme Personality, 231
Supreme Personality of Godhead, 303,339
Supreme Primal Cause, 231
Supreme Primal State, 277
supreme proprietor, 228,312
Supreme Soul, 409
Supreme Spirit, 101,312
Surendra, 294
surface, 393
surrender to Krishna, 245
survival, 479
suspended existence, 367
suspended individuality, 284
svabhāva, 157
svabhāvajā, 487
svacakṣuṣā, 348
Svārga angelic world, 67,207,294,327,
svarga, 294
swami accomplice, 531
swindler, 338
synopsis, 533

synthesis, 413

T

T. Lobsang Rampa, 426
Tandi, 92
tanum, 285
tat tvam asi, 16
Tat, 502
tattvavit, 154
teacher, 11,44
teen rebellion, 38
teenager comparison, 490
Tejomaya, 370
terrain, 152
territories, 152,312
texture of being, 487
texture of existence, 257
They-are-impersonalists, 488
thighs, 476
thinking stopped, 172,187
Third Eye book, 426
third eye focus, 138,201,406,426,260,261
throwing tridents, 438
throw—offs, 488
thumb, 409
thunderbolt, 331
thunderstormer, 326
Tibetan monasteries, 426
tides, 274
tiger skin, 189
tigers, 480
time cycles, 265,332,514
tortoise comparison, 78
towns, 395
tradition, 35, 36,495,540
trance states, 26
transcendental energy, 260
transcendental experience, 186
transmigration,
automatic, 50,55
ceased, 204
forceful, 395
scary, 395
subtle body based, 163
uncertain, 283
uncontrolled, 391
transmutation, 334
tree of existence, 434
trend, 487
tridents, 438
truthfulness, 458
tusks, 232
Tvaṣṭā, 326
twice born, 15
twilight of consciousness, 283
twist of fate, 168
tyāga, 505

U

Uchchaihshravah, 330
Uddhava, 149,242,418,509
ultimate man, 354
ultimate reference, 354
ultimate shelter, 354
ultimatum, 306
Umā,
——see also Durgā
93,94,319,322,429,454,
unconscious, 393
United States, 272
Universal Form,
art work, 350
author saw, 346
cooperation with, 537
Durga's, 448
eyes, 407
fearful, 346
harsh?, 361
puppets, 407
reformatory energies, 407
seers of, 355
Shiva's, 448
vision required, 81
universal teacher, 407
university, 334
unmanifest energy, 393
Upamanyu, Mahayogin, 92,93,319,346,389,455
Upanishads, 50,52,91, 164,231,253,403
urination, 465
Urukrāma, 326
user of living space, 416
Ushana, 338
utility of the individual, 15

V

Vachnamrut, 448
vagina, 418
Vaikuntha, 266
vairāgyena, 216
Vaishnavism, 342
vaishvanara, 444
Vajra, 330
Vāk, 336
Valmiki Rāmāyaṇa, 392
varṇaśrām, 37
Varuṇa, 326, 332
Vasava, 327
Vasiṣṭha, 313
Vasudeva, 286,301,338, 351,373,379
Vāsuki, 331
Veda, 101,139
Vedanta, 445
Vedas,
Arjuna quoted, 67
best production, 434
brahmin property, 69
incentives, 222
Om supreme, 231
on God, 447
scope of, 69
Vedic culture, 306
Vedic priests, 67
Vedic rituals, 292
Vedic study, 375
vegetarian diet, 256
vegetation, 434
vetti, 410
victory, 338,339
Vidhātā, 326
Vidura, 536
vigor, 468
vijñānam, 185
Vikarṇa, 16
villages, 395
Vimūḍhḍātma, 109
Vinata, 332
violence,
Bābāji on, 466
described, 398
sponsorship, 212
supernatural type, 457
Supreme Spirit's, 212
Vishnu Murti, 382
Vishnu Purana, 326
Vishnu, Lord,
Central Figure, 407
cosmic energy producer, 233
descent as Icon, 202
four—handed, 374
greatest person, 442
orders Arjuna, 362
Prahlāda, 332
Urukrāma, 326
yogi parents, 221
Vishnudevananda, 431

Vishvamitra, 470
vision of reality, 441
vision of similarity, 214
vision,
internal, 202
inverted, 288
psychic, 27
spiritual spiritual forms, 376
types, 426
Vittesha, 328
Vivasvān, 326,447
Vivekananda, 334
Vivsvāt, 120
vocal cord, 393
vows, 289,290
Vrishni clan, 338
vrittis, 169,289,468
Vṛndāvana, 198,227,291, 292,373,536
Vyaghrapāda, 93
Vyasadeva, Krishna Dvaipayana, 27,206,207,221 233,241,268,294,300, 319,338,392,418,482

W

waiver, 149,178
war, internal, 80
water, subtle, 38
wealth, 13
weapons, 331
weapons, sound producing type, 135
we—are—devotees, 488
weather personality, 326
weight, psychological, 183
Western Civilization, 454
wheel, 296
wind, 282,333
windless place, 199
womb, 418
women,
—see also females
focusing power, 524
insecurity, 13
Vedic status, 305
workers comparison, 213
work—prone people, 425
world of light, 233
world savior, 407
World War II, 465
world,
purpose, 255
utilization, 140
worries,
freedom from, 77
puberty onset, 477
worship ceremony, 453
worship procedures, 98
worship, system, 298

XY

yajñārtha, 97
Yajur Veda, 292,447
yama, 26,117
Yama,
astral pioneer, 92
judge of departed souls, 332
spirit realized, 50
yati, 217
yatra, 204
yoga practice,
——see kriyā yoga practice
yoga siddha body, 29,174
Yoga Sūtras, 26,174,199,203,289,468
yogadhāraṇām, 261
Yogananda, Paramhansa Mahayogin, 202,213,243, 244,271,272,334, 404,437,438,461,551
yogārūḍhas, 179
yoga—siddha body, 427
yogavittamah, 378
Yogeshwara, 345
Yogeshwarananda,Yogiraj Mahayogin,213,231,300, 311-313,394,418,425, 426,439,448,465,469
brahmarandra entry, 244
causal perception, 182
causal plane, 268
on low rebirth, 223
on posture, 192
writer trained by, 201
Yogi Bhajan, Harbhajan Singh, Mahayogin 461,546
yogi,
——see kriyā yogi
you are that, 164
Yudhiṣṭhira, 22,206,207,294,319, 320,339,433,457,536
yugavatar, 433
Yuktesvara Swami, Giri, 438

Z

zone—bound, 274

LIST OF TEACHERS

Gaudiya Vaishnava teacher:
Srila Bhaktivedanta Swami Prabhupada
Haṭha yoga teacher:
Swami Vishnudevananda
Kundalini yoga teacher:
Mahayogi Sri Harbhajan Singh
Celibacy yoga teachers:
Swami Shivananda,
Srila Yogiraj Yogeshwarananda
Purity—of—the—psyche yoga teacher:
Srila Yogiraj Yogeshwarananda
Kriyā yoga teachers:
Srila Babaji Mahasaya,
Siddha Swami Muktananda
Brahma yoga teacher:
Siddha Swami Nityananda

About the Author

Michael Beloved (Yogi Madhvāchārya) took his current body in 1951 in Guyana. In 1965, while living in Trinidad, he instinctively began doing yoga postures and trying to make sense of the supernatural side of life.

Later on, in 1970, in the Philippines, he approached a Martial Arts Master named Mr. Arthur Beverford, explaining to the teacher that he was seeking a yoga instructor. Mr. Beverford identified himself as an advanced disciple of Rishi Singh Gherwal, an astanga yoga master.

Mr. Beverford taught the traditional Astanga Yoga with stress on postures, attentive breathing and brow chakra centering meditation. In 1972, Madhvāchārya entered the Denver Colorado Ashram of Kundalini Yoga Master Sri Harbhajan Singh. There he took instruction in Bhastrika Prāṇāyāma and its application to yoga postures. He was supervised mostly by Yogi Bhajan's disciple named Prem Kaur.

In 1979 Madhvāchārya formally entered the disciplic succession of the Brahma—Madhava Gaudiya Sampradaya through Swami Kirtanananda, who was a prominent sannyasi disciple of the Great Vaishnava Authority Sri Swami Bhaktivedanta Prabhupada, the exponent of devotion to Sri Krishna.

After carefully studying and practicing the devotional process introduced by Sri Swami Bhaktivedanta Prabhupada, Madhvacharya was inspired to do a translation of the Bhagavād—gītā, which is published without Sanskrit as ***Bhagavad Gītā English*** *and with Sanskrit word—for—word as* ***Bhagavad Gītā Revealed****. Thereafter he published an explanatory commentary titled* ***Bhagavad Gītā Explained****. This* ***Kriyā Yoga Bhagavad Gita*** *is his 2nd commentary, specifically for showing the kriyā yoga techniques given by Sri Krishna to Arjuna This commentary was inspired by Sri Babaji Mahasaya of the Kriyā lineage*

It may free a reader from ineffective kriyā techniques. For practicing yogis, it would confirm valid kriyās and show new ones. And most of all, this would reveal the kriyās which were directly taught by Lord Krishna.

This translation does not concern making or controlling disciples. It is designed to give readers insight to what Sri Krishna and Arjuna discussed in the discourse, without any effort to convince or convert. It is free of missionary overtones.

Regarding the kriyā yogi devotees, Sri Krishna said this:

तेषां सततयुक्तानां भजतां प्रीतिपूर्वकम् । ददामि बुद्धियोगं तं येन मामुपयान्ति ते ॥१०.१०॥
तेषामेवानुकम्पार्थम् अहमज्ञानजं तमः । नाशयाम्यात्मभावस्थो ज्ञानदीपेन भास्वता ॥१०.११॥

teṣāṁ satatayuktānāṁ bhajatāṁ prītipūrvakam
dadāmi buddhiyogaṁ taṁ yena māmupayānti te (10.10)
teṣāmevānukampārtham ahamajñānajaṁ tamaḥ
nāśayāmyātmabhāvastho jñānadīpena bhāsvatā (10.11)

Of those who are constantly disciplined, who worship with affection, I give the technique by which they draw near to Me. (10.10)

In the interest of assisting them, I who am situated within their beings, cause the ignorance, produced by the stupefying influence of material nature to be banished by their clear realized insight (10.11)

Publications

English Series

Bhagavad Gita English

Anu Gita English

Markandeya Samasya English

Yoga Sutras English

Uddhava Gita English

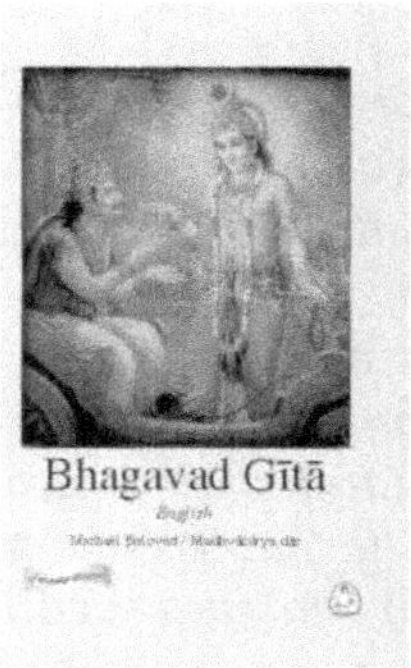

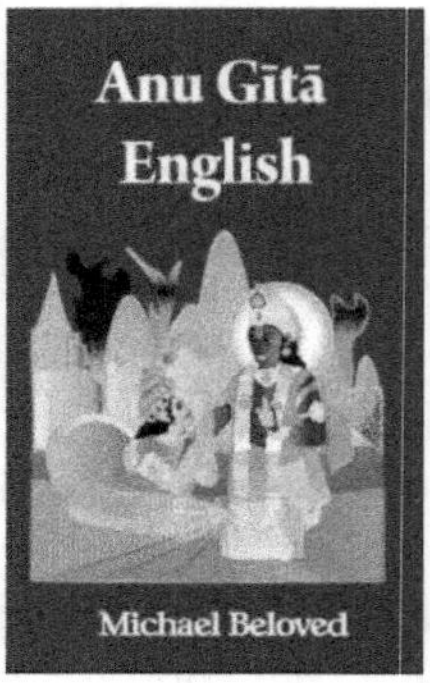

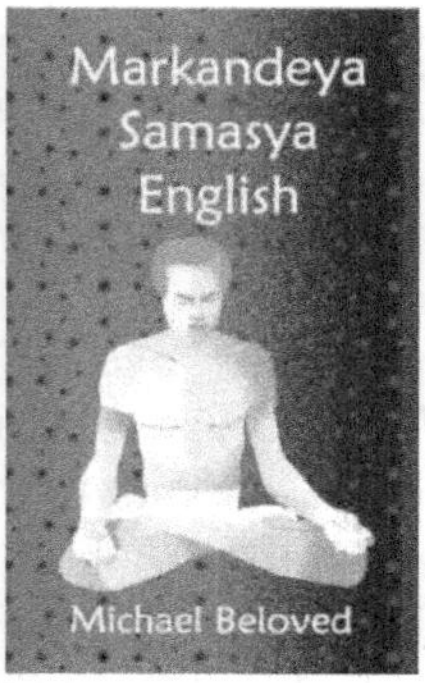

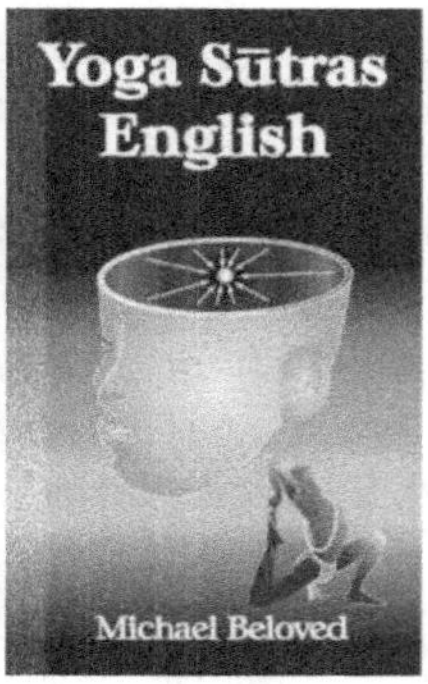

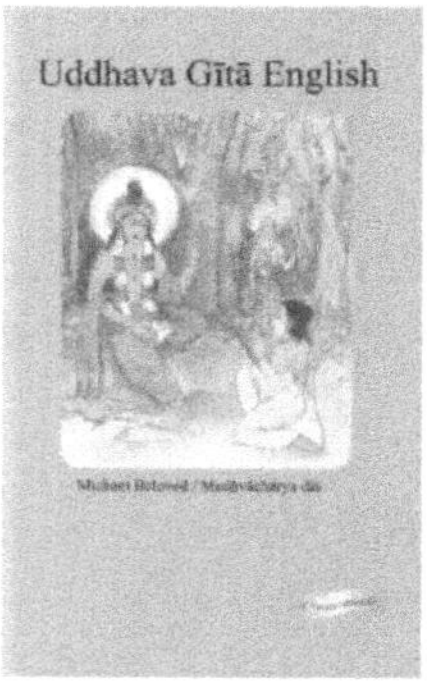

These are in 21st Century English, very precise and exacting. Many Sanskrit words which were considered untranslatable into a Western language are rendered in precise, expressive and modern English, due to the English language becoming the world's universal means of concept conveyance.

Three of these books are instructions from Krishna. **In Bhagavad Gita English** and **Anu Gita English**, the instructions were for Arjuna. In the **Uddhava Gita English,** it was for Uddhava. Bhagavad Gita and Anu Gita are extracted from the Mahabharata. Uddhava Gita was extracted from the 11th Canto of the Srimad Bhagavatam (Bhagavata Purana). One of these books, the **Markandeya Samasya English** is about Krishna, as described by Yogi Markandeya, who survived the cosmic collapse and reached a divine child in whose transcendental body, the collapsed world was existing. Another of these books, the **Yoga Sutras English,** is the detailed syllabus about yoga practice.

My suggestion is that you read **Bhagavad Gita English**, the **Anu Gita English, the Markandeya Samasya English,** the **Yoga Sutras English** and lastly the **Uddhava Gita English**, which is much more complicated and detailed.

For each of these books we have at least one commentary, which is published separately. Thus your particular interest can be researched further in the commentaries.

The smallest of these commentaries and perhaps the simplest is the one for the Anu Gita. We published its commentary as the Anu Gita Explained. The Bhagavad Gita explanations were published in three distinct targeted commentaries. The first is Bhagavad Gita Explained, which sheds lights on how people in the time of Krishna and Arjuna regarded the information and applied it. Bhagavad Gita is an exposition of the application of yoga practice to cultural activities, which is known in the Sanskrit language as karma yoga.

Interestingly, Bhagavad Gita was spoken on a battlefield just before one of the greatest battles in the ancient world. A warrior, Arjuna, lost his wits and had no idea that he could apply his training in yoga to political dealings. Krishna, his charioteer, lectured on the spur of the moment to give Arjuna the skill of using yoga proficiency in cultural dealings including how to deal with corrupt officials on a battlefield.

The second commentary is the Kriya Yoga Bhagavad Gita. This clears the air about Krishna's information on the science of kriya yoga, showing that its techniques are clearly described free of charge to anyone who takes the time to read Bhagavad Gita. Kriya yoga concerns the battlefield which is the psyche of the living being. The internal war and the mental and emotional forces which are hostile to self-realization are dealt with in the kriya yoga practice.

The third commentary is the Brahma Yoga Bhagavad Gita. This shows what Krishna had to say outright and what he hinted about which concerns the brahma yoga practice, a mystic process for those who mastered kriya yoga.

There is one commentary for the **Markandeya Samasya English**. The title of that publication is Krishna Cosmic Body.

There are two commentaries to the Yoga Sutras. One is the Yoga Sutras of Patanjali and the other is the Meditation Expertise. These give detailed explanations of the process of Yoga.

For the Uddhava Gita, we published the Uddhava Gita Explained. This is a large book and requires concentration and study for integration of the information. Of the books which deal with transcendental topics, my opinion is that the discourse between Krishna and Uddhava has the complete information about the realities in existence. This book is the one which removes massive existential ignorance.

Meditation Series

Meditation Pictorial

Meditation Expertise

Core-Self Discovery

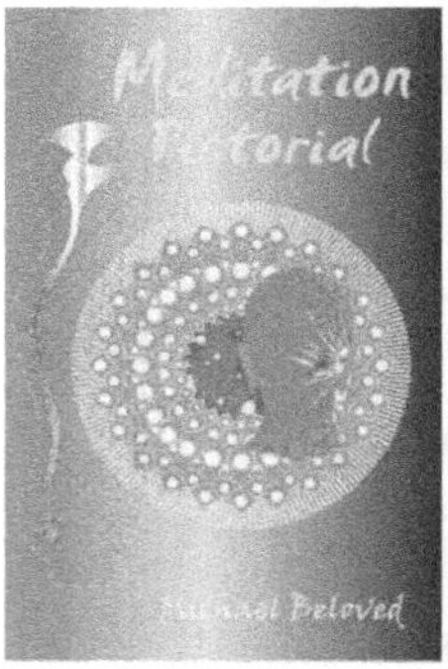

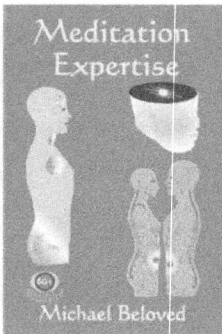

The specialty of these books is the mind diagrams which profusely illustrate what is written. This shows exactly what one has to do mentally to develop and then sustain a meditation practice.

In the **Meditation Pictorial**, one is shown how to develop psychic insight, a feature without which meditation is imagination and visualization, without any mystic experience per se.

In the **Meditation Expertise**, one is shown how to corral one's practice to bring it in line with the classic syllabus of yoga which Patanjali lays out as the ashtanga yoga eight-staged practice.

In **Core-Self Discovery**, one is taken though the course of pratyahar sensual energy withdrawal which is the 5th stage of yoga in the Patanjali ashtanga eight-process complete system of yoga practice. These events lead to the discovery of a core-self which is surrounded by psychic organs in the head of the subtle body. This product has a DVD component for teachers and self-teaching students.

These books are profusely illustrated with mind diagrams showing the components of psychic consciousness and the inner design of the subtle body.

Explained Series

Bhagavad Gita Explained

Uddhava Gita Explained

Anu Gita Explained

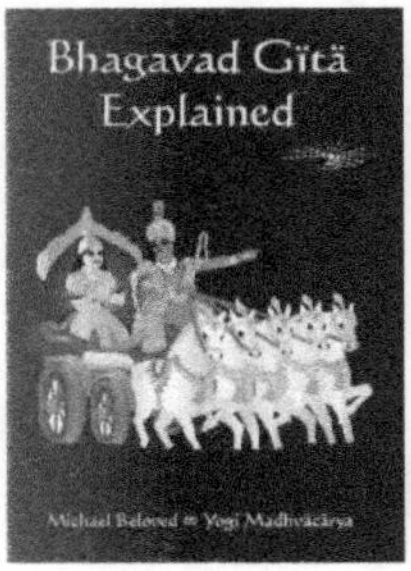

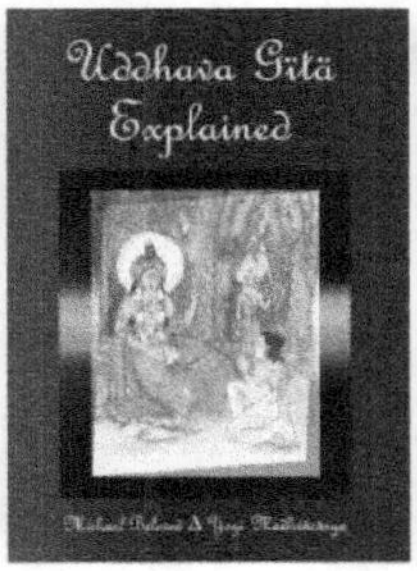

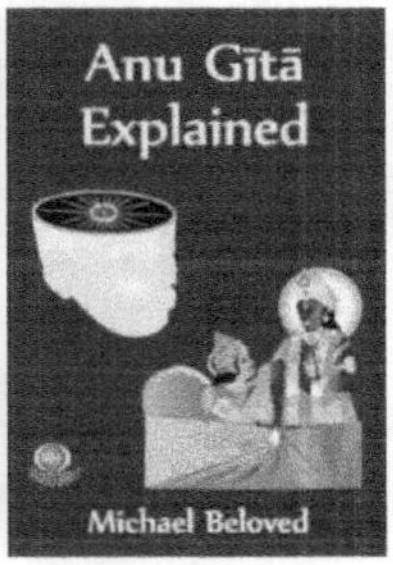

The specialty of these books is that they are free of missionary intentions, cult tactics and philosophical distortion. Instead of using these books to add credence to a philosophy, meditation process, belief or plea for followers, I spread the information out so that a reader can look through this literature and freely take or leave anything as desired.

When Krishna stressed himself as God, I stated that. When Krishna laid no claims for supremacy, I showed that. The reader is left to form an independent opinion about the validity of the information and the credibility of Krishna.

There is a difference in the discourse with Arjuna in the Bhagavad Gita and the one with Uddhava in the Uddhava Gita. In fact these two books may appear to contradict each other. In the Bhagavad Gita, Krishna pressured Arjuna to complete social duties. In the Uddhava Gita, Krishna insisted that Uddhava should abandon the same.

The Anu Gita is not as popular as the Bhagavad Gita but it is the conclusion of that text. Anu means what is to follow, what proceeds. In this discourse, an anxious Arjuna request that Krishna should repeat the Bhagavad Gita and again show His supernatural and divine forms.

However Krishna refuses to do so and chastises Arjuna for being a disappointment in forgetting what was revealed. Krishna then cites a celestial yogi, a near-perfected being, who explained the process of transmigration in vivid detail.

Commentaries

Yoga Sutras of Patanjali

Meditation Expertise

Krishna Cosmic Body

Anu Gita Explained

Bhagavad Gita Explained

Kriya Yoga Bhagavad Gita

Brahma Yoga Bhagavad Gita

Uddhava Gita Explained

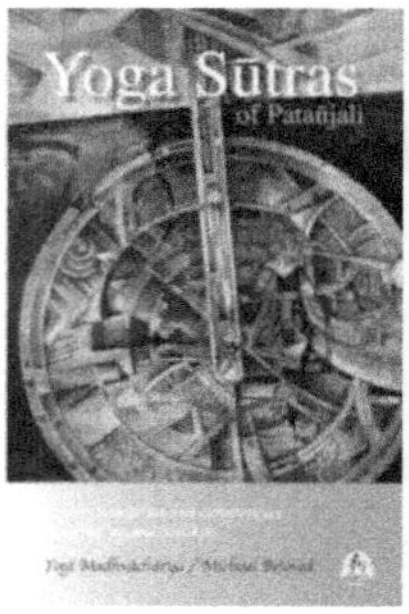

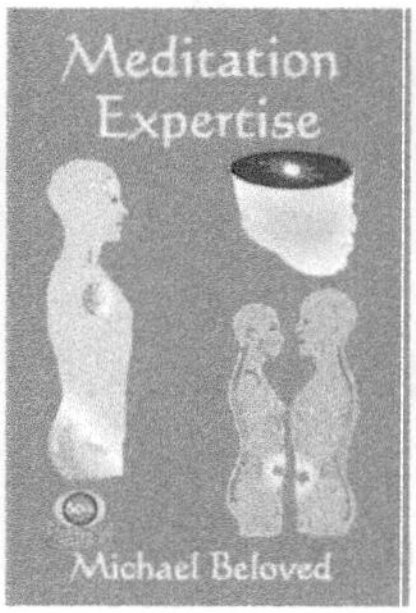

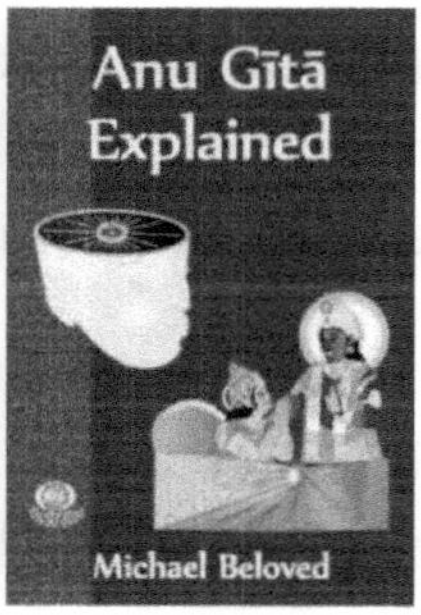

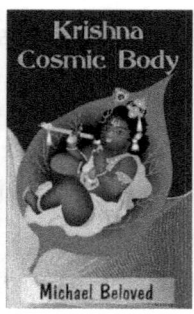

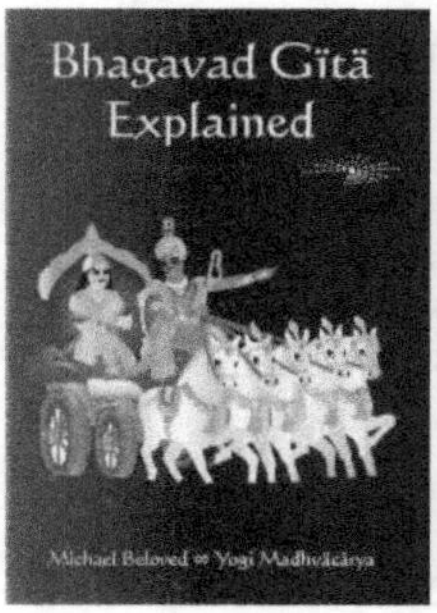

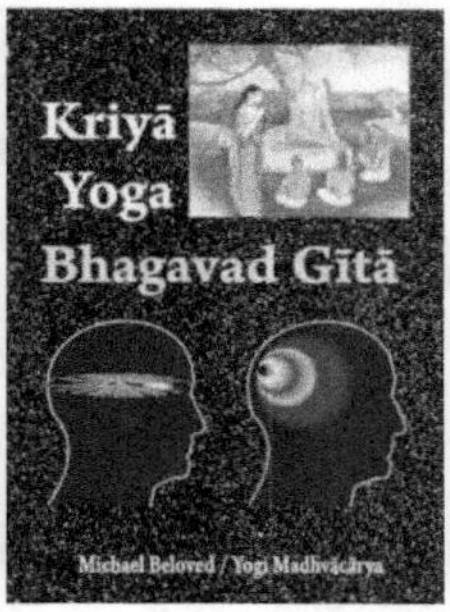

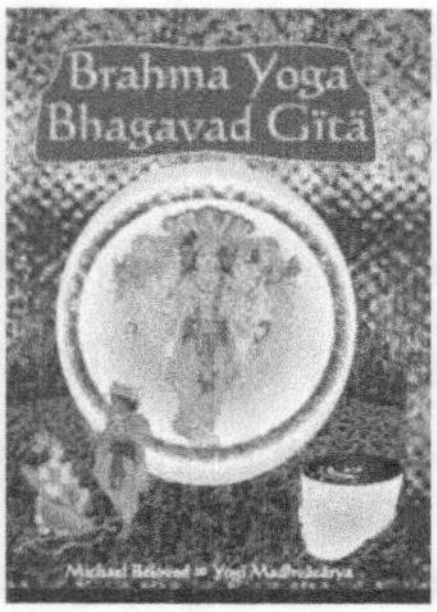

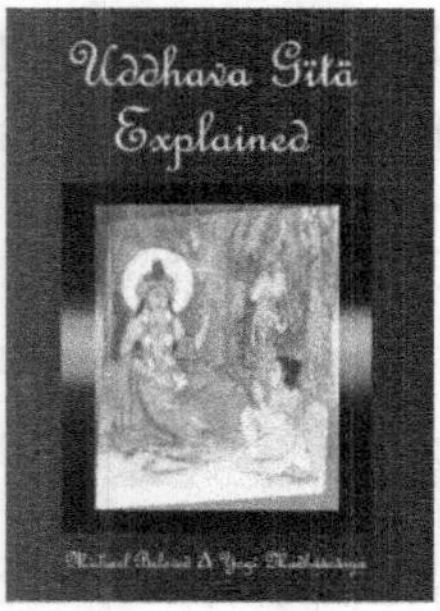

Yoga Sutras of Patanjali is the globally acclaimed text book of yoga. This has detailed expositions of yoga techniques. Many kriya techniques are vividly described in the commentary.

Meditation Expertise is an analysis and application of the Yoga Sutras. This book is loaded with illustrations and has detailed explanations of secretive advanced meditation techniques which are called kriyas in the Sanskrit language.

Krishna Cosmic Body is a narrative commentary on the Markandeya Samasya portion of the Aranyaka Parva of the Mahabharata. This is the detailed description of the dissolution of the world, as experienced by the great yogin Markandeya who transcended the cosmic deity, Brahma, and reached Brahma's source who is the divine infant, Krishna.

Anu Gita Explained is a detailed explanation of how we endure many material bodies in the course of transmigrating through various life-forms. This is a discourse between Krishna and Arjuna. Arjuna requested of Krishna a display of the Universal Form and a repeat narration of the Bhagavad Gita but Krishna declined and explained what a siddha perfected being told the Yadu family about the sequence of existences one endures and the systematic flow of those lives at the convenience of material nature.

Bhagavad Gita Explained shows what was said in the Gita without religious overtones and sectarian biases.

Kriya Yoga Bhagavad Gita shows the instructions for those who are doing kriya yoga.

Brahma Yoga Bhagavad Gita shows the instructions for those who are doing brahma yoga.

Uddhava Gita Explained shows the instructions to Uddhava which are more advanced than the ones given to Arjuna.

Bhagavad Gita is an instruction for applying the expertise of yoga in the cultural field. This is why the process taught to Arjuna is called karma yoga which means karma + yoga or cultural activities done with a yogic demeanor.

Uddhava Gita is an instruction for apply the expertise of yoga to attaining spiritual status. This is why it is explains jnana yoga and bhakti yoga in detail. Jnana yoga is using mystic skill for knowing the spiritual part of existence. Bhakti yoga is for developing affectionate relationships with divine beings.

Karma yoga is for negotiating the social concerns in the material world and therefore it is inferior to bhakti yoga which concerns negotiating the social concerns in the spiritual world.

This world has a social environment and the spiritual world has one too.

Right now Uddhava Gita is the most advanced informative spiritual book on the planet. There is nothing anywhere which is superior to it or which goes into so much detail as it. It verified that historically Krishna is the most advanced human being to ever have left literary instructions on this planet. Even Patanjali Yoga Sutras which I translated and gave an application for in my book, **Meditation Expertise**, does not go as far as the Uddhava Gita.

Some of the information of these two books is identical but while the Yoga Sutras are concerned with the personal spiritual emancipation (kaivalyam) of the individual spirits, the Uddhava Gita explains that and also explains the situations in the spiritual universes.

Bhagavad Gita is from the Mahabharata which is the history of the Pandavas. Arjuna, the student of the Gita, is one of the Pandavas brothers. He was in a social hassle and did not know how to apply yoga expertise to solve it. Krishna gave him a crash-course on the battlefield about that.

Uddhava Gita is from the Srimad Bhagavatam (Bhagavata Purana), which is a history of the incarnations of Krishna. Uddhava was a relative of Krishna. He was concerned about the situation of the deaths of many of his relatives but Krishna diverted Uddhava's attention to the practice of yoga for the purpose of successfully migrating to the spiritual environment.

Specialty

These books are based on the author's experiences in meditation, yoga practice and participation in spiritual groups:

Spiritual Master

sex you!

Sleep **Paralysis**

Astral Projection

Masturbation Psychic Details

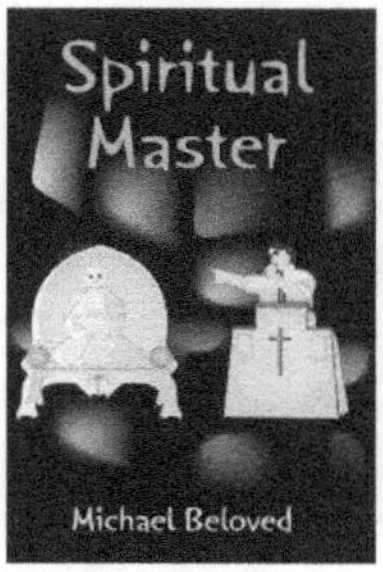

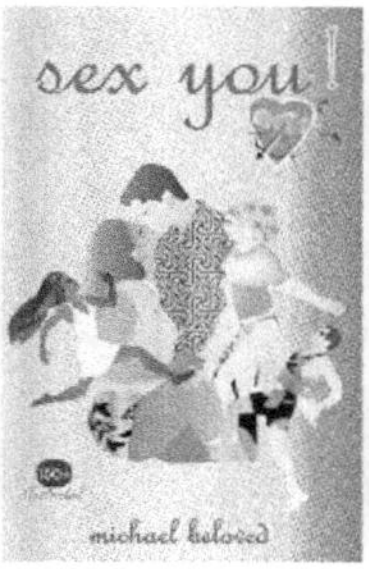

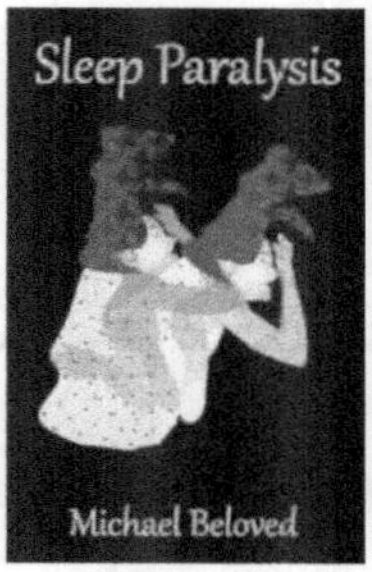

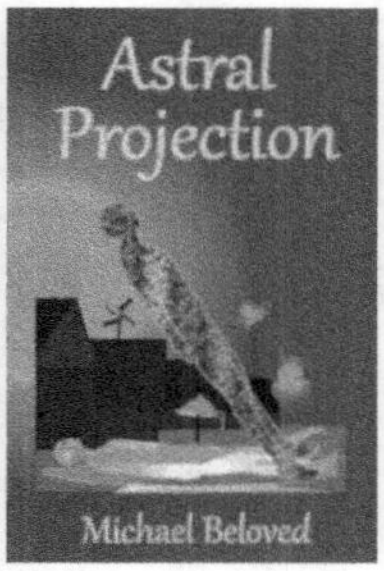

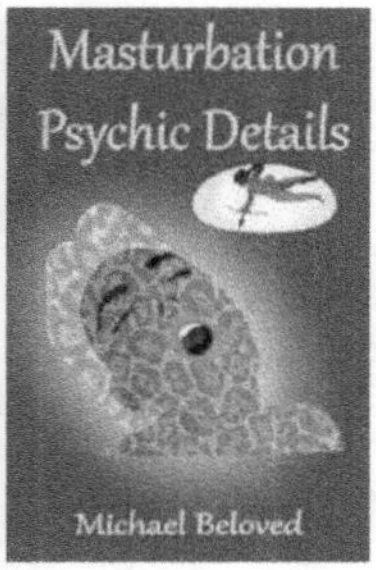

In **Spiritual Master**, Michael draws from experience with gurus or with their senior students. His contact with astral gurus is rated. He walks you through the avenue of gurus showing what you should do and what you should not do, so as to gain proficiency in whatever area of spirituality the guru has proficiency.

sex you! is a masterpiece about the adventures of an individual spirit's passage through the parents' psyches. The conversion of a departed soul into a sexual urge is described. The transit from the afterlife to residency in the emotions of the parents is detailed. This is about sex and you; learn about how much of you comprises the romantic energy of your would-be parents!

Sleep Paralysis clears misconceptions so that one can see what sleep paralysis is and what frightening astral experience occurs while the paralysis is being experienced. This disempowerment has great value in giving you confidence that you can and do exist even if you are unable to operate the physical body. The implication is that one can exist apart from and will survive the loss of the material body.

Astral Projection details experiences Michael had even in childhood, where he assumed incorrectly that everyone was astrally conversant. He discusses the life force psychic mechanism which operates the sleep-wake cycle of the physical form, and which budgets energy into the separated astral form which determines if the individual will have dream recall or no objective awareness during the projections. Astral travel happens on every occasion when the physical body sleeps. What is missing in awareness is the observer status while the astral body is separated.

Masturbation Psychic Details is a surprise presentation which relates what happens on the psychic plane during a masturbation event. This does not tackle moral issues or even addictions but shows the involvement of memory and the sure but hidden subconscious mind which operates many features of the psyche irrespective of the desire or approval of the self-conscious personality.

Online Resources

Visit The Website And Forum

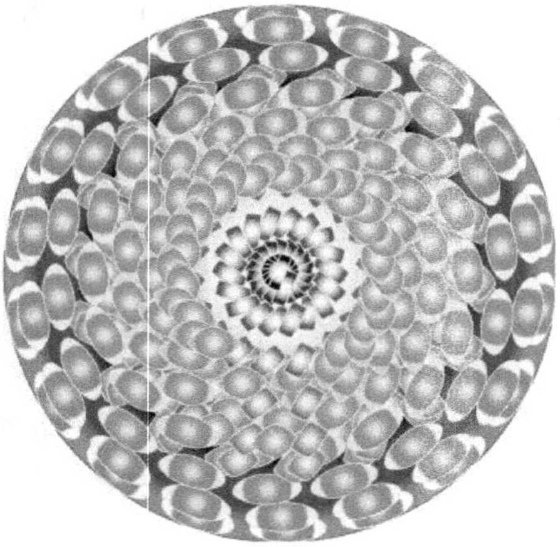

Email:	michaelbelovedbooks@gmail.com axisnexus@gmail.com
Website Forum:	michaelbeloved.com inselfyoga.com

www.ingramcontent.com/pod-product-compliance
Lightning Source LLC
Chambersburg PA
CBHW082141230426
43672CB00016B/2927
* 9 7 8 0 9 7 9 3 9 1 6 4 4 *